Cognition and Occupation in Rehabilitation

Cognitive Models for Intervention in Occupational Therapy

Noomi Katz, PhD, OTR, Editor

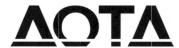 The American Occupational Therapy Association, Inc.

The American Occupational Therapy Association, Inc. Mission Statement

The mission of the American Occupational Therapy Association is to support a professional community for members, and to develop and preserve the viability and relevance of the profession. The organization serves the interest of its members, represents the profession to the public, and promotes access to occupational therapy services.

Disclaimers

"This publication is designed to provide accurate and authoritative information in regard to the subject matter covered. It is sold or distributed with the understanding that the publisher is not engaged in rendering legal, accounting, or other professional services. If legal advice or other expert assistance is required, the services of a competent professional should be sought."

—*From the Declaration of Principles jointly adopted by the American Bar Association and a Committee of Publishers and Associations*

It is the objective of the American Occupational Therapy Association to be a forum for free expression and interchange of ideas. The opinions expressed by the contributors to this work are their own and not necessarily those of either the editors or the American Occupational Therapy Association.

AOTA Director of Nonperiodical Publications: Frances E. McCarrey
AOTA Managing Editor of Nonperiodical Publications: Mary C. Fisk
Text Design by World Composition Services, Inc.
Cover design by Paul A. Platosh

ISBN 1-56900-085-9

Printed in the United States of America

Contents

Contributors

Beatriz C. Abreu, PhD, OTR, FAOTA
Clinical Professor
University of Texas Medical Branch,
    and Director of Occupational Therapy,
Transitional Learning Community
Galveston, TX

Claudia K. Allen, MA, OTR/L, FAOTA
Chief, Occupational Therapy Department,
    Los Angeles
and Clinical Assistant Professor, University of
    Southern California, Los Angeles, CA

Sara Averbuch, MA, OTR
Instructor, Department of Occupational Therapy
Tel Aviv University, Tel Aviv
and Senior Therapist Loewenstein Rehabilitation
    Hospital, Rannana, Israel

Tina Blue, OTR/L
The Veranda Nursing and Rehabilitation Center,
    Orlando, FL

Elizabeth DePoy, PhD, MSW, OTR/L
Professor of Social Work
and Coordinator of Research and Evaluation,
    Center for Community Inclusion,
University of Maine, Orono, ME

Linda Duncombe, MSc, OTR
Clinical Associate Professor
Department of Occupational Therapy
Boston University Sargent College
Boston, MA

Gordon Giles, MA, DipCot, OTR
Director of Clinical Services
Neurobehavioral Program at Highview
and Associate Professor at Samuel Merrit College
Oakland, CA

Lynn Gitlow, MEd, OTR/L
Assistant Research Professor
Center for Community Inclusion, University of
    Maine, Orone, ME

Naomi Hadas-Lidor, MA, OTR
Instructor and Doctoral Candidate
Department of Occupational Therapy
Tel Aviv University Ramat Aviv
Tel Aviv, Israel

Adina Hartman-Maier, MSc, OTR
Doctoral Student
School of Occupational Therapy
Hebrew University, Jerusalem, Israel

Naomi Josman, PhD, OTR
Assistant Professor
Department of Occupational Therapy
Haifa University, Mount Carmel, Israel

Noomi Katz, PhD, OTR
Associate Professor
Chairperson Graduate Program
School of Occupational Therapy
Hebrew University, Jerusalem, Israel

Linda Levy, MA, OTR/L, FAOTA
Associate Professor
Department of Occupational Therapy
Temple University, Philadelphia, PA

Joan P. Toglia, MA, OTR
Chairperson, Occupational Therapy Program
Mercy College, Dobbs Ferry, NY

Foreword

Cognitive rehabilitation is marked by significant shifts in the locus, focus, and modus of treatment. Within the field of rehabilitation (modus), there is an increasing attention to functional capabilities (focus) and community adaptation (locus). As therapists, we can no longer be satisfied with the amelioration of symptoms and improvement on test scores as objectives of rehabilitation. Emphasis and resources must be given instead to improving occupational functions and facilitating the quality of life for the individual and his or her family.

The contributors to *Cognition and Occupation* present a multidimensional perspective of cognition and cognitive deficits needed to provide effective rehabilitation. Individual, social, and cultural factors that contribute to the assessment and intervention strategies for cognitive rehabilitation are discussed. Treatment is considered from an individual, task, and environmental perspective, with increasing attention given to the importance of the physical, social, and cultural environments (contexts) to the intervention process. There is also increasing recognition that the interactions among the brain, behavior, and environment are dynamic and represent an open system. Thus, therapeutic interventions can derive from one or a combination of these aspects.

The necessity to use and further define theoretical models to guide the use of intervention techniques is emphasized in each chapter of this eminently readable book. Different theoretical models and/or applications of a model to clinical populations are presented and richly illustrated with case studies. Common to each of the models is the goal of intervention—to enable occupational performance and to improve the quality of life for the client and his or her family and caregivers.

Assessment is considered from several perspectives. In addition to discussing traditional assessment of cognitive abilities, several chapters examine the assessment of processes or strategies used by a client as he or she performs tasks. This focus on process rather than product reflects current trends in assessment in many disciplines. Based on the work of Luria, Vygotsky, and Feuerstein, this approach identifies those variables that facilitate better performance and enables a clearer linkage between assessment and intervention. There is also an increasing use of inquiry strategies such as narratives incorporated into occupational therapy assessment.

In developing this text, Dr. Katz responded to the need to examine issues and theories in assessment and intervention in cognitive rehabilitation as evidenced by the organization of this book and the selection of contributors. Issues that confront occupational therapists as they work with individuals with cognitive impairments are comprehensively examined. The role of factors such as pathophysiology, spontaneous recovery, preexisting cognitive and personality issues, aging and life span cognitive changes, the client's personal reaction to his or her deficits, the multifactorial nature of tests, the relevance of test content for the client, the ecological validity of tests and intervention procedures, learning potential, and psychosocial factors are discussed relative to assessment, intervention, and outcome.

Clinical application for adolescents through the elderly and for various diagnostic groups are presented. The case examples provided in the chapters enhance our understanding of the intervention process and the complex relationship among the individual, the task, and the environment.

This text includes a critical review of cognitive rehabilitation research in occupational therapy, and authors of several chapters articulate the need for further research. In fact, the questions that are raised in this book will likely direct future research in cognitive rehabilitation in occupational therapy. Many of the chapter authors acknowledge that, at this time, there is not sufficient research to identify the most effective approach to cognitive rehabilitation. The current state of the field includes a place for both the macro and the micro approaches to rehabilitation. Both the top-down treatments and the bottom-up treatments should be considered.

However, as emphasized throughout the text, the focus must remain on occupational performance in the context of the daily lives of our clients and their families or caregivers.

Cognition and Occupation is a much needed resource. Without question, this book succeeds in its purpose of providing a comprehensive state of the art view of cognitive rehabilitation in occupational therapy from theoretical, practical, and research perspectives. This text represents a major contribution to the field of cognitive rehabilitation and is likely to be regarded as the authoritative book about cognitive rehabilitation in occupational therapy.

Sharon A. Cermak, EdD, OTR/L, FAOTA
Professor of Occupational Therapy
Boston University
Sargent College of Health and Rehabilitation Sciences

Preface

This current work is a new and updated book on cognition and occupation in rehabilitation. The purpose of the first book in occupational therapy on cognitive rehabilitation (Katz, 1992) was to provide a comprehensive state-of-the-art "knowledge base" on cognitive theoretical models in occupational therapy for adolescent and adult clients with cognitive dysfunction. The current book expands on the original ideas and models of intervention and adds new ones, providing a comprehensive view on cognitive rehabilitation in occupational therapy for theoretical, practical, and research perspectives.

Cognition is conceived as a basic universal human trait that underlies every human occupation, crossing over all specialty areas within occupational therapy. The development of cognitive theoretical models for practice in occupational therapy, which integrate knowledge on cognition from different scientific disciplines with occupational therapy tenets and principles regarding occupational performance, was and still is relatively new and unique.

In the past 5 years since the publication of the previous book, the profession witnessed the beginning of the occupational science discipline (Clark et al., 1991; Yerxa et al., 1989; Yerxa, 1993)—the development of a basic science that will provide an additional knowledge base for occupational therapy intervention. The purpose of this science, according to Zemke and Clark (1996), is to generate knowledge about the form, function, and meaning of human occupation in all contexts, including the therapeutic context that makes the link to occupational therapy practice. Yerxa et al. (1989) stress the need for understanding the relationship between engagement in occupation and an individual's health. Yerxa (1993) poses further questions about the relationship between engagement in daily activities and the quality of life and healthfulness. Yerxa and her colleagues propose that knowledge generated in basic research inquiry leads to occupational therapy intervention with people with disabilities. I agree with that assertion and concur with Kielhofner (1992) that we need both levels of inquiry, basic and applied, to enlarge and deepen the scientific basis of our models of interventions in general and in cognitive intervention specifically.

The current book continues the premise put forward previously that the ideas and applications provided in the various models contribute to the knowledge base of occupational science in exploring and conceptualizing the role cognition or information processing plays in the interaction between occupation and health. Information processing is conceived within the occupational science model as a "subsystem which deals with the cognitive operations that are used by humans to organize behavior" (Clark et al., 1991, p. 303).

Making the link to the occupational therapy domain of concern as defined by Mosey (1981, 1986) and Katz (1985), occupational performance or human occupations were considered the core of the domain, and performance or competence components its parameters along with age, environment, and time parameters. Using further the third edition of the *AOTA Uniform Terminology* (1994) performance areas, performance components, and performance contexts are regarded as the parameters of the domain of concern. However, as stated, "function in performance areas (i.e., *occupational performance added*) is the ultimate concern of occupational therapy, with performance components considered as they relate to participation in performance areas" (p. 1047). Accepting the above conceptualizations, the current book and the models presented in it look through the lenses of the cognitive performance component as it relates to occupational performance within different contexts. Trombly (1995) recently discussed ways to conceptualize occupation: occupation-as-an-end and occupation-as-means. The first way includes the performance areas, human occupations that are the goal of occupational therapy intervention. The second way is the use of occupation as therapy or therapeutic occupations (Nelson, 1996) to bring about changes in performance components (Trombly, 1995), among them cognitive components. Thus, through occupations the therapeutic process to remediate cognitive impairments and/or adapt and compensate for cognitive disabilities is undertaken to enable occupational performance.

Focus on cognition is almost an unnecessary question, as human beings have the most developed brain among the species; by that we mean the most developed intellectual capacities to acquire, process, and apply information in daily functioning and to adapt to environmental demands (Diller, 1993; Lidz, 1987). Cognitive abilities enable the "doing" of human beings and define the level and limits of the individual's occupational performance. Metacognitive skills—knowledge and control—include awareness of abilities and disabilities and executive functions that consist of initiation, planning, problems solving, self-regulation, and self-correction. Cognitive skills comprise such areas as attention, orientation, perception, praxis, visual-motor organization, memory, and thinking operations. Disturbance in any of these skills may cause disabilities in daily performance, the extent of which is determined by premorbid level of development, the severity of central nervous system damage or changes, and the demands and contexts of the daily tasks. Therefore, according to Diller (1993), cognitive rehabilitation goals are to reduce the disturbance and its consequences in daily functioning and to increase the quality of life both for people who have cognitive deficits and their caregivers.

The relationships between occupational performance areas and the cognitive performance component are complex and multi-interactional and are influenced of course by additional performance components (sensorimotor, psychosocial) and by the performance contexts (temporal, environ-

ment) (*Uniform Terminology*, 1994). However, metacognitive skills have far reaching global influences over all performance areas and components: without awareness we do not know what and how much we can or cannot do, and if executive functions are impaired we will not initiate occupational performance or plan appropriately and monitor performance of any task (Katz & Hartman-Maier, in this book). The cognitive perspective is applied to individuals who have cognitive deficits for various reasons; however, it is also appropriate for intervention with individuals in any other dysfunctional situation.

Abreu (in this book) exemplifies the conceptualization depicted above by developing her original quadraphonic approach into a holistic system that combines analysis of performance components with human occupations from a macro and micro perspective. Abreu provides a well-thought theoretical and practical cognitive functional rehabilitation system that focuses on both the occupational performance (macro perspective) and performance components, the underlying skills (micro perspective). Through her work, as well as in the other cognitive models presented in this book, the direction of growth and change since the original writings is in defining the unique occupational therapy perspective in cognitive rehabilitation, namely *cognitive rehabilitation through occupation*, with the ultimate goal being optimal occupational performance.

Organization of the Book

The book is organized into two parts. The first part includes nine chapters that present seven cognitive models for intervention in occupational therapy. The second part consists of three different general chapters that relate in one way or another to all models and to the subject area of cognition and occupation in rehabilitation.

Part One: Cognitive Models for Intervention

Each of the cognitive models for practice in occupational therapy described in this book includes

1) a theoretical base—integrating various scientific concepts with occupational therapy principles and postulates; 2) intervention—including evaluation procedures, assessment instruments, and treatment methods; 3) research to support the model; 4) case studies illustrating the intervention process to a variety of clients; and 5) implications for further knowledge development.

In the past, two general approaches in cognitive rehabilitation were traditionally discussed, namely, remedial versus functional/adaptive with different underlying assumptions (Katz, 1994; Neistadt, 1990; Toglia, 1992). However, it became more and more clear that we are not referring to a dichotomy but to a continuum. This continuum extends from a remedial approach in the first stages of the client illness to a more adaptive/compensatory approach in the long-term, stable residual stage of the client's condition. Severity of the dysfunction and the causes, the target populations and their age, as well as environmental context are major determinants of the approach taken. Hence, the focus of the various models presented in this book differs on this continuum according to the parameters outlined above. It is, however, important to stress that all models focus on the clients' occupational performance as the goal of intervention and that is what establishes them as occupational therapy cognitive models.

Another aspect that differentiates the models is their client population. I will use this aspect to organize the order of the chapters into four sections that may help clinicians, educators, and students to focus first in their area of interest. These four sections relate to models for individuals with brain injuries, mental health problems, elderly with dementia, and generic for all populations. However, I would like to emphasize that the order of the chapters in the book is of no major importance in itself. Each chapter (excluding chapters 5 and 7 which should be read in conjunction with the original model) is complete on its own; thus, the chapters can be read in any sequence the reader chooses. On the other hand, to choose a model *for intervention,* a therapist has to consider the specific problems of the individual client and the context in which the client will have to function.

Section One: Brain injuries

Four of the models were developed originally for clients following brain injuries. Toglia (in chapter 1) presents a Dynamic Interactional Model to cognitive rehabilitation. Cognition is viewed as a dynamic interaction between the individual, the task, and the environment. Dynamic instruments for assessment are presented, and a multicontent treatment approach is outlined that reflects the dynamic view of cognition.

Abreu (chapter 2) presents a holistic view in rehabilitation that integrates a macro occupational performance perspective and a micro performance components perspective through her Quadrophonic Model. Evaluation and treatment from both perspectives are combined in this model, and an elaborate case study is provided to exemplify the intervention process.

Averbuch and Katz's (chapter 3) Cognitive Retraining Model is based on the assumptions that learned skills generalize and can be transferred to functional areas. In this sense it is a remedial approach. The theoretical base is grounded in neuropsychological and cognitive psychology theories. Instruments to assess cognitive skills with research data to support them as well as training methods are described along with case studies.

Giles (chapter 4) presents a Neurofunctional Model to rehabilitation with emphasis on clients with severe brain injury. The focus of this model is the retraining of real world skills in natural situations, namely, using an adaptive/compensatory approach based on neuropsychological and behavioral theories.

Section Two: Mental Health

Josman (chapter 5) applies the Dynamic Interactional Model by Toglia (chapter 1) to clients who have schizophrenia. She shows how this model can be used with individuals who have mental health problems and specifically for clients with schizophrenia.

Duncombe (chapter 6) presents a Cognitive-Behavioral Model that is based on theories in mental health and their adaptation in occupational therapy. This model can be applied to various clients who have mental health dysfunctions.

These two chapters are new in this book and are an important addition. In chapter 5 Josman shows how to extend a model developed for brain injury to the psychiatric population, while in chapter 6 Duncombe shows the integration of theories from psychology and their application as a model in occupational therapy.

Section Three: Elderly with Dementia

Levy (chapter 7) discusses the application of Allen's model in the rehabilitation of the older adult with dementia. Levy disseminates the extensive gerontological literature with her theoretical work on the adaptation of activities and cognitive disability model for the aged population and the caregivers. This is the only chapter that provides direct application to the elderly population, which makes it unique and important for therapists working with these clients.

Section Four: Generic for all Populations

Allen and Blue (chapter 8) present the current stage of the Cognitive Disabilities Model originated by Allen. The model was developed for psychiatric clients and was for many years applied to these clients and to the elderly only. Since 1992 the authors elaborated the model in more general terms, applying it to all populations with brain dysfunction causing disabilities in daily functioning. An extensive process of evaluation with the Allen Battery is described, and case studies are presented for various client populations.

Hadas-Lidor and Katz (chapter 9) describe the application of Feuerestein's Dynamic Theory for Cognitive Modifiability and Mediated learning Experience in occupational therapy. Application to clients with cognitive, emotional and/or adaptational dysfunction is presented; thus, this model is intended for any client who has cognitive dysfunctions, irrespective of the cause, illness, or cultural deprivation.

These two models exemplify both ends of the continuum, one an adaptive approach and the second a remedial one.

Part Two: General Topics

The three chapters in this part are an important addition to this book. Dissemination of the literature on cognitive changes in later life by Levy (chapter 10) provides essential knowledge on a difficult issue that must always be considered when working with elderly individuals.

Normal age-related changes that occur in later life have to be taken into account when evaluating clients and comparing their performance to what is expected from healthy persons, as well as when planning intervention. Therefore, the information in this chapter can be beneficial for the application of any model to the elderly population.

Chapter 11 on metacognition by Katz and Hartman-Maier was intended to highlight this aspect of cognition, which has far-reaching implications for any occupational performance with every client population whether having cognitive skill dysfunctions, sensorimotor, or psychosocial dysfunctions.

Chapter 12 by DePoy and Gitlow provides a critical review of cognitive rehabilitation research in occupational therapy in general and related examples taken from the models in the book. More importantly, they suggest a framework for doing research in this area that should be very beneficial for further knowledge development.

Finally, all chapters together provide a broad knowledge base and clinical applications in occupational therapy for adolescent, adult, and elderly populations with cognitive dysfunctions. The authors who collaborated in this book make an important contribution to our knowledge on the interaction between cognition and occupation in influencing clients' state of health. They provide multiple ways to approach the problem of cognitive dysfunctions and to intervene with various client populations. It is my hope that the book will inspire further study and intervention in the area of cognition and occupation in rehabilitation.

Noomi Katz

References

AOTA Uniform Terminology for Occupational Therapy (3rd ed.) (1994). *American Journal of Occupational Therapy, 48,* 1047–1054.

Clark, F.A., Parham, D., Carlson, M.E., Frank, G., Jackson, J., Pierce, D., Wolfe, R.J., & Zemke, R. (1991). Occupational Science: Academic innovation in the service of occupational therapy's future. *American Journal of Occupational Therapy, 45,* 300–310.

Diller, L. (1993). Introduction to cognitive rehabilitation. In C.B Royeen *AOTA Self-Study Series: Cognitive rehabilitation.* Bethesda, MD: American Occupational Therapy Association

Katz, N. (1985). Domain of concern: Reconsidered. *American Journal of Occupational Therapy, 39,* 518–524.

Katz, N. (1992). *Cognitive rehabilitation: Models for intervention in occupational therapy.* Stoneham, MA: Butterworth-Heinemann.

Katz, N. (1994). Cognitive rehabilitation: Intervention and research on cognition. *Occupational Therapy International, I,* 49–63.

Kielhofner, G. (1992). *Conceptual foundations of occupational therapy.* Philadelphia: Davis.

Kielhofner, G. (1995). *A model of human occupation: Theory and application* (2nd Ed.) Baltimore: Williams and Wilkins.

Lidz, C.S. (1987). *Dynamic assessment.* New York: Guilford Press.

Mosey, A.C. (1981). *Occupational therapy: Configuration of a profession.* New York: Raven Press.

Mosey, A.C. (1986). *Psychosocial components of occupational therapy.* New York: Raven Press.

Neistadt, M.E. (1990). A critical analysis of occupational therapy approaches for perceptual deficits in adults with brain injury. *American Journal of Occupational Therapy, 44,* 299–304.

Nelson, D.L. (1996). Therapeutic occupation: A definition. *American Journal of Occupational Therapy, 50,* 775–782.

Toglia, J.P. (1992). A dynamic interactional approach to cognitive rehabilitation. In N. Katz, (Ed.), *Cognitive rehabilitation: Models for intervention in occupational therapy.* Stoneham, MA: Butterworth-Heinemann.

Trombly, C.A. (1995). Occupation: Purposefulness and meaningfulness as therapeutic mechanisms. *American Journal of Occupational Therapy, 49,* 960–972.

Yerxa, E.J., Clark, F.A., Frank, G., Jackson, J., Parham, D., Pierce, D., Stein, C., & Zemke, R. (1989). An introduction to occupational science: A foundation for occupational therapy in the 21st century. *Occupational Therapy in Health Care, 6,* 1–17.

Yerxa, E. J. (1993). Occupational science: A new source of power for participants in occupational therapy. *Occupational Science: Australia, I,* 3–10.

Zemke, R., & Clark, F. (1996). *Occupational science: The evolving discipline.* Philadelphia: Davis.

Cognitive Models for Intervention

Brain Injuries

CHAPTER 1

A Dynamic Interactional Model to Cognitive Rehabilitation

Joan P. Toglia, MA, OTR

What one addresses in cognitive rehabilitation depends to a large extent upon how one conceptualizes cognition and the scope of cognitive functioning. Traditional cognitive rehabilitation approaches have been guided by the assumption that cognition can be divided into distinct subskills (Trexler, 1987). In this chapter, I propose a dynamic interactional view of cognition as an alternative to traditional deficit and syndrome-specific approaches. In this dynamic approach, the clinician is urged to abandon classical taxonomies of dysfunction and instead to investigate dynamically the underlying conditions and processing strategies that influence performance. Assessment uses cues and task alterations to identify the individual's potential for change. Treatment incorporates a number of components: strategy training, practice in multiple situations, establishment of criteria for transfer, metacognitive training, and consideration of learner characteristics to facilitate transfer of learning.

Until now, cognitive psychology theories have not been used as a guide for cognitive rehabilitation assessment and treatment. This chapter represents an attempt to integrate the cognitive psychology theories of how normal people learn and generalize information with the rehabilitation of clients with cognitive dysfunction.

Cognitive dysfunction can be seen in people with developmental, neurologic, or psychiatric dysfunction. The theoretical concepts presented in this chapter are broad and apply to all populations. However, the specific assessment and treatment techniques described later have been developed for

the brain-injured adult. Some of these techniques have recently been used with schizophrenic clients who manifest negative symptoms (see chapter 5).

The Scope of Cognition in the Traditional Approach

Traditionally, cognition has been viewed as a higher-level cortical function that can be divided into separate subskills such as attention, memory, organization, reasoning, and problem solving (Pedretti, 1981; Trexler, 1982). This view of cognition did not originate from theory of cognition; it was derived from psychometric models of intelligence testing and from localization approaches. Psychometric approaches in intelligence testing used techniques (such as factor analysis) to identify tests that tapped different mental abilities (Sternberg, 1986). Deficits were derived from performance analyses on specific tests. A poor performance on a specific test (such as a memory test) was assumed to reflect a deficiency in the specific skill (e.g., memory) that the test was designed to measure. Localization approaches emphasized the correlation of specific skills and/or syndrome types to the location of the brain lesion (Trexler, 1982). This approach, in combination with the traditional psychometric testing, reinforced the assumption that cognition could be divided into distinct entities. In addition, stage-specific models that proposed that the brain processes first simple then complex information provided support for the view that cognitive subskills are hierarchically arranged. The assumption that cognition is composed of separate hierarchical subskills and that cognitive dysfunction is defined according to separate syndromes or deficits is reflected in most current cognitive perceptual treatment programs (Trexler, 1987). The terms "deficit specific" (cognitive deficits defined according to performance on specific tests), "reductionistic" (cognition reduced to separate skills), and "transfer training" have all been used to describe treatment approaches based on this view of cognition.

Deficit Specific Approaches

Trexler (1987) describes the characteristics of a reductionistic or deficit-specific approach as follows:

1. Cognitive subskills are hierarchical in nature; for example, more basic skills such as attention and memory are requisite to higher-order skills such as logical reasoning.
2. Treatment involves repetitive practice on a specific tabletop or computer task until the client reaches some identified criteria.
3. The remediation program is organized into activities that address specific deficits, which are derived from test performance.

For example, if the client does poorly on a test that measures attention, his or her treatment is based on receiving a graded sequence of attentional activities. The parameters and methods of training are closely related to the materials used to evaluate the client. This approach is similar to the transfer training approach used by Frostig & Home (1973) in the early 1970s to treat perceptual motor problems in learning disabled children. In both approaches it is assumed that any improvements observed with a specific skill will affect performance on other tasks that involve the same underlying skill.

In some cases, the cognitive remediation program is organized around modules (such as an attentional module or a reasoning module). All clients receive the same type of treatment activities within each module. The client progresses from one module to another until a specific performance criterion is reached or until progress has plateaued (Ben-Yishay & Diller, 1983). Ready-made exercises or training modules have the advantage of being practical and easy to use by a beginning therapist. They also assure that each client with a similar problem (as defined by standardized testing) receives the same treatment in the same way. This type of program lends itself readily to empirical research methods and outcome studies. Most of the literature on cognitive rehabilitation emphasizes deficit-specific or reductionistic approaches (Trexler, 1987).

Limitations of the Deficit-Specific Approach

The deficit-specific approach does not describe how specific skills interrelate during cognitive processing and task performance. Factors such as reasoning, verbal comprehension, and visual spatial skills are useful in describing broad areas of strengths and weaknesses; however, as Sternberg (1985) points out, "the information conveyed by factors is not specific enough for training" (p. 218). For example, labels such as "visual spatial" or "reasoning" do not specify what characteristics of visual spatial abilities or reasoning contribute to either high or low performance. Additionally, in the clinical setting one never observes isolated cognitive deficits. Cognitive problems often overlap and correlate with one another, which leads one to question the usefulness of this division (Toglia & Golisz, 1990). Seron & Deloche (1989) have urged clinicians to abandon the classical syndrome-oriented approach used in classifying cognitive dysfunction. There is strong evidence that syndrome approaches are not sufficiently precise. Many classical syndromes such as visual agnosia, Broca's aphasia, and constructional apraxia group clients together who present highly heterogeneous deficits (Seron & Deloche, 1989).

The Dynamic Approach

Another approach to cognitive rehabilitation has been described by Trexler (1987) as the dynamic approach. In this approach, cognition is defined in terms of global capacities. Characteristics of a dynamic approach include the following:

1. Treatment is delivered in a reactive mode; the individual's response determines how and what kinds of therapy will be administered.
2. There is little emphasis placed on the absolute level of performance on specific tests.
3. There is no predetermined or prescribed sequence of treatment activities.

Specific skills such as spatial analysis and recall are not addressed separately. The clinician operates as a detective with each individual case and analyzes common underlying behaviors to account for difficulty on a number of different tasks. This approach abandons classical taxonomies of dysfunction.

One of the inherent limitations with the dynamic approach is the difficulty of performing empirical research when no two clients receive the same treatment in the same way. This method is also time-consuming and requires an experienced clinician. Very little has been written about the dynamic approach. The following represents an attempt to further define and expand the dynamic approach.

Theoretical Foundations for a Dynamic Interactional Model of Cognition

Cognition is generally defined as the individual's capacity to acquire and use information in order to adapt to environmental demands (Lidz, 1987). This definition encompasses information processing skills, learning, and generalization. The capacity to acquire information involves information processing skills or the ability to take in, organize, assimilate, and integrate new information with previous experiences (Adamovich, Henderson, & Averbuch, 1985). Environmental adaptation involves using information that has been previously acquired to plan and structure behavior for goal attainment. Thus the ability to apply what has been learned to a variety of different situations is inherent within the concept of cognition (Lidz,

1987). This description of cognition cuts across specific domains. Cognition is not divided into distinct entities nor is it localized to the cortex. Instead cognitive abilities and deficiencies are analyzed according to underlying strategies and potential for learning.

Essential to the conceptualization of cognition is the idea that cognition is an ongoing product of the dynamic interaction between the individual, the task, and the environment (see Figure 1-1). Cognition is not static; it changes with our interaction with the external world (Lidz, 1987).

The dynamic nature of cognition is reflected in the way that information processing resources are allocated and used. Normally, we can only process a limited amount of information at any one time. Although there is a fixed or structural limit in the capacity to process information (structural capacity), there are differences in the way that this fixed capacity can be used. The same task can require different amounts of information processing capacity depending on how one goes about performing it. The term "functional capacity" refers to the ability to use our limited information processing capacity efficiently. The efficient allocation of limited processing resources is central to learning and cognition. Functional capacity is modifiable and varies with characteristics of the task, the environment, and the individual (Flavell, 1985). For example, an individual who is cooking an old recipe in a familiar environment and/or easily organizes the task components will use fewer processing resources in making dinner than one who is in an unfamiliar kitchen making a recipe for the first time and/or who is approaching the task in a haphazard and disorganized manner. The information processing resources required for a task are determined by the interaction among individual components such as processing strategies, metacognition, and learner characteristics (e.g., previous experience, motivation, personality, and emotions) and the task and environment (Bransford, 1979; Brown, Bransford, Ferrara, & Campione, 1983). Each of these three components (involving the individual, the task, and the environment) of the dynamic interactional model and their influence on learning and information processing will be discussed in following sections.

Figure 1-1

Dynamic Interactional Model of Cognition

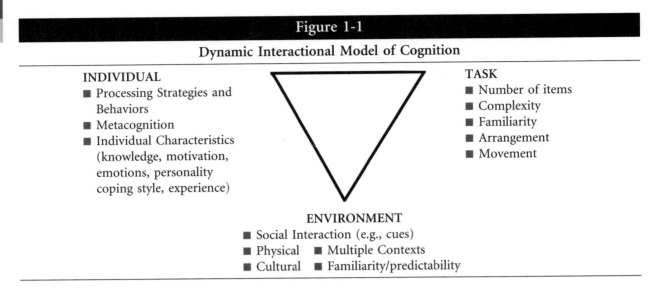

INDIVIDUAL
- Processing Strategies and Behaviors
- Metacognition
- Individual Characteristics (knowledge, motivation, emotions, personality coping style, experience)

TASK
- Number of items
- Complexity
- Familiarity
- Arrangement
- Movement

ENVIRONMENT
- Social Interaction (e.g., cues)
- Physical
- Cultural
- Multiple Contexts
- Familiarity/predictability

Individual Components

Processing Strategies

Processing strategies and behaviors are defined globally as organized approaches, routines, or tactics that operate to select and guide the processing of information (Abreu & Toglia, 1987; Lidz, 1987). The appropriate selection of processing strategies increases efficient use of information processing resources. For example, when confronted with a large amount of information we may automatically prioritize information and decide where to start, what to do first, second, and so on. We may select the most important stimuli and ignore the unimportant stimuli. We may organize or cluster related information together or decide to shift our attention among various stimuli (Abreu & Toglia, 1987). All of these strategies enhance our ability to take in and assimilate information.

The types of processing strategies employed by the individual determine the depth at which information is processed. Deep processing strategies are characterized by active elaboration, organization, and attempts to relate new information to previous experiences or knowledge. The more one attends to an item and actively thinks about its meaning in relation to other concepts, the more deeply the information will be processed (Toglia, 1993a). Surface-level strategies include memorizing words without actively elaborating or reorganizing the material to obtain meaning (Nolen, 1988). Information that is processed at deep levels is more easily understood and retained than information processed at shallow levels (Anderson, 1985). Thus the types of processing strategies used are a critical variable in learning and retention. Evidence suggests that by modifying processing strategies one can increase performance and that, unlike poor learners, good learners spontaneously apply deep processing strategies (Lidz, 1987).

Processing strategies and behaviors are the most observable aspects of a learner's performance and the aspects most accessible to intervention and modification. They have been defined broadly to encompass underlying processing behaviors and cognitive styles. Processing strategies includes behaviors that cut across specific cognitive domains. Table 1-1 includes some of the observable processing strategies and behaviors that can underlie task performance in cognitive skill areas. There are too many possible strategies to include them all. As one can see, there is considerable overlap between the different areas. Attention to detail (or the spontaneous comparison of stimuli) underlies performance in attention tasks, memory tasks, and visual processing tasks. The same underlying processing strategies and behaviors can influence performance in a number of different skill areas.

Processing strategies can be external or internal in nature. External strategies involve interaction with external items, aids, or cues while internal strategies involve mental rehearsal, self-reminders,

Table 1-1

Cognitive Function: Underlying Elements

Structure	Processing Strategies and Behaviors
Attention	■ Reacts to a gross change in the environment ■ Detects subtle changes in task conditions ■ Initiates exploration (search of the environment) ■ Searches for information in a planned, systematic manner ■ Inhibits automatic responses ■ Maintains goal-directed behavior ■ Is unhindered by internal or external distractions peripheral to the task ■ Sustains focus of attention on task (eye contact) ■ Persists with a repetitive activity over time ■ Paces and monitors speed of response ■ Reduces stimuli/Identifies irrelevant information (cross out, sort, remove what is unnecessary) ■ Identifies relevant information (highlights, distinguishes critical details spontaneously, compares stimuli and chooses important facts) ■ Simultaneously attends to overall stimulus as well as details ■ Keeps track of rules, facts, pieces of information (external vs. internal methods) ■ Allocates resources by placing greater effort and concentration on more critical aspects of the task ■ Easily disengages focus of attention when necessary ■ Follows changes in task, stimuli, or rules without error, withdrawal, or resistance
Visual Processing	■ Initiates active visual search ■ Plans and systematically explores the visual display ■ Sustains visual fixation on stimuli for appropriate length of time ■ Distinguishes critical features of the object or picture ■ Detects and compares subtle visual details ■ Attends to the overall configuration ■ Shifts scanning approach with different stimuli arrangements ■ Localizes information in space ■ Pays equal attention to all parts of the visual field or stimulus figure ■ Paces and monitors speed of response to visual information ■ Simultaneously keeps track of what is seen ■ Looks at the whole and divides it into parts ■ Recognizes the stimulus from different perspectives (involves identifying critical attributes, visual imagery, and abstract thinking) ■ Can use visual imagery to describe objects or pictures that are not present ■ Simultaneously attends to the parts and whole
Memory	■ Recognizes overall context ■ Recognizes most important details or information ■ Focuses, fixates on stimulus to be recalled ■ Sustains focus of attention on material to be remembered ■ Spontaneously shifts focus of attention to the different stimuli to be remembered ■ Uses stimuli reduction methods (e.g., studies only a limited portion at one time and breaks the large amount into smaller, more manageable units) ■ Summarizes or identifies the main points or theme ■ Uses rehearsal (requires sustained repetitive activity)

continued

Table 1-1—*Continued.*

Cognitive Function: Underlying Elements

Structure	Processing Strategies and Behaviors
Memory	■ Uses association (requires ability to recognize similarities and differences between stimuli and organize information into concept categories)
	■ Uses elaboration (the ability to link meaningless with meaningful information)
	■ Has the ability to access previous knowledge and relate new information to old information
	■ Uses visual imagery
	■ Initiates use of memory strategy (e.g., if unable to spontaneously recall, does not give up but persists in trying to use active retrieval strategies to trigger memory)
	■ Spontaneously uses external aids to assist in recall
Problem Solving	■ Recognizes that an obstacle or problem exists
	■ Predicts the consequences of an obstacle or action
	■ Analyzes the conditions of the problem
	■ Recognizes when information is incomplete and actively searches for needed information
	■ Attends to relevant details, highlights or lists critical information
	■ Prioritizes information
	■ Distinguishes critical facts, assumptions, and irrelevant information
	■ Summarizes the main issues
	■ Simultaneously keeps track of all the relevant information; uses external aids when appropriate
	■ Narrows down range of possibilities
	■ Has ability to hypothesize (goes beyond "here and now" and anticipates events, or plan future goals)
	■ When problem is large, breaks problem up into two or more manageable subproblems
	■ When stuck, reexamines the problem in a different way, reorganizes information differently, asks questions for clarification, talks aloud through each step, or brainstorms
	■ Is able to view situation or problem from different vantage points
	■ Formulates a plan (sequence of action)
	■ Shifts to alternative strategies, plans when needed
	■ Classifies or groups related information together
	■ Initiates the plan of action
	■ Shows flexibility and reversibility in thinking
	■ Simultaneously holds in mind all the qualities of a situation, object or experience
	■ Monitors speed or pace as carrying out the task.
	■ Persists with the task in searching for a solution
	■ Spontaneously checks work

self-cues, or self-questions. External and internal strategies can be further described by their range of application. Situational strategies are effective in specific tasks or environments while nonsituational strategies are applicable in a wide range of tasks and environments (Toglia, 1989a). One example of a situational strategy is rehearsal or repeating information to oneself over and over. This strategy may be useful when the amount of information to be remembered is small; it is not effective in situations where the amount to be recalled is large. Nonsituational strategies are nonspecific in nature and include pacing the speed of response, visualizing oneself performing a task prior to actual performance, and verbalizing the task steps or rules during task performance. Processing strategies are overseen and managed by metacognitive processes. Strategy use requires the ability to anticipate difficulties and accurately judge task difficulty in relationship to one's current abilities (Brown et al., 1983). If one does not understand the full extent of his or her limitations, he or she will not perceive the need to approach the task in a more efficient way.

Metacognition

Metacognition refers to knowledge and regulation of one's own cognitive processes and capacities. It includes two interrelated aspects: awareness of one's own cognitive processes and capacities, and the ability to monitor performance (Flavell, 1985). Awareness has been further differentiated by Crosson et al. (1989) into three independent aspects:

1. Intellectual awareness, which refers to the client's ability to understand that at some level a particular function is impaired.
2. Emergent awareness, which is the ability to recognize a problem when it is actually happening.
3. Anticipatory awareness, or the ability to anticipate that a problem may occur.

Thus, awareness is not all or none. There are different aspects of awareness that may be observed before, during, and immediately after performing a task. The metacognitive skills involved within awareness and self-monitoring include the ability to evaluate task difficulty in relationship to one's own strengths and weaknesses; to predict or anticipate the likelihood of problems or the consequences of action; to plan ahead; to choose appropriate strategies; to recognize errors as they are occurring; to verify the accuracy of performance; and to revise solutions (Toglia, 1991). These skills have been demonstrated to be critical components in the learning and generalization process (Belmont, Butterfield, & Ferretti, 1982). They also influence the individuals degree of self-efficacy and motivation.

Self-efficacy is described as judgments and beliefs of one's performance capabilities with respect to a task. It includes the beliefs a person has regarding his or her control over a situation (Gage & Polatajko, 1994). Impairments in metacognitive skills result in errors of judgment regarding one's performance. This inevitably leads to a perceived lack of predictability and loss of control over performance. The individual who is unable to anticipate or recognize errors is taken by surprise with unexpected task outcomes or performance. Overly optimistic predictions of performance results in an inability to establish realistic goals. The individual experiences repeated failures without understanding why and eventually gives up. A strong sense of self-efficacy is related to persistence and effort in an activity, commitment to goals, high self-esteem, psychological well-being and motivation (Gage & Polatajko, 1994). The more an individual believes he or she has control over a situation, the better he or she will perform (Bandura, 1986). Thus metacognition is closely related to self-efficacy, motivation, and learning.

Learner Characteristics

The ability to maximize use of our limited information processing capacity depends on our ability to link new information with previous experience. Past knowledge influences the strategy selection, organization, representation, and processing speed of new information (Bransford, Sherwood, Vye, & Rieser, 1986). There are two types of knowledge. Procedural knowledge, or knowing how to perform, is acquired through practice and feedback. It is activated when the individual recognizes patterns associated with a given action sequence. Declarative knowledge, or knowing about facts and things, is acquired when new information stimulates the activation of relevant prior knowledge. Organization and elaboration of new information are required to activate declarative knowledge (Gange, 1985). When people are presented with information in a way that helps them activate appropriate knowledge, it can have a powerful effect on their abilities to process information (Bransford, 1979). Information that is recognized as familiar is easier to organize and is processed with less effort and less stress on the capacity limitations of the system. Thus the amount of information that can be taken in at any one time varies with the meaningfulness and familiarity of the stimulus (Toglia, 1993a).

The use of strategies, metacognitive skills, and previous knowledge to process information requires the individual's active participation. The individual's emotional state, personality characteristics, and motivation will significantly influence the extent to which information is processed deeply and is monitored (Brown, 1988). For example, anxiety, depression, and boredom will decrease the ability to process information deeply and use effective strategies. Likewise, an individual who believes that he or she will not get better no matter how hard they try may not persist or actively participate in task performance (Gage & Polatajko, 1994). Premorbid personality characteristics such as a lifelong pattern of resistance to change or a tendency to be set in one's own ways of doings things may also influence the way in which information is processed and perceived.

Environment

The type of environment (social, physical, cultural) an individual is in can influence his or her ability to process information and adapt to demands.

The social environment has occupied a central place in some theories of cognitive development and includes the people with whom the individual interacts (Feuerstein, 1979; Vygotsky, 1978). Vygotsky (1978) and Feuerstein (1979) have argued that much of learning and higher cognitive skills are mediated through social interaction. For example in child development, an experienced adult guides the child through problem-solving activities and structures the child's learning environment by selecting, focusing, and organizing incoming stimuli. Social interactions can transform or mediate incoming information either to enhance or to impede information processing (Jensen & Feuerstein, 1987). An adult may speak rapidly and present the child with complex directions to a task. The child may become overwhelmed by the information, and withdraw or refuse to participate. Another adult may present the same information in a slow, simplified, and structured manner and the child may readily participate in the task. In one case information processing is inhibited, whereas in the other case it is enhanced. When another person successfully structures incoming information, the individual may begin to internalize this external structuring and adopt regulatory activities on his or her own (Brown & Ferrara, 1985). Vygotsky (1978) describes the distance between the level of a child's unaided performance and the level that can be accomplished through guidance or collaboration with a more knowledgeable participant as the "zone of proximal development." Solving tasks with the assistance of a more knowledgeable person creates the zone of proximal development by tapping processes that "will mature tomorrow but are in the embryonic state" (Vygotsky, 1978, p. 86). The level of performance the child can reach unaided characterizes the cognitive skills that have already developed, while the zone of proximal development characterizes cognitive skills that are in the developmental stage (Brown & French, 1979). Vygotsky's (1978) and Feuerstein's (1979) theories imply that what an individual can accomplish with guidance or external aid from a more capable peer indicates the individual's learning potential. This concept has direct implications for assessment and treatment of brain-injured adults. Cicerone and Tupper (1986) propose that Vygotsky's definition of the zone of proximal development can be adopted as a guiding principle in the dynamic assessment of rehabilitation potential.

The physical environment includes the materials and objects that surround an individual. The cultural environment involves the values and expectations accepted by the person's cultural group. More familiar physical and cultural environments can influence the individual's ability to process information (Abreu & Toglia, 1987). Familiar environments provide contextual cues that can facilitate the access of previous knowledge and skills and guide in the selection and processing of new information.

Features of the physical environment such as the degree of auditory and visual distractions, and the organization and arrangement of objects, can affect the ability to perform a task. For example, a client may be asked to make cereal and toast for breakfast. In one situation, the kitchen may be familiar, quiet, and neatly organized. The refrigerator and cabinets may have only a few items on each shelf and the counter may contain only a toaster oven. In another situation, the kitchen may be unfamiliar, cluttered, and disorganized. The refrigerator and cabinets may be visually overcrowded with a large assortment of items. The counter may contain a number of different appliances and unfamiliar gadgets. In addition, auditory distractions such as the telephone ringing, sirens, and busy traffic from the street may be present. Although the task instructions and goal remain the same, the strategies needed to perform the task are very different. In the latter example, the physical environment places greater demands on attention, visual discrimination, ability to keep track of information, and organization. The abilities of the client need to be matched with the features of both the task and the environment.

The Task

The self-monitoring skills and processing strategies needed to perform the task are partially determined by parameters of the task. Table 1-2 illustrates how the manipulation of individual features of a task can place different demands on the underlying skills and strategies required to perform a figure ground task or visual discrimination. In assessment and treatment one or two task parameters are systematically changed while the others are held constant to determine its effect on performance. For example, in a figure ground task, differences in the familiarity of the stimuli, number of stimuli, contrast, and degree of detail, determine the skills and strategies required to perform the task. Difficulty on a figure ground task can occur for many different reasons. The extent to which cognitive perceptual symptoms are observed depends on the task parameters. An individual may be able to choose one object out of 10 familiar objects lined up on a shelf but may be unable to accurately locate an abstract shape embedded in an unfamiliar design pattern. Both can be considered figure ground tasks but the demands of the tasks and the strategies needed to perform them are very different.

The task parameters under which performance breaks down can be analyzed during assessment and treatment by systematically varying individual task parameters while simultaneously holding other parameters constant. This provides insight into the client's underlying difficulties. This concept can also be illustrated within the context of a categorization task. For example, a client may be unable to accurately sort 35 cards into meaningful categories; however, when the number of cards is reduced to 15, the client may have no difficulty. The ability to categorize or to recognize the objects' similarities and differences may be intact. However, difficulty recalling which cards have been placed in which categories may interfere with the client's ability to perform the task when a larger number of stimuli are involved. A larger number of stimuli requires additional strategies for keeping track of and organizing the material. It also requires closer self-monitoring skills.

Additional task parameters such as the body alignment, positioning, and active movement patterns required during an activity can also influence the selection of different processing strategies (Abreu & Toglia, 1987). By analyzing the task parameters, one can understand the conditions that cause information processing to break down. This contrasts to the deficit-specific approach, where the deficit is defined by the task. Thus, if the client cannot do a categorization task or a figure ground task, he or she is assumed to have a categorization or figure ground deficit. The task parameters that influence performance are not analyzed.

In addition to influencing the ability to process information, task characteristics can also influence the ability to transfer learning. Tasks can be divided into surface characteristics and conceptual characteristics. The surface characteristics of a task are easily observed. They include the type of stimuli, their spatial arrangement and presentation mode, directions needed for the task, and/or active movement and postural requirements. The conceptual characteristics of a task cannot be directly observed. These include the underlying skills and strategies used to perform the task as well as the underlying meaning of the task to the individual (Toglia, 1991). The closer two tasks are physically (or the more they share surface characteristics), the easier it is to transfer learning (Gange, 1970; Gick & Holyoak, 1983).

Transfer of learning can occur at different distances along a continuum and is defined according

	Table 1-2		
Visual Discrimination and/or Figure Ground Tasks—Task Grading			
Task Parameters	**Simple** Less attention and effort $\rightarrow$	**Complex** Greater attention and effort	**Demands with Increased Complexity**
Familiarity of stimuli	Familiar stimuli, e.g., simple shapes, everyday objects, letters, words	$\rightarrow$ Less familiar, e.g., unusual objects, abstract unfamiliar shapes	More difficult to pick up distinctive features
Directions	Structured, e.g., matching or point to specific items	$\rightarrow$ Unstructured, e.g., "Tell me what you see." "Find all the food items."	Requires initiation and organized visual search strategies, persistence
Distinctive features	Readily apparent, e.g., regular pen. The pen point is the distinctive feature.	$\rightarrow$ Obscure or partially hidden features, e.g., novelty pen that looks like a candy cane	Greater part-whole synthesis, visual attention. More difficult to pick of critical features and recognize items—Increased likelihood of misperception.
Degree of detail	Little to no detail	$\rightarrow$ Fine detail	Greater demands on visual acuity, scanning, and attention
Contrast	High contrast, e.g., red sock with white socks	$\rightarrow$ Low contrast, e.g., light beige and white socks	Harder to determine where one item ends and another begins; greater demands on visual acuity and selective attention
Background	Soft backgrounds, solids, nonpatterned	$\rightarrow$ Confusing and distracting backgrounds, patterns	Greater selective attention
Context	Within environmental context, e.g., grooming item in bathroom	$\rightarrow$ Outside of context, e.g., grooming item in therapy area	Greater visual attention to critical features. Less cues for recognition
Amount	Less than 10 items are presented at any one time	$\rightarrow$ 25–50 items are presented simultaneously	Greater demands on selective attention, and strategies to keep track of visual stimuli
Arrangement	Organized into predictable format such as horizontal rows	$\rightarrow$ Randomly scattered and/or overlapping so that some features of objects are partially obscured	Greater demands on saccadic eye movements, part-whole synthesis, strategies to keep track of visual stimuli, ability to change search pattern

In treatment, some task parameters are held constant, while others are varied to emphasize particular skills and strategies.

Adapted from Toglia (in press). Cognitive retraining and rehabilitation. In M. E. Neistadt & E. B. Crepeau (Eds.), Willard & Spackman's occupational therapy (9th ed.). Philadelphia: Lippincott.

to task characteristics (Toglia, 1991). For example, near transfer is an alternative form of the same task (only one or two surface task parameters are changed). Intermediate transfer occurs when the new task shares some physical features with the original task, but they are less obvious (three to six surface task parameters are changed). Far transfer occurs when the task is conceptually the same, but physically different (all task parameters are changed except for one or two). Very far transfer occurs when what has been learned in treatment is transferred to everyday functions.

Summary of the Dynamic Interactional Model of Cognition

In this model, cognition is viewed as a dynamic interaction between the individual (strategies, metacognition, learner characteristics), the task, and the environment (social, physical, and cultural) (Bransford, 1979; Brown et al., 1983; Lidz, 1987). The environment can mediate processing between the task and the individual. In some situations the task parameters may be the primary influence on information processing; in other situations the environment or individual characteristics may be the most influential. To understand cognitive function, one must analyze the interaction between all three components. Assessment and treatment reflect this dynamic view of cognition.

Redefining Cognitive Function and Dysfunction

Cognitive function, as previously described, requires the ability to receive, elaborate, and monitor incoming information. It involves the ability to flexibly use and apply information across task boundaries. Cognitive function includes the spontaneous selection and use of efficient processing strategies, the ability to access previous knowledge when needed, and awareness of one's cognitive capacity (Lidz, 1987). It is described by defining the task parameters and environment as well as the underlying processing strategies that are needed to perform the task. Cognitive symptoms are observed when there is a mismatch between the abilities of the client and the features of the task and environment.

This approach emphasizes the global capacities of cognition. Inefficient use and/or limits in information processing resources underlie many different cognitive symptoms. Cognitive dysfunction is conceptualized in terms of deficiencies in processing strategies and metacognitive strategies rather than by deficits in specific cognitive skills (Toglia, 1993a). Brain-injured individuals often display inflexible and inefficient strategy use. There is a failure to initiate and apply use of self-regulatory or metacognitive behaviors such as anticipating, monitoring, checking, and revising solutions. Difficulties in a wide range of attention, memory, visual processing, and problem-solving tasks may be reflective of the same underlying behavior or inefficient strategy. For example, a tendency to overfocus on irrelevant details may interfere with a memory task, a visual processing task, and a problem-solving task. The common behaviors that interfere with performance on a number of different tasks are analyzed rather than deficits in specific cognitive skills. In addition, the task parameters and the environmental characteristics that increase and decrease the cognitive perceptual symptoms are specified when describing cognitive dysfunction.

Cognitive dysfunction can affect functioning in all spheres of life: social and interpersonal, work, leisure, and daily living. Individual tasks may be performed inefficiently. The client may be unable to decide what to attend to first, how to prioritize, or how to break the task into steps. Excessive time may be spent processing nonessential details, and the client may have difficulty keeping track of previous events or associating related information (Toglia & Golisz, 1990). A significant number of brain-injured clients are unaware of their limitations in task performance (Anderson & Tranel, 1989). Individuals who are unable to accurately judge the difficulty of a task in relationship to their own abilities tend to go beyond what they are capable of and show impairments in judgment and safety. Diminished awareness affects the ability to learn from one's mistakes and use feedback to modify behavior (Barco et al., 1991).

In social situations, cognitive dysfunction may interfere with the individual's ability to accurately take in and integrate all parts of a situation. The client may have decreased awareness of another person's verbal and nonverbal reactions and may have difficulty following conversations. His or her behavior may, therefore, be inappropriate to the context of the situation (Toglia & Golisz, 1990). In addition, difficulty in shifting one's attention or viewing information from different perspectives may interfere with the ability to compromise and understand another person's point of view. Diminished social skills result in social isolation and depression, which further inhibit cognitive functioning (Fine, 1993).

Cognitive problems reflect a reduced capacity to acquire and use new information. Cognitive dysfunction can be summarized as representing core deficiencies in the following areas:

1. The ability to select and use efficient processing strategies to organize and structure incoming information (Bolger, 1982; Melamed, Rahmani, Greenstein, Groswasser, & Najenson, 1985)
2. The ability to anticipate, monitor, and verify the accuracy of performance
3. The ability to access previous knowledge when needed
4. Flexible application of knowledge and skills to a variety of situations (Toglia, 1991).

These deficits may be observed in localized areas such as in visual processing, or they may exist regardless of the modality involved. Deficient functions are not completely absent but represent areas of weakness and vulnerability (Groverman, Brown, & Miller, 1985). The extent to which these deficiencies are observed depends on the parameters of the task (e.g., number of stimuli, complexity, familiarity), the environment, and the learner's characteristics (emotional status, motivation, personality). For example, a client's tendency to overfocus on irrelevant details or to recognize and anticipate errors may only emerge under certain task and environmental conditions. The underlying processes and behaviors that are interfering with the client's performance in the majority of tasks are the components that are analyzed during assessment and targeted as priorities for treatment.

Different Types of Assessment Methods

Assessment methods can be described as static, qualitative, or dynamic. Each type of assessment addresses a different set of questions. Static assessments such as standardized cognitive screening instruments and neuropsychological tests are based on traditional psychometric models. They define "here and now" performance. The objective of static assessments is to identify and quantify cognitive deficits. This information is necessary for diagnosis, monitoring progress, discharge planning, and client or caregiver education regarding ex-

pected behaviors (Toglia, 1989b). In static assessments, the end product of performance is often viewed as more important than clinical observations and it can be difficult to determine what contributed to the final results. Qualitative assessment methods emphasize the process of observing how an individual goes about performing a task. Sometimes the approach to a task or the way in which an individual accomplishes a task provides more information than the end result. The same quantitative score may be interpreted in two different ways when combined with qualitative information (Golisz & Toglia, in press). Dynamic methods seek to identify and specify the conditions that have the greatest influence on performance. Dynamic assessment incorporates qualitative methods but it goes beyond them by using methods that attempt to facilitate or change performance. The extent to which performance can be changed through cues or task modifications is directly related to choosing and planning interventions. Table 1-3 summarizes the different questions that each method addresses. An example that illustrates the use of each method is given within the context of a cancellation task. In a cancellation task, a client is asked to cross out a target letter or number on a page out of an array of other letters or numbers. Quantitative methods emphasize the number of target items that are omitted. A qualitative approach is interested in observing where the individual begins and how he proceeds, whereas a dynamic method provides cues to attempt to facilitate performance. The different testing methods may be used alone or in combination. The emphasis and extent of testing depends on the purpose of assessment.

In many cases, the first step in assessment is problem identification. In cases where it is unclear whether the client has cognitive perceptual deficits, or to what extent they are present, a static assessment is most appropriate. However, in some cases, quantification and identification of cognitive perceptual deficits may have already been established through a neuropsychological evaluation. Once general deficits are identified, the role of the occupational therapist is to explore these deficits further. The therapist needs to specify which conditions increase or decrease symptoms and investigate the client's use of processing strategies. This information is a necessary prerequisite for treat-

Table 1-3		
Different Assessment Methods		
Static	**Qualitative**	**Dynamic**
Is there a problem?	What is the underlying nature of the problem?	Can performance be facilitated or changed?
What is the problem?	Why is the person having difficulty?	What cues/conditions increase or decrease the symptoms?
What is the severity of the problem?		What is the individual's potential for learning?
Example: Cancellation test The number of items omitted on the right and left side is scored.	*Example: Cancellation test* Different colored pencils are given every 10 seconds to document the pattern of scanning; where it began, how it proceeded.	*Example: Cancellation test* Graded cues are given during or after the task to determine if the client can improve or self-correct performance.

Adapted from Toglia, J. P. (1996, June). *The Multicontext Approach to cognitive rehabilitation.* [Supplement manual to workshop conducted at New York Hospital, New York.]

ment. In situations where cognitive deficits have already been objectively identified by another discipline, it is not time- or cost-efficient for the occupational therapist to assess all areas of cognitive perceptual function. For example, if the neuropsychological report indicates that visual perceptual skills are intact while memory, organization, and problem-solving skills are impaired, the occupational therapy evaluation does not need to address visual spatial skills.

Dynamic Interactional Assessment

Dynamic assessment is based on Vygotsky's (1978) concept of the zone of proximal development. The principles of dynamic assessment have been used in standard assessments with learning disabled, mentally retarded, and normal children (Campione, Brown, 1987; Jensen & Feuerstein, 1987). Dynamic Interactional Assessment (DIA), also termed *dynamic investigative assessment,* uses principles of dynamic assessment that have been adapted for use with brain-injured individuals. Dynamic assessment procedures are combined with investigation of strategy use and awareness in DIA.

DIA is based on the dynamic interactional model of cognition described earlier. In this approach,

the ability to learn and generalize information is central to the concept of cognition. Therefore, the assessment of cognitive abilities includes estimates of the potential for learning and looks at how an individual goes about solving problems and dealing with situations. An observed problem with a specific task is often the result of interactions among multiple components including personality and emotional factors, task and environment variables, as well as deficiencies in processing strategies and metacognitive skills. DIA attempts to specify how external (task, environment) and internal (processing strategies, metacognition, motivation) components influence the ability to process information.

DIA consists of three components that are integrated during assessment: (1) awareness questioning, (2) cueing and task grading, (3) strategy investigation (Toglia, 1993a). Theses components of dynamic interactional assessment are described below and summarized in Table 1-4.

Awareness questioning

DIA begins with an awareness interview that is designed to differentiate among different aspects of awareness (intellectual, anticipatory, emergent). The individual is asked general questions regarding

Table 1-4

Components of Dynamic Interactional Assessment (DIA)

1. **Awareness Interview**
   a) Prior to Task
   —General Questioning
   —Prediction

   b) Immediately After Task
   —General Questioning
   —Estimation

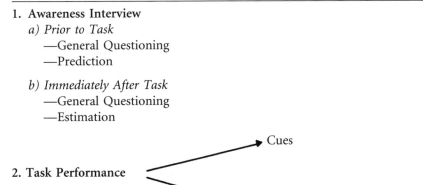

2. **Task Performance**

   Cues

   Changes in Task Parameters

3. **Strategy Investigation and Probing of Responses**

Adapted from Toglia, J. P. (1996, June). The Multicontext Approach to cognitive rehabilitation. [Supplement manual to workshop conducted at New York Hospital, New York.]

his or her cognitive perceptual functioning to assess intellectual awareness. The questions gradually become more specific and require the client to predict his or her performance (anticipatory awareness). During task performance, the therapist observes emergent awareness or the extent to which the client is able to self-detect and correct errors. Immediately following task performance, the individual is once again asked to rate his or her overall performance and specifically estimate performance or score. There is evidence that indicates that awareness can be differentiated by the type and timing of awareness questions (Schacter, 1991). An awareness interview that is currently being tested with stroke clients who have unilateral inattention is illustrated in Table 1-5. The interview is divided into questions that are asked before and then after the task. Within each section both general and specific questions are asked. This format is being used and tested in other areas of cognition as well.

Cueing and Task Grading

If the client has difficulty during a task, the clinician attempts to facilitate performance by providing a series of cues and/or reducing the demands of the task. A sample sequence of graded cues used in a cancellation task to facilitate attention to the left side is presented in Table 1-6. Performance may also be facilitated by gradually changing one parameter of the task at a time (e.g., decreasing the number of items or simplifying the instructions). If an individual's initial attempt at a task is completely unsuccessful (no partially accurate responses), task modifications should be used rather than verbal cues.

Strategy Investigation

Strategy investigation involves probing the individual's responses without suggesting the answers. For example, the individual may be asked to explain why he or she chose a particular answer, using such "questions" as, "Tell me how you chose this solution. Tell me how you know these items are the same. Tell me how you kept track of everything that you needed to do." In addition, techniques such as reflection or repeating the client's answer may be used (Toglia 1989b).

DIA is individually focused, flexible, interactionist, and process-oriented. The examiner does not

Table 1-5

Sample Items from Unilateral Inattention Awareness Interview

Prior to the Task (general and specific questions)

Are you having any trouble locating or seeing all the objects around you since your stroke?
4 I'm certain, I don't have any difficulties
3 I don't think I have any difficulties
2 I think I may have difficulties
1 I'm certain I have difficulties

Are you having any trouble finding things on the left side?
(same choices as above)

If ans 2 or 1 ask: *How frequently is this difficulty interfering with your ability to function?*
5 Not at all
4 Occasionally (1 to 3 times a month)
3 One or two times a week
2 Several times a week (3 to 6 times a week)
1 Daily

Prediction (sample items)
I am going to ask you to read this paragraph. Do you think you will have any difficulty?
4 I'm certain I don't have any difficulties
3 I don't think I have any difficulties
2 I think I may have difficulties
1 I'm certain I have difficulties

What kind of difficulty do you think you would have?

If ans 2 or 1 ask: *Do you think you would miss any words?*
5 No
4 I could miss a couple of words—1 or 2
3 I could miss a few—Less than 25%
2 I could miss a several—Up to one-half
1 I could miss many words—more than one-half

After Task: Estimation of Performance (general and specific questions)

How did you do on this task?
4 I'm certain I didn't have any difficulties
3 I don't think I had any difficulties
2 I think I may have had difficulties
1 I'm certain I had difficulties

Do you think you would have performed any differently on this task before your stroke/injury?
    1. Yes   2. No

What was your accuracy on this task?
5 I did not miss any words or numbers
4 I may have missed 1 or 2
3 I may have missed a few—Less than 25%
2 I may have missed—Up to one-half
1 I may have missed many words or numbers—More than one-half

Adapted from Toglia, J. P. (1996, June). The Multicontext Approach to cognitive rehabilitation. [Supplement manual to workshop conducted at New York Hospital, New York.]

Table 1-6	
Sample Graded Cue Sequence	
Rationale	**Example of Cues**
Check and verify answer	Are you sure you found all the letter As?
General feedback	There are still some left. Can you find them?
Specific feedback	There are still some on the left side.
Provide alternative approach	Try: beginning here. Go slower and use your finger to point to each letter.
Task modification	Change one task parameter (e.g., number of items on the page are reduced; bright red line is placed in the left margin).

From Toglia, J. P. (1996, June). The Multicontext Approach to cognitive rehabilitation. [Supplement manual to workshop conducted at New York Hospital, New York.]

simply observe behavior but attempts to change behavior. The assessment analyzes the use of processing strategies and metacognitive skills (self-monitoring, awareness) during task performance. DIA seeks to estimate the degree of change that is possible as well as to specify the means by which changes in performance can be produced (Toglia, 1989b). Assessment focuses on the individual's best performance or maximum level of function. It taps on weakened skills that lie beneath the surface but have the potential for function. Assessment within the zone of proximal development has been thought to discriminate differences in abilities not identified using conventional methods (Brown & Ferrara, 1985; Brown & French, 1979). Affected functions may exhibit a differing potential for change. Not all functions that are impaired show equal potential for restitution (Cicerone & Tupper, 1986).

In DIA, the examiner–examinee relationship is considered crucial. In standardized tests, the procedures are designed to provide the same environment for each examinee. Examiners are trained to remain neutral, not to question or add to the individual's response and not to help the individual in any way. They have avoided the use of cues, questioning task modifications, and interaction with the examinee in standardized testing because they can influence reliability and validity. DIA seeks to measure cognitive modifiability or the change that is possible under different conditions. Classical psychometric procedures cannot be accommodated easily for the measurement of

change. Therefore, DIA requires use of a nontraditional measurement model (Embretson, 1987).

There are several different test designs that can incorporate the use of dynamic testing procedures (Embretson, 1987; Toglia, 1989b). I am currently working on developing a number of different types of DIAs for the brain-injured adult. Some of the assessments have also been piloted with chronic schizophrenic clients. The individual assessments cover a range of tasks including sorting cards into categories, the Contextual Memory Test (Toglia, 1989b; 1993b), and copying designs. Four examples—the Contextual Memory Test, Dynamic Visual Processing Assessment, Toglia Category Assessment, and Deductive Reasoning Test—are presented in the following section. Each assessment was developed through videotape analysis of clients performing tasks with unstandardized cues and questions. From the videotape analysis, guidelines and sequences of cues and questioning were developed.

One limitation of DIAs is that the use of cues prevents the test from being used to measure progress or change over time. Another limitation is that extensive examiner training is required to use and interpret the assessments proficiently. In addition, most of the dynamic assessments described in the following section require use of language skills. However, the principles of DIA can easily be adapted for aphasic clients by using tactile or visual cues. An example of the application of dynamic assessment principles to functional tasks and individuals with aphasia and apraxia follows.

Examples of Dynamic Interactional Assessment

The Contextual Memory Test

The Contextual Memory Test (CMT) (Toglia, 1993b) investigates awareness of memory capacity, recall performance, and strategy use. The test begins by asking the individual general questions about his or her memory functioning and then asking the individual to predict his or her score. The individual is asked to study a picture card containing 20 line drawings of items for 90 seconds. The pictures are related to a restaurant theme or to a morning theme. In part I the individual is not told that the items pictured on the card are related to a theme (see Table 1-7). The individual is asked to recall the items immediately after presentation and then again after 15 to 20 minutes. After immediate recall, the individual is asked to estimate his or her performance and the use of strategies are probed with standard questions. Table 1-7 presents an illustration of the morning scene as well as sample questions used to probe awareness and strategy use.

If the individual demonstrates poor recall and poor strategy use in part I, part II is administered. Part II involves repeating the recall section with an equivalent form of the test. The major difference between part I and part II is that the instructions for the test in part II provide information on the theme or context of the pictures. The purpose is to determine whether recall performance can be influenced by giving the individual a cue to help

---

Table 1-7

Sample Items from the Contextual Memory Test

Awareness and Strategy Questions	Morning Scene
Prior to the Task: Have you noticed any changes in your memory? If you studied 20 objects for a minute and a half, how many do you think you would be able to remember? *After the Task:* How difficult was this task for you? Estimate the number of objects that you remembered. When you were studying the information, what did you do to help you remember?	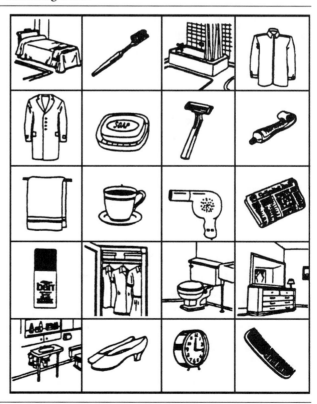

From Toglia, J. P. (1993b). *The Contextual Memory Test.* Tucson: Therapy Skill Builders. © 1993 Joan Toglia. Reprinted with Permission.

in categorizing items and utilizing the background theme of the items. If recall performance is not facilitated with cues, then recognition memory may be tested by presenting 40 cards, one at a time, and asking the individual to choose the target stimulus items (Toglia, 1993b).

The CMT has both static and dynamic qualities. Part I may be used alone to screen individuals for memory impairments. Part II provides a dynamic component to the assessment. One task parameter is changed to examine the effect on recall performance. An individual can have difficulty on the CMT for a variety of different reasons. An individual may perform poorly because of difficulty in shifting visual attention to different items, tendency to overfocus on irrelevant details, poor attention span, decreased ability to recognize categories or create relationships and associations between items, or decreased ability to initiate active strategy use. The order of recall as well as the response to strategy investigation questions and cues given in part II provide insight into the underlying difficulties. Performance is analyzed by looking at the combination of results in the areas of awareness, recall, and strategy use. The test manual describes how different patterns of performance provide different implications for treatment (Toglia, 1993b).

Normative data have been collected on 375 adults in the New York area ranging in age from 18 to 86 with a mean age of 46. In addition, Hartman-Maeir & Josman (unpublished) have recently completed the collection of normative data on 217 adults in Israel, ages 18 to 86. Preliminary analysis of the Israeli data suggests that items such as a cash register, sandwich, and bathtub were confusing and may need to be modified for this population. Average recall scores in the Israeli population were similar to that of the New York group (within less than one raw score point) within the exception of the above-60 age group. The average recall scores in this age group appear to be slightly lower than the New York group (within less than two raw score points). These data need to be further analyzed and may be related to differences within the two populations in educational background, familiarity of the items, and/or criteria for inclusion. Additional normative data are being collected

on the above-60 age group in the New York area. Normative data are also being collected on the pediatric population (ages 7 to 18). In general, pilot data on the pediatric population suggest that individuals age 12 and above perform similarly to the adult population while those under the age of 12 show a tendency to overestimate their scores, use poor strategies, and perform lower on recall measures. This is consistent with literature on the development of strategy use and metamemory skills.

Reliability and validity studies have been conducted on the CMT with brain-injured subjects and are described in the test manual. Concurrent validity was established by examining the correlation between the recall scores of the CMT and the Rivermead Behavioral Memory Test (Wilson, Cockburn, & Baddeley, 1985). Correlations ranged from .80 to .84. In addition, it was found that the two tests were similar in rating the severity of the memory disorder (e.g., normal, mild, moderate, severe) in the majority of clients (Toglia, 1993b).

Performances of 112 brain-injured subjects were compared with normal subjects on several different measures of the CMT. For example, in the area of awareness, brain-injured and normal individuals demonstrated significant differences in both the direction and the magnitude of predicted scores. Normal individuals tended to underestimate their scores by one or two items. Brain-injured individuals tended to overestimate their actual scores by an average of six items. An interesting finding was that the brain-injured individuals' actual predictions were similar to the scores of normal individuals. Thus it seems that brain-injured subjects tend to estimate their abilities based on their premorbid capacities (Toglia, 1993b).

Recently, responses to different aspects of awareness questions were examined. The results support the hypothesis that different aspects of awareness may be tapped by differences in the type and timing of the questions. For example, the correlation between general awareness questions and the ability to predict one's memory score was low, indicating little relationship between the two scores. The ability to generally acknowledge a memory problem does not seem to be related to the ability to predict memory capacity. Many clients readily admitted to and described memory problems but could not use this knowledge to accurately estimate the difficulty of a task or anticipate problems. In addition, there was little relationship between responses prior to the memory task and responses after the memory task, indicating that the questions asked before and after a task may measure different aspects of awareness. The results suggest that awareness may be differentiated by systematic and objective assessment.

Responses to awareness questions provide important implications for treatment. For example, an individual who has a tendency to considerably overestimate his or her score may have difficulty initiating memory compensatory techniques because he or she may be unable to anticipate when they might be needed. On the other hand, individuals who show good prediction scores may be good candidates for training in memory compensatory strategies. Several authors have observed a positive relationship between awareness and treatment outcome. Objective measurements of awareness may be helpful in predicting functional outcome.

The Dynamic Visual Processing Assessment

The Dynamic Visual Processing Assessment (DVPA) (Toglia & Finkelstein, 1991) consists of line drawings of objects that are presented under different task conditions. Object perception, unilateral inattention, the ability to keep track of what is seen, and organization of scanning are analyzed as each of four task conditions (number, arrangement, rotation, and familiarity) are independently changed. The test seeks to identify the specific task variables that influence the ability to process information. For example, it can determine the effect the number of items has on an examinee's unilateral inattention or his or her ability to keep track of what is seen. The test is progressively graded from simple to complex. Simple visual processing tasks are relatively automatic in nature and require little attention or effort. Complex visual processing tasks require effort, analysis, attention, and comparison of detail. The test begins at a middle level and moves up or down depending on the client's responses. In addition, a cueing sequence is incorporated into testing to determine the amount and type of assistance that enhance performance. There are two types of cueing sequences: cues for errors of omission and cues for errors of misperception (see Table 1-8). The use of cues and level of cueing indicates a lower ability.

Although the DVPA is in the research phase and is not yet commercially available, the concept can be used in the clinic by systematically varying task dimensions while presenting self-related and non-self-related objects. A sample worksheet is presented in Table 1-8. The first step is to collect self-related and non-self-related objects or pictures of objects (about 16 to 25 in each category). It is recommended that the therapist begin with 8 to 10 non–self-related objects that are scattered, overlapping each other, and rotated in varying positions on a table. The client is then asked, "Tell me what you see." Depending on the client's response, the task demands can be increased or decreased in difficulty by changing the number of items, the arrangement, or the type of items. The clinician observes where and how the client begins, the organization of scanning, and the ability to keep track of items that are named. If the client accurately names or describes an item, a check mark is placed next to it. An "O" or "M" is used to indicate an item that was omitted or misperceived. After the client is finished naming all the items, omission cues and/or misperception cues are given if errors were made. A matching format can be used with clients who have language difficulties. Table 1-8 illustrates a client who did not exhibit symptoms of neglect when eight self-related items were presented in an horizontal format. However, when eight non–self-related items were scattered and rotated, symptoms of left-sided neglect were observed.

The DVPA is designed to explain the task conditions that influence the identification and organization of visual information. It was hypothesized that a test that analyzes difficulty level according to the task parameters rather than according to specific items may show closer correlation with function. Kline (1997) investigated the relationship between the Modified DVPA and functional performance and found that the Modified DVPA demonstrated a stronger relationship to IADL skills

Table 1-8

Dynamic Visual Processing Assessment: Sample Assessment Worksheet

Dynamic Visual Processing Cue Sequence

Omission Cues	Score	Misperception Cues
Are you sure you have seen all the objects on the page? Could there be more?	4	Tell me how you know it is a _____. Could it be anything else?
There are still some that you didn't mention. Can you find them?	3	No, it is not a _____. Look again. or Describe what it looks like.
Look on the right/left/upper/middle of the page. Can you think of a way to help you keep track of the objects? Try it.	2	What category do you think it belongs to (present 5 choices)?
Try moving your eyes all the way over here (place red line). Try pointing like this to each object you mention in an organized way.	1	Look here (point to specific features).

From: Toglia, J.P., & Finkelstein, N. (1991). Test Protocol: The Dynamic Visual Processing Assessment. New York: New York Hospital Cornell Medical Center.

Dynamic Visual Processing Assessment of Objects

Fill out the form as outlined below:

Parameters: Specify any of the following: Horizontal row, Vertical row, Scattered, Overlapping, and Rotated or Nonrotated.

Object Type: Indicate self-related or non–self-related. Indicate the number of objects presented at one time.

Cues: Provide the below cues in graded order and document the cue score that facilitates a response. If the individual does not mention an item, omission cues are given. If the individual misnames an item or inaccurately describes the function of the item, misperception cues are given.

Client Performance

1. **Parameters:** Horizontal, 8, self-related				
Objects Type and # : 8 Non–self-related	Result	Omission Cues	Misperception Cues	Comments
Fork	√			
Toothbrush	√			
Comb	√			
Razor	√			
Spoon	√			
Watch	√			
Knife	√			
Hairbrush	√			

2. **Parameters:** Scattered, overlapping, rotated				
Objects Type and # : 8 Non–self-related	Result	Omission Cues	Misperception Cues	Comments
Battery	O	3		Missed items in left corner
Key	√			
Roll of camera film	√			
Can opener	√			
Screw driver	O	2		Missed item on left
Letter opener	M		4	Perseverated "screwdriver"
Roll of tape	√			Bracelet
Scissors	√			

√ = WNL;   O = omitted;   M = misperceived

Adapted from Toglia, J. P. (1996, June). The Multicontext Approach to cognitive rehabilitation. [Supplement manual to workshop conducted at New York Hospital, New York.]

than another standardized test of visual perception. This supports the validity of the tool and the theoretical foundation of the DVPA.

The Toglia Category Assessment

The Toglia Category Assessment (TCA) was designed to examine the ability to establish categories or switch conceptual sets. Awareness is investigated by asking the client standard questions designed to investigate awareness before and after task performance. The test uses 18 plastic utensils that can be sorted according to size (small or large), color (red, yellow, and green), and utensil type (knife, fork, or spoon). The examiner asks the client to sort the 18 utensils into different groups so that the items in one group are different in one way from those of the other groups. Once the client correctly classifies the items according to one attribute (size, color, or type), he or she is then asked to sort the items again in a different way and then again in a third way. Strategy use is investigated by asking the client to explain how the groups are different after each classification. Standard sequences of cues are provided if the client has difficulty (Toglia, 1994). Use of the cues helps to differentiate clients and their underlying problems. An individual can have difficulty with the TCA for a variety of reasons, such as a tendency to become stuck or preservative in one category or solution, a tendency to lose track of the sorting principle or categories, a concrete approach such as only grouping utensils according to use or function, or a disorganized approach to searching and sorting.

For example, one brain-injured client sorted the utensils into spoons, forks, and knives. When asked to sort the utensils a different way, the client shuffled the utensils around but ended up with the same three categories. Again the procedure was repeated and the client did the same thing. However, when he was cued to attend to the individual attributes (size and color), he immediately sorted them in different ways. This indicated that the client's underlying problem was a tendency to become stuck in one response. Another client was able to sort the utensils into two separate groups (first color and then type of utensil) but could not think of a third way to sort them. Although he

was provided with maximum cues, the client insisted there were only the two ways to sort the utensils and stated that "size was not a good category." These two clients' responses to cues provide differential implications for treatment that are described in the test manual (Toglia, 1994).

The test results are interpreted by examining responses to awareness questions in combination with the individual's responsiveness to cues. The extent to which awareness can be facilitated during task performance, and the individual's ability to benefit from cues and show a learning curve, are analyzed.

Josman (1993) conducted reliability and validity studies on the TCA with 35 brain-injured subjects and 35 chronic schizophrenic subjects. An interrater reliability of .87 was found. Performance on the TCA was compared to performance on the Riska Object Classification Test (ROC) (Riska & Allen, 1985) to establish concurrent validity. A moderate positive correlation was found between the two tests, which was statistically significant. Josman (1993) also investigated the ability to estimate performance immediately following the tasks and found that there was a significant difference between the mean awareness scores of the brain-injured and psychiatric populations. These results suggest that awareness questions may be useful in differentiating between populations. She also found that brain-injured clients who estimated that the task would be easy tended to have more difficulty than those who estimated that the test was hard. This is consistent with other studies that have found that a failure to recognize the difficulty of a task is associated with poorer task performance. Normative studies are currently in progress with the pediatric, elderly, and adult populations.

The Deductive Reasoning Test

The TCA utensils may also be used to dynamically assess deductive reasoning. In using the test for deductive reasoning, a question game is used to investigate the ability to formulate and test different hypotheses. In this task the examiner tells the client that he or she has to determine which utensil the examiner is thinking of, with the least amount of guessing and the fewest number of questions as possible. The client has to ask questions that can be answered as "yes" or "no." The examiner does not actually think of an item but answers "no" to all the questions (whenever possible) until there is only one possibility left. The answer is obtainable with five questions when 18 utensils of different colors (red, yellow, green), size (big, small), and type (fork, spoon, knife) are used. For example, if the following five questions are asked, the answer can be easily deduced: Is it red? yellow? spoon? fork? small? The answer must be a large green knife. If the client does not solve the problem with five questions, another trial is given with a maximum of up to three trials. The examiner gives a standard sequence of prompts when the client is unable to solve the problem with four questions. Preliminary analysis has revealed interesting patterns of responses. Two clients asked about each utensil, one by one: Is it this fork? Is it this spoon? When cued to narrow down the questions, one client immediately generated an efficient set of questions. The other client required maximum cues and still could not generate a different set of questions. In both cases the clients had the same initial baseline response, but again there were significant differences in the way they responded to cues. These differences have different implications for treatment planning. In one case, the client requires only a general cue to think of an alternative approach to the task. In the other case, treatment needs to focus on helping the client to attend to and discriminate between the various attributes before attempting to solve a problem.

Application of Dynamic Assessment Concepts to Aphasia and Apraxia

Dynamic assessment concepts may also be applied to individuals with aphasia and apraxia. Table 1-9 illustrates five sample items from a functional dynamic assessment. Each task is divided into substeps. The tasks range from those that are simple and include only three substeps (e.g., peel the banana) to those that are more complex (e.g., make a bowl of cereal). Each task is presented to the client with three to four unnecessary items. For example, in the cereal task, extra items such as a can opener, scissors, fork, and knife are placed on

the table along with the cereal items. The ability to perform each substep is documented in the result section by using the codes on the bottom of the form. For example, if the individual requires cues, a "C" is placed next to the substep. If the individual is unable to perform the substep with cues, the examiner performs that particular substep for the client and records an "E" next to that substep. The number of cues and type of cues required are recorded in the next two columns. Cues include visual gesturing or demonstration of the action by the examiner with or without the intended object, tapping or pointing to selected items, placing the correct item in the individual's hand, and providing partial tactile guidance if necessary. Table 1-9 illustrates a client who was globally aphasic and apraxic following bilateral strokes. The test results indicate that performance was consistently facilitated by selecting the relevant items and initiating the task by placing the appropriate item in the client's hand. This information was used in training the caregiver to enhance the individual's function. Rather than attempting to give the client verbal instructions, the caregiver was instructed to limit the number of items presented to the client at one time. The caregiver was also trained to place the initial item in the client's hand and provide a visual gesture depicting the action of the item if needed.

Linking Assessment to Treatment

In DIA, individuals are not classified as having deficits in separate cognitive areas. An individual may have difficulty on a memory task, a visual processing task, and a problem-solving task, but DIA focuses on the common behaviors that influence task performance. For example, difficulty in pacing speed of response or in considering all aspects of a situation can interfere with performance on a memory task and a visual processing task. DIA provides a starting point for treatment. It specifies the task parameters (e.g., number of items, arrangement of items) under which cognitive perceptual symptoms are most likely to emerge. These task parameters represent the starting point of treatment activities. In addition, the behaviors or symptoms that are observed on a wide range of

Table 1-9

Sample Dynamic Assessment of Clients with Aphasia and Apraxia

Task Direction	Objects on Table	Task Steps	Results	Cues	Type of Cues
Peel the banana	banana, orange, apple	Selects banana Orients banana Peels all sides	E √ √	0	
Butter the bread and cut it in half	knife, spoon, fork, plate, butter, bread cream cheese, sugar	Selects knife Holds knife properly Opens butter Butter on knife Spreads butter on bread Repeats spreading Cuts bread	E √- c √ √- √ C	2 3	P/G P/A/G
Pour the soda into the glass and drink it with the straw	soda can, glass, straw, fork, can opener, coffee mug, bowl	Selects can Opens can Pours into glass Opens straw Places straw in glass Drinks	E √- √ C √ C	1 3	G P/T/G
Fit the letter into the envelope, put a stamp on it	letter (8.5 × 11), envelope, stamp, letter opener, scissors, pen	Selects paper Folds paper Selects envelope Puts paper in envelope Takes stamp off packet Places stamp properly	E C E C C E	2 3 2	Gestures/ P P/T/G T/G
Make yourself a bowl of cereal	cereal, milk, bowl, spoon, fork, knife can of soda, box of pancake mix, orange juice, can opener, scissors	Selects cereal Opens cereal box Pours into bowl Selects milk Opens milk Pours milk Selects spoon Holds spoon properly Eats cereal	E E C C C* C C C	1 2 1 2 1 1	G-gestures A/T G G P G

Results

√   Client performs step without cues.
√- Client performs step in an awkward and clumsy manner without cues.
C   Client performs step with cues.
E   Examiner performs this step. Even with cues, client is unable to perform this step.
*   Step occurred out of sequence.

Cues may include but are not limited to:

V   = Verbal cues: Repeating/ rephrasing, simplifying directions, stating name of key object
SR = Stimuli reduction - Remove the unnecessary items
P   = Visually focusing attention by pointing
A   = Auditorily focusing attention by tapping
G   = Visually gesturing action without object
G/0 = Visually gesturing action with object
T   = Tactile cues to initiate movement
TS = Task segmentation—Remove all items. Present one item at a time in the order in which it is used.

Note: If examiner places object in client's hand, then a E is used for item selection, because the examiner performed this step.

Adapted from Toglia, J. (Dec, 1993). Treatment of individuals with limb apraxia. Presented at AOTA Neuroscience Institute: Treating Adults with Apraxia, Denver, Co.

tasks and are *most* responsive to cues are targeted for intervention using a multicontext approach. It is important to note that the areas that are most responsive to cues are not always the most observable deficits. They represent weakened skills that lie just below the surface and emerge inconsistently and/or with guidance. Cognitive perceptual difficulties can be conceptualized in layers. Once the layer that is functioning just beneath the surface emerges consistently, the next layer of difficulties may become ready for intervention.

Treatment

The Dynamic Interactional Model of Cognition provides a framework for simultaneously using and integrating different treatment approaches. It proposes that a mismatch among the individual's capabilities, the task, and the environment results in the expression of cognitive symptoms. Treatment needs to use activities that meet the abilities of the individual. This may require breaking down some components of a task or adapting some features of the environment and task while simultaneously training the individual to use a targeted strategy or cognitive subskill. The person's strategies or behaviors that are most responsive to cues are targeted for change using a multicontext approach. At the same time, treatment may seek to adapt features of the task or environment to maximize function in those areas that show less responsiveness to change. Different approaches to treatment such as adaptation, functional skill training, compensation, and remediation inherently contain different assumptions regarding the individual's awareness and ability to learn (Toglia, in press), but they are not mutually exclusive. In clinical practice they are often used simultaneously, although in some cases treatment emphasizes one approach more than another. The clinician needs to carefully match the individual's capabilities with assumptions and expectations regarding change. In planning treatment, the clinician needs to ask the following questions: To what extent is change expected from the individual? What is the individual's potential for change or learning? To what extent should others change the task and/or environment?

Therapists should remember that decisions regarding the client's rehabilitation potential are based on a number of additional factors, including the nature and expected course of the illness or injury, the length of time since onset, and the assessment results of other multidisciplinary team members.

The Multicontext Treatment Approach

The multicontext treatment approach is based on the Dynamic Interactional Model of Cognition. Treatment systematically changes task and environmental variables to enhance the person's ability to process, monitor, and use information across new tasks and situations. The same strategy and self-monitoring techniques remain constant in treatment while the task and environment gradually change (Toglia, 1991). This approach encompasses both compensatory and remedial methods.

Remedial treatment aims to improve or restore the areas impaired by the injury; compensatory treatment focuses on areas of strength (Neistadt, 1990). Although remediation and compensation appear to target different areas of treatment, the line between them is questionable. For example, is a residual skill that has been weakened by brain injury an impairment or an intact area of strength? At times the skills that are considered to be impaired and the skills that are considered to be residual strengths may overlap or even be identical. Furthermore, in both remediation and compensation, the focus of change is the person. The person is required to learn a technique or strategy that needs to be applied across different situations. Neistadt (1994a) reviewed neuroscience research on learning and concluded that since both approaches involve learning, "neither approach can be said to take advantage of neural plasticity more than the other; both approaches can facilitate neural plasticity" (p. 428).

In addition to learning and generalization, awareness is required from the client in both remediation and compensation. A client who is unable to recognize his or her errors, or predict when they are likely to occur, will not initiate the use of compensatory strategies and will not actively participate in remedial interventions. The multicontext approach simultaneously integrates both compensatory and/or remedial strategies with awareness training techniques. There is an emphasis on changing the person's use of strategies and self-monitoring skills, within tasks and environments that may need to be adapted to meet the information processing level of the client.

The components of the multicontext approach include an emphasis on processing strategies; task analysis, establishment of criteria for transfer, and practice in multiple environments; metacognitive training; and consideration of learner characteristics (Toglia, 1991). Each of these components will be discussed below.

Processing Strategies

Treatment teaches the individual to use targeted processing strategies under certain task conditions to control cognitive perceptual symptoms (such as distractibility, impulsivity, inability to shift attention, disorganization, inattention to one side of the environment, or tendency to overfocus on parts of an item or task). In treatment, the individual learns to recognize the task conditions under which symptoms are least likely and most likely to emerge. This assists the individual in identifying situations in which a particular strategy is needed. The treatment samples below illustrate an emphasis on training use of processing strategies within the task parameters that the client can function.

Strategy Training and Unilateral Inattention

Mr. Jones tended to miss items on the left side whenever 10 or more objects were close together, similar in shape, and randomly scattered. When familiar objects with obvious differences were arranged horizontally and evenly spaced, he had no difficulty. Treatment helped Mr. Jones learn to identify the task situations in which he was most likely to have success and those in which he was most vulnerable to error. For example, prior to each task, Mr. Jones was asked to predict the difficulty level of the task and to anticipate whether he would need to use special strategies such as an anchor. Strategies that were predicted in situations

where 10 or more items were randomly scattered included rearranging items prior to scanning, tactile exploration of space (eyes closed) to get an internal image of the size of the space to be explored prior to a visual search, and placing a particular object on the left side to help him know when he was at the left side. An emphasis was placed on accurately anticipating task difficulty and the need to use a particular strategy rather than emphasizing the task results. In addition, the frequency with which strategies such as tactile exploration and anchoring were initiated by Mr. Jones was recorded and graphed to provide feedback.

The next example describes how treatment emphasizes the use of strategies to control impulsivity under specified task parameters.

Strategy Training for Impulsivity and Selective Attention

Gary demonstrated difficulty monitoring and adjusting his speed of response when 5 to 10 items were presented simultaneously and slight attention to detail was required. He tended to make numerous errors because he chose items quickly without fully attending to them. For example, when asked to make cereal, he quickly reached for a carton of orange juice in the refrigerator and did not realize his error until he had poured the orange juice into his cereal. When one or two items were presented at a time, Gary did not make errors. When he was cued to slow down his responses, performance was significantly improved. Treatment involved teaching Gary to monitor and pace his speed of response in a variety of different tasks. Prior to tasks, he was asked to predict the number of responses that would be performed with "good timing" (e.g., looking around at all the items prior to making a choice) and the number of responses that would be "too quick" (e.g., reaching haphazardly without attending to all the choices and making errors). Gary was also asked to visualize himself performing the task with good timing and timing that was too quick. During the task, he was encouraged to use his finger to point to each item to assist him in slowing down his responses. A chart was kept to record the number of responses that demonstrated good timing. This same strategy and self-monitoring system was emphasized in other card tasks, games, computer activities, and functional tasks such as choosing all the items needed to make a sandwich. The motor demands of the tasks varied from tabletop tasks to tasks that involved standing, reaching, and weight shifting. Although the context of the task and the environment were varied, the strategy and self-monitoring system remained consistent throughout treatment. When Gary demonstrated improved ability to pace his speed of response under the task conditions described above, the tasks were then graded in difficulty and the number of items presented simultaneously were increased to 15 to 20.

Analyzing Strategy Training Examples

In each case example, treatment began by specifying the task conditions at which the client could function. The client was taught to apply targeted processing strategies across different situations that stayed within specified task parameters. The processing strategies were aimed at inhibiting or controlling the appearance of cognitive perceptual symptoms such as impulsivity and the tendency to miss information.

The case example involving unilateral inattention described use of external strategies such as tactile exploration of space, rearrangment of items, and use of an anchor. Examples of internal strategies for unilateral inattention include remembering to begin the task at the left margin, remembering to move his or her eyes to the left, or remembering to ask himself the same question periodically, "Am I remembering to look to the left?" The case example involving impulsivity included use of both an internal strategy (visualization prior to actual performance) and external strategy (finger pointing). Additional internal strategies that may be used to assist the individual in monitoring impulsivity include counting silently to 10 before providing a response or verbalizing the rules/stimuli silently to oneself before responding. Additional external strategies include using an external timer to assist the individual in slowing down his or her responses (e.g., "Take your time and wait until you hear the buzzer before you respond.").

Other examples of external strategies include blocking out or reducing the amount of information; task reorganization; and using task checklists, timers, alarm reminders, organizers, tape recorders, notebooks, and highlighters to focus attention on relevant stimuli, and rulers or measuring devices to ensure proper spacing or arrangement of items. Additional examples of internal strategies include using elaboration and association techniques, self-questioning, setting priorities, and remembering to attend to details before responding. Table 1-10 summarizes additional examples of various processing strategies that may be emphasized in treatment (Toglia, 1991). In addition, the processing strategies and behaviors listed in Table 1-2 are further examples of areas that may be targeted for treatment.

During all treatment sessions, the therapist analyzes client's behaviors and the processing strategies that the client is or is not using. Improvements in the ability to initiate use of a processing strategy should be reflected in a number of different tasks.

Task Analysis, Establishment of Criteria for Transfer, and Practice in Multiple Tasks and Environments

Processing strategies are practiced in a variety of different situations during treatment to demonstrate the range of the strategy's applicability and to assist the client in understanding the conditions in which it is useful (Brown & Kane, 1988; Brown et al., 1983). The therapist avoids exclusive use of either functional activities or tabletop activities because if what is taught is embedded in one context, the skills learned may be accessible only in relation to that specific context. Several authors have emphasized the importance of using a variety of situations and examples to promote generalization (Gick & Holyoak, 1987; Sohlberg & Raskin, 1996). In the multicontext approach, the same processing strategies are practiced in a variety of tabletop, computer, gross motor, and functional activities, although the range and variety of tasks are not randomly chosen. Task and movement parameters are carefully analyzed and graded on a horizontal continuum to progressively place more demands

Table 1-10

Sample Processing Strategies

Sample Problem Behaviors/Symptoms	Sample Strategy	Description
Poor planning, attention, self-control	Verbal mediation or self-instructional procedures	Client is taught to say self-cues, task goals, plans, or task instructions out loud or silently before and/or during execution of a task.
Distracted by irrelevant information; difficulty selecting the main point	Underline, circle, or highlight critical details or facts.	Client is taught to highlight, circle, or list information most critical to the task or problem.
Tendency to become overwhelmed by the amount of information	Stimuli removal	Client is taught to remove, cover, or visually block out information.
Loses track of steps; performs tasks incompletely; performs unnecessary steps	Visual imagery prior to task performance	Client imagines self-performing task in an accurate and smooth manner; vividly imagines achieving the desired outcome; or imagines performing task with possible obstacles and imagine effective coping strategies.
Poor visual object recognition	Verbalization of object characteristics	Client is taught to silently verbalize the characteristics of an object prior to determining what the object is.
Difficulty recognizing and locating objects	Visual imagery prior to visual search	Vividly imagines the target item or object before searching for it.
Difficulty finding items; haphazard, disorganized approach	Categorization	Client is taught to rearrange similar items into meaningful clusters or smaller groups (e.g., grocery list; items in a closet or shelf).
Haphazard approach, difficulty focusing on task; does not know where to begin; appears overwhelmed by the amount of information	Task segmentation	Client is taught to simplify a task by breaking it down into smaller, more manageable components; dealing with one step or component of the task at a time.
Difficulty locating and finding items; tendency to omit items or steps during a task	Rearrangement of items	Client is taught to rearrange items prior to starting a task so that they are organized according to the sequence of use; there are spaces between them; they are arranged in a linear rather then scattered arrangement.
Tendency to overfocus on the parts of a visual scene or stimulus	Look all over before responding	Client is taught to gain an impression of the whole before attending to the parts. Look all over; actively scan the entire visual display from different perspectives prior to attending to pieces.
Impulsive, tendency to miss details, disorganized visual scanning	Point or use finger to help focus on details	Client is taught to point to stimuli prior to responding to focus attention on details and/or slow down responses. Finger pointing may also assist in facilitating an organized pattern of visual scanning.

on the ability to transfer and generalize use of the targeted strategies (Toglia, 1991).

Transfer of learning is not all or none. There are different degrees of transfer as defined earlier in this chapter. However, it is best to conceptualize the concept of transfer on a horizontal continuum (see Figure 1-2) rather than in absolute categories. In treatment, the physical similarity of tasks or environments is gradually reduced while the underlying strategies required remain constant (Toglia, 1991). Near transfer involves tasks and environments that are physically similar or share surface characteristics (Toglia, 1991). When two situations are physically different, transfer becomes more difficult because the similarities of the two situations may not be recognized. It is harder to recognize that the targeted strategy may be of use. Near and far transfer tasks look very different from each other and lie at opposite ends of the same continuum. However, the underlying skills and strategies needed to perform both near and far transfer tasks are the same and the level of task difficulty is equivalent.

Treatment involves analyzing an activity to identify which parameters will stay constant in treatment and which parameters will change. The observable or physical features of a task and/or environment are those that are changed while the underlying skill or strategy required stays constant. The same task and strategy can be practiced in different environments and/or with different types of people. Examples of parameters that are likely to increase the difficulty of an activity include the number of items in the task, the degree of detail, the number of task steps or rules, the number of possible choices, the discriminability of the task and environmental stimuli, the degree of distractions in the environment, and the unpredictability or unfamiliarity of the environmental context. The parameters that are not likely to increase task difficulty include the type of stimuli and the attributes of the stimuli such as color, size, shape, the task category, and the familiarity of the environment (Toglia, in press).

In many cases the parameters that increase the difficulty of the activity depend on the client's problem areas. For example, if a client has visual scanning problems, then increasing the size of the space to be explored and randomly scattering the items will significantly increase difficulty. On the other hand, if the client has difficulty in problem-solving tasks and in generating alternative hypotheses, then increasing the size of space in which the task is performed is not likely to increase difficulty level. The task is only graded in difficulty when there is evidence that the individual can apply use of the targeted strategy and self-monitoring skill across the transfer continuum (from near transfer to far transfer tasks).

The multicontext treatment planning forms in Case Examples 1 and 2 illustrate application of the multicontext treatment approach to two sample cases. In the first case example, the client, Rose, performs tasks in the incorrect sequence. The strategy to be emphasized in a variety of different tasks is pregathering needed items prior to the task and using a checklist. Treatment tasks that involve four to six objects and approximately five to seven task steps are chosen to match the difficulty of the task to the client's functional level. Task parameters that either remain constant or vary are delineated, and a variety of tasks that range from near to far transfer are identified. Treatment tasks move from making beverages and simple snacks to nonfood kitchen tasks and then to simple household tasks. Figure 1-2 illustrates how the surface similarity between treatment tasks is gradually reduced along a horizontal continuum.

Treatment tasks are only graded in difficulty when the individual demonstrates the ability to use the same strategy across a variety of situations that range from near to far transfer. For example, in the Case Example 1, the tasks could be graded in difficulty by requiring Rose to perform tasks with a greater number of steps (e.g., making cereal, toast, and coffee). It should be kept in mind that the client's ability to effectively use a strategy depends on the level of task difficulty. An individual may apply a targeted strategy to far transfer tasks when the number of items is limited to fewer than five and there are no more than five to seven task steps. As soon as the task is increased in difficulty (e.g., number of objects and/or steps are increased), the individual may once again have difficulty using the same strategy beyond the near transfer level. Thus, the ability to transfer strategies to different situations may be observed within a specified level of task difficulty. The multicontext

Case Example 1

Application of the Multicontext Treatment Approach

Rose is a 68-year-old female, 6 weeks post left CVA.

Daily life problem: Rose tends to either omit steps during task performance or performs the task steps out of sequence. For example, when attempting to make a grilled cheese sandwich, she placed the cheese in the toaster oven and left the bread outside; when making instant coffee, she put the pot on the stove without filling it up with water; when making ice tea, she filled the glass with water, stirred, then put in the ice tea mix. In all tasks, Rose demonstrates a vague notion that something is wrong but cannot identify her errors.

Previous activity interests: Housewife; enjoys cooking, crafts, reading. Her goal is to be able to independently make simple snacks and meals and perform simple household tasks.

Highest physical level: Ambulates with quad cane.

Strategy/ Behavior to be emphasized in all activities: Pregather all objects and place them in order of use prior to performing a task and use a checklist (provided by therapist) to keep track of each task step.

Constant Surface Task Parameters: The task parameters that will remain the same in all treatment tasks include the following:
Arrangement: Kitchen closets and refrigerator neatly organized
  Number of task objects: Approximately 4–6 objects
  Number of task steps: Maximum of 5–7 task substeps
  Task context: Familiar kitchen or household tasks

Variable Task Parameters: the following task parameters were gradually varied:
  Environment: Vary—kitchen in clinic, kitchen at home, stovetop counter on unit, prepare beverage or snack at counter or tabletop
  Movement requirements: Performed in standing, sitting at counter, vary need for reaching, bending
  Location of items: Place in different cabinets, different locations within refrigerator or on counter
  Type of stimuli: Different types of pots, spoons, cups, packages, jars
  Task category: Different types of beverages, snacks, nonfood kitchen tasks, other household tasks
  Type of task steps: Move from task steps involving boiling water, mixing, or stirring to steps that involve spreading, cutting, assembly, or arrangement of items

Initial Task: Make instant coffee.

Near Transfer (change 1–2 task parameters)
■ Making instant coffee with a different cup, pot, or premeasured packages. Other near transfer tasks include making tea or hot chocolate.

Intermediate Transfer (change 3–6 task parameters)
■ Making instant soup, oatmeal, jello, pudding, frozen vegetables or pasta using different types of boxes, packages, pots, and bowls placed in different locations within the kitchen. Tasks may be performed at a table or countertop; sitting on stool or standing; in different kitchens (home and clinic).
■ Change type of task steps, stimuli within the same environment: Making two slices of toast with butter and jelly; peanut butter and jelly sandwich.

Far Transfer (change all or nearly all task parameters)
■ Change task category within the same environment: Loading and starting the dishwasher, setting a table for two.
■ Change environment and task category; e.g., making a bed, doing a small load of laundry.

Self-Monitoring Techniques: Every 5 minutes Rose is asked to read a cue card that asks : "Am I using the checklist, am I crossing out each step as it is completed?" Rose is also encouraged to stop and ask for assistance when she has a vague feeling that something may be wrong.

Use of charts, graphs, scores for each task: Charts are used during treatment to keep track of the number of times Rose (1) initiates use of the targeted strategies (checklist, pregathers needed items) with and without assistance, (2) appropriately stops and recognizes that "something is wrong" during performance of the task.

Figure 1-2

The Transfer Continuum

Same strategy emphasized across different tasks and situations

←——→

	NEAR		INTERMEDIATE		FAR		
Initial task: Instant coffee-jar	Making instant coffee with premeasured packages; different cup, pot; different location of items	Making tea or hot chocolate	Making instant oatmeal or soup, pudding or jello performed at the counter, table, different kitchens	Making pasta, frozen vegetables, using different pots	Making toast with butter and jelly, or a peanut butter and jelly sandwich	Loading and starting the dishwasher; or setting a table for two	Making the bed; or doing a small load of laundry

approach suggests that the process of transfer may be enhanced in some clients by gradually changing the appearance of the task and environment while emphasizing the same underlying behavior or strategy so that the client learns that it is not the task or the environment that is important but the behavior (Toglia, 1991). Attention is drawn to the core similarity of the tasks and away from the surface similarities and differences.

Case Example 2 also illustrates these principles. In this case Ann confuses objects of similar size and shape. Treatment is focused on training Ann to monitor and improve her ability to visually attend to detail. The targeted strategy is using finger pointing during visual search to assist her in attending to subtle differences between everyday objects. In addition, the strategy of stimuli reduction or visually covering some of the visual information and systematically attending to one part of the visual display is practiced when finger pointing is impractical or insufficient. Motor goals of weight shifting to the left, weight bearing on the left upper extremity during reaching, and isolated shoulder movement are reinforced within different activities. Once the ability to successfully initiate finger pointing and stimuli reduction strategies is observed in different contexts with everyday objects, the treatment activities can be increased in diffi-

Case Example 2

Application of the Multicontext Treatment Approach

Ann is a 66-year-old female s/p Rt CVA 3 months ago. She was at a rehabilitation center for 9 weeks and is now receiving home care OT and PT.

Daily life problem: Ann has difficulty attending to critical visual details and makes frequent misinterpretations when there are 10 or more objects. For example, she frequently confuses items that are similar in shape (e.g., chooses tube of hand cream instead of toothpaste during brushing teeth, chooses a bottle of shampoo instead of liquid detergent). Requires occasional min. assist in dressing. Has difficulty locating arm hole, collar, etc. when clothing has a busy design or pattern. Has difficulty finding needed items, particularly in cluttered closets, drawers, or shelves. Ann can no longer follow a pattern in sewing or knitting. Ann is aware that she is having visual difficulties but attributes it to needing new eyeglasses. Her near acuity is 20/30 with her corrective lenses.

Previous activity interests: Housewife; enjoyed cooking, entertaining, sewing, knitting; playing cards with friends; attending local senior citizens' center.

Highest physical level: Ambulates 10 feet with a quad cane and close supervision. Demonstrates decreased weight shift to L in unsupported dynamic reaching activities. Standing tolerance is limited to 5 minutes. LUE—Shoulder partially isolated; distally—gross pinch and grasp.

continued

Case Example 2—*Continued.*
Application of the Multicontext Treatment Approach

Strategy/Behavior to be emphasized in all activities: Attention to critical visual details using finger pointing. Stimuli reduction—blocking or covering part of the visual display.

Constant Task Parameters:
Type of stimuli: Basic, familiar objects that are similar in size and shape
Presentation mode: 3D
Arrangement: Scattered/overlapping
Amount: 10–20
Rules: Involve choosing target stimuli

Variable Task Parameters:
Type of stimuli: Vary type of objects
Movement requirements: Vary—standing, sitting, bending, reaching, weight bearing
Space: Vary—confined spaces, e.g., draw to larger spaces—floor, entire table, etc.
Task category: Varied: e.g., different functional tasks, crafts, games
Environment: Vary kitchen, clinic, bedroom, gift shop, bathroom, etc.

Initial Task: 20 spoons scattered on the kitchen counter. Find all the teaspoons out of scattered tablespoons, soupspoons, measuring spoons, teaspoons. Place each type of spoon in a drawer with an organizer.

Near Transfer (change 1-2 task parameters)
■ Find all the butter knives in a drawer full of steak knives, dinner knives, butter knives. Find the utensils with a certain handle or pattern.

Intermediate Transfer (change 3-6 task parameters)
■ Kitchen—While standing, empty the dishwasher and place saucers in one cabinet, dessert plates in another cabinet or sort dishes, bowls, and cups into different cabinets according to the pattern (requires weight shifting).
■ Kitchen—Cabinet full of various types of canned goods; while standing remove all the canned soups or all the canned vegetables.
■ Buttons—Find all the matching buttons scattered in a bin.
■ Sitting at edge of mat, cards scattered on mat and on floor—Find all the red even numbers.
■ Standing at a table, find matching fabric squares with similar patterns/designs scattered across a table.

Far Transfer (change all or nearly all task parameters)
■ Laundry—Sort white socks according to the size and pattern.
■ Craft—Find specific items spread across the table (shell, tile, bead) within the context of a craft task.
■ Gift shop shelf—Find different items (tube of hand cream, toothpaste, or birthday card for a child).
■ Standing at a closet—Choose all the short sleeve shirts;

Self-Monitoring Techniques: Prior to and during initial searching for specific items Ann was instructed to say aloud "I must remember to pay attention to details." At 5-minute intervals she was asked to rate herself on the following: Am I using my finger to help me? Am I paying careful attention to the details? Am I removing/covering other objects if they are distracting to me?

Use of charts, graphs, scores: The number of times Ann spontaneously used her finger during visual search or covered/removed other distracting visual stimuli was recorded on a chart.

culty by using less familiar objects or by requiring Ann to locate specific details in crowded pictures, catalogs, food circulars, bills, schedules, calendars, charts, recipes, menus, maps, newspapers, and sewing and knitting catalogs. When the treatment activities are upgraded, a decreased ability to apply and use a previously learned strategy may be observed.

The transfer continuum represents a guideline for treatment planning, but it does not need to be strictly adhered to for all clients. For example, in situations where the strategy to be trained is general or nonsituational (e.g., check work, plan ahead), and the deficits are mild, the individual may be able to recognize the similarity between near and far transfer tasks. Treatment may consist of practicing the targeted strategy within a variety of far transfer tasks. However, when the individual has difficulty recognizing the similarity between two situations, the multicontext approach suggests that gradually changing the surface features of the task and moving treatment along the transfer continuum may increase the probability that transfer will occur in some individuals.

Metacognitive Training

The client can move from a cued to an uncued condition only when he or she has internalized the ability to estimate and self-monitor performance. If the client does not understand the full extent of the deficit, he or she will be unable to accurately estimate the difficulty of tasks and will not perceive the need to approach the task in a more efficient way. Lawson and Rice (1989) report a case in which an individual was able to successfully use strategies when prompted, but he did not spontaneously use these strategies. Training that included self-questioning techniques, error monitoring, and self-instructional procedures were effective in increasing strategy initiation. This supports the view that specific strategy training needs to be combined with metacognitive training.

Metacognitive training involves rebuilding a sense of self. It helps individuals redefine their knowledge of their own capabilities and limitations through systematic feedback and self-monitoring techniques. Metacognitive training promotes self-efficacy or a perceived sense of control over task performance. Clients are taught how to anticipate and evaluate their own performance (Toglia, in press). The ability to recognize and monitor errors prevents surprises in task outcome. During metacognitive training, the responsibility of cueing and structuring tasks is gradually transferred from the therapist to the client. The therapist is challenged to creatively think of ways to assist the client in using internal strategies or cues in the environment to enhance task performance. Every external cue that is effective in enhancing performance should

be carefully analyzed. The therapist has the responsibility of thinking of ways to help the client initiate the same cue by himself or herself.

Metacognitive or awareness training techniques can be integrated into all treatment activities including practice in functional tasks. If the individual is unaware of his or her deficit, treatment may need to begin at a level considerably above the level of breakdown to help the client recognize that a problem exists. Strategies such as self-prediction, role reversal, self-questioning, self-evaluation, structured error monitoring systems, and videotape feedback (Toglia, 1991; in press) are used to address different aspects of metacognitive function. Table 1-11 provides several examples of specific metacognitive strategies.

Learner Characteristics

When planning and selecting treatment activities, the therapist needs to consider the learner characteristics of the client, including motivation and individual personality characteristics. In the multicontext approach, treatment activities are not predetermined. The activities chosen depend to some extent on the client's premorbid personality and interests. If the client enjoyed competitive situations, then competitive gamelike situations would be used in treatment. If the client previously worked with numbers and finance, then treatment activities that involved numbers and money would be integrated into the total treatment program. Both functional and remedial activities are used in treatment. There are advantages and disadvantages to both.

Functional activities require the integration of all performance components. Although they may be more meaningful for the client, such activities do not easily lend themselves to strategy analysis, didactic interruptions, or manipulation of specific task parameters, all of which are characteristic of treatment. Remedial activities, on the other hand, can be easily controlled and manipulated to emphasize different strategies and skills (Ben-Yishay & Diller, 1983). Remedial tasks do not have to be limited to parquetry block activities or peg designs. They can incorporate the use of meaningful and relevant stimuli such as stamps, coins, utensils,

	Table 1-11	
	Metacognitive Strategies and Training Techniques	
Behavior	**Metacognitive Strategy or Technique**	**Description**
Client uses strategies when cued but does not initiate use of a strategy	Anticipation	Client is asked to anticipate any of the following: a) the types of obstacles that might be encountered prior to performing the task, b) the possible outcomes or consequences, c) the need to choose a strategy.
Client overestimates his or her abilities	Self-prediction	Client is asked to predict the general difficulty level of the task on a rating scale or predict specific aspects of performance such as accuracy score, time score. Predictions are compared with actual performance.
Client does not spontaneously check work	Self-checking and self-evaluation	After every 5 or 10 minutes, client is asked to self-check his work and fill out a self-evaluation form.
Client does not self-monitor performance during a task	Self-Questioning	Client is taught to ask self key questions during a task. The questions may be written on cue cards. External aids such as an alarm or buzzer may be used to remind the individual to read the cue card in the initial stages: Examples of questions include: ■ Do I understand the problem? ■ Am I getting sidetracked by irrelevant details? ■ Do I need more information? ■ Am I getting stuck?
Unable to monitor time during a task. Requires excessive time to perform tasks; performs unnecessary steps, gets caught up in unnecessary details, becomes sidetracked	Time monitoring	Estimate time; set time limits prior to initiation of the task and compare or evaluate results. Prior to performing the task, visualize oneself performing the task with and without getting sidetracked.
Client has poor error monitoring and detection skills	Role reversal	The therapist performs a task and makes errors due to distractibility, impulsivity etc. The client observes the therapist's performance and gives the therapist feedback (points out errors and states why they may have occurred).

pencils, and pens. Because the activities are outside the realm of everyday function, therefore, they require the therapist to make an extra effort to actively engage and motivate the client. The therapist needs to create an atmosphere of challenge and support. The therapist's tone of voice and the man- ner in which he or she presents the activities is important in engaging the client in treatment. For example, the therapist can enthusiastically say, "Let's see if you can keep your attention strong and steady so that you will get a score of 90%. If you feel your attention withering away, stop and take a break. Ready? Let's give it all you've got." The therapist needs to clearly define the goals of each activity in concrete terms that the client can understand (Ben-Yishay & Diller, 1983). Feedback in the form of charts, graphs, or point systems can be used to reinforce the extent to which the targeted strategy and self-monitoring techniques are used. It can also enhance motivation and assist the client in understanding the goals of the individual treatment session. In Case Example 1, the therapist could record a check mark on a chart each time the client, Rose, initiates use of the checklist. Emphasis is not on the task outcome but on reinforcing the use of targeted behaviors or strategies. Behaviors such as initiating use of a targeted strategy, spontaneously checking work, or recognizing errors as they are occurring can be reinforced by objectively recording and charting the frequency of desired behaviors. Clients lose interest when they do not understand the purpose of the activity or see any progress. If the client cannot understand the relevance of an activity, or the purpose of the treatment session, change is not likely to occur.

Group Treatment

It is important to keep in mind that individual treatment needs to be combined with group treatment activities. The same self-monitoring or task strategies that are emphasized in individual sessions can be reinforced within a group treatment session. Group activities can include problem solving and role-playing activities. For example, differences of opinion or conflicts between two people can be role-played in front of the group. Group members can be asked to think about a response to the situation, view the problem from different perspectives, and offer alternative solutions (Toglia & Golisz, 1990). Grattan and Eslinger (1989) found a significant correlation between flexibility of thinking and empathy and have suggested that treatment of brain-injured clients with frontal lobe damage include training in social skills and social sensitivity. In addition to role-playing activities, tasks that involve cooperative effort, planning, and organization can be done. Examples include putting together a newsletter, interviewing various people within the facility, or planning and organiz-

ing a bake sale, a holiday party, a raffle, or group outing. Each group session can end by asking members to complete a self-evaluation rating form that includes questions such as: Did I listen to other group members? Did I compromise? Was I open and receptive to other opinions? Did I remain calm, even when I did not agree? Did I communicate my thoughts effectively? Did I help the group stay focused on the goal? The self-rating form can be discussed openly and each member can receive feedback on his or her behavior from other group members. Strategies emphasized in individual treatment sessions such as monitoring the tendency to get stuck in one perspective or viewpoint, listing or prioritizing task steps prior to beginning an activity, estimating a time goal, and summarizing the main points of a conversation can all be emphasized within the group context.

Treatment Planning

The multicontext treatment approach is individualized and flexible. The sequence of treatment is not predetermined. The client's response to activities determines the subsequent course of treatment. Therefore, a clinician needs to have a large repertoire of treatment activities. One limitation of the multicontext treatment approach is the time required for treatment planning. To use the multicontext approach within a clinic, treatment activities and materials that are relevant to everyday life need to be well organized and accessible. Table 1-12 lists sample materials that can be organized and used to generate a wide variety of treatment activities. Computer tasks that can be easily structured or graded by the therapist, such as Print Shop or Calendar Creator, are also recommended. Computer programs that present drills of the same exercise, graded in difficulty, are generally avoided unless they require initiation and application of a targeted strategy and are used within the context of a variety of other activities. The treatment planning forms illustrated in Case Examples 1 and 2 should be used as a guide in planning treatment. Once this form is practiced with several clients, the process of generating a variety of activities along the transfer continuum becomes easier.

Table 1-12

Treatment Materials for Cognitive Rehabilitation

Cards
- Cards—numbers (single), combination: match the winning tickets, match the telephone numbers
- Cards—letters
- Cards—objects
- Cards—sports teams
- Playing cards

Can use magnetic strips on the back of cards

Object Boxes
- Unusual objects (novelty shops)
- Exact matches
- Nonexact matches
- Picture to object, nonexact
- Objects with subtle differences
  Stamps
  Coins
  Utensils (teaspoons, soupspoons, different handles, dessert forks, dinner forks, etc.)
  Keys
  Pencils (different colors, lengths, erasers, points)
  Screws and bolts
  Paper clips—different sizes, colors, shapes

Schedules / Lists / Grids (Enlarge schedules to decrease demands on scanning and attention or retype to decrease amount)
- Schedule of sporting events
- Schedule of concerts, plays
- Schedule of classes
- Schedule of children's activities
- TV shows
- List of different birthdays
- List of different appointments; things to do
- Airplane, train, bus schedules (Group Games and Activities book has sample simple and complex schedules)
- Magnetic schedule board—copy schedule onto board
- Blank calendars—fill in calendar; appointment book—make schedules

Price Comparison
- Different magazine subscription offers
- Banks and checking accounts
- College tuition
- Credit card offers
- Vacations—plane tickets; hotel prices, apartments with specifications
- Travel brochures, advertisements, AAA travel book, Club Med books
- Coupons for local stores (dry cleaners, airport service, rug cleaners, etc.)

Different Reading Materials for Scanning and Problem Solving
Get a variety of different sizes, print, and formats: Enlarge and reduce information to place less demands on scanning or attention
- Circulars
- Newspapers; classified sections, movies, TV listings, stocks
- Magazines
- Brochures

continued

Table 1-12—*Continued.*

Treatment Materials for Cognitive Rehabilitation

Different Reading Materials for Scanning and Problem Solving—*Continued*
- Paragraphs: Different-size print and spacing—paragraphs to summarize main idea
- Coupons
- Catalogs (stationery; clothing, household etc.)
- Spreadsheets (different sizes and types (can be generated from the computer)
- Telephone book: Company telephone directory, List of telephone numbers
- Menus
- Bills—different types
- Store receipts (scanning)
- Store price tags
- Cookbook; recipe box

Forms
- Credit card (charge) slips
- Subscription to magazine
- Bank deposit slips, etc.
- Order forms to catalogs
- Applications for membership, jobs
- Paragraphs with errors; misspelled words; different-sized print and spacing
- Tax forms
- Blank receipts

Directions
- Casio programmable watch and directions or directions for an electronic diary
- Card game or board game
- Directions for a magic trick
- Directions to offices or locations within building
- Directions for use with maps
- Directions for an appliance

Miscellaneous
- Medication bottles with different instructions (for scanning or scheduling)
- Letter or telegram writing situations (limited number of words)
- Organization of drawer, bulletin board, schedule board, closet
- Sorting mail task—Mail—junk mail, bills, advertisements
- Collating task (and photocopying) and/or filing task
- Take inventory in a closet for a list of particular items/linen, inventory of books, videos
- Interview another person and take notes simultaneously
- Role-play taking telephone message while simultaneously talking
- Given a situation and list—fill out invitations and mail list
- Interpret graphs, charts—months of low sales, identify patterns, trends in numbers, sales
- Tape recorder—tape of conversations, new reports, interview for summary; to take notes

From Toglia, J. P. (1996, June). The Multicontext Approach to cognitive rehabilitation. [Supplement manual to workshop conducted at New York Hospital, New York.]

Case Presentation

Marge is a 45-year-old female status post closed head injury 10 months ago. She has two children, ages 8 and 10, and previously worked full time as an executive secretary in a large corporation. She was hospitalized in an acute care hospital for 4 weeks and in an inpatient rehabilitation center for a total of 3½ months. She received home-based therapy for 6 months prior to attending an outpatient rehabilitation center for assessment and treatment. Marge states that everything she does re-

Table 1-13

Sample Items from Daily Living Questionnaire

Place a check if your ability to do this activity has changed:

Part I

_____ Cross the street
_____ Compose a letter or report
_____ Follow a recipe
_____ Remember appointments

_____ Read
_____ Schedule daily activities
_____ Find items in a crowded closet or shelf
_____ Drive

Part II

_____ Solve problems
_____ Perform daily activities at a normal speed
_____ Take initiative to start a new activity
_____ Resume an activity without difficulty after being interrupted
_____ Understand new instructions
_____ Keep track of time
_____ Stay focused on the task to be accomplished

Adapted from Toglia, J. P. (1996, June). The Multicontext Approach to cognitive rehabilitation. [Supplement manual to workshop conducted at New York Hospital, New York.]

quires excessive time. Her husband reports that she is able to perform routine self-care and household tasks but has difficulty coping with minor unexpected events (unexpected telephone call, interruptions, inability to find a particular item). Although she is able to prepare a sandwich or simple meal, she often takes out unnecessary items and easily becomes sidetracked. Her husband states that she completes about 10% of what she sets out to do during the day.

A neuropsychological assessment revealed deficits in the areas of attention, memory, and executive functions. The occupational therapy assessment began by examining the congruence between the husband's and client's perception of her difficulties by using a structured checklist (see Table 1-13). Marge and her husband had similar perceptions of her functional difficulties. Although Marge was able to describe the tasks she had difficulty performing, she could not explain why they were so difficult.

Dynamic Interactional Assessment

Awareness. Upon general questioning, Marge readily admits to difficulties in the areas of mem-

ory, organization, and problem solving and describes functional difficulties. However, she was unable to use this intellectual knowledge to accurately predict task difficulty. On nearly all tasks, she demonstrated a tendency to considerably overestimate her abilities. She recognized errors immediately after performance on three out of five tasks.

Processing Strategies and Task Conditions. Marge was able to perform tasks that had a limited number of items or steps and did not require her to impose an organizational structure. For example, she was able to quickly identify and keep track of eight items that were scattered and rotated on a page and sort 25 pictures of objects into preestablished categories. Tasks that involved dealing with more than 16 items simultaneously and/or in which she was required to impose an organizational structure were characterized by a tendency to become sidetracked by irrelevant information and/or overfocused on details. For example, performance on a visual processing task (DVPA) involving identification of 16 items that were scattered and rotated was characterized by a tendency to describe unnecessary details. This caused her to visually lose track of the items she had already named. A memory task (CMT) involving recalling

20 items related to a theme was characterized by a tendency to recall unnecessary details and to recall items in pairs or small clusters, e.g., spoon–fork; coat–ashtray, rather then recall items in large groups. A task that required sorting a stack of bills according to the due date was characterized by a tendency to become sidetracked by reading the type of items bought and the prices. She lost track of the original goal. Likewise, during a task involving prioritizing a list of errands, Marge overfocused on the amount of time each task would take and lost track of the need to prioritize and sequence the errands.

Responsiveness to cues.   Once Marge became side-tracked or stuck in one approach to a task, she had difficulty recognizing her error and required specific cues to switch attention back to the original plan or goal. For example, on a task that required her to generate different methods in sorting uten-sils (TCA), she fixated on one particular sorting pattern and required moderate cues to generate the last category. Marge was most responsive to cues in situations where she visually omitted or missed relevant items because of a haphazard ap-proach or in which she was cued to visually attend to broader categories.

Functional Implications.   Functional tasks that re-quired visually selecting relevant items from 16 or more scattered items, such as locating relevant items in an unorganized drawer, closet, or refriger-ator, are likely to present some difficulty. Marge is extremely vulnerable to errors in unstructured tasks that require organization and planning, such as paying bills, shopping, and cooking multistep meals. In addition, tasks that require generating different methods or hypotheses present the most difficulty for her.

Treatment

In the initial phase of outpatient treatment, the therapist assisted Marge in adapting features of her environment by reorganizing closets, cabinets, and drawers and having her husband prioritize errands for the day and preorganize tasks she needed to complete. These adaptations assisted her in attend-ing to relevant information and reduced her ten-dency to become sidetracked by choosing unneces-sary items during functional tasks.

At the same time, treatment incorporated strate-gies that required Marge to visually attend to all relevant stimuli by using organizational strategies as this was the area most responsive to cues. Marge's difficulty in shifting the task method or approach was less responsive to cues and therefore was not a target for change in the beginning of treatment. Initially, Marge was provided with a list of items that needed to be reorganized or re-arranged for efficient task performance (see Case Example 3). As a prerequisite to independence in tasks such as meal preparation, Marge was asked to demonstrate the following behaviors within tasks that require organization of preselected items.

1. Spontaneously rearrange or reorganize lists or items 75% of the time
2. Recognize the tendency to become sidetracked 90% of the time
3. Check work and recognize errors with the assis-tance of a self-evaluation form 90% of the time
4. Accurately anticipate task difficulty 75% of the time.

Within 8 to 10 weeks, Marge had met all of the above goals and demonstrated the ability to use strategies to organize items that were preselected. Treatment tasks were then graded by requiring Marge to internally make decisions about what was relevant to include within a task (e.g., make a list of the items needed for a trip; make a list of the items needed for a recipe; identify the key steps to a task; identify information that would be rele-vant to include in a complaint letter, a want ad, or a party invitation). These activities involved making choices and decisions. Gradually, Marge was required to generate different methods for organizing these same tasks. Finally, treatment pro-gressed to activities that emphasized identifying, choosing, and carrying out the relevant steps to an unstructured task or problem. Examples of ac-tivities included planning a monthly calendar and determining alternative methods for organizing and scheduling a variety of appointments, planning a picnic or lunch, and designing her daughter's birthday invitation on the computer. At this point,

Application of the Multicontext Treatment Approach

Marge is a 45-year-old female s/p closed head trauma. Currently receiving outpatient rehabilitation.

Daily life problem: Marge requires excessive time to complete activities. Becomes easily sidetracked or distracted by irrelevant visual stimuli.

Previous activity interests: Worked as a executive secretary prior to accident. Used a computer at work and home; 2 girls ages 9 and 11. Enjoyed cooking.

Highest physical level: Ambulatory without assistive device.

Constant Task Parameters:
Presentation mode: written (2D) / objects
Arrangement: Preselected list of items are disorganized
Amount: 16–25 items
Rules: Involve reorganizing items prior to gathering them or initiating task

Variable Task Parameters:
Type of stimuli: Vary—lists, objects, cards, books, catalogs, schedules
Environment: Vary, e.g., kitchen, different type of stores (supermarket, stationery store), clinic
Space: Vary
Task category: Varies: kitchen tasks, shopping, computer, tabletop
Movement requirements: Varies

Strategy/Behavior to be emphasized in all activities: Rearrangement or reorganization of items prior to task. Monitor tendency to become sidetracked and to gather unnecessary items.

Initial Task: Marge is given a list of items needed for a particular recipe. The list is disorganized and randomly lists different types of items (baking dish, salt, milk, mixer) located in different places in the kitchen. Marge is asked to think of a way to reorganize the items on the list prior to selecting them.

Near Transfer (change 1-2 task parameters): Same as above only a completely different recipe and list of items are used.

Intermediate Transfer (change 3-6 task parameters)
- Marge is given a disorganized list of items to find in a catalog or store circular.
- Given a disorganized shopping list of items, select relevant coupons from a food circular.
- Given a random list of recipes, find the specified recipes in a recipe box or cookbook. (requires rearranging the list into desserts, side dishes, etc.).
- Reorganize a supermarket shopping list prior to shopping.

Far Transfer (change all or nearly all task parameters)
- Given a disorganized shopping list of supplies her daughters need for the first day of school, reorganize the list prior to choosing them in a store.
- Given a random list of errands (including things that need to be done today vs. next week), rearrange the list according to order of priority.
- Rearrange a disorganized list of different appointments and things to do on a calendar.
- Rearrange given items within a drawer or shelf, bedroom closet, bookshelf, desk, coupon, or recipe box.
- Rearrange a disorganized list of files on the computer.

Self-Monitoring Techniques:
- Self-Prediction: Marge was asked to predict on a scale of 1 to 5 whether she would be able to stay completely focused on the task and whether she thought she needed to use special strategies such as task rearrangement methods. Her predictions were compared with her actual performance.
- Self-Questioning: At 5–10 minute intervals, Marge was asked to rate herself on the following questions, which were written on index cards : Did I rearrange items efficiently? Am I using the list? Am I crossing off each item after I retrieve it? Am I staying focused? Am I getting sidetracked? Am I sticking to what I need to do? Am I systematically dealing with one part at a time?

Use of Charts, graphs, scores:
- The number of times that Marge accurately anticipates the need to use strategy and spontaneously initiates rearrangement of items prior to beginning the task is recorded. The number of times Marge spontaneously uses the reorganized list to cross off items is also recorded.

treatment focused on additional strategies such as mentally rehearsing performing the steps, visualizing the task outcome, writing down the key steps of the task and establishing time goals. At times, Marge had difficulty taking the time out to preplan because her previous style involved "jumping into things." Treatment involved a process of helping Marge to let go of her previous style and accept a new style of approaching tasks.

At 23 months post injury, Marge is now managing the majority of everyday household tasks with only occasional difficulties. She continues to receive occupational therapy services privately with a short-term goal of beginning to plan a dinner party for friends and volunteering to assist with an event in her daughter's school. Although her intellectual awareness is good, she still overestimates her abilities about 25% of the time during unstructured tasks, partially because she is unable to let go of the desire to do things the way she used to. However, her ability to monitor ongoing performance has significantly improved so that she is able to recognize errors as they are occurring the majority of time.

Marge's case illustrates the use of a combination of approaches and different types of strategies. Methods of adaptation, compensation, internal strategy training, and self-monitoring strategies were used simultaneously throughout treatment. In treatment, it is most efficient to use a combination of approaches. The multicontext approach should be used only for those areas that show potential to change or readiness for function. This may not be the client's most obvious deficit, but it may assist the client in functioning at a slightly higher level under certain conditions.

Marge's case also illustrates the struggle that some clients have in letting go of their previous cognitive style and accepting different methods for task performance. The ability to effectively use strategies requires acceptance as well as awareness.

Research

Although the multicontext treatment approach has not been systematically studied and compared with other treatment approaches, there is a growing number of case reports that demonstrates the effi-

cacy of individual components of the approach such as strategy training, metacognitive training, and practice in different contexts.

Strategy Training

Several case reports in the literature document the effectiveness of strategy training in the areas of problem solving, attention, memory, unilateral inattention, and visual processing. For example, verbal mediation and self-instructional strategies have been reported to be effective in improving concentration (Webster & Scott, 1983), planning and self-regulation skills (Cicerone & Wood, 1987), and unilateral inattention (Robertson, Tegner, Tham, Lo, & Nimmo-Smith, 1995). Self-instructional procedures involve saying self-cues, task goals, plans, or task instructions out loud before and/or during execution of a task. The technique may also include talking aloud each step of a task to focus attention on the task and inhibit distractions and stereotypic behaviors. The overt verbalization is gradually faded to a whisper and eventually the client is asked to "talk silently to himself."

Freeman, Mittenburg, Dicowden, and Bat-Ami (1992) describes effective use of a combination of memory strategies and self-monitoring strategies to improve paragraph retention. The techniques used included use of visual imagery during reading, notetaking while reading, and use of a key word list at the end of each paragraph. Individuals were also asked to restate the material or summarize information at the end of each page, pick out the main idea of the paragraph, and ask themselves questions such as "Am I keeping track of everything? Am I following the story? Does it all make sense?" The effectiveness of training in a memory retrieval strategy using retrospection and self-questioning techniques has been described by Deelman, Berg, and Koning-Haanstra (1990). A 32-year-old head trauma client was trained 9 months post injury to use a systematic approach to retrieving information. First, she was taught to try to think back to the input situation and try to find a context by asking herself general questions such as "Which activities are usual on that day?" Second, she was trained to search within the context by asking herself more specific questions such as "Were other people involved in the activities?" Finally, she was trained to verify her answers.

Training in problem-solving strategies has been described by Van Cramon, Matthes-Von Cramon, and Mai (1991). They taught brain-injured subjects to simplify a multistage problem by breaking it down into smaller and more manageable components. Treatment improved performance on problem-solving tasks and reduced the client's tendency to jump to conclusions without considering all the relevant facts. Results appeared to generalize to everyday activities in some of the clients. Toglia (1989a) described the effective use of self-monitoring strategies and situational strategies in a 66-year-old businessman with severe visual perceptual deficits. Several strategies were trained including stimulus reduction, visual imagery, and organization. Recently Nelson and Lenhart (1996) described effective use of organizational and planning strategies such as categorizing items by location in the supermarket in a head trauma client who was 5 years post injury. The use of strategies was only possible after the client became aware of her deficits.

Practice in Different Tasks and Environments

In general, the studies that have shown greater success in cognitive rehabilitation are those that have employed a broader range of treatment tasks while those that have used only one or two graded training tasks have tended to produce task specific effects (Neistadt, 1994b; Sohlberg & Raskin, 1996). Lloyd and Cuvo (1994) reviewed 15 studies of traumatically brain-injured adults and found that those studies reporting more successful outcomes included training in a variety of examples. Likewise, in a review of 14 studies on remediation of attentional deficits, Mateer, Sohlberg, and Young-man (1990) found that those studies reporting positive outcomes used a wider variety of training tasks. In Neistadt's (1994b) review of studies on perceptual retraining, she concluded that intermediate and far transfer "will only occur for clients with localized brain lesions and good cognitive skills who have been trained with a variety of treatment tasks" (p.232). Raskin and Gordon (1992)

describe three case studies of brain-injured adults with cognitive deficits. Treatment included remedial and compensation training. Generalization was addressed in each treatment program by using a variety of different treatment tasks including those relevant to everyday life. They reported positive outcomes and argued that "no matter what approach one uses to treat cognitive deficits (remedial or compensation), generalization is only achieved when it is built into the training program" (p.44).

Metacognitive Training

The area of metacognitive training in the brain-injured adult is still a relatively new area of investigation. The cases that have been reported in the literature show promising results and suggest that awareness and self-monitoring may be enhanced through training in at least some brain-injured clients. Cicerone and Giacino (1992) report success in the use of self-prediction in two head-injured clients with executive dysfunction. Clients were required to predict how many moves it would take them to complete the Tower of London puzzle. The authors observed that one of the clients was able to spontaneously apply the strategy of prediction to his time management of daily activities. They suggest that the use of self-predictions may be effective in assisting clients to anticipate the effects of their own behavior. Soderback, Bengtsson, Ginsburg, and Ekholm (1992) described the success of videotape feedback in four clients with right hemispheric stroke and unilateral neglect. In videotape feedback, a videotape is stopped at different points and aspects of the client's behavior are discussed and reviewed. Increased awareness as well as increased ability to use compensatory strategies were observed. Structured error monitoring has been described by Cicerone and Giacino (1992). In this procedure, the client's performance was stopped immediately when an error was made and the client's attention was focused on the error. The client was required to keep a record of his own errors and systematically compare his responses on subsequent trials. The authors observed the ability of the client to apply the error monitoring routine to a clerical task, although the client continued to require some prompts.

Summary and Implications for Future Research

In this chapter, I have presented a dynamic interactional model of cognition as a foundation for occupational therapy assessment and treatment of cognitive dysfunction. This model was contrasted to traditional deficit-specific and syndrome-specific approaches that have been guided by a narrow conceptualization of cognition. In the dynamic interactional model of cognition, learning and the ability to transfer information flexibly across task boundaries are seen as integral components of cognition. Therefore, learning potential and learning transfer are directly addressed in assessment and treatment. This dynamic approach to cognitive rehabilitation is still in its initial stages of development. In this chapter, samples of assessment and treatment techniques that have been developed for the brain-injured adult were presented. The DIA uses cues and task modifications to determine the conditions under which the client is likely to succeed as well as those under which he or she is likely to fail. This information is directly related to treatment planning.

The multicontext treatment approach involves practicing the same processing strategy with a variety of selected tasks, movement patterns, and environments. Learning transfer occurs at different levels, and treatment attempts to facilitate the transfer process by combining training in multiple situations with strategy training and metacognitive training. The ability to transfer skills learned in one situation to another situation is constantly observed and worked for within a specific level of task difficulty. The multicontext approach is used to address behaviors that show potential for change. The client is expected to learn to apply a targeted strategy within a variety of situations; thus, change is expected from the person. In cases where the individual does not demonstrate the potential to learn or apply information across situations, adaptation or functional skill training may be a more appropriate treatment emphasis. Treatment

is most efficient when various approaches are integrated and used simultaneously whenever possible. The task and environment may be adapted to meet the information processing level of the client by adjusting environmental and task demands (reduced number of items or task steps) while the individual is taught to apply a targeted strategy.

Although case reports have supported the effectiveness of the components of the multicontext approach such as strategy training, metacognitive training, and practice in multiple situations, the multicontext approach needs to be systematically tested and compared to other approaches developed for the brain-injured adult. Different brain-injured adults may respond differently to various approaches. The level of severity, stage of recovery, and type of cognitive dysfunction may influence the technique or approach that is most effective in enhancing function.

This approach needs be explored further with other populations such as the developmentally disabled, psychiatric populations, and individuals with language impairment. The specific assessment and treatment techniques presented in this chapter rely heavily on verbal mediation. Clients with significant language impairment may not be capable of responding to verbal cues. In these cases, the same theoretical concepts described in this chapter can be applied, but the specific assessment and treatment techniques must be adapted. An example of an informal assessment that analyzes a client's response to nonverbal cues and changes in task parameters was presented, but needs further development. While awareness training techniques and self-monitoring strategies described in this chapter would not be appropriate for these clients, awareness of cognitive capacity and the ability to recognize and correct errors could be promoted through tactile, kinesthetic, or visual feedback.

Many of the assessment and treatment issues I have touched on have not been well investigated in the adult brain-injured or psychiatric populations. The principles of dynamic assessment have been researched with learning disabled, mentally retarded, and normal children, but they have not been well tested with adult populations. The reliability and validity of DIA methods in measuring learning potential and cognitive modifiability needs to be established in the adult brain-injured population. The extent to which DIA methods measure task-specific learning versus generalized learning potential is debatable. Transfer probes, or tasks that differ in surface characteristics but require the same underlying skills, could eventually be added to DIAs. In addition, the measurement models used in dynamic assessment are being refined and expanded. Some controversy exists over how standardized the cues need to be and whether traditional measurement models of reliability and validity should be used. Other areas of future research include the utility of DIA in planning treatment, predicting the client's response to intervention, and predicting the client's performance on functional tasks.

There are also some questions surrounding the treatment issues addressed in this chapter. For example, the concept of awareness of cognitive capacity and self-monitoring skills, despite its importance, has just begun to be researched in clinical practice. Most standardized test measures do not even include an assessment of this function. Although the question of whether awareness and self-monitoring skills can be improved in the brain-injured adult has been addressed within scattered case reports, there has been a lack of empirical studies. No one has attempted to analyze the awareness training techniques that are most effective with different brain-injured populations.

The effect of the nature of the environment and the activity on learning have also been virtually unexplored in the brain-injured adult. Comparing treatment that takes place in the same environment versus multiple environments needs further investigation. In addition, research that directly compares treatment that is conducted with the same graded tabletop or computer activity to treatment consisting of a variety of different types of activities needs to be done. Currently a review of the literature indicates that studies that have found task-specific effects used a narrow range of treatment tasks while studies that have documented more positive outcomes have used a wider variety of treatment activities, but there have been no studies of direct comparison. The conditions that promote and facilitate learning transfer have been investigated in normal adults and children but, again,

this area has not been adequately investigated with the brain-injured population. Strategy use and strategy training also need further investigation. Can brain-injured adults be taught to use processing strategies efficiently? Which strategies are hardest and which are easiest for different types of brain-injured clients to use? Are there qualitative differences in the processing strategies used or not used among different clients? Finally, treatment conducted in a predetermined hierarchical sequence needs to be contrasted with programs that are not conducted in a fixed sequence. In other words, the reductionistic approach to cognitive rehabilitation needs to be compared to the DIA approach.

This chapter provided a theoretical foundation as a guide for assessment, treatment, and future research. In it, I touched upon many issues that need further exploration with the cognitively disabled population. In the absence of evidence that demonstrates that one cognitive rehabilitation approach is better than another, clinicians should continue to keep a broad perspective, critically analyze the results of their treatment, and ask many questions.

References

Abreu, B. C., & Toglia, J. P. (1987). Cognitive rehabilitation: A model for occupational therapy. *American Journal of Occupational Therapy, 41,* 439–448.

Adamovich, B., Henderson, J., & Averbach, S. (1985). *Rehabilitation of closed head-injured clients.* San Diego: College-Hill Press.

Anderson, J. (1985). *Cognitive psychology and its implications.* New York: Freeman.

Anderson, S. W., & Tranel, D. (1989). Awareness of disease states following cerebral infarction, dementia and head trauma: Standardized assessment. *Clinical Neuropsychologist, 3,* 327–339.

Bandura, A. (1986). *Social foundations of thought and action: A social cognitive theory.* Englewood Cliffs, NJ: Prentice-Hall.

Barco, P. P., Crosson, B., Bolesta, M. M., Werts, D., & Stout, R. (1991). Training awareness and compensation in postacute head injury rehabilitation. In J. S. Kreutzer & P. H. Wehman (Eds.), *Cognitive rehabilitation for persons with traumatic brain injury: A functional approach.* Baltimore: Brookes.

Belmont, J. M., Butterfield, E. C., & Ferretti, R. P. (1982). To secure transfer of training: Instruct self-management skills.

In D. K. Detterman & R. J. Stemberg (Eds.), *How and how much can intelligence be increased.* Norwood, NJ: ABLEX.

Ben-Yishay, Y., & Diller, L. (1983). Cognitive remediation. In M. Rosenthal, E. Griffith, M. Bond, & J. Miller (Eds.), *Rehabilitation of the head injured adult.* Philadelphia: Davis.

Bolger, J. P. (1982). Cognitive retraining: A developmental approach. *Clinical Neuropsychology, 4,* 66–70.

Bransford, J. (1979). *Human cognition: Learning, understanding and remembering.* Belmont, CA: Wadsworth.

Bransford, J., Sherwood, R., Vye, N., & Rieser, J. (1986). Teaching thinking and problem solving: Research foundations. *American Psychologist, 41,* 1078–1089.

Brown, A. (1988). Motivation to learn and understand: On taking charge of one's own learning. *Cognition and Instruction, 5,* 311–321.

Brown, A., Bransford, J., Ferrara, R., & Campione, J. (1983). Learning, remembering and understanding. In J. Flavell & E. Markman (Eds.). *Handbook of child psychology* (vol. 3, pp. 77–158). New York: Wiley.

Brown, A. L., & Ferrara, R. A. (1985). Diagnosing zones of proximal development. In J. V. Wertsch (Ed.), *Culture, communication, and cognition: Vygotskian perspectives.* New York: Cambridge University Press.

Brown, A. L., & French, L. A. (1979). The zone of proximal development: Implications for intelligence testing in the year 2000. *Intelligence, 3,* 253–271.

Brown, A. L., & Kane, M. J. (1988). Preschool children can learn to transfer: Learning to learn and learning from example. *Cognitive Psychology, 20,* 493–523.

Campione, J. C., & Brown, A. L. (1987). Linking dynamic assessment with school achievement. In C. Lidz (Ed.), *Dynamic Assessment.* New York: Guilford Press.

Cicerone, D. K., & Giacino, T. J. (1992). Remediation of executive function deficits after traumatic brain injury. *NeuroRehabilitation, 2*(3), 12–22.

Cicerone, K. D., & Tupper, D. E. (1986). Cognitive assessment in the neuropsychological rehabilitation of head injured adults. In B. P. Uzzell & Y. Gross (Eds.), *Clinical neuropsychology of intervention..* Boston: Martinus-Nijhoff.

Cicerone, K. D., & Wood, J. C. (1987). Planning disorder after closed head injury: A case study. *Archives of Physical Medicine and Rehabilitation, 68,* 111–115.

Crossan, C., Barco, P. P., Velozo, C., Bolesta, M. M., Cooper, P. V., Werts, D., & Brobeck, T. C. (1989). Awareness and compensation in postacute head injury rehabilitation. *Journal of Head Trauma Rehabilitation, 4,* 46–54.

Deelman, B. G., Berg, I. J., & Koning-Haanstra, M. (1990). Memory strategies for closed head-injured patients. Do lessons in cognitive psychology help? In R.Wood & I. Fussy (Eds.), *Cognitive rehabilitation in perspective.* London: Taylor & Francis.

Embretson, S. (1987). Toward development of a psychometric approach. In C. S. Lidz (Ed.), *Dynamic assessment.* New York: Guilford Press.

Feuerstein, R. (1979). *The dynamic assessment of retarded performers: The learning potential device, theory, instruments and techniques.* Baltimore: University Park Press.

Fine, S. (1993). Lesson 3: Interaction between psychosocial variables and cognitive function. In C. B. Royeen (Ed.), *AOTA Self-Study Series: Cognitive rehabilitation.* Bethesda, MD: American Occupational Therapy Association.

Flavell, J. H. (1985). *Cognitive development.* Englewood Cliffs, NJ: Prentice-Hall.

Freeman, M. R., Mittenberg, G., Dicowden, M., & Bat-Ami, M. (1992). Executive and compensatory memory retraining in traumatic brain injury. *Brain Injury, 6,* 65–70.

Frostig, M., & Home, D. (1973). *Frostig program for the development of visual perception* (rev. ed.). Chicago: Follett.

Gage, M., & Polatajko, H. (1994). Enhancing occupational performance through an understanding of perceived self-efficacy. *American Journal of Occupational Therapy, 48,* 452–461.

Gange, E. (l985). *The cognitive psychology of school learning.* Boston: Little, Brown.

Gange, R. M. (1970). *The conditions of learning* (2nd ed.). New York: Holt, Rinehart, & Winston.

Gick, M. L., & Holyoak, K. J. (1983). Schema induction and analogical transfer. *Cognitive Psychology, 15,* 1–38.

Gick, M. L., & Holyoak, K. J. (1987). The cognitive basis of knowledge transfer. In S.M. Cormier & J. D. Hagman (Eds.), *Transfer of learning: Contemporary research and applications.* London: Academic Press.

Golisz, K. G. & Toglia, J. P. (in press). Evaluation of perception and cognition. In M. E. Neistadt & E. B. Crepeau (Eds.), *Willard & Spackman's occupational therapy* (9th ed.). Philadelphia: Lippincott.

Grattan, L. M., & Eslinger, P. J. (1989). Higher cognition and social behavior: Changes in cognitive flexibility and empathy after cerebral lesions. *Neuropsychologia, 3,* 175–185.

Groverman, A. M., Brown, E. W., & Miller, M. H. (1985). Moving toward common ground: Utilizing Feuerstein's model in cognitive rehabilitation. *Cognitive Rehabilitation,* 28–30.

Jensen, M. R., & Feuerstein, R. (1987). The learning potential assessment device: From philosophy to practice. In C. S. Lidz (Ed.), *Dynamic assessment.* New York: Guilford Press.

Josman, N. (1993). Assessment of categorization skills in brain injured and schizophrenic persons: Validation of the Toglia Category Assessment (TCA). Doctoral dissertation, New York University.

Kline, N. F. (1997). The Modified Dynamic Visual Processing Assessment (Modified DVPA): Its relationship to function. Doctoral dissertation, New York University, New York.

Kline, N. F., & Toglia, J. (1994*). Manual for the Modified DVPA.* Unpublished manual.

Lawson, M., & Rice, D. (1989). Effects of training in use of executive strategies on a verbal memory problem resulting from closed head injury. *Journal of Clinical & Experimental Neuropsychology, 11,* 842–854.

Lidz, C. S. (1987). Cognitive deficiencies revisited. In C. S. Lidz (Ed.), *Dynamic assessment.* New York: Guilford Press.

Lloyd, L. F., & Cuvo, A.J. (1994). Maintenance and generalization of behaviors after treatment of persons with traumatic brain injury. *Brain Injury, 8,* 529–540.

Mateer, C., Sohlberg, M., & Youngman, P. (1990). The management of acquired attention and memory deficits. In R. Wood & I. Fussey (Eds.), *Cognitive rehabilitation in perspective.* London: Taylor & Francis.

Melamed, L., Rahmani, L., Greenstein, Y., Groswasser, Z., & Najenson, T. (1985). Divided attention in brain-injured clients. *Scandinavian Journal of Rehabilitation Medicine, 12,* 16–20.

Neistadt, M. E (1990). A critical analysis of occupational therapy approaches for perceptual deficits in adults with brain injury. *American Journal of Occupational Therapy, 44,* 299–304.

Neistadt, M. E. (1994a). The neurobiology of learning: Implications for treatment of adults with brain injury. *American Journal of Occupational Therapy, 48,* 421–430.

Neistadt, M. E. (1994b). Perceptual retraining for adults with diffuse brain injury. *American Journal of Occupational Therapy, 48,* 225–233.

Nelson, D. L., & Lenhart, D. A. (1996). Resumption of outpatient occupational therapy for a young woman five years after traumatic brain injury. *American Journal of Occupational Therapy, 50,* 223–228.

Nolen, S. B. (1988). Reasons for studying: Motivational orientations and study strategies. *Cognition and Instruction, 5,* 269–287.

Pedretti, L. W. (1981). *Occupational therapy: Practice skills for physical dysfunction.* St. Louis: Mosby.

Raskin, S. A., & Gordon, W.A. (1992). The impact of different approaches to cognitive remediation on generalization. *NeuroRehabilitation, 2,* 38–45.

Riska, L.W. & Allen, C. K. (1985). Research with a nondisabled population. In C. K. Allen, *Occupational therapy for psychiatric diseases: Measurement and management of cognitive disabilities.* Boston: Little, Brown.

Robertson, I. H., Tegner, R., Tham, K., Lo, A., & Nimmo-Smith, N. I. (1995). Sustained attention training for unilateral neglect: Theoretical and rehabilitation implications. *Journal of Clinical Neuropsychology, 17*(3), 416–430.

Schacter, D. L.(1991). Unawareness of deficit and unawareness of knowledge in patients with memory disorders. In G. P. Prigatano & D. Schacter (Eds.), *Awareness of deficit after brain injury: Clinical and theoretical issues.* New York: Oxford University Press.

Seron, X., & Deloche, G. (1989). Introduction. In X. Seron & G. Deloche (Eds.), *Cognitive approaches in neuropsychological rehabilitation.* Hillsdale, NJ: Erlbaum.

Soderback, I., Bengtsson, I., Ginsburg, E., & Ekholm, J. (1992). Video feedback in occupational therapy: Its effect in patients with neglect syndrome. *Archives of Physical Medicine & Rehabilitation, 73,* 1140–1146.

Sohlberg, M. M., & Raskin, S. A. (1996). Priniciples of generalization applied to attention and memory interventions. *Journal of Head Trauma Rehabilitation, 11,* 65–78.

Sternberg, R. J. (1985). Instrumental and componential approaches to the nature and training of intelligence. In S. F. Chipman, J. W. Segal & R. Glaser (Eds.), *Thinking and learning skills,* Vol. 2. Hillsdale, NJ: Erlbaum.

Sternberg, R. J. (1986). *Intelligence applied: Understanding and increasing your intellectual skills.* Orlando, FL: Harcourt Brace Jovanovich.

Toglia, J. P. (1989a). Visual perception of objects: An approach to assessment and intervention. *American Journal of Occupational Therapy, 44,* 587–595.

Toglia, J. P. (1989b). Approaches to cognitive assessment of the brain-injured adult: Traditional methods and dynamic investigation. *Occupational Therapy Practice, 1,* 36–57.

Toglia, J. P. (1991). Generalization of treatment: A multicontextual approach to cognitive perceptual impairment in the brain injured adult. *American Journal of Occupational Therapy, 45,* 6, 505–516.

Toglia, J. P. (1993a). Lesson 4: Attention and memory. In C. B. Royeen (Ed.), *AOTA Self-Study Series: Cognitive rehabilitation.* Bethesda, MD: American Occupational Therapy Association.

Toglia, J. P. (1993b). *The Contextual Memory Test.* Tucson: Therapy Skill Builders.

Toglia J. P. (1994). *Dynamic assessment of categorization skills: The Toglia Category Assessment.* Pequannock, NJ: Maddak.

Toglia, J. P. (1996, June). A Multicontext Approach to cognitive rehabilitation (Supplement manual to workshop conducted at New York Hospital, New York.)

Toglia, J.P. (in press). Cognitive Perceptual Retraining and Rehabilitation. In M. E. Neistadt & E. B. Crepeau (Eds.), *Willard & Spackman's occupational therapy* (9th ed.). Philadelphia: Lippincott.

Toglia, J. P. & Finkelstein, N. (1991). *Test protocol: The Dynamic Visual Processing Assessment.* New York: New York Hospital-Cornell Medical Center.

Toglia, J. P., & Golisz, K. (1990). *Cognitive rehabilitation: Group games and activities.* Tucson: Therapy Skill Builders.

Trexler, L. (1982). Introduction. In L. Trexler (Ed.), *Cognitive rehabilitation conceptualization and intervention).* New York: Plenum Press.

Trexler, L. (1987). Neuropsychological rehabilitation in the United States. In M. Meier, A. Benton, & L. Diller (Eds.), *Neuropsychological rehabilitation.* New York: Guilford Press.

Trexler, L. E., Webb, P. M., & Zappala, G. (1994). Strategic aspects of neuropsychological rehabilitation. In A. L. Christensen & B. P. Uzzell (Eds.), *Brain injury and neuropsycho-*

logical rehabilitation: International perspectives. Hillsdale, NJ: Erbaum.

Von Cramon, D. Y., Matthes-Von Cramon, G., & Mai, N. (1991). Problem solving deficits in brain injured patients: A therapeutic approach. *Neuropsychological Rehabilitation, 1,* 45–64.

Vygotsky, L. S. (1978). *Mind in society: The development of higher psychological processes.* Cambridge: Harvard University Press.

Webster, J. S., & Scott, R. R. (1983). The effects of self-instructional training on attentional deficits following head injury. *Clinical Neuropsychology, 5,* 69–74.

Wilson, B., Cockburn, J., & Baddeley, A. (1985). *The Rivermead Behavioral Memory Test.* Reading, England: Thames Valley Test.

CHAPTER 2

The Quadraphonic Approach: Holistic Rehabilitation for Brain Injury

Beatriz C. Abreu, PhD, OTR, FAOTA

In this chapter, I propose a holistic system of cognitive and functional rehabilitation in which the therapist combines an analysis of performance components and their underlying skills with a synthesis of meaningful human occupations from both a macro and a micro perspective. The use of this dual perspective emerged from my reflection on over 3 decades of clinical practice in cognitive rehabilitation with a broad spectrum of clients from coma to community reentry.

I originally introduced the Quadraphonic Approach in 1990 and designed it to integrate four theoretical perspectives for the evaluation and treatment of cognitive rehabilitation and postural control primarily from a micro perspective (Krinsky, 1990). The four theories used were information processing, teaching/learning, neurodevelopmental, and biomechanical (Abreu, 1981; 1990; 1992; 1994). Although the original version of the Quadraphonic Approach focused on the micro perspective, it did include some qualitative assessments in addition to standard quantitative methods. Therapists, using traditional and dynamic interactive cognitive rehabilitation methods, have generally interpreted learning within a cognitive framework (Abreu & Hinojosa, 1992; Katz, 1992). Over the past 6 years, I have expanded the Quadraphonic Approach in a holistic fashion through the introduction of a macro perspective that uses narrative and functional analysis of occupational performance as well as qualitative and quantitative methods. This chapter is a summary of the Quadraphonic Approach and is presented in five sections: (1) Refocusing Cognitive Rehabilitation; (2) Evaluation: The Macro Perspective; (3) Evaluation: The Micro Perspective; (4) Holistic and Confluent Treatment: Edgar's Case; and (5) Scientific Inquiry.

Refocusing Cognitive Rehabilitation

Despite the prominent place of holism in occupational therapy practice, practitioners in cognitive rehabilitation have shown difficulty in harmonizing the scope of cognitive retraining with the characteristics of a holistic practice. In the Quadraphonic Approach, I present a holistic and confluent rehabilitation process that includes the reductionism necessary to practice cognitive retraining. To implement this integration of holistic principles with reductionism, the practitioner might reflect on three considerations prompted by Yerxa (1992) in her foreword to the text entitled *Cognitive Rehabilitation: Models for Intervention in Occupational Therapy.*

First, Yerxa suggested that cognitive rehabilitation should be a synthesis of the values, beliefs, and assumptions of occupational therapy practice. Second, she suggested that cognitive rehabilitation should be grounded in the broad interdisciplinary knowledge required to test clients who will use both body and mind to interact with the environment. Third, she argued that cognitive rehabilitation should be made individual by individuals and within the real environments that create occupational challenges and demands. The Quadraphonic Approach proposes a fluid movement back and forth between macro and micro perspectives—a dual consideration that attends to performance components and whole-person functioning.

Peloquin's (1996) articulation of confluent education provided guidelines that assist practitioners to refocus cognitive rehabilitation in the manner that Yerxa (1992) suggested. Confluence is the flowing together of two or more streams of thought, and confluent education is the deliberate and purposeful evocation by responsible agents of knowledge, skills, attitudes, and feelings that flow together to produce wholeness in the person (Brown, 1971). Peloquin (1996) suggested that such integration of the affective and cognitive elements in individual and group learning is advantageous in helping students to cultivate desirable knowledge, attitudes, and behavior. I propose that the confluent educational model is also appropriate for a holistic clinical practice. If cognitive rehabilitation must include a reductionistic focus on performance components such as memory, that focus does not preclude a confluent approach to the treatment of memory problems, wherein affective considerations are integrated into cognitive rehabilitation strategies.

A holistic practice recognizes that individuals are meaningfully interconnected within a societal context and are capable of maintaining and restoring equilibrium in a global health environment (McColl, 1994; McColl, Gerein, & Valentine, 1997; Miller, 1992). Adherence to these beliefs can energize occupational therapists to refocus cognitive rehabilitation along functional lines by changing the manner in which they relate to their clients (Peloquin, 1993a; 1993b). Changes can occur through an expanded focus on the client-therapist relationship to include explicit reciprocity, the surrender of treatment control, the establishment of authentic interactions, the acceptance of a client's responsibility for choice, and ultimately the acceptance of both the client and therapist as thinking-feeling individuals (Peloquin, 1990a; 1990b; 1993a; 1993b; 1995; 1996). Given this expanded focus, a therapist will include in rehabilitation those issues that relate to the affective domain: emotion, motivation, satisfaction, intuition, imagi-

nation, creativity, interpersonal capacities, values, norms, spirituality, ethics, and culture. A holistic practice will deliberately use methods, actions, and interactions that develop the affective domain. The environmental design of such a practice is nurturing and supports the interconnectedness of cognition, function, and affect in both teachers and learners.

In confluent practice, the teaching/learning partners engage in the adventure of cognitive-functional rehabilitation with the goal of health and optimal adaptation through which clients adjust behaviors, attitudes, and values to make them more congruent with the new external and internal demands subsequent to disease or trauma (Abreu, 1994; 1992). Given this refocusing of cognitive-functional rehabilitation, let us proceed to consider a client/learner-centered model of therapy and a holistic and confluent practice.

Cognition and learning have been traditionally interpreted within a cognitive framework (Katz, 1992). In contrast, I propose that cognition and learning should be viewed within an occupations framework that supports the inclusion of a macro or functional analysis and synthesis of a client's occupational story (Abreu, 1994; Wood, Abreu, Duval, & Gerber, 1994). The macro perspective is based on the use of narrative and functional analysis to explain and predict the behavior of an individual based on four characteristics that define behavior. The four characteristics are lifestyle, lifestage, health, and disadvantage status. Lifestyle status describes and predicts the individual's manner of expressing, producing, and performing day-to-day occupations. Examples of lifestyle status include the client's personal characteristics and use of economic resources. Lifestage status describes the individual's physical, emotional, and spiritual periods of growth and development—turning points and lifemarkers. Examples of lifestage status include childhood, adolescence, adulthood as well as marriage, divorce, death, accomplishments, and failures. Health status describes the presence of premorbid conditions such as arthritis or back pain as well as any changes in behaviors, values, or attitudes after the illness or injury. Disadvantage status describes the degree of functional restriction that results from impairment, including personal as well as social disadvantage. One example of

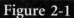

Figure 2-1

The Quadraphonic Approach

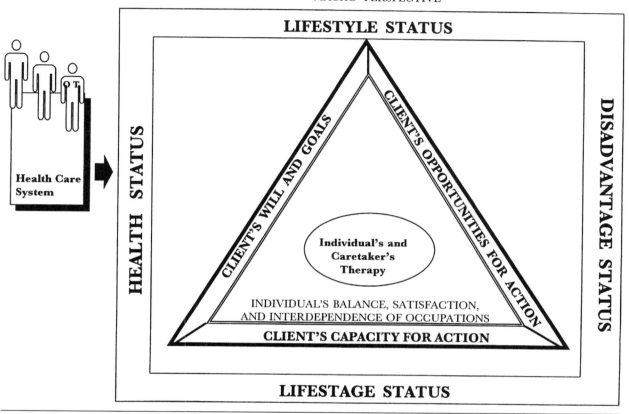

From: Abreu, B.C. (1994). The Quadraphonic Approach: Evaluation and Treatment of the Brain Injured Patient. New York, NY: Therapeutic Service Systems.

disadvantage status is a client's inability to go to the movies, shop, or cook because of physical, cognitive, or psychosocial impairments. Another example is a client's inability to be a financial provider, spouse, parent, or caretaker as a result of disability. Figure 2-1 is a depiction of the four characteristics in the macro perspective.

Evaluation: The Macro Perspective

From the macro perspective, therapists may use a wide range of functional assessment tools that are appropriate for evaluation. Standardized functional outcome scales are specific tools used in evaluation to compare the results of individual assessments to national standards. The determina-

tion of which scale to use in the evaluation process is a clinical judgment. In addition to these scales, the therapist may want to survey clients and their families regarding their perception of outcome and satisfaction with achievement (Ottenbacher & Christiansen, 1997). Two such surveys are the Craig Handicap Assessment and Reporting Teaching (Segal & Schall, 1995) and the Community Integration Questionnaire (Willer, Ottenbacher, & Coad, 1994). The importance of maintaining a focus on functional outcomes is underscored by the recent development of classifications known as Functional Related Groups (FRGs) (Stineman, Hamilton, Granger, Goin, Escarce, & Williams, 1994).

Cognitive and functional evaluations from the macro perspective are based on an examination of the individual's subjective sense of satisfaction and adaptation after a breach in health (Abreu, 1994; Trombly, 1993). For this element of the evaluation, the therapist will rely on narrative communications from the client and from family members as well as functional assessments of the client's real life occupations. Occupations have been described as the meaningful ordinary and familiar things that people do every day for personal and/or cultural reasons (Clark, 1993; Zemke & Clark, 1996a). These activities undergo constant change according to the individual's lifestyle, lifestage, health, and disadvantage. Chunks of meaningful activities are orchestrated in a nonlinear progression from day to day (Clark, 1993).

Through interview questions that prompt personal sharing, the therapist seeks to better understand the client's personal story; the client might be asked to bring personal documents, photographs, or meaningful objects that can enhance communication (Clark, 1993). Because brain injury can cause expressive and receptive disorders of communication, flexible methods of eliciting information are quite important. The use of narrative for the macro evaluation assists the therapist to discover the way in which the client makes sense of his or her life experiences (Polkinghorne, 1988; Riessman, 1993).

In the Quadraphonic Approach, I provide a system of six assessment strips for the cognitive and functional classification of each client (see Table 2-1). Four of the strips are based on a macro perspective and two strips on the micro. The strips are used to classify each client on one of seven functional performance levels listed in Table 2-2. Based on this functional performance classification, the therapist works with the client to design functional treatment guidelines that enable advancement to the next functional level. There are six treatment guidelines leading from coma to community reentry, which will be discussed later in this chapter.

The Narrative

Storytelling and narrative modes of analysis have been used by Mattingly and Fleming (1993) as a way to help therapists reflect on their practice.

These researchers used an interpretative strategy of asking participating therapists to view segments of videotapes of occupational therapy practice and to analyze the viewing and categorize the results as if they were chapters of a story. One outcome of these studies was that participant-therapists became more conscious of their assumptions as opposed to what actually mattered to the client. Narrative reflections also increased the therapists' awareness that practice is only partially shaped by a therapist's original evaluation and treatment plan. The occupational therapy process unfolds with interferences, surprises, improvisations, and dynamic interactions among a variety of team players, two of whom are the occupational therapist and the client.

One of the goals of the Quadraphonic Approach is to increase the awareness of both the therapist and the client with regard to the affective domain of the therapeutic experience. Narrative thinking can guide the therapist toward a focus on the experience of adaptation after disease, injury, or trauma for more effective cognitive and functional rehabilitation. The humanistic orientation provided by the use of narrative enhances the capacity of the occupational therapist to consider the client's experience of brain injury and the manner in which personal restrictions and social disadvantages affect a life. Examples of narrative strategies in occupational therapy are the interview, occupational storytelling, and occupational storymaking (Clark, 1993; Clark, Ennevor, & Richardson, 1996; Mattingly & Fleming, 1993). Bateson (1989) described how narratives or personal stories provide a framework for reflecting about the unique shape, relationships, and commitments of individual lives (Krefting & Krefting, 1990). Nachmanovitch (1990) emphasized the power of improvisation in life and the arts. That same power can be tapped in cognitive rehabilitation.

The use of the narrative in the macro framework for occupation yields a client-centered therapeutic orientation in which the therapist functions as a professional consultant who advises on the management of various aspects of the client's life (Bridge & Twible, in press; Herzberg, 1990; Patterson & Marks, 1992). This macro framework is also influenced by recent changes in the health care delivery system such as demedicalization and consumerism, both of which place the patient in a more central role in rehabilitation (Bridge & Twible, in press; Holyoke & Elkan, 1995; Pollock, 1993). The interview is a tool used to elicit information. Storytelling considers a client's short- and long-term memories, while storymaking involves the creation or playing out of rehabilitation outcomes—what the client and rehabilitation team would like to accomplish or see happen. Progression toward planned cognitive and functional outcomes is not linear but full of tricks, reversals, and surprises. The predicted outcomes are uncertain and not predetermined by critical pathways. Because the main character in the rehabilitation process is the client who has suffered the brain injury, the narrative, in addition to the medical diagnosis, is an important factor in developing a holistic treatment plan.

The Quadraphonic Approach uses narrative to embrace a real life occupations framework from both the macro and micro perspective to maximize the performance and satisfaction of clients in a holistic and confluent manner. Wood et al. (1994) defined the macro framework for cognitive rehabilitation as a clinical orientation that relies upon daily living, leisure, recreation, work, and other ordinary occupations as primary therapeutic modalities. Effective adaptation and optimal health are identified as outcomes. The macro perspective has also been referred to as adaptive, functional, and top-down (Abreu, 1994; Siev, Frieshtat, & Zoltan, 1986; Trombly, 1993).

In contrast, the micro perspective of occupational functioning focuses on the foundational subskills or performance components including attention, memory, categorization, and problem solving. These subskills can be further broken down; memory can be broken down into visual and auditory memory or categories such as short-term and long-term memory. The micro perspective has also been called restorative and/or bottom-up (Abreu, 1994; Trombly, 1993; Wood et al., 1994). I propose that practitioners reject the underlying assumptions that support a treatment dichotomy within which therapists must choose between either macro or micro, or between functional or restorative perspectives. The dual system of rehabilitation proposed herein facilitates a free-flowing movement between macro and micro perspectives

embracing both remediation and compensation techniques.

The Interview, Storytelling, and Storymaking

The interview is one of the assessment tools used to elicit the narrative. The interview is conducted in a face-to-face meeting during which the therapist documents information reported by the client. The interview process can be expanded by including the client's family members as well as significant others and may also include a written survey that does not involve a face-to-face meeting. The interview should be a dynamic and interactive process during which the therapist documents direct observation of the client's social experiences together with the client's descriptions of personal behaviors in an effort to guide and engage the client in meaningful communication about every day experiences (Holstein & Gubrium, 1995). This process assists in the discovery of an individual's patterns of interaction and self-organization within society (Psathas, 1995). The individual's cognitive and functional skills can be better understood with reference to the social milieu within which the individual is embedded (Vygotsky, 1978).

Facilitating storytelling can shed light on the personal and social disadvantages that emerge from the individual's societal embeddedness (Josselson & Lieblich, 1995). To study a whole person, one cannot rely exclusively on logical numerical methods and objective descriptions. The interview allows for the search and discovery of the individual's real life setting, the significance to the client of the everyday, and the manner in which the client achieves an "underlife" (those behaviors that may not be typical of the individual but that characterize functioning in the treatment facility or in the institutions that provide rehabilitation services).

Stories that emerge during an active interview can be triggered either by something that is said or done by the client or by the therapist's pursuit of a comment that is not topically coherent. The active interview is an improvisational production that is structured and focused yet allows for spontaneity and responsivity within parameters provided

Table 2-1

Six Assessment Strips

Occupational Therapy Department   DOA: Evaluation/Discharge Form

Client: Initial Date: Discharge Date:

SCALE:

7.0=Independent	100%	3.0=Moderate Assistance 50%
6.0=Modified Independence	90%	2.0=Maximum Assistance 25%
5.0=Supervised Assistance	80%	1.0=Dependent
4.0=Minimal Assistance	75%	

CODE:
IL=Initial Level
DL=Discharge Level

2/96

SUBJECTIVE: (Individual client story-expressed Client and/or Family Goals)

OBJECTIVE: (Identify the IPP Goal objective for client month by month–Patient and/or Family Education Instructional Training)

1. Personal Management:

Scale IL DL — Basic ADL #1 | Basic ADL #2 | Housekeeping | Laundry | Apartment Check | Awareness/Satisfaction

(Scale: 7 6 5 4 3 2 1)

Initial Goals/Plans:

Discharge Goals/Plans:

2. Shopping/Cooking/Independent Meal Preparation

Scale IL DL — Menu Planning | Grocery Shopping | Cooking Group | Cold Prep/Clean Up | Micro Prep/Clean Up | Stove Prep/Clean Up | Apt. Trial Group/Management Grp | Awareness/Satisfaction

(Scale: 7 6 5 4 3 2 1)

Initial Goals/Plans:

Discharge Goals/Plans:

3. Mobility Planning/Mobility:

Scale IL DL — Basic Mobility Subskills Ground | Basic Mobility TLC Block | Mobility Planning | Specified Mobility #1 N | Specified Mobility #2 C | Advanced Mobility Community | Awareness/Satisfaction

(Scale: 7 6 5 4 3 2 1)

Initial Goals/Plans:

Discharge Goals/Plans:

Initial Evaluation Therapist: Date:

Discharge Evaluation Therapist: Date:

Table 2-1—*Continued.*

Six Assessment Strips

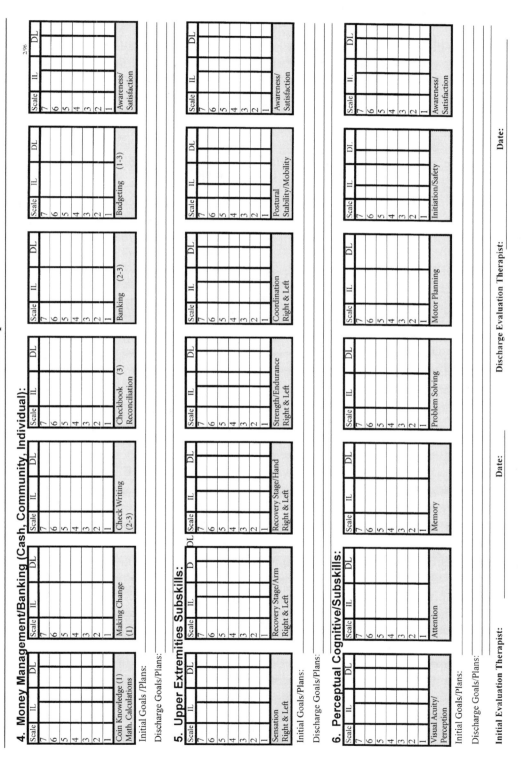

Table 2-2
Seven Functional Levels

Totally dependent

Goal: To increase the performance level and satisfy to 25%. Increase awareness of relevant environmental characteristics and inhibit irrelevant characteristics.

Environmental Conditions:

At this level, clients require a stable therapeutic environment with minimal processing demands. The instructions are simple with one-step commands. Continuous cuing is required. Objects should be familiar and nonrotated. The duration of engagement in the activity should be brief and the speed of presentation slow. Treatment emphasizes a multisensory approach using a variety of limited stimuli and movement patterns. The focus should be on functional outcome. The therapist must determine when breakdown occurs. Cues are generated primarily by the therapist and are task and goal specific. Performance may not increase with cuing. A feedback program is used to provide information on performance and results. Emphasis on micro-match functional context.

Maximum Dependence:

Goal: To increase the performance level to 50%. Increase error detection in performance guided by external cues.

Environmental conditions:

Exposure to predictable and unpredictable conditions. At this stage, the environmental regulations require a higher processing demand. The instructions are short and simple with two-step commands. Continuous cuing may be required. Objects remain familiar and nonrotated. The duration and speed of the presentation is increased. Treatment emphasizes cortical and subcortical strategies. Cues are generated primarily by the therapist and are task, goal, and strategy specific. A feedback program is used to provide information on performance and results. Once client is able to perform task/activity over 50% of the time (not chance), a variation of mix-match and adapt environments can follow.

Moderate Dependence:

Goal: To increase performance level and satisfaction to 75%. Facilitate client's error detection and error correction performance, guided by external cues and self-monitoring.

Environmental conditions:

Combine a variety of environments, postural supports, and body positions. Continue to increase processing demands. The instructions are short and simple with two-step commands. Unfamiliar objects are used and rotated. The duration and speed of the activity are again increased. The duration of activities is 45 minutes. Treatment emphasizes cortical and subcortical strategies. Cues are encouraged to be self-generated and are task, goal, and strategy specific. Performance may increase with cues. A feedback program is used to provide information on performance and results.

continued

Table 2-2—*Continued*

Seven Functional Levels

Minimal Assistance:

Goal: To increase performance level and satisfaction above 75%. Promote client's ability to set up and restructure the environment.

Environmental Conditions Mix-Match and Adapt:

Combine a variety of environments, postural supports, and body positions; high processing demands. The instructions are given with two or more step commands. Objects are similar, unfamiliar, and abstract, rotated, and nonrotated. The duration is lengthened to 1 hour. Treatment emphasizes strategies and self-monitoring. Cues are generated and performance may increase. A feedback frequency program is used to change, diminish, or delete external feedback.

Supervised Assistance:

Goal: To increase performance and satisfaction above 80%. Promote client's ability to function and control in structured and unstructured environments.

Environmental Conditions Mix-Match and Adapt:

Combine a variety of environments, postural supports, and body positions; high processing demands. The instructions are given with three or more step commands. Objects are similar, unfamiliar, and abstract, rotated and nonrotated. The duration is greater than 1 hour. Treatment emphasizes the client's control and decision making. Performance may not be dependent on cues. A feedback frequency program is used to change, diminish, or delete external feedback.

Independent with modification:

Goal: To increase performance level to above 90% so that the client is able to perform with minimal modification, promote client's selection and control in a variety of environments.

Environmental Conditions Mix Match and Adapt:

Combine and match a variety of environments, postural supports, and body positions; high processing demands. The instructions are with three or more step commands. Objects are similar, unfamiliar, and abstract, rotated and nonrotated. The duration of the activity is for 1.5 hours or more. Cues should be self-generated. A feedback frequency program is used to change, diminish, or delete external feedback.

Client is independent without modification. Client does not need OT services.

No modifications required in physical, social or cultural context.

From Abreu, B. (1990). The quadraphonic approach: Management of cognitive and postural dysfunction. New York: Therapeutic Service Systems. Reprinted with permission.

by the interviewer (Holstein & Gubrium, 1995). Considerations that affect the framework of the interview include:

■ the client's competency as narrator given his/her state of impairment, disability, and disadvantage
■ the client's capacity to demonstrate and communicate what is meaningful and what societal interactions are like

■ the opportunity to evaluate the client's satisfaction with personal roles (i.e., mother, brother, client) as well as satisfaction with the occupational therapy services being provided
■ the facilitation of ordinary exchanges that rely on mutual attentiveness, monitoring, and responsiveness (i.e., being sensitive to turn-taking in the conversation)
■ the climate of mutual disclosure

- the emphasis on sentiment and emotion that is the core of human experience
- the acceptance that the interview is biased and multidirectional
- the employment of improvisation during the interview process.

Storytelling also may be influenced by the client's reduced ability to acquire, store, and recall information about personally experienced events (episodic memory) and/or general world knowledge (semantic memory). An example of episodic memory is a client's recollection of what he or she ate for breakfast or how he or she participated in the high school graduation ceremony. By comparison, an example of semantic memory is the client's recollection of what Americans eat for breakfast or what type of celebrations they have when they complete high school.

Individuals who have experienced brain injury show a diversity of symptoms that reflect different aspects of cognition. Impairment is reported in almost every aspect of cognitive functioning following brain injury: general cognitive ability (Duchek & Abreu, 1997; Lezak, 1983), attention (Toglia, 1993; Van Zomeren & Brouwer, 1994), memory (Toglia, 1993; Wilson, 1987), visual-spatial perception and integration (Gianutsos & Matheson, 1987; Warren, 1993), and language (Hartley, 1995). All of these impairments contribute to a decrease in the capacity to communicate. The characteristics of the client's social communication may also vary depending on the location and extent of the lesion. For example, if the posterior region of the right hemisphere or the frontal lobes is affected, the therapist may have difficulty obtaining information that requires visual-spatial processing such as making/reading facial expressions, visual scanning, respecting personal space, and interpreting complex visual information (Braun, Baribeau, Ethier, Daigneault, & Proulx, 1989).

Such impairments may affect the client's storytelling abilities, diminishing the ability to relate personal history and reconstructions. Specific examples may include:

- reduced mastery of vocabulary
- diminished capacity to name words and speak fluently

- reduced comprehension of lengthy and complex visual and auditory information
- inability to follow three or more step instructions
- decreased ability to make social connections necessary for politeness and courteous conversation (Coelho, Liles, & Duffy, 1991; Hartley, 1995; Hartley & Jensen, 1992; Rehak, Kaplan, Weylman, Kelly, Brownell, & Gardner, 1992).

The client's comprehension and fluidity may fluctuate because of lapses in alertness and attention, decreased empathy, and reduced initiation or motivation. The net effect of the client's difficulties may be the production of a broken story. The story will warrant a therapist's increased sensitivity and trust in the client's capacity to communicate what is meaningful. The client's impairments are not static; they are context- and goal-dependent and they may vary depending on where and when the therapist conducts the interview. For example, if a therapist chooses to conduct a portion of the interview in a restaurant favored by the client, this environment will change the client's affect, tone, and fluidity.

The goal of the interview and its associated storytelling is to create a partnership that helps clients to share their messages about morals and beliefs and the meaning that they find in their lives and social worlds. These messages are sometimes more important than the specific events or details uncovered in the interview. The therapist may discover, through communicative improvisations, information about a client's norms and values that may not be apparent in his or her institutional underlife. See Table 2-3 for a list of sample questions that can be included in the interview done from the macro perspective. The result of the narrative process is a summary of the client's story that can be used as a basis for the evaluation.

Guidelines for Evaluation from the Macro Perspective

After the narrative information has been collected, the evaluation process continues with the classification of the client's performance through the use of the six cognitive and functional evaluation strips

Table 2-3
Sample Questions for the Interview

Content (WHAT TO ASK—The wording)	Process (HOW TO ASK—The way to ask)	Context (WHERE TO ASK—The place to ask)
1. Describe your life as if it were a book. Describe this stage of your life as a chapter.	1. Attend to the content.	1. Change the locations of the interview to evoke the story.
2. How did you feel about being admitted to this institution?	2. Attend to the flow of the topic.	2. Restaurants.
3. Let's talk about how it feels to be diagnosed with a brain injury.	3. Encourage elaboration.	3. Churches, Synagogues, Religious Institutions.
4. Let's talk about how it feels to have a cognitive impairment.	4. Provide self-disclosing incidents.	4. Schools.
5. What happened to your life when you decided to be admitted to this institution?	5. Provide clarification of the collaborative role.	5. Theaters/Movies.
6. Overall, what has been your experience after your incident (tumor, accident, stroke, illness)?	6. Discuss events at length.	6. Outdoor Areas.
7. Teach me about dressing with one hand.	7. Cultivate the art of hearing.	7. Other personally meaningful locations.
8. Could you tell me what happened to your family after your brain injury?	8. Recognize the gestalt of the story.	
9. What was your role in your family?	9. Analyze and narrow the themes of the story (verbal/non-verbal).	
10. Could you tell me how different your role as a (father, sister, wife, worker...) is now?	10. Interview until saturation: nothing new comes out.	
11. After the rehabilitation program ends what happens next?		

From: Abreu, B.C. (1994). The Quadraphonic Approach: Evaluation and Treatment of the Brain Injured Patient. New York, NY: Therapeutic Service Systems.

mentioned earlier. The six strips are personal management; shopping, cooking, and independent meal preparation; mobility planning/mobility; money management; upper extremities subskills; and cognitive perceptual subskills (see Table 2-1). The first four of the evaluation strips view occupation from the macro perspective. Each time a strip is used in the macro perspective, the therapist must consider the following guidelines:

- an examination of the characteristics that affect the client's behavior including lifestyle, lifestage, health, and disability status
- a precise operational definition of the assessment area
- a consideration of the client's choices and degree of control within the evaluation process
- documentation of the results that include commentary about the client's personal awareness

and responsivity as well as his or her interaction with therapist, task, and environment

■ a consideration of the psychometric character of the evaluation and whether it yields both qualitative and quantitative performance data.

The use of the four evaluation strips in the macro perspective will depend on the individual circumstances of each client. The therapist will seek to understand the big picture of a client's lifestyle by eliciting a detailed discussion of individual circumstances in an interview that is structured around open-ended questions. In an effort to focus the evaluation, the therapist may ask a client questions about personal status such as "How much help would you like to contribute to managing the household?" or "What are some of the more frustrating aspects of your present situation?" Given a response that suggests the client wants to continue helping with shopping and food preparation but is having problems being efficient in the grocery store, the therapist might offer to assess these areas.

For example, a client named Edgar who has a diagnosis of brain injury and records a moderate memory deficit has been admitted into a community reentry facility from a rehabilitation hospital. In the initial interview, Edgar indicates that his primary goals are to return home to his wife, Daisy, to contribute to the management of the household, and to return to work as a chemical engineer. By stating these goals, Edgar determines the point at which the therapist starts the assessment. In an effort to focus the assessment, the therapist may ask Edgar questions about his goals, such as: What skills do you need in order to return home? How much help were you giving Daisy at home? What are the skills required as a chemical engineer? What do you do for fun? The answers to these questions will lead to the introduction of the cognitive and functional macro evaluation strips.

During the evaluation, the therapist and Edgar decide to use grocery shopping as one of the skills to be tested. The shopping task is divided into four components, each valued at 25%: plan a shopping list, plan a budget, plan how to get to the store, and go to the store and shop. During the evaluation, the therapist assesses the four components and records the score. If the client is unable to perform any function, the therapist uses a tutoring approach

that includes questions, cues, prompts, and repetition to determine if the client can improve his or her performance. For example, the therapist may use a hierarchical cue procedure that would include awareness cues ("Look carefully"), general directives ("Look in the frozen food section"), specific directives ("Look for ice cream"), or answers ("Here is the ice cream"). This procedure will show if a client can benefit from cues and therefore benefit from further rehabilitation. Some clients will be able to benefit from remediation and others will require compensatory techniques.

In this case, the therapist will test Edgar's planning skills and accompany him to the store to assess and document his performance. The therapist and Edgar will establish the targeted performance level and supplement the assessment with narrative information. Prior to shopping, Edgar might be asked how well he anticipates doing; after completing the task, he might be asked how well he thought he did. During the shopping test, the therapist will observe Edgar's response to other shoppers and his effectiveness with the cashier. The therapist will also note the strategies Edgar uses to remember, the responses he gives, and the results of any suggestions or modifications given to him. This information will contribute to the qualitative aspects of the evaluation. Throughout the evaluation process, Edgar will be a collaborator and thus continually learn about his performance. When the therapist completes the macro evaluation of those functions identified as important by Edgar and Daisy, focus can then shift to the micro perspective.

Evaluation: The Micro Perspective

Evaluation from the micro perspective provides a biomedical orientation in which the occupational therapist functions as a professional offering specialized services for the management of cognitive and functional rehabilitation (Bridge & Twible, 1997; McColl et al., 1997; McColl, Law, & Stewart, 1993; WHO, 1980). The micro perspective is an affirmation of the need for the detection, identification, and measurement of impairments that cause disability; it is important because the therapist may need to assume responsibility for the client until the medical situation stabilizes and the client's cognitive and functional capacities improve (Bridge & Twible, 1997; McColl et al., 1997).

From the micro perspective, the Quadraphonic Approach provides a frame of reference that integrates four theoretical foundations to guide the evaluation and treatment of cognitive-perceptual and postural control dysfunction. When considering such impairments, the therapist must be aware that they do not occur in isolation but are influenced by factors such as the client's mood and motivational dynamics (Diller, 1993). The format used for the development of this particular micro frame of reference (Abreu, 1994; 1992) includes three components:

- a theoretical base
- a function/dysfunction continuum
- applications to practice that describe examples of evaluation and treatment.

The three assumptions for this frame of reference are:

1. That continuous analysis of the components of occupational performance (bottom-up approach) combined with analysis of total performance or occupations (top-down approach) is critical for rehabilitation and that cognitive impairment has an effect on perceptual motor function.
2. That the integration of the cognitive-perceptual and postural control systems is required in cognitive rehabilitation because their separation excludes the role of cognition in movement.
3. That applied phenomenology (Fleming, 1991) is necessary to understand the meaning that clients attribute to their illnesses and other life experiences. The narrative process is critical in order to individualize treatment so that it will be optimally useful to clients who need to improve adaptive strategies after brain injury or trauma (Clark, 1993).

The micro perspective of the Quadraphonic Approach uses four complementary functional theories that facilitate the collaborative design of therapeutic interventions to improve a client's adaptive strategies. The four theories that can be used to

explain and predict behaviors are information processing, teaching/learning, neurodevelopmental, and biomechanical.

Information Processing Theory

Information processing theory is used to explain how an individual's mind functions, that is, how people perceive and react to the environment. One segment of information processing theory views persons as analogous to computers. This segment postulates that there are three successive processing stages within the nervous system: detection of the stimulus, discrimination and analysis of the stimulus, and response selection and determination based on hypotheses derived from the relationship between sensory stimuli and past experience (Abreu, 1992; Klatzy, 1980; Light, 1990).

The detection stage entails the discovery, registration, and/or recognition of sensory cues. The discrimination and analysis stage includes the interpretation and organization of raw sensory information into a code. This code, or new communication system, is used by the individual's nervous system to determine a response. Discrimination and analysis also depend on the integrity of the sensory receptors (i.e., tactile, vestibular, and ocular). The clarity of the stimulus as well as its intensity, pattern, complexity, and significance for the individual affect the discrimination and analysis of stimuli (Abreu, 1981). The response selection and determination stage involves comparing the stimulus with experiences in long-term memory and relating the stimulus to the overall purpose and goal of the response. In this stage, the response is planned, structured, and activated. The complexity and the duration of the activity will affect the response. The three successive stages of information processing occur at various levels within the central nervous system and at rates faster than a millisecond. The stages are fully interactive and interdependent in nature.

A response can be data-driven and/or conceptually driven (Norman, 1969; 1979). A data-driven response is dependent on a client's analysis of incoming data. When a client is given, as a test, an unfamiliar drawing to reproduce, he or she may focus on all the details in order to understand what

Figure 2-2

The Quadraphonic Approach

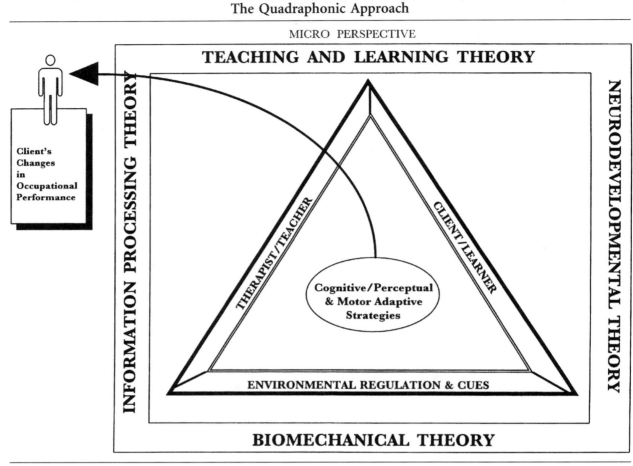

From: Abreu, B.C. (1990). The Quadraphonic Approach: Evaluation and Treatment of the Brain Injured Patient. New York, NY: Therapeutic Service Systems.

to do. That response can be said to be data-driven. A conceptually driven response is more dependent on the environmental context of the stimulus event and is shaped by the individual's memories, personality, and culture (Norman 1969; 1979). When a client is given a drawing of an object that resembles a childhood toy or game, he or she may say, "I'm not doing this test; it's for kids." That response is more conceptually driven.

Brain trauma or disease reduces information processing skills. The dysfunction can occur at any stage of processing—stimulus detection, stimulus discrimination and analysis, or response selection and determination. Although information processing theory can be used to explain some behaviors seen after brain injury and to identify the process-

ing stages, the theory does not explain how an individual evaluates or uses cues gathered from the environment. Therefore, a theory that addresses the process of capturing information from the environment is needed to complement information processing.

Teaching/Learning Theory

Explanations for the manner in which a client might use cues to facilitate information processing can be drawn from teaching/learning theory. This theory explains how individuals use cues to alter their capacity and methods of response to increase cognitive awareness and enhance control. There are several teaching/learning theories. Two that relate to the capturing of information from the environment are self-generated or natural learning, and externally generated or mediated learning (Schwartz, 1991).

Self-generated or natural learning refers to the inherent ability of an individual to learn skills, tasks, or behaviors without external mediation (Schwartz, 1991). Examples are the ability to learn how to sit, walk, and manipulate objects spontaneously using natural strategies for gathering cues from the environment without the aid of an external resource such as a therapist. By comparison, externally generated or mediated learning requires input from an outside source such as a therapist, computer, or self-instructional packet. Although cognitive and functional rehabilitation relies heavily on externally-generated learning, therapists must remember that some of their clients are also capable of self-generated learning (Zimmerman, 1995). According to Schwartz (1991), therapists and clients who use external mediators predetermine

1. The structure of the learning environment
2. The nature of the learning material
3. The type of learning activity, role, and task
4. The type of feedback
5. The manner of evaluation of the learning experience.

Two types of strategies, behavioral and cognitive, can be used for either self-generated or externally generated learning in cognitive-functional rehabilitation (Jacobs, 1993; Schwartz, 1985). A comparison of the behavioral and cognitive learning strategies is provided in Table 2-4.

Metacognitive theory is a part of teaching/learning theory that has particular relevance for clients who function at higher levels and have competence in communication. Metacognitive theory explains the conscious thinking and feeling that accompany and pertain to problem solving (Berry, 1983; Bewick, Raymond, Malia, & Bennett, 1995; Brown & Palincsar, 1989; Paris & Winograd, 1990; Winne, 1995). An individual who uses metacognitive strategies will engage in a conscious prediction, monitoring, and planning that considers the capacities of the self, the demands of the task, and the param-

eters of the strategy (Brown, 1988; Flavell, 1979; Flavell, 1985). Metacognitive strategies can be either self-generated or externally generated. Metacognitive training uses language to influence the degree of interaction that the client has with the environment (Abreu, 1992). Language gives meaning to objects and allows individuals to know what objects are and what objects do or allow an individual to do (Gibson, 1979; Luria, 1973). Language is used as an interactive means of influencing new and more effective learning strategies that increase independence and life satisfaction after the challenge of brain injury. Language cues are words, phrases, or signals used as part of the learning strategy. An example of a client's use of metacognitive theory might be when he or she uses self-talk in analyzing a problem before engaging in its solution. ("If I slow down I am more apt to succeed.")

The theoretical foundations provided by information processing and teaching/learning serve to explain cognition from "the eyebrows up" as if this function resided only in the brain. The rest of the body, including head, neck, trunk, and limb functioning, represents the biomechanical and neuromuscular systems that have a close relationship with the cognitive-perceptual system. The artificial separation of the brain from the rest of the body does not give credit to the relationship between body and mind. Our bodies are the biomechanical expression of a nervous system that shapes postural control. The control and posture gained through the ability to pre-position, position, and maintain body alignment are critical for functional activity. Treatments that address movement also need to consider their influences on cognition. The next two theories are used to provide an explanation of movement as it relates to brain injury.

Neurodevelopmental Theory

Neurodevelopmental theory is concerned with the quality of movement as it relates to the client with developmental or acquired brain injury. Historically, this theory has explained techniques based on a "hard-wired" hierarchical view of the nervous system and has encouraged a genetic-reflex constraint model in rehabilitation. The genetic-reflex

Table 2-4
Behavioral and Cognitive Strategies

Behavioral Learning Strategies	Cognitive Learning Strategies
Based on behavior modification	Are based on information-processing from cognitive psychology
Analyze observable behavior	Analyze behavior that cannot be directly observed
Identify functional relationships	Describe how information is processed, structured, and modified.
Prescribe cause-effect and reward-punishment guidelines in order to gain better control of specified behavior in treatment	Prescribe person-specific tasks, situations, and strategies in order to increase information-processing capabilities.
Assume that consequences influence behavior	Assume that conscious awareness and prediction of outcomes influence behavior.
Do not include ideation, imagery, or meaning	Include ideation, imagery, and meaning
Use positive and negative behaviors as reinforcement	Use self-esteem and a sense of mastery as reinforcement

From Abreu, B.C. (1990). The Quadraphonic Approach: Evaluation and Treatment of the Brain Injured Patient. New York, NY: Therapeutic Service Systems.

constraint model is used to explain the individual's inherent capacities to develop normal movement patterns based on genetic endowment and a fixed hierarchical reflex control mechanism. The current view is that the nervous system is more flexible and adaptive. This newer environmental (physical-social-cultural) constraint model does not deny the hard-wired and hierarchical nature of some structures within the nervous system, but it also explains and supports the nervous system's variability. This variability is shown when different movements in different circumstances activate a variety of nervous system structures and communication strategies (Reed, 1989a; 1989b). The communication functions within the nervous system rely on redundancy wherein a variety of multi-modal sensory receptors generate the same information guaranteeing an effective interaction with the environment (Nashner, 1982). For example, when a client with a brain injury moves around in a given environment, he or she derives overlapping visual, vestibular, and proprioceptive information relative to position in space. Success in his or her mobility is possible given this multimodal input even if one or more receptors are impaired.

The environment includes the aggregate of all relevant characteristics derived from people, objects, circumstances, and conditions that surround the individual (Gentile, 1987). Characteristics that influence action are called environmental regulators because they direct and organize (regulate) an individual's movement for action. Gentile (1987) describes three types of critical environmental regulators that relate to perceptual motor skills: stationary, moving, and intervariable.

Stationary regulators do not move. They include supportive surfaces for clients in both standing and seated positions as well as stationary objects that surround the client in the environment. To be included as regulators such objects must influence the client's actions; an example of a stationary regulator is a piece of furniture around which a client must walk. A stationary environment allows for self-paced actions (Gentile, 1987).

Moving regulators are people, support surfaces, and objects that move within the individual's environment. One example of a moving regulator is an escalator. The speed of movement of such a regulator can vary and affect the ability of the individual to achieve goals. In a slow-moving environment, an individual is better able to self-pace. In a fast-moving environment, the individual must predict and anticipate what to do and thus demonstrate more response diversification. In this context, the moving environment also requires external timing and faster reaction-time responses (Gentile, 1987).

Intervariable regulators are people, support surfaces, and objects that move at variable speeds and/or in changing directions; they fluctuate from one encounter to the next. An example of an intervariable regulator is a bouncing ball. When dealing with intervariable regulators, the individual must perform as many response variations as there are changes in the environmental regulator. The individual must maintain vigilance in order to detect changes.

Developmental or acquired brain injury can reduce an individual's capacity to detect and discriminate stimuli, as well as to respond to relevant environmental regulators (Abreu, 1992; Abreu, 1994; Abreu, 1995; Lee, 1989). Brain injury can affect environmental interactions and may hinder the formulation of postural control strategies during the experience of external and internal perturbations or disturbances of balance (Abreu, 1995; Nashner, 1982; Newton, 1995). A client may, for example, be hampered in formulating a postural control response because of a preoccupying thought (internal perturbation), the sound of a siren (auditory external perturbation), or being jostled in a crowd (physical external perturbation). Most of the regulators discussed to this point are purely physical. Social and cultural regulators are also critical, and these will be discussed later in this chapter.

Biomechanical Theory

The ability of an individual to adapt to the demands of environmental regulators depends on the integrity of the central and peripheral nervous system that is expressed through the musculoskeletal system of the body. The body is the biomechanical effector of centrally and peripherally determined motor plans. Biomechanical theory is useful in explaining and analyzing a client's movement; it enables the therapist to better understand the integration of the nervous and musculoskeletal systems with perceptual motor skills. The individual's musculoskeletal system expresses the generation, scaling, and coordination of movement but can also be a movement regulator or constraint. The integrity and function of bone, tendons, ligaments, and muscles may facilitate or frustrate movement strategies.

Biomechanics relates to the laws and principles of human movement and assists in understanding the client with brain injury. Mechanical kinesiology is the study and analysis of movement from two perspectives that are important in cognitive and functional rehabilitation: kinematics and kinetics. Kinematics describes the mechanical components of the body without consideration of the balanced and unbalanced forces that cause motion. Examples of kinematics are the therapist's naming a motion such as flexion and counting and measuring the movements. This process is similar to that which occurs in goniometry. Kinetics, on the other hand, describes the causal analysis of motion with consideration of the interacting forces that cause motion. Kinetics is divided into static and dynamic analysis. An example of kinetics is the therapist's determination that the client cannot flex because extensor tone is high and flexors are weak.

Brain injury can affect head and trunk movements and lead to a biomechanical disarrangement sometimes associated with the disappearance of symmetrical motor behaviors. Body displacement, velocity, and angular joint movements may be adversely affected after brain injury thereby causing deterioration of the quality and quantity of the client's movement dynamics. Therefore, evaluation of client performance using kinetics to analyze the mechanical components and kinematics to analyze interactive forces can provide guidelines for practice.

Three Interactive Forces for the Micro Perspective

Guided by the four theoretical foundations just described, the therapist and client develop strategies for evaluation and intervention from the micro perspective while analyzing the effect of three interactive forces and their affective elements: the client/

Table 2-5

Three Interactive Forces for Micro Evaluation

The Client/Learner	The Environment	The Therapist/Teacher
(1) Story of the client's adaptation and losses.	(1) Physical	(1) Procedural
(2) The client's stages of awareness of impairment, disability, and restrictions.	(2) Social	(2) Interactive
(3) The client's stages of motor learning or relearning.	(3) Cultural	(3) Conditional
(4) The stage of recovery and acceptance.		

From: Abreu, B.C. (1990). The Quadraphonic Approach: Evaluation and Treatment of the Brain Injured Patient. New York, NY: Therapeutic Service Systems.

learner, the environment, and the therapist/teacher. Table 2-5 outlines these forces.

The Client/Learner

Four significant factors contribute to the client/learner's agency as the first interactive force. These factors offer a comprehensive view of the client and include

- the client's story of adaptation and losses
- stage of awareness
- the stage of motor learning
- stage of recovery and acceptance.

The story of the client is the narrative of the incidents, events, and changes leading up to the current time. Told by the client and significant others, documented by the therapist, and used as a basis for evaluation and treatment, this narrative can reveal the strategies for adaptation used by the client both before and after the injury. Adaptation is the process by which clients adjust their behaviors, attitudes, and values to make themselves more congruent with the new external and internal demands subsequent to disease or trauma. The client's ability to deal with loss is a significant strategy to consider in treatment of brain injury.

The client's stage of awareness also contributes to his or her agency as an interactive force (Gasquoine, 1992; Prigatano, Altman, & O'Brien,

1990). I combined information from two sources to describe the relative stages of awareness. One view holds that the various stages of awareness can occur at any point from coma to community reentry (Bottcher, 1989). A second view identifies three types of awareness that occur among clients with brain injury: intellectual, emergent, and anticipatory (Crosson, Barco, Velozo, Bolesta, Cooper, Werts, & Brobeck, 1989). Intellectual awareness is defined as some level of understanding on the part of the client that a particular function is impaired. Emergent awareness is the client's recognition of a problem as it happens. Anticipatory awareness is the client's ability to predict that a problem will occur based on a solid awareness of the impairment (Crosson et al., 1989). Although optimal community reintegration requires anticipatory awareness, clients with brain injury may also reenter their environments at different stages. A client's disposition at reentry depends on multiple factors, including recovery of function, social support systems, and insurance coverage.

The third important factor that shapes the manner in which the client will act as an interactive force is the client's motor learning stage. Motor learning is the acquisition of skilled movements as a result of practice. In cognitive rehabilitation, the requisite motor skills are considered new skills because they have been lost because of disease or trauma. According to Fitts and Posner (1967), the three stages of motor learning are cognitive, associative, and autonomous. In the cognitive stage,

Figure 2-3				
An Awareness and Motor Learning Continuum				
Coma	Wakefulness without Awareness	Intellectual Awareness	Emergent Awareness	Anticipatory Awareness	Community Re-entry skills
		Cognitive Learning Stage	Associative Learning Stage	Autonomous Learning Stage	

After Crosson et al (1989); Fitts and Posner (1967)

the client's processing of task requirements is variable and full of errors. In the associative stage, the client begins to develop an internal reference of correctness and a capacity to detect errors. The feedback requirements are minimal and the client learns through trial and error. Performance is less variable and more accurate. During the final autonomous stage, a client pays minimal attention to performance because of the presence of full error detection capabilities and a very stable performance. The continuum that is represented in figure 2-3 illustrates an interface between the stages of awareness and the stages of motor learning.

I propose that the continuum is flexible, interdependent, and a dynamic interface between awareness and motor learning. Furthermore, the client's response to any test, activity, task, or role depends on personal ability, developmental history, emotional condition, and perception of meaning (Nelson, 1987).

The final factor related to the client's role as an interactive force is his or her ability to accept and cope with each stage of recovery. This ability depends to a great extent on an individual's motivation, hope, and commitment to reshape lifestyle and personal identity (Corbin & Strauss, 1988).

The Environment

The second major interactive force at the micro level is the environment. There are three types of environments—physical, social, and cultural. In cognitive and functional rehabilitation, the physical environment has historically received the most emphasis (Abreu, 1981; Abreu, 1992; Abreu & Toglia, 1987). The physical environment includes the characteristics, both relevant and irrelevant, that are associated with the activities, conditions, circumstances, objects, and people surrounding the client (Gentile, 1987). These characteristics include the quantity, size, spatial orientation, speed, and duration of the stimuli as well as whether they are stationary or moving. All of these characteristics or task parameters interact to regulate a client's movement and posture; this interaction was discussed at length in the section on neurodevelopmental and biomechanical theory.

The social environment includes the client's voluntary relationships or social networks, the family structure, and community resources (Mosey, 1986). Additionally, the social environment includes the client's perception of personal roles, rights, duties, and privileges (Mosey, 1986). These aspects of the environment are critical in guiding the client's discharge plans and in formulating adaptive strategies for community reentry. These adaptations are greatly affected by the actions of the client, family, and friends with regard to the rehabilitation process (Corbin & Strauss, 1988). Any adaptation includes both the personal context (the client's function) and the social context (the client's support systems) (Pierce & Frank, 1992).

The cultural environment is a complex subject that includes the traditions, values, norms, language, and symbolic meanings that are shared as cultural agreements between the client and any group (Mosey, 1986). These agreements describe how things should be done in ethical and/or aesthetic terms. Cultural environment regulates the types of activities, tasks, roles in which a client will participate, and the people with whom he or she will engage.

The Therapist/Teacher

The third force to consider at the micro level is the therapist/teacher who must use clinical reasoning and the principles of therapeutic relationships to make clinical judgments. This type of reasoning, based on a series of analytical steps, may be represented by clinical pathways, flowcharts, mathematical models, or judgmental formulations. Clinical reasoning helps the therapist formulate an educated evaluation, plan an effective treatment plan, and reevaluate the plan as required.

Fleming (1991) describes three types of reasoning that influence clinical judgments: procedural, interactive, and conditional. Procedural reasoning can be described as the way in which therapists think about the diagnosis and impairment and the manner in which they initially interact with a client. Interactive reasoning is the way therapists think about and interact with clients in order to determine their current needs and values. Conditional reasoning occurs when the therapist engages in the acts of thinking about, interpreting, and interacting while considering brain injury in a broader social and temporal context that goes beyond disability to the client's view of the future (Fleming, 1991).

The therapist must be aware that all clinical decision-making processes are based on imperfect measurements that are subject to some degree of ambiguity, contain some possibility of error, and need to be continually reevaluated.

Guidelines for Evaluation from the Micro Perspective

Evaluation from the micro perspective is characterized by five guidelines that parallel those used with the macro perspective:

- an examination of the client's cognition (mind) and postural control (body strategies)
- a precise determination and definition of those processes that will be assessed (such as attention,

memory, problem solving, motor planning), and a selection of the evaluative strategies that correspond with these definitions
- a consideration of the client's choices and degree of control within the evaluation process
- a scoring and documentation of results that includes commentary about the client's personal awareness and responsivity as well as his or her interaction with therapist, task, and environment
- a consideration of the psychometric character of the evaluation and whether it yields both qualitative and quantitative data about the client's performance.

These factors guide the therapist when selecting which assessments or activities to use for evaluation. For example, the client named Edgar reports a moderate memory deficit and indicates that his primary aim is to return home to his wife, Daisy, and to continue working as a chemical engineer. By stating this impairment, Edgar determines the therapist's starting point. From this point, the therapist will move more deeply into an evaluation attending to the five guidelines as they relate to Edgar's use of memory strategies.

The micro evaluation uses a cuing system to aid in the development of treatment plans for adults with brain injury (Abreu, 1992; Abreu & Toglia, 1987). Throughout the evaluation the therapist uses questions and probes in an attempt to clarify whether the client understood instructions and to investigate more deeply the performance and responses given during the task or test. This investigation is conducted in order to specify the factors contributing to the client's use of inefficient strategies and to identify the contextual modifications that may improve his or her performance. Tables 2-6 and 2-7 show examples of evaluations that might have been used with Edgar.

Holistic and Confluent Treatment: Edgar's Case

Upon completion of the macro and micro evaluation, the therapist is ready to work with the client to develop a holistic and confluent treatment plan. As previously stated, holistic treatment is based on

Table 2-6
Micro Evaluation Samples—Coma and Minimally Responsive

The four theories are the statements that describe and predict the micro-perspective evaluation guidelines.

Information Processing Evaluation	Teaching/Learning Evaluation	Neurodevelopmental Evaluation	Biomechanical Evaluation
1-Coma-Near Coma Scale (CNS) 2-Coma Recovery Scale (CRS) 3-Sensory Stimulation Assessment Measure (SSAM) 4-Western Neuro-sensory Stimulation (WNSS) 5-Quadraphonic Evaluation System (QES)-personalized form tracking a 24 hour spectrum. *Determine arousal patterns and changes in response in arousal and attention as a result of interventions.	1-Stimulus-response transfer or carry-over 2-Personalized target stimulation such as a-gustatory memories b-tactile memories c-auditory memories d-visual memories	1-Modified tasks based on neurodevelopmental analysis 2-Observational findings such as a-balance and postural control b-musculoskeletal tone c-symmetry d-movement disassociations e-reaction and movement time f-mobility and stability	1-Modified tasks based on kinematic and kinetic analysis 2-Observational findings such as a-active range of motion b-passive range of motion c-muscle power d-joint-play movements e-endurance f-coordination

The three forces are the regulators of the evaluation micro-perspective. It predicts the evaluation interaction process.

The Client/Learner	The Therapist/Teacher	The Training/Compensatory Environment
Losses ■ Could you tell me how Edgar handled previous losses? ■ How are you handling the loss of Edgar as you know him? *Awareness* Edgar most likely will not have a general sense that there is a problem (intellectual awareness), be unable to recognize a problem exists (emergent awareness) and/or be unable to predict problems in the future (anticipatory awareness). *Motor Learning* Edgar's motor re-learning actions and sequences at this stage are full of error and variable performance. The actions are reflexive and/or conscious. *Stage of Acceptance* ■ Could you tell me how Edgar may accept or cope with illness as he recovers?	1. Are you primarily controlling the evaluation/treatment session? 2. Are your judgements focused or driven primarily by the protocols, procedures, test and measurement methods, and/or Edgar's diagnosis? 3. Are your judgements focused or driven primarily by Edgar's needs and values (what Edgar feels is good, meaningful, and important)? 4. Are your judgements focused or driven primarily by Edgar's social support system and the timing of his disadvantage?	1. Are the physical traits of the environment stable, unchangeable, and as familiar as possible to provide a close fit to the minimal processing Edgar has at this stage? 2. Are Edgar's cultural and personal system traits represented and included during the intervention process? 3. Are Edgar's social personal support systems represented and included during the intervention process?

From Abreu, B. C. (1990). The Quadraphonic Approach: Evaluation and Treatment of the Brain Injured Patient. New York, NY: Therapeutic Service Systems.

Table 2-7

Micro Evaluation Samples—Acute and Community Reentry

The four theories are the statements that describe and predict the micro-perspective evaluation guidelines.

Information Processing Evaluation	Teaching/Learning Evaluation	Neurodevelopmental Evaluation	Biomechanical Evaluation
1-Attentional battery=modified tests, eye fixations, visual scanning, modified stroop, and modified trailmaking. 2-Visual perception battery=visual acuity, visual analysis, visual spatial, visual motor. 3-Recognition and recall battery=storytelling, visual action picture, 20 associated photos, 20 associated words, repeating story, belonging item. 4-Problem solving battery=list to make shopping easier, categorize in groups, functional hypothetical, discovery photograph rules. 5-Motor planning battery=gesture imitations, metronome movement patterns, object manipulation, blocks construction. 6-Postural control battery=asymmetry assessment, theoretical base of support assessment, self-perturbation, external perturbations -T form.		1-Modified task based on neurodevelopmental analysis 2-Observational findings such as a-balance and postural control b-musculoskeletal tone c-symmetry d-movement disassociations e-reaction and movement time f-mobility and stability	1-Modified tasks based on kinematic and kinetic analysis 2-Observational findings such as a-active range of motion b-passive range of motion c-muscle power d-joint-play movements e-endurance f-coordination

*Performance versus learning effects.

The three forces are the regulators of the evaluation micro-perspective. It predicts the evaluation interaction process.

The Client/Learner	The Therapist/Teacher	The Training/Compensatory Environment
Losses ■ Could you tell me how you handled previous losses? ■ Let's talk about how you are different now from before the injury/accident/illness. *Awareness* *Before you test:* ■ Why are you taking these type of tests before? ■ Do you remember what the results of tests like these were? ■ Why are you taking these tests? ■ How well do you think you will do on this test/task/activity?	1. Are you primarily controlling the evaluation/treatment session? 2. Are your judgements focused or driven primarily by the protocols, procedures, test and measurement methods, and/or Edgar's diagnosis? 3. Are your judgements focused or driven primarily by Edgar's needs and values (what Edgar feels is good, meaningful, and important)? 4. Are your judgements focused or driven primarily by Edgar's social support system and the timing of his disadvantage?	1. Are the physical traits of the environment an additional task demand, which tends to inhibit initial acquisition of task competency but ultimately to facilitate transfer? 2. Are Edgar's cultural and personal systems' traits represented and included during the intervention process? 3. Are Edgar's social personal support systems represented and included during the intervention process.

During:
- How are you doing with this test/task/activity?
- Can you tell me what just happened? (error/ problem recognition)

After test:
- How well did you do?
- Did you perform better or worse than you expected?
- How may this problem affect your plans to go back to live/work/school independently? (Specify areas.)

Motor Learning
- Are your motor actions and sequences conscious, full of errors, and variable performance requiring constant feedback?
- Are motor actions and sequences associative with less errors and requiring less feedback?
- Are motor actions automatic with no errors and independent?

Stage of Acceptance
- Describe your life as it were a book?
- Describe how well you have accepted changes and illnesses in the past. Let's talk about how it feels to be at this stage of your recovery.

From Abreu, B. C. (1990). The Quadraphonic Approach: Evaluation and Treatment of the Brain Injured Patient. New York, NY: Therapeutic Service Systems.

a global health notion that clients are capable of maintaining and restoring equilibrium in their lives (McColl,1994). Holistic treatment will use confluent methods, actions, and interactions that develop the affective domain. The holistic and confluent approach is particularly important if one aims to preserve the personalization of the rehabilitation process in a managed care environment (Abreu & Price-Lackey, 1994; Peloquin, 1996).

In the current managed care environment, critical pathways can be used to organize treatment plans in a holistic fashion, avoiding duplication of services and maximizing interdisciplinary cooperation. These pathways are the blueprint created by a health care team (including client and family) based on the diagnosis and desired functional outcomes (Abreu, Seale, Podlesak, & Hartley, 1996). The efficiency and effectiveness of the critical pathway is measured by functional outcomes that match the client's goals and satisfaction with the services rendered (Abreu et al., 1996).

The case study of Edgar will be used to demonstrate selective methods of a treatment approach that is holistic and confluent. The reader is reminded that, in the Quadraphonic Approach, there is always a free-flowing movement between the macro and micro perspectives. I designed six treatment environments to match seven cognitive and functional levels. (The seventh level, that of independence, warrants no therapeutic intervention.) The six treatment environments are total dependence, maximum dependence, moderate dependence, minimal assistance, supervised assistance, and independence with no modification. In the story of Edgar's recovery, total dependence, moderate dependence, and supervised assistance will be highlighted in three practice settings: a coma unit, a rehabilitation unit, and a community reentry setting.

Treatment Guidelines for Functional Levels

During treatment, therapists tutor, coach, and encourage the client and his or her social support systems (family and friends) to develop strategies for dealing with the impairments, disabilities, and disadvantages resulting from brain injury. If a client is evaluated with a functional performance level below 50%, the therapist may use traditional as well as more affective approaches in order to encourage the client with both verbal and nonverbal exchanges that communicate support (Peloquin, 1995).

On the other hand, for those clients who have shown functional performance ranging from 50 to 90% independence, the most beneficial therapeutic environment is variable and with increasing task demands. These additional task demands create contextual interference that facilitates successful performance (Druckman & Bjork, 1991; Druckman & Bjork, 1994; Schmidt & Bjork, 1992). For a more detailed delineation of the suggested therapeutic environment for each level of client function see Table 2-2.

Phases of Treatment

In addition to the functional performance guidelines, I propose three phases for every treatment level: preparatory, performance, and post-performance.

Preparatory Phase

The preparatory phase addresses four treatment techniques that precede the demand for performance: emotional and mental, attentional recruitment, organizational and reorganizational, and practice schedule and feedback plan.

By using emotional and mental techniques in the preparatory phase, the therapist is better able to engage the client as a partner in the treatment process. This is accomplished through the use of the macro assessment tools that are used to establish a connection with the client's story and personal goals. Through specific explanations of the purpose of treatment and through body language that communicates interest and empathy, the therapist invites the client into a critical collaborative relationship. The preparatory phase may also include relaxation techniques. Quiet and stable environments are recommended and the use of meditation and subliminal self-help techniques may help some clients.

Attentional recruitment techniques include a wide range of strategies for increasing the client's readiness and capacity to gather and retain information. These techniques also facilitate the client in letting go of irrelevant information so it will not interfere with his or her functional performance. The therapist can invite the client to describe aloud what to do and how to do it as a technique for awareness and self-monitoring. For visual acuity and perception training, I recommend increasing luminance and the use of large print. In addition, the therapist can increase background contrast, increase light, and decrease shadows (Lampert & Lapolice, 1995; Warren, 1995). A multimodal approach to instructions (visual, auditory, kinesthetic, verbal, and nonverbal) is recommended.

Neurodevelopmental and biomechanical techniques are also used as attentional motor recruitment techniques in order to provide the client with sufficient trunk control or trunk support to assure postural readiness. Poor bodily alignment because of muscle tone and musculoskeletal changes can rob the client of the appropriate postural support required to attend to incoming information. The client may not be able to simultaneously focus on controlling posture (sitting or standing) while gathering visual and auditory information. Therefore, the clinician either provides facilitation/inhibition motor techniques for postural control/support or uses external support devices to compensate for the impaired postural control.

In addition, the therapist can use traditional information processing techniques and cognitive rehabilitation techniques that help the client notice the critical traits of the activity, task, or role: verbal repetitions, cues to initiate, simplifications through concrete instructions, and changes in the pace or duration of instructions and stimuli presented.

The third set of treatment techniques in the preparation phase are organizational and reorganizational techniques. These include a wide variety of strategies for planning and arranging information and procedures in an orderly fashion so that the client will gain more understanding and develop more skills from any training session. Organization is the act of thinking about what one is going to do or is doing. Organizational strategies help us to consciously monitor and control the way in which we plan to execute instructions for unified action with coherent relations among steps. This

conscious self-awareness and self-monitoring about how to organize learning before it happens and while it happens is also called metacognition or reflection.

Organizational strategies help clients to monitor and control behavior through reflection about the factual knowledge given about the skill or task, its components, its controls, and its functions. Factual knowledge is called declarative knowledge and is known as *declarative memory* when retained or stored in memory. Organizational strategies can also be used to help clients monitor and control behavior through reflection on procedural knowledge or the rules given regarding how to perform a task. When rule-based or procedural knowledge is retained or stored it is called *procedural memory*. Finally, organizational strategies help with a client's introspection about his or her ability to handle a task that is actually being attempted.

Psychologists and educators, particularly Chi and colleagues (1982; 1985; 1989; 1994), have supported the idea that self-regulation of cognitive skills in the classroom can help individuals solving mathematics and physics problems and playing chess (Dreyfus & Dreyfus, 1986; Gagne & Smith, 1962; Kluwe, 1987; Paris & Winograd, 1990; Schoenfield, 1987; Silver, 1987; Swanson, 1990). Other studies, with special populations, support the use of self-regulation to assist in speech and language (Blackmer & Mitton, 1991; Dabbs, Evans, Hopper, & Purvis, 1980; Koegel, Koegel, & Ingham, 1986; Schloss & Wood, 1990; Shriberg & Kwiatkowski, 1990; Whitney & Goldstein, 1989). The use of self-regulation in cognitive rehabilitation after acquired brain injury is growing and further studies are needed to establish validation and efficacy (Abreu, 1992; Abreu & Toglia, 1987; Bewick, Raymond, Malia, & Bennett, 1995; Toglia, 1991; Webster & Scott, 1983; Ylvisaker & Szekeres, 1989).

The value of reflective problem solving using metacognitive and affective techniques has been advocated by several occupational therapists for use in both the clinic and the classroom (Abreu, 1992; Abreu, 1994; Abreu & Toglia, 1987; Neistadt, 1992; Parham, 1987; Peloquin, 1996; Schon, 1987; Toglia, 1991; Toglia, 1993). Introspective analysis that allows individuals to understand the reasons for their failures is a process of learning to learn (Stuss, 1992).

Good learners comprehend the problem, represent the principles of the problem in formal terms, plan a solution, execute the plan, and interpret and evaluate the solution (Posner, 1988). Metacognitive techniques include developing a plan of action, maintaining and monitoring the plan, and evaluating the plan before, during, and after the action (Brown, 1978; Brown, 1987; Flavell, 1985; Flavell, 1987). The metacognitive approach uses questions, cues, and prompts to bring awareness to the client's rules of behavior, task performance, and use of strategies. The client is encouraged to engage in self-explanation and self-monitoring through talk-aloud or think-aloud methods. However, if a client is unable to self-explain and monitor, the therapist can cue with questions and prompts. The four basic questions that a client can ask about any task are:

1. What should I do *before* I start this training session?
2. What should I do *during* this training session?
3. What should I do *after* this training session?
4. Do I need to do *anything else* to perform better during training?

The educational literature suggests that good students use more self-talk about actions that exemplify the solutions. They also use more self-monitoring for evaluating their accuracy than other students (Chi & Bassok, 1989; Chi, Leeuw, Chiu, & LaVancher, 1994; VanLehn, Jones, & Chi, 1991; VanLehn, Jones, & Chi, 1992). Similar procedures have been described in the rehabilitation literature of occupational therapy with a head-injured client (Abreu, 1992; Abreu & Toglia, 1987; Toglia, 1993; Webster & Scott, 1983).

The fourth set of techniques used in the preparatory phase include the practice schedule and feedback plan. A practice schedule defines the type and quantity of the repeated performances needed by the client for learning to occur. The therapist proposes the best practice schedule for a client depending on the level of recovery and the physical and cognitive tolerance for training. There is no evidence in the literature to support one particular schedule over another. Therefore, therapists must use clinical judgment to decide which type and

order of practice training to use. The training can be an intense practice process or more distributed (spread out). Training can be designed to include partial or complete tasks and can use forward or backward chaining. In clinical retrospect, I have not perceived a proportional relationship between the number of practice performances and the mastery or retention of a skill. Practice does not guarantee performance with brain injury. During the preparatory phase, the client/learner helps the therapist to establish a timeline for the achievement of outcome goals.

A feedback plan defines the type and quantity of the responses that will be given to modify, correct, and/or strengthen a behavior displayed by the client during the practice session. In the Quadraphonic Approach, I advocate the use of consistent feedback with clients who perform at a level of independence from 0 to 49%. On the other hand, for clients who are performing at a level of independence above 50%, the use of random feedback is highly recommended (Abreu, 1994).

Certain motor learning and action system theorists have stated that using variability in practice improves the retention and transfer of motor skills (Druckman & Bjork; 1991, Druckman & Bjork, 1994; Reed, 1982; Schmidt, 1988; Schmidt & Bjork, 1992). I have noted that not all clients benefit from random and less frequent feedback and that clients with low cognitive levels and those in early recovery stages perform better with the use of constant and amplified feedback. But as soon as the clients show understanding of the goal and some stability in their responses that is not attributable to chance (i.e., above 50% accuracy), I implement a lower frequency feedback schedule.

Performance Phase

The performance phase is the stage in treatment during which the client/learner executes, does, or creates something for purposes of learning or relearning, and for satisfaction. For me, the performance phase of treatment includes an improvisation by the therapist to spontaneously create a caring and effective bond with the client. In this phase, the client who has recently become a novice in ordinary occupations in which he or she was previously an expert, must regain expertise. The literature on tutoring individuals to progress from novice to expert levels has given me guidelines for the performance phase of treatment.

Information on identifying effective strategies that move learners toward expertise has been the subject of investigation in cognitive psychology and artificial intelligence (Chi, Glaser, & Rees, 1982). Research in artificial intelligence attempts to simulate human capacities in a mechanized environment via expert systems. The characteristics of an expert, whether human or machine, can be considered as broad guidelines for engaging the client in ordinary occupations. In general experts:

■ excel in their own domain
■ perceive larger meaningful patterns and conceptual frames and have vast organizational strategies
■ can process information and problem solve faster
■ have superior short-term and long-term memory
■ use more associations with more principles
■ spend a great deal of time analyzing a problem qualitatively
■ have strong self-monitoring skills (Chi & Glaser, 1985).

Experts must explicity know how to use effective strategies in conjunction with their content knowledge for mastery of any skill/knowledge (Glaser & Chi, 1988; Posner, 1988). The use of strategies can enhance problem solving through the discovery of better ways to express, recognize, and use diverse and particular forms of knowledge.

In collaboration with an interdisciplinary rehabilitation team, I created a list of contextual modifiers that can enhance client success during the performance phase. Contextual modifications are cues that can originate from three primary sources—the therapist, the task/environment, and the client as well as the interplay among them that occurs during task performance. Although these modifications interact closely, it is important to articulate and distinguish them for purposes of evaluation, treatment, and research.

The contextual modifiers listed in Table 2-8 are recommended for use as treatment tools and for documenting the qualitative aspects of the client's performance. The first column describes the contextual dimension or type of modifier. Some of these modifiers are not totally exclusive or discrete; they may be nested or embedded in others. Because the modifiers are qualitative tools, their goal is to identify, describe, and analyze the patterns of a client's changes in performance. These tools are classified as soft and they enhance the therapist's awareness of interactional considerations essential for treatment and aid in the identification of the kind of strategy that improves performance. Therapists must remember that improved performance does not always correlate with client satisfaction.

The second column lists the standard approach or the first strategy in treatment: After giving standard instructions, the therapist observes the client's behavior without modification. Wait and see what happens. The therapist should then repeat the instructions and modify the environment. This step is represented with various recommendations for modifications or contextual modifiers listed in column three. Notice that these items specify either training or compensatory techniques. For example, consider error detection/correction technique as it relates to the case of Edgar.

Edgar was unable to detect or correct errors in money management when balancing his checking account. With verbal and visual cueing, Edgar was able to increase his functional performance level and balance the account accurately. Even so, Daisy was taught to supervise Edgar because after eight 1-hour therapy sessions, there was no generalization of performance. Edgar was successful only with cueing given to initiate, increased illumination, and concrete explanations. Use of pictorial representations did not help him. Edgar was aware that he was cue-dependent and needed external monitoring. He was able to perform all cash transactions using self-generated cues like "count your change twice" before putting it in your pocket. The contextual modifiers listed in column three include both self-specific and task-specific strategies.

The fourth column, outcome, is a guide used to indicate performance. The outcome results can

Table 2-8

Contextual Modifiers

CONTEXTUAL DIMENSION	STANDARD APPROACH	CONTEXTUAL MODIFICATIONS [Therapist/ Client / Task]	*OUTCOME* Successful Unsuccessful	
1. **Sensory modality:** The visual, verbal, tactile, or movement cues provided.	☐ Standard No modification of sensory input	☐ Give verbal repetition ☐ Give verbal cues [includes questions / probes] ☐ Give visual cue / non-verbal feedback ☐ Give tactile / kinesthetic cue ☐ Give pictorial represen-tation ☐ Give written cues ☐ Increase illumination, contrast, brightness ☐ Other [e.g. enlarge]	*Given:* ☐ *Verbal repetition* ☐ *Verbal cues* ☐ *Visual cue / non-verbal feedback* ☐ *Tactile / kinesthetic cue* ☐ *Pictorial representation* ☐ *Written cues* ☐ *Increased illumination, contrast, brightness* ☐ *Other [e.g. enlarge]*	☐ ☐ ☐ ☐ ☐ ☐ ☐ ☐
2. **Amount of Information:** The number of instruc-tion steps, choices, or pieces of information presented.	☐ Standard No modification to amount of information	☐ Cue to initiate ☐ Give one step at a time ☐ Reduce the number of steps ☐ Shorten the task ☐ Other	*Given:* ☐ *Cueing to initiate* ☐ *One step at a time* ☐ *Reduced number of steps* ☐ *Shortening of the task* ☐ *Other*	☐ ☐ ☐ ☐ ☐
3. **Complexity:** The level of difficulty of the pieces of information given.	☐ Standard No modification of level of difficulty	☐ Simplify by using concrete explanations ☐ Simplify by demonstra-ting ☐ Simplify by using familiar tasks ☐ Simplify by using self-related items ☐ Simplify by increasing the spacing between items or objects [non-scattered] ☐ Simplify by decreasing spatial traits or position of objects ☐ Other	*Given:* ☐ *Concrete explanations* ☐ *Demonstrations* ☐ *Familiar tasks only* ☐ *Self-related items* ☐ *Increased spacing between items or objects [non-scattered]* ☐ *Decreased spatial traits or position of objects* ☐ *Other*	☐ ☐ ☐ ☐ ☐ ☐ ☐
4. **Pace:** The speed and consistency with which information is presented.	☐ Standard No modification of pace	☐ Give slow presentation ☐ Give fast presentation ☐ Give predictable / stable presentation ☐ Give random / unpre-dictable presentation ☐ Other	*Given:* ☐ *Slow presentation* ☐ *Fast presentation* ☐ *Predictable / stable presentation* ☐ *Random / unpre-dictable presentation* ☐ *Other*	☐ ☐ ☐ ☐ ☐
5. **Duration:** The interval of time that the client is given in which to respond to an instruction.	☐ Standard No modification of duration of time	☐ Give 15 seconds ☐ Give 30 seconds ☐ Give 1 minute	*Given:* ☐ *15 seconds* ☐ *30 seconds* ☐ *1 minute*	☐ ☐ ☐
6. **Activity Phase:** The phase during an activity when the client's functioning breaks down and the therapist offers feedback.	☐ Standard No modification through-out any phase of the test, task, or activity	Give feedback: ☐ At preparatory stage ☐ At initiation stage ☐ At middle stage ☐ At end stage ☐ After completion	*Given feedback:* ☐ *At preparatory stage* ☐ *At initiation stage* ☐ *At middle stage* ☐ *At end stage* ☐ *After completion*	☐ ☐ ☐ ☐ ☐

Page 1

Table 2-8—*Continued.*

Contextual Modifiers

CONTEXTUAL DIMENSION	STANDARD APPROACH	CONTEXTUAL MODIFICATIONS [Therapist/ Client / Task]	OUTCOME Successful	Unsuccessful
7. **Postural Readiness:** The bodily positions that facilitate the client's execution of a task.	☐ Standard position assumed by client	Cue the client to position the: ☐ Eyes ☐ Head / neck ☐ Limbs ☐ Hand ☐ Hips ☐ None ☐ Other	Given cueing to position: *Eyes Head / neck Limbs Hand Hips None Other*	☐ ☐ ☐ ☐ ☐ ☐ ☐
8. **Expectations for Accuracy / Correctness:** The therapist's anticipation / expectation relative to the client's success or failure.	☐ Standard expectations	☐ Therapist anticipates task failure ☐ Therapist anticipates task success ☐ No anticipation ☐ Other	*But therapist's expectation was a failure And therapist's expectation was a success In the absence of any particular expectation Other*	☐ ☐ ☐ ☐
9. **Error Detection / Correction:** Information provided the client relative to the presence of error.	☐ Standard Client initiates response to error in the absence of observable cueing.	☐ Cue for error detection ☐ Cue for error correction ☐ Client self cues for error detection ☐ Client self-cues for error correction ☐ Other	*Given:* *Therapist cueing for error detection Therapist cueing for error correction Client self-cueing for error detection Client self-cueing for error correction Other*	☐ ☐ ☐ ☐ ☐
10. **Organizational Strategy:** Organizational methods / guidelines provided.	☐ Standard organization offered	☐ Provide guidelines about where to start / end ☐ Provide guidelines about where to look ☐ Provide guidelines about what to say ☐ Provide rules and guidelines for behavior ☐ Reorganize information ☐ Client self-initiates strategy: ☐ Other	*Given:* *Guidelines about where to start / end Guidelines about where to look Guidelines about what to say Rules and guidelines for behavior Reorganized information Self initiated strategy:* *Other*	☐ ☐ ☐ ☐ ☐ ☐ ☐
11. **Therapy Set:** Information given the client about the goal / performance of the task or therapy.	☐ Standard request to perform	☐ Explain goal / purpose of task ☐ Explain goal / purpose of therapy ☐ Explain role of the therapist ☐ Other	*Given:* *Explanation of the goal / purpose of task Explanation of the goal / purpose of therapy Explanation of the role of the therapist Other*	☐ ☐ ☐ ☐
12. **Personal History:** References to the client's needs, values, interests, or preferences.	☐ Standard request to perform	☐ Connect task with the client's interests / preferences ☐ Connect task with the client's hobbies ☐ Refer to client's needs / goals ☐ Refer to client's values ☐ Use personally relevant task ☐ Use personally concrete task ☐ Other	*Given:* *A connection made with the client's interests / preferences A connection made with the client's hobbies Reference to client's needs / goals Reference to client's values Use of a personally relevant task Use of a personally concrete task Other*	☐ ☐ ☐ ☐ ☐ ☐ ☐

Table 2-8—*Continued.*

Contextual Modifiers

CONTEXTUAL DIMENSION	STANDARD APPROACH	CONTEXTUAL MODIFICATIONS [Therapist/ Client / Task]	*OUTCOME* Successful *Unsuccessful*	
13. **Social Milieu:** Manipulation made to the client's social environment: Client's family, friends, social, and institutional support system.	☐ Standard No modification of social milieu.	☐ Seat the client near a friend ☐ Ask the client to help another ☐ Ask a client-helper to work with the client ☐ Ask a question to elicit interaction ☐ Encourage group bonding in spite of individual variation	*Given:* ☐ *Seating near a friend* ☐ *A request to help another* ☐ *A client-helper* ☐ *A question to elicit interaction* ☐ *Other* _____	☐ ☐ ☐ ☐ *[e.g. claims no fit]*
14. **Safety:** The information that the client requires in order to perform safely.	☐ Standard No modification of set up, equipment, and safety demands	☐ Explain safety measures ☐ Explain preventive measures ☐ Explain dangerous consequences ☐ Explain emergency procedures ☐ Repeat preventive measure ☐ Other	*Given:* ☐ *Explanation of safety measures* ☐ *Explanation of preventative measures* ☐ *Explanation of dangerous consequences* ☐ *Explanation of emergency procedures* ☐ *Repetition of preventive measure* ☐ *Other*	☐ ☐ ☐ ☐ ☐
15. **Awareness of a Problem:** Awareness of impairment, dysfunction, restriction, and/or personal or social disadvantage.	☐ Standard No modification secondary to awareness capacities and limitations	☐ Give general cues that a problem exists ☐ Give specific cues when error happens or problem exists ☐ Give specific cues after error happens or problem occurs ☐ Give gentle confrontation about the undetected problem ☐ Give away the answer / solution ☐ Other	*Given:* ☐ *General cues that a problem exists* ☐ *Specific cues when error happened or problem existed* ☐ *Specific cues after error happened or problem occurred.* ☐ *Gentle confrontation about undetected problem* ☐ *An answer / solution* ☐ *Other*	☐ ☐ ☐ ☐ ☐ ☐
16. **Feedback Type:** The structuring of corrective verbal information that the client is given with which to respond to an instruction.	☐ Standard No modification of feedback	☐ Give Knowledge of performance feedback [KP]: Corrective information about a component or part of task, test, or movement ☐ Give Knowledge of results feedback [KR]: Corrective information about the total or whole task, test, or movement goal ☐ Give positive feedback: Corrective information in form of approvals, assurances, reinforcers ☐ Give negative feedback: Corrective information in form of disapprovals or negative reinforcers	*Given:* ☐ *Knowledge of performance feedback* ☐ *Knowledge of results feedback* ☐ *Positive feedback* ☐ *Negative feedback*	☐ ☐ ☐ ☐

Page 3

Table 2-8—Continued.

Contextual Modifiers

CONTEXTUAL DIMENSION	STANDARD APPROACH	CONTEXTUAL MODIFICATIONS [Therapist/ Client / Task]	OUTCOME Successful / Unsuccessful
(continued) 16. **Feedback Type:** The structuring of corrective verbal information that the client is given with which to respond to an instruction.		☐ Give private feedback: Corrective information in a confidential or private environment ☐ Give public feedback: Corrective information provided in a group view or community environment	Given: ☐ Private feedback ☐ ☐ Public feedback ☐
17. **Voice Tone Changes:** The modification of verbal tone used to address the client.	☐ Standard No modification in voice	☐ Use a therapy voice: formal therapeutic language ☐ Use a directive voice: inter-personally controlling, commanding ☐ Use a sympathetic voice: calm, confident, yet gentle ☐ Use a modulated voice: modified to increase understanding [i.e., slower, louder, shorter statements] or cooperation	Given: ☐ Formal tone ☐ ☐ Commanding tone ☐ ☐ Calm and gentle tone ☐ ☐ Modulated tone to increase understanding or cooperation ☐ ☐ Other ☐
18. **Medications:** Substances used to affect client's cognitive function.	☐ Standard No medications	Names ☐ _____ ☐ _____ ☐ _____ ☐ _____	Given: _____ medication ☐ _____ medication ☐ _____ medication ☐ _____ medication ☐
19. **Therapist's use of self:** The conscious use of personal strengths and interpersonal capacities.	☐ Standard No deliberate use of personal interventions	☐ Given expressive touch ☐ Use gentle humor ☐ Move closer to the client ☐ Actively listen to a client's concern ☐ Use encouraging words or gestures ☐ Give power of choice	Given: ☐ Expressive touch ☐ ☐ Gentle humor ☐ ☐ Proximity of the therapist ☐ ☐ Active listening ☐ ☐ Encouragement ☐ ☐ Choices/control ☐

From: Abreu, B.C. (1994). The Quadraphonic Approach: Evaluation and Treatment of the Brain Injured Patient. New York, NY: Therapeutic Service Systems.

Note : A Formula
Client's performance was successful in _____ when given _____ .
(Indicate the task / module)   (Indicate the contextual modifiers that helped)
Use of _____ did not help. Client's level of awareness of his or her problems was
(Indicate other modifiers used that were not successful)

_____ .
(State client 's level of awareness)

be further developed to frame a narrative that describes the task and the successful and unsuccessful modifications.

The contextual modifier tools are used to gather data that can be stored and analyzed through a variety of methods. Computer software, such as the Nonnumerical Unstructured Data Indexing, Searching, and Theorizing (Weitzman & Miles, 1995) can be used to analyze the qualitative data provided by the use of contextual modifiers (Scolari Sage Publications). The results can show which learning patterns and compensation techniques are best used for cognitive rehabilitation. A pilot study of these modifiers is underway at the Transitional Learning Community at Galveston, including the occupational therapy, physical therapy, and neuropsychology departments (Abreu, Peloquin, & Reed, 1997). A second pilot study is also being conducted at the same location, comparing the use of these modifiers in a virtual reality environment with a real life clinical environment (Christiansen, Abreu, & Huffman, 1996).

Post-Performance Phase

The post-performance phase is reflective and consists of an intense post-performance review of the training session. The review includes an evaluation of the training strategies used, the actions used to reinforce client confidence, and the client's and therapist's reactions to personal performance including mutual satisfaction or dissatisfaction, self-confidence, and goal readjustment. Examples of post-performance reflective questions are: What kind of reminders or help did you give Edgar? Was the type and amount of help provided to Edgar successful and satisfying for him and you?

Many of the contextual modifiers used are based on cognitive apprenticeship as well as information processing and teaching/learning techniques. These teaching-learning techniques focus on the qualitative analysis of both verbal and nonverbal instructions. One example, scaffolding, is used to refer to the guided learning techniques generated by the therapist/teacher to provide support in the form of cues, reminders, and other help necessary for the apprentice to perform an approximation of the training goal/task.

The therapist/teacher acts as a guide, shaping the learning and relearning efforts of the client with brain injury until the adjustable and temporary support is no longer needed. Many times, however, this support cannot be removed either because clients cannot generalize their training from clinic to environment or because they have not been able to achieve performance levels that are safe and do not require supervision. Self-efficacy judgments are decisions based on what people believe they can do in varied circumstances. A client's self-efficacy beliefs can change through occupational therapy interventions that offer direct mastery experiences and opportunities to make inferences from social comparisons, influences, and physiological states (Bandura, 1977). The post-performance phase of reflection includes inquiry into the effects of social learning during the occupational therapy.

Edgar's Case: Sample Interventions

Following is a brief discussion of three stages of Edgar's recovery with samples of treatment plans. For didactic purposes, the case of Edgar is a based on a composite of many cases I encountered over the years. Remember that the Quadraphonic Approach advocates that the therapist should act as a collaborator in treatment freely moving between the macro and micro perspectives.

Stage 1. The Coma Stage—Low Arousal.

Had it not been for recent medical advances, Edgar, like many other clients with head injury, might have died secondary to metabolic imbalance and/or secondary complications from urinary tract and respiratory infections (Bartkowski & Lovely, 1986; O'Dell & Riggs, 1996). In addition, medical technology now allows clients like Edgar to both survive and prosper. Medical practitioners involved with the rehabilitation of brain injury are faced with therapeutic and ethical challenges for those involved in their care (O'Dell, Jasin, Lyons, Stivers, & Meszaros, 1996; O'Dell & Riggs, 1996; Rosenberg & Ashwal, 1996).

Edgar is a 25-year-old traffic accident victim who was in coma for 1 week. He was recorded as Glascow scale (7) and and his multimodal evoked potential data were considered good predictors of his recovery and mortality (Bartkowski & Lovely, 1986; O'Dell & Riggs, 1996). During coma, Edgar lacked meaningful interaction with people and the environment; however, he showed sleep and wake rhythms (Shaw, 1986). His decerebrate motor reactions began to fade after seven days, and prehension, chewing, sucking, and postural adjustment reflexes began to emerge. He moved from coma to resumption of vegetative functions in 1 month entering a persistent vegetative state (PVS). In this new state, he was able to control his respiration, blood pressure, digestive, and excretory functions (Rappaport, 1986). During PVS the therapist and the other team members instructed Edgar's family and social support system to evaluate and track the length of arousal time, the presence of volitional versus coincidental movement, and the nature of the multimodal stimuli required to elicit appropriate responses. The family's participation in the treatment process provided Edgar's family with some opportunity for control and responsibility and for the expression of their love.

During PVS stage, the occupational therapist used both the macro and micro perspectives for rehabilitation. Tactile stimulation, so essential for the eliciting of arousal responses, became a form of expressive touch and part of the attempt to communicate with and encourage Edgar during this stage of his recovery. The therapist's verbal communication with Edgar, both words and interactions, reflected respect for and sensitivity to the image of Edgar that was constructed through interviews with Daisy. Family and friends also contributed through narratives, pictures, and visits to the intensive care unit. Time use is a constraint that can enhance occupational therapy practice at the coma level and throughout recovery (Christiansen, 1996; Kielhofner, 1977; Kielhofner, 1985; Neville, 1980; White, 1996). The therapist and the members of the coma rehabilitation team each made an attempt to simulate and facilitate the functioning of Edgar's internal time clock with cues related to external time.

While treating Edgar in the coma phase, the therapist would greet him a resounding "Good morning, Edgar," and a team member added the specific time of day such as "it's 7:00 a.m." or "it's 8:00 a.m." In addition, when greeting those other individuals who may also be present, the therapist used the same approach. Other external cues designed to help Edgar regulate his internal clock were putting the television or radio on with Edgar's favorite programs; reading the newspaper; and turning on the news or weather channels (White, 1996). Each of these actions aimed to influence Edgar's internal time clocks so that he could regain a sense of sleep-wake time or a rest-activity cycle (Christiansen, 1996). The internal time clocks such as the sleep-wake cycle, hormonal activity, and variations in blood pressure and body temperature as well as the external time clocks such as daylight, noise, and social rituals resemble the increase or decrease in social activity and interaction associated with the start and end of daily occupations (Christiansen, 1996).

The occupational therapist working with the allied health team and the family monitored, collected, analyzed, and reported the rate of Edgar's recovery in order to predict outcomes during this minimally responsive stage. The "minimally responsive state" should be differentiated from "coma." The minimally responsive patient demonstrates some evidence of consciousness while the patient in coma does not. At this stage, it is extremely important to monitor such changes precisely (Abreu, 1992 ; Giacino, Kezmarsky, DeLuca, & Cicerone, 1991a). A monitoring form was used to track daily changes in Edgar's responsiveness (see Table 2-9). This form was kept at Edgar's bedside in a binder. All team members were instructed in how to use the monitoring system and each team member was given a different-colored pencil with which to check and record observable responses. The occupational therapist summarized the findings daily and noted them in the medical record. The 24-hour monitoring chart proved effective and useful in revealing Edgar's individual pattern of arousal. Edgar showed progress in corneal reflexes, pupillary reactivity, oculomotor responses, and spontaneous eye opening (Giacino et al., 1991a). He also improved in the duration of time of his arousal, the presence of volitional versus coincidental movement, and a lessened degree of intensity of the multimodal stimuli required to elicit his responses.

Table 2-9

Quadrophonic Approach Evaluation System Behavioral Hourly Chart

Behavioral Hourly Chart   Occupational Therapy

Patient:	Handedness:
Date:	Lesion Site:
Age:	Education:
Dx:	Native Lang.:
Onset:	Therapist:

Period of Observation:
From: a.m./p.m.   To: a.m.p.m.   Observation Location:

Characteristics of   Behavior

Indicate whether each behavior was present, present = P or absent = A.

1a 2 3 4 5 6 7 8 9 10 11 12m 1 2 3 4 5 6 7 8 9 10 11 12m

1.
2.
3.
4.

1a 2 3 4 5 6 7 8 9 10 11 12m 1 2 3 4 5 6 7 8 9 10 11 12m

5.
6.
7.
8.
9.
10.

1a 2 3 4 5 6 7 8 9 10 11 12m 1 2 3 4 5 6 7 8 9 10 11 12m

11.
12.
13.
14.
15.
16.
17.

1a 2 3 4 5 6 7 8 9 10 11 12m 1 2 3 4 5 6 7 8 9 10 11 12m

18.
19.
20.

Test for Pupillary Constriction: 1) Darken the room to enlarge the pupils. 2) Shine the light from a small penlite directly into the pupil of the eye. 3) Note whether the pupil constricts briskly or sluggishly. 4) Repeat the procedure for the the other eye. 5) Shine the light into both eyes simultaneously so that the same amount of light reaches both. Turn the light on and off. 6) Note whether the two pupils dilate and constrict together and simultaneously, to the same degree. The chart above is a guide for determining pupil size.

From: Abreu, B. C. (1990). The Quadraphonic Approach: Evaluation and Treatment of the Brain Injured Patient. New York, NY: Therapeutic Service Systems.

A second tracking system based on the coma intervention program treatment procedures used at the JFK Johnson Rehabilitation Institute designed by Giacino and colleagues (1991a; 1991b; 1996) was also used with Edgar. This progress tracking chart can be used to record progress on a monthly basis. The baseline response relates to two commands chosen from a list of 10 (close eyes, move arm, move leg, move fingers, open mouth, look away from me, look at me, look up, look down, touch my hand) observed over four consecutive trials (estimated at 15, 30, 45, and 60 seconds) then translated into percentages.

In the process, every time a team member interacted with Edgar, he was oriented to the name of the team member, the time of day, the reason for the visit, and the protocol being used. Closing remarks were also provided at the end of the visit with statements indicating when the team member would see Edgar again. The team members changed the instructions given in order to distinguish whether Edgar's corresponding movements were voluntary or incidental. For example, "Edgar, move your right arm" was alternated with "Edgar, stop moving your right arm." All stimuli, whether tactile, visual, or auditory, were followed by ample processing time. Stimuli were also manipulated to allow for Edgar's maximally efficient manual exploration, visual location, and fixation.

The team was encouraged to systematically record Edgar's response 15 seconds after stimulation. They asked Edgar to use two different movements in communicating (i.e., one for "yes" and another for "no") rather than relying on the execution of a single movement. Arousal was measured by the wakefulness revealed by eye opening; attention was determined by the number of times Edgar responded each time a stimulus was presented. The stimulus was personalized by using symbolic items such as Daisy's perfume or an audiotaped message from his family and friends.

Stage 2. The Rehabilitation Stage

After emerging from coma, Edgar was ready for more dynamic interventions. Edgar's capacity for independent living, work, and leisure occupations was predictably limited by the sequelae of brain injury. This capacity was limited by impairments in attention, memory, capacity to learn, and postural control (Abreu, 1981; Abreu, 1995; Sohlberg & Mateer, 1989; Sunderland, Harris, & Gleave, 1984). These sequelae are treated clinically in two manners: retraining and compensation. Although the effectiveness or either technique has yet to be fully supported in the literature, both techniques are used in the clinic. Retraining programs involve the use of exercises, repetitive practice, or drills (Sohlberg & Mateer, 1989). Compensatory pro-

grams involve the use of externally and internally based rule-behaviors such as mnemonic devices, memory notebooks, and electronic watches (Harrell, Parente, Bellingrath, & Lisicia, 1992). Another example of compensation is the use of systematic training that specifies the establishment of routines and the development of procedural strategies or rule-based actions (Bewick, Raymond, Malia, & Bennett, 1995; Sohlberg & Mateer, 1989).

Edgar benefited from the use of these mechanistic organizational strategies. For example, an enlarged laminated instruction card placed near the equipment Edgar used served as a compensatory memory strategy. Enlarged simplified instructions were used in a very systematic manner. Edgar initially read the instructions aloud and, when questioned, answered why he was reading them aloud. Later, he was able to read instructions silently. Many times Edgar did not remember doing specific actions but he continued to perform accurately, in a timely manner, and safely while depending on cues.

Given his moderate memory loss, Edgar also used a compensatory memory notebook divided into sections that provided a rich repository of information to help reconstruct his life after brain injury. The notebook was divided into sections different from those more traditionally used (Sohlberg & Mateer, 1989) in cognitive rehabilitation. The sections reflected a more holistic and confluent approach to rehabilitation. They included the following: (1) "My story"—This section included photographs, pictures, and names with brief descriptions of family members, friends, pets, coworkers, favorite occupations and hobbies, and occupations and happy moments before the injury. (2) "My time use"—This section contained Edgar's schedule of therapies, meals, and to-do lists of more personal projects with their times and dates (a page that allowed reflection about time use was filled in weekly). (3) "My temporary support system"—This section included photographs and names with brief descriptions of therapists, doctors, nurses, dietician, and aides who worked with Edgar on a daily basis. The brief descriptions identified each person by role, function, and participation in Edgar's rehabilitation program. A page that allowed reflections about Edgar's satisfaction with services was filled in weekly. (4) "My private thoughts"—This section contained feelings, reactions, and responses that Edgar shared during his psychosocial support interventions with the psychologist. This section was shared with others only at Edgar's initiation, thus providing Edgar with a sense of privacy and control over self-disclosure.

For postural control issues Edgar engaged in a motor work-up program in occupational therapy. Edgar engaged in relaxation and breathing exercises for 10 minutes before starting the motor work-up module. The therapist performed these exercises with Edgar in a quiet room assigned for individual therapy. The therapist also engaged Edgar in neurodevelopmental and biomechanical maneuvers for the improvement of his more affected hemiparetic side, upper and lower extremities, and neck and trunk. The therapist started with the scapular and shoulder muscle and joint complex, as well as wrist and hand muscle and joint complex to free these of limitations and to establish a better balance between flexor and extensor muscles, adductors and abductors, and supinators and pronators. Weight shifting and weight bearing exercises for scapula, elbow, hand, hip, knee, and feet were also performed. The therapist used landmarks on Edgar's body prominences such as the inferior angle of the scapula and the superior anterior posterior iliac crest to visualize whether Edgar's body asymmetry improved after the manual maneuver. To monitor weight distribution bilaterally, the therapist used videotaping with reflectors and sensors taped on the joint, as well as T-foam (dense foam that registers bodily indentations) before and after the session. I noted that realigning Edgar's body using key points of control resulted in an increase in Edgar's symmetry, a disassociation of movements or an ability to move each individual body segment in isolation, improved joint mobility, and increased awareness.

After the motor work-up, Edgar chose tasks and occupations that he enjoyed so as to provide him with an opportunity to increase his endurance and coordination and control his posture. These activities were monitored with the goal of increasing his coordination in timed tasks from 10- to 7-second response rates in one week (a subskill goal). Another goal was for Edgar to engage in some of his favorite activities, carpentry and antiquing, within a 3 week period for a 2-hour standing session. Edgar's long-term goal for postural control was to be able to dance with Daisy within 8 weeks.

Some of Edgar's postural control issues were related to his mild attentional problems. While standing, Edgar was unable to attend to all aspects of the environment without missing information. Postural control demands were interfering with his attentional capacity and his strategy was to respond too quickly or slowly. He was taught to self-monitor and self-talk through the activity so that he could concentrate and maintain his focus while working on his tolerance for standing. Organizations and metacognitive strategies reflecting on person, task, and strategy were facilitated. Edgar was able to accomplish his goal and danced with Daisy at a friend's wedding.

Edgar had a general awareness about his strength and limitations. He was able to recognize and appraise the difficulties he was having as he did a task and when cued, but he was unable to foresee potential limitations secondary to his disability in the future.

Stage 3. The Community Reentry Stage

After receiving rehabilitation services in a hospital and after achieving medical stability, Edgar was discharged even though he had not reached his optimal potential. At this time he was admitted to a transitional living community. Many clients achieve maximum benefit from training and/or compensation strategies at such community reentry centers that bridge hospitals, nursing homes, and long-term centers with the community. The interventions that Edgar received in the acute hospital were limited by time constraints as well as by the nature of the rehab techniques that could be effieiently administered. Documentation indicated that Edgar had reached independence in basic personal management (ADL) and that although he improved in the use of self-mediated learning strategies, he was still unable to return home. Daisy was working full time as a teacher and she felt Edgar would not be safe at home alone.

Edgar previously worked as a high-salaried chemical engineer who supervised seven other engineers in a water purification plant. At the community reentry level, the focus is primarily on functional outcomes and, in Edgar's case, transition to the highest degree of independence using community-based services as well as community resources for medical needs was the goal. Daisy complained about Edgar's memory and reported problems with Edgar's getting lost. Edgar dismissed the memory issue claiming it was not that bad and saying, "I was forgetful before." Daisy was also concerned with changes in Edgar's social behaviors. Previously gregarious, Edgar now preferred to be only with her and discouraged visitors.

By the third month at the transitional center, Edgar and Daisy had both received extensive training in memory and compensatory strategies from the entire rehabilitation team. The memory book that he brought from the hospital was reduced in size and Daisy and Edgar were taught how to keep personal memory books that included a section called "my private thoughts." This section was set up differently from the one that Edgar had used in the hospital. The pages were divided in half. On one half, Edgar and Daisy were instructed to track positive and negative feelings experienced during the day. Once a week they were to each go back and analyze their logs, clustering the themes that emerged from their notes. They were both taught this process in order to increase their affective communication and increase their awareness of patterns of behavior that invited encouragement or compliments from their partner.

As noted earlier, Edgar could not attend to all aspects of a task or situation without missing information. Therefore, the kitchen at home was rearranged and reorganized with labels and pictures that made it easier for Edgar to recognize where utensils and food were located instead of having to use his memory. Many of the foods were kept in see-through containers or plastic bags rather than opaque containers for easier detection and recognition.

Edgar showed moderate impairment in free recall of visual and auditory information during short-term and long-term memory tasks. His performance improved when the task involved recognition and retrieval of auditory and visual information. In naturalistic environments Edgar performed more poorly. He got lost moving from building to building or office to office in the center. He did not seem to recognize the impact that this

impairment would have on his goal of returning to work. He stated, "I'll do better in my office. I have worked there for years." He showed low anticipatory awareness of his disability. I have seen a high degree of inaccuracy when individuals give personal accounts of their abilities to remember everyday items. Some clinicians question the reliability of self-report techniques because they correlate only minimally with performance on memory tests (Bennett-Levy, Polkey, & Powell, 1980; Sunderland, Harris & Gleave, 1984).

Edgar was unable to categorize information based on many characteristics. He was unable to understand jokes; he showed decreased empathy and reflection. His ability to reason deductively from general abstractions to specific rules of thumb, and to inductively go beyond the obvious or specific evidence, was also impaired (Johnson-Laird, 1995; Pellegrino, 1995).

Edgar brought some of his personal projects to occupational therapy treatment sessions and, with moderate assistance, completed several of these. He identified the type of work project that he was managing before the accident: purifying the water for a small city in Texas. Prior to the start of training, the internal case manager contacted Edgar's employer to verify Edgar's previous workload and responsibilities. At the transitional living center, the internal case manager monitors communication with employer, family, and external case managers (third-party payers). Edgar's employer supported the high degree of responsibility required of his position and this information was passed to the occupational therapist and the rest of the team by the case manager. Following two individual simulated work sessions, a situational assessment in Edgar's work place was performed. The results confirmed Edgar's dependency on external cues, mediation, and supervision. Edgar was unable to perform the work tasks that he did before the injury.

In addition to individual therapy sessions Edgar engaged in group interventions. One of the interventions was the "relax and have fun" group. The group was given this name by former clients because they found that it helped them relax and have fun during evenings and weekends when therapy schedules addressed leisure and recreational activities. As its central focus, the group planned two or three community outings each week. Edgar's participation and behaviors were evaluated and documented according to the skills required to plan and enact the "rest and fun" activities. Edgar took great pleasure in planning and participating in fishing and sailing outings.

Clients at transitional centers are given opportunities to participate in community rituals including an induction ceremony and a graduation ceremony. Edgar participated in both. The induction ceremony was performed by the clients with staff guidance as needed so as to identify and support the individual goals of each new client. Such a ritual fosters solidarity among the clients and the rehab team. The graduation ceremony celebrates the achievement of the clients when they are ready for community reentry.

Graduation was a very powerful and emotional treatment tool for Edgar, Daisy, and the rehabilitation community as a whole. This ritualized social encounter gave increased meaning and legitimacy to the completion of his rehabilitation experience (Crepeau, 1995). The graduation ceremony also represented Edgar's reclamation of membership in the community at large rather than a sustained membership in a group of clients living an "underlife" in an institution of care. Edgar regained his status as husband, lover, and friend, and found employment with his company in a different capacity.

Following is a review of quantitative and qualitative methodologies and an examination of selected pilot studies presented to support some of the postulates of the Quadraphonic Approach.

Scientific Inquiry

Science is the systematized knowledge of nature and the physical world. Chalmers (1990) describes science as having both cognitive and social dimensions. The cognitive dimension refers to the system of methods and procedures of investigation used to generate knowledge. The social dimension relates to the scientific community's political influence in the promotion of science (Chalmers, 1990; Zemke & Clark, 1996b).

Occupational therapists as well as occupational scientists use systematic methods of investigation to expand and/or generate new knowledge and test applications in practice through extrapolation from theories and empirical data (Mosey, 1989; 1992; Zemke, 1989; Zemke & Clark, 1996a; Zemke & Clark, 1996b). All scientific inquiry includes logical reasoning, speculation, and interpretation. There are two types of scientific inquiry: (1) basic, which is concerned with the development of theories in cognition, and (2) applied, which relates to frames of references and practical guidelines in cognitive rehabilitation. Both types of scientific inquiry reflect the political bias of the therapist/scientist who is investigating and the community that accepts and promotes the findings (Clark, Zemke, Frank, Parham, Neville-Jan, Hedricks, Carson, Fazio, & Abreu, 1993; Mosey, 1993). With this biased perspective in mind, I advocate the need for critical thinking and for logical and creative scientific inquiry that will reshape cognitive rehabilitation for a holistic practice.

Scientific inquiry in cognitive rehabilitation includes the capacity for reflection that comes from the realm of ideation and imagination with a focus on the nature of the person and his or her dynamic and symbolic interactions. I believe that therapists need to focus on the nature of persons and the manner through which they derive meaning from the world in order to enhance cognitive rehabilitation techniques.

Qualitative Findings and Implications for a Holistic Practice

Qualitative research is a type of scientific inquiry, also known as naturalistic or interpretative, that includes a variety of social research methods such as ethnography, phenomenology, and grounded theory (Hasselkus, 1995; Krefting, 1991). Such research methods are used in the macro perspective of cognitive rehabilitation.

The purpose of ethnography is to examine people from another culture or subculture, relying on participant or client observation (Atkinson & Hammersley, 1994). Phenomenology is a type of qualitative research design used to examine what it is like to have a particular experience and belong to a given social order relying on participant descriptions and interpretations (Holstein & Gubrium, 1994). Grounded theory is the general qualitative methodology used to develop and construct social theory using inductive reasoning (Strauss & Corbin, 1994). Grounded theories are used to describe and explain changes in the patterns of actions, interactions, and relationships that occur among the phenomena under study. I propose the use of these three methodoligies as a requirement for education, practice, and research in cognitive rehabilitation.

The major assumptions of therapists and researchers using qualitative methodologies are that (1) as researchers they have a bias, (2) they are nonauthorative because they have not experienced brain injury, and (3) they are a politically loaded observer because they advocate or support a particular type of therapy (Bruner, 1993; Spencer, Krefting, & Mattingly, 1993). In qualitative research, conceptual understanding is pluralistic, open to a variety of interpretations, and shaped by the perspective of the researcher (Bruner, 1993). This is important to remember when comparing methodologies. All research studies reflect the beliefs, assumptions, and purposes of the researcher (Hasselkus, 1995).

Qualitative methodologies enable us to examine the social interdependence that exists between individuals and their families, communities, ethnic traditions, and national cultures (Frank, 1996; Kielhofner, 1982). Occupational therapists and occupational scientists must look carefully at the individual patterns of occupational selection and orchestration beyond a client-centered perspective (Frank, 1996). In addition, researchers using qualitative methodologies can study occupational habits, perseverance, engrossment, flow, and termination (Carlson, 1996) to understand cognitive rehabilitation from a macro perspective beyond the narrow confines of a cognitive framework.

Some researchers have explored the experiences of therapists who treat individuals with brain injury. Abreu (1990) studied the interaction of one occupational therapist with two clients, one post stroke and one head injury. The study was conducted in a cognitive rehabilitation setting for a period of three months. Four major themes emerged from the interaction of the therapist with the clients. (1) There were communication differences depending on the diagnosis, with the therapist interacting more dynamically with a young male client with head injury than with an older female who had had a stroke. (2) The therapist saw both clients as having little cognitive and physical control or personal power. (3) The cognitive rehabilitation specialty is draining. (4) The physical therapist's role in cognitive rehabilitation seems much more easily described and understood than that of the occupational therapist.

A second qualitative study, by Allison & Strong (1994), supported the complexity and personalization of verbal strategies required for effective rehabilitation. The researchers discovered four major categories of verbal strategies used by the therapist in their interaction with the client: therapy voice, modified information, directive voice, and sympathetic voice. A third study, by Crepeau (1993), explored the interactions within interdisciplinary team meetings and interpreted these interactions as reflecting two major strategies: (1) a ritualistic identification of images that signified the development of a collective health care identity, and (2) the construction of acts aimed to understand the client and achieve consensus.

Krefting (1989) explored and interpreted the client's coping with loss of self-identity through concealment strategies such as describing oneself as being the silent versus the talkative type rather than openly declaring difficulty participating in a conversation. In addition, she reinterpreted lack of awareness of disability as a "blind spot." She stated that the concept of a blind spot was less reductionistic than a lack of awareness. Schwartzberg (1994) researched high-level brain-injured clients participating in self-help groups and discovered that this therapeutic intervention helped in the legitimization of the experience of brain injury. Clark (1993) used narrative analysis to explore direct clinical practice with an individual post stroke by:

- reconstructing childhood occupations
- storytelling
- interpreting acute rehabilitation as a right of passage that moved a person from identity to abandonment

- using storymaking
- facilitating occupational storytelling.

This is an example of an occupational therapy practice embedded in real life. All of these qualitative studies demonstrate the contribution that interpretative analysis can make in cognitive rehabilitation.

Quantitative Findings and Implications for Holistic Practice

Quantitative methodologies is a second type of scientific inquiry that encompasses a variety of research approaches including experimental, evaluative, heuristic, correlational, survey, historical, and others (Stein, 1989). Such methodologies enable therapists to examine cognitive rehabilitation in order to develop new theories and to apply them to clinical practice. Quantitative research involves the enumeration of data on individuals, phenomena, or units being studied. Limited quantitative research on the efficacy of cognitive rehabilitation has been conducted but needs further development. The heterogenity of brain injury and the complexity of cognitive rehabilitation limit the ability of researchers to evaluate comprehensive frames of reference. Only portions of a particular frame of reference can be assessed to support adequacy or efficacy (Mosey, 1992).

I conducted several pilot studies using attention tests to investigate the behaviors of brain-injured clients. One study used eye fixation to study attention to static stimuli. Fixation is the ability to maintain the center of vision or fovea. In the eye fixation test, the client was asked to fixate on a penlight for 20 seconds. The results were that many clients with low cognitive levels were unable to fixate for more than 10 seconds. In a second pilot study, I examined the performance effect in clients with stroke or brain tumor in an acute rehabilitation unit by having them repeat the same paper-pencil task three consecutive times. This task required that clients cancel 60 targets in a field of 300 stimuli. The targets were equally divided and distributed in four quadrants so that each quadrant had a total of 15 targets. Each cancellation task varied

one surface characteristic. The target and stimulus field first consisted of numbers, then letters, and finally shapes. The results showed that there were differences in the speed of response and accuracy depending on their diagnoses. Clients with stroke tended to show a performance effect of increasing accuracy and speed. On the other hand, clients with brain tumor diagnosis tended to show a decreasing accuracy and speed (Abreu, 1992).

In a third study, I evaluated 15 children with severe learning disabilities. A fixation test and a visual scanning test were administered. The results of the fixation test showed that the majority of the children who could not read were able to fixate only for 3 seconds. The results of the scanning test showed that, for all of the children, performance was inconsistent and severe impairment in accuracy, speed, and organizational strategy was present.

Using a modified Stroop test, I examined the performance of a variety of clients with brain injury and found that some of those with speech and language impairments could not understand the test instructions. The clients who could comprehend the instructions were given the test. One of the performance components evaluated using this method was self-correction. Low-level cognitive clients were unable to self-correct while higher-level clients could correct. The ability to self-correct has been proposed as a possible predictor of functional outcomes.

I also coordinated two quality improvement projects related to awareness of disability among clients with head injury. In the first project, the therapists asked the clients if they had any problems with self-care, money management, and menu planning. Then the clients were asked the same question while an actual problem was occurring. Finally, the clients were asked if these problems were going to have an effect on their life after community reentry. The answers were compared with the therapists' observations and the findings were that

- The clients all agreed that they had problems with self-care, money management, and menu planning.
- They showed decreased awareness of disability even while problems were occurring.

■ Most of the clients did not think that these problems were going to have a substantial effect on their real life performance, which resulted in an overestimation of ability.

I observed that many clients who have suffered a stroke or head injury have selective awareness of their disabilities. They are aware of specific deficits such as being unable to walk or speak in the same manner as they did before the injury, but they are not aware of memory or money management problems. The lack of anticipatory awareness is a good predictor for the level of supervison required for community reentry because compensatory strategies require that the client recognize that there is a problem with functional performance.

In addition, I conducted a study on the effects of spatial and temporal parameters of a reaching task on postural control after stroke (Abreu, 1995). Spatial parameters included the position and direction of a task; temporal parameters included the time, sequencing, and chronology of action. The degree of variability of these parameters determined the degree of predictability of the environmental regulator. Therapists believe that tasks and activities used in cognitive-perceptual training should go from simple to complex, starting in a predictable environment and proceeding to an unpredictable environment. The findings of this study were that there was greater postural control stability when completing a reaching tasks in an unpredictable, multicontext, or variable environment in both the anterior-posterior and medial-lateral planes as opposed to the same reaching task conducted in a predictable, fixed environment. I concluded that training should include the concurrent use of both predictable and unpredictable conditions rather than using them sequentially (Abreu, 1995).

The quantitative studies summarized in this section highlight some of the subskills evaluated from the micro perspective. Integration of these methods with qualitative methods will yield a holistic practice. This will require a team approach in a family and community-centered cognitive rehabilitation model. The focus of cognitive rehabilitation is undergoing a paradigm shift from teaching to learning in much the same way as education (Barr & Tagg, 1995). I propose that occupational therapist should incorporate the affective domain, intuition, and inspirational variables based on culture and individual differences.

Conclusion

In the Quadraphonic Approach, I attempt to integrate macro and micro rehabilitation perspectives because this dual system reflects the recognition of the complexity of human occupation and cognitive impairment. The influence of the affective domain has been a factor in the development of the Quadraphonic Approach since its inception but has only been recently delineated.

Acknowledgment

To Suzanne M. Peloquin, PhD, OTR, for her numerous writings and help as a resource person offering inspiration for confluent practice. To Dr. Brent Masel and the Moody Foundation for their support of this work, and Jane Keel for assisting with this project. This chapter is based on The Quadraphonic Approach workshops formatted here in condensed form. Portions of the microperspective appeared in Lesson 8 in the 12-lesson AOTA Self-Study Series: *Cognitive Rehabilitation.*

References

Abreu, B. C. (1981). Interdisciplinary approach to adult visual perceptual function: Dysfunction continuum. In B. C. Abreu (Ed.), *Physical disabilities manual.* New York: Raven Press.

Abreu, B. C. (1990). *The quadraphonic approach: Management of cognitive and postural dysfunction.* New York: Therapeutic Service Systems.

Abreu, B. C. (1992). The quadraphonic approach: Management of cognitive-perceptual and postural control dysfunction. *Occupational Therapy Practice, 3*(4), 12–29.

Abreu, B. C. (1994). Perceptual motor skills. In C. B. Royeen, *AOTA self-study series: Cognitive rehabilitation.* Bethesda, MD: American Occupational Therapy Association.

Abreu, B. C. (1995). The effect of environmental regulations on postural control after stroke. *American Journal of Occupational Therapy, 49,* 517–525.

Abreu, B. C., & Hinojosa, J. (1992). Process approach for cognitive-perceptual and postural control dysfunction for adults with brain injury. In N. Katz (Ed.), *Cognitive rehabilitation: Models for intervention in occupational therapy.* Stoneham, MA: Butterworth-Heinemann.

Abreu, B., Peloquin, S., Reed, K. (1997). Contextual modifications: Cognitive rehabilitation and occupational therapy education. The American Occupational Therapy Annual Conference. April 13, Orlando, Florida.

Abreu, B., & Price-Lackey, P. (1994). Documentation and additional considerations. In C. B. Royeen (Ed.), *AOTA self-study series: Cognitive rehabilitation.* Bethesda, MD: American Occupational Therapy Association.

Abreu, B. C., Seale, G., Podlesak, J., & Hartley, L. (1996). Development of critical paths for postacute brain injury rehabilitation: Lesson learned. *American Journal of Occupational Therapy, 50,* 417–427.

Abreu, B. C., & Toglia, J. P. (1987). Cognitive rehabilitation: An occupational therapy model. *American Journal of Occupational Therapy, 41,* 439–448.

Allison, H., & Strong, J. (1994). Verbal strategies used by occupational therapists in direct client encounters. *Occupational Therapy Journal of Research, 14* (2), 112–129.

Atkinson, P., & Hammersley, M. (1994). Ethnography and paticipant observation. In N. K. Denzin & Y. S. Lincoln (Eds.), *Handbook of qualitative research.* California: Sage.

Bandura, A. (1977). Self-efficacy: Toward a unifying theory of behavioral change. *Psychological Review, 84* (2), 191–215.

Barr, R. B., & Tagg, J. (1995). From teaching to learning— A new paradigm for undergraduate education. *Change,* 13–25.

Bartkowski, H. M., & Lovely, M. P. (1986). Prognosis in coma and the persistent vegetative state. *Head Trauma Rehabilitation, 1* (1), 1–5.

Bateson, M. C. (Ed.). (1989). *Composing a life.* New York: Atlantic Monthly Press.

Bennett-Levy, J., Polkey, C. E., & Powell, G. E. (1980). Self-report of memory skills after temporal lobectomy: The effect of clinical variables. *Cortex, 15,* 543–557.

Berry, D. C. (1983). Metacognitive experience and transfer of logical reasoning. *Quarterly Journal of Experimental Psychology, 35A,* 39–49.

Bewick, K. C., Raymond, M. J., Malia, K. B., & Bennett, T. L. (1995). Metacognition as the ultimate executive: Techniques and tasks to facilitate executive functions. *Neuro-Rehabilitation, 5,* 367–375.

Blackmer, E. R., & Mitton, J. L. (1991). Theories of monitoring and the timing of repairs in spontaneous speech. *Cognition, 39,* 173–194.

Bottcher, S. A. (1989). Cognitive retraining: A nursing approach to rehabilitation of the brain injured. *Nursing Clinics of North America, 24,* 193–208.

Braun, C. M., Baribeau, J. M., Ethier, M., Daigneault, S., & Proulx, R. (1989). Processing of pragmatic and facial affective information by patients with closed-head injuries. *Brain Injury, 3* (1), 5–17.

Bridge, C., & Twible, R. (1997). Clinical reasoning. In C. Christiansen, & C. Baum (Eds.). *Occupational therapy: Enabling function and well-being.* Thorofare, NJ: Slack.

Brown, A. (1987). Metacognition, executive control, self-regulation, and other more mysterious mechanisms. In F. E. Weinert & R. H. Kluwe (Eds.), *Metacognition, motivation, and understanding.* Hillsdale, NJ: Erlbaum.

Brown, A. (1988). Motivation to learn and understand: On taking charge of one's own learning. *Cognition and Instruction, 5,* 311–321.

Brown, A. L. (1978). Knowing when, where, and how to remember: A problem of metacognition. In R. Glaser (Ed.), *Advances in instructional psychology* (Vol. 1). Hillsdale, NJ: Erlbaum.

Brown, A. L., & Palincsar, A. S. (1989). Guided, cooperative learning and individual knowledge acquisition. In L. B. Resnick (Ed.), *Knowing, learning and instruction: Essays in honor of Robert Glaser.* Hillsdale, NJ: Erlbaum.

Brown, G. (1971). *Human teaching for human learning.* New York: Viking.

Bruner, E. M. (1993). Introduction: The ethnographic self and the personal self. In P. Benson (Ed.), *Anthropology and literature.* Urbana: University of Illinois Press.

Carlson, M. (1996). The self-perpetuation of occupations. In R. Zemke & F. Clark (Eds.), *Occupational science: The evolving discipline.* Philadelphia: Davis.

Chalmers, A. F. (1990). *Science and its fabrication.* Minneapolis: University of Minneapolis Press.

Chi, M. T. H., & Bassok, M. (1989). Learning from examples via self-explanations. In L. B. Resnick (Ed.), *Knowing, learning, and instruction: Essays in honor of Robert Glaser.* Hillsdale, NJ: Erlbaum.

Chi, M. T. H., & Glaser, R. (1985). Problem-solving ability. In R. J. Sternberg (Ed.), *Human abilities—an information-processing approach.* New York: Freeman.

Chi, M. T. H., Glaser, R., & Rees, E. (1982). Expertise in problem solving. In R. Sternberg (Ed.), *Advances in psychology of human intelligence* (Vol. 1.) Hillsdale, NJ: Erlbaum.

Chi, M. T. H., Leeuw, N. D., Chiu, M. H., & LaVancher, C. (1994). Eliciting self-explanations improves understanding. *Cognitive Science, 18,* 439–477.

Christiansen, C. H. (1996). Three perspectives on balance in occupation. In R. Zemke & F. Clark (Eds.), *Occupational science—The evolving discipline.* Philadelphia: Davis.

Christiansen, C., Abreu, B. C., & Huffman, K. (1996). Creating a virtual environment for brain injury rehabilitation and research a preliminary report. *Journal of Medicine and Virtual Reality,* 6–9.

Clark, F. (1993). Occupation embedded in a real life: Interweaving occupational science and occupational therapy. Eleanor Clark Slagle Lecture. *American Journal of Occupational Therapy, 47,* 1067–1078.

Clark, F., Ennevor, B. L., & Richardson, P. L. (1996). A grounded theory of techniques for occupational storytelling and occupational storymaking. In R. Zemke & F. Clark (Eds.), *Occupational science—The evolving discipline*. Philadelphia: Davis.

Clark, F., Zemke, R., Frank, G., Parham, D., Neville-Jan, A., Hedricks, C., Carson, M., Fazio, L., & Abreu, B. (1993). The issue is—Dangers inherent in the partition of occupational therapy and occupational science. *American Journal of Occupational Therapy, 47*, 184–186.

Coelho, C. A., Liles, B. Z., & Duffy, R. J. (1991). Discourse analyses with closed head injured adults: Evidence for differing patterns of deficits. *Archives of Physical Medicine and Rehabilitation, 72*, 465–468.

Corbin, J. M., & Strauss, A. (1988). *Unending work and care: Managing chronic illness at home*. San Francisco: Jossey-Bass.

Crepeau, E. B. (1993). Three images of interdisciplinary team meetings. *American Journal of Occupational Therapy, 48* (8), 717–722.

Crepeau, E. B. (1995). The practice of the future: Putting occupation back into therapy. In C. B. Royeen (Ed.), *AOTA self-study series: Rituals*. Bethesda, MD: American Occupational Therapy Association.

Crosson, B., Barco, P. P., Velozo, C. A., Bolesta, M. M., Cooper, P. V., Werts, D., & Brobeck, T. C. (1989). Awareness and compensation in postacute head injury rehabilitation. *Journal of Head Trauma Rehabilitation, 4* (3), 46–54.

Dabbs, J. M., Evans, M. S., Hopper, C. H., & Purvis, J. A. (1980). Self-monitors in conversation: What do they monitor? *Journal of Personality and Social Psychology, 39* (2), 278–284.

Diller, L. (1993). Introduction to cognitive rehabilitation. In C. B. Royeen (Ed.), *AOTA self-study series: Cognitive rehabilitation*. Bethesda, MD: American Occupational Therapy Association.

Dreyfus, H., & Dreyfus, S. (Eds.). (1986). *Mind over machine*. New York: Free Press.

Druckman, D., & Bjork, R. A. (Eds.). (1991). *In the mind's eye: Enhancing human performance*. Washington, DC: National Academy Press.

Druckman, D., & Bjork, R. A. (Eds.). (1994). *Learning, remembering, believing: Enhancing human performance*. Washington, DC: National Academy Press.

Duchek, J. M., & Abreu, B. C. (1997). Meeting the challenges of cognitive disabilities. In C. Christiansen & C. Baum (Eds.), *Occupational therapy: Enabling function and well-being*. Thorofare, NJ: Slack.

Fitts, P. M., & Posner, M. I. (1967). *Human performance*. Belmont, CA: Brooks/Cole.

Flavell, J. H. (1979). Metacognition and cognitive monitoring: A new area of cognitive-developmental inquiry. *American Psychologist, 34*, 906–911.

Flavell, J. H. (1985). *Cognitive development*. Englewood Cliffs, NJ: Prentice-Hall.

Flavell, J. H. (1987). Speculations about the nature and development of metacognition. In F. E. Weinert & R. H. Kluwe (Eds.), *Metacognition, motivation and understanding*. Hillsdale, NJ: Erlbaum.

Fleming, M. H. (1991). The therapist with the three-track mind. *American Journal of Occupational Therapy, 45*, 1007–1014.

Frank, G. (1996). Life histories in occupational therapy clinical practice. *American Journal of Occupational Therapy, 50*, 251–254.

Gagne, R. M., & Smith, E. C. (1962). A study of the effects of verbalization on problem solving. *Journal of Experimental Psychology, 63* (1), 12–18.

Gasquoine, P. G. (1992). Affective state and awareness of sensory and cognitive effects after closed head injury. *Neuropsychology, 6* (3), 187–196.

Gentile, A. M. (1987). Skill acquisition: Action, movement, and neuromotor processes. In J. H. Carr, R. B. Shepherd, J. Gordon, A. M. Gentile, & J. M. Held (Eds.), *Movement science foundations for physical therapy in rehabilitation*. Rockville, MD: Aspen.

Giacino, J. T. (1996). Sensory stimulation: Theoretical perspectives and the evidence for effectiveness. *Neurorehabilitation, 6*, 69–78.

Giacino, J. T., Kezmarsky, M. A., DeLuca, J., & Cicerone, K. D. (1991a). Monitoring rate of recovery to predict outcome in minimally responsive patients. *Archives of Physical Medicine and Rehabilitation, 72*, 897–900.

Giacino, J. T., Sharlow-Galella, M., Kezmarsky, M. A., McKenna, K., Nelson, P., King, M., Brown, A. C., & Cicerone, K. D. (1991b). *JFK coma recovery scale and coma intervention program treatment procedures*. Edison, NJ: JFK Medical Center.

Gibson, J. J. (1979). *The ecological approach to visual perception*. Boston: Houghton Mifflin.

Gianutsos, R., & Matheson, P. (1987). The rehabilitation of visual perceptual disorders attributable to brain injury. In Meier, M. J., Benton, A. L., & Diller, L. (Eds.), *Neuropsychological Rehabilitation*. New York: Guilford Press.

Glaser, R., & Chi, M. T. H. (1988). Overview. In M. T. H. Chi, R. Glaser, & M. J. Farr (Eds.), *The nature of expertise*. Hillsdale, NJ: Erlbaum.

Harrell, M., Parente, F., Bellingrath, E., & Lisicia, K. (1992). *Cognitive rehabilitation of memory: A practical guide*. Gaithersberg, MD: Aspen.

Hartley, L. L. (1995). *Cognitive-communicative abilities following brain injury: A functional approach*. San Diego: Singular.

Hartley, L. L., & Jensen, P. J. (1992). Three discourse profiles of closed-head-injury speakers: Theoretical and clinical implications. *Brain Injury, 6* (3), 271–282.

Hasselkus, B. R. (1995). Beyond ethnography: Expanding our understanding and criteria for qualitative research. *Occupational Therapy Journal of Research, 15* (2), 75–84.

Herzberg, S. R. (1990). Client or patient: Which term is more appropriate for use in occupational therapy? *American Journal of Occupational Therapy, 44,* 561–565.

Holstein, J. A., & Gubrium, J. F. (1994). Phenomenology, ethnomethodology, and interpretive practice. In N. K. Denzin & Y. S. Lincoln (Eds.), *Handbook of qualitative research* (pp. 262–272). California: Sage.

Holstein, J. A., & Gubrium, J. F. (1995). *The active interview.* (Qualitative Research Methods Series 37) Thousand Oaks, CA: Sage Publications.

Holyoke, P., & Elkan, L. (1995). *Rehabilitation services inventory and quality.* Toronto: Institute for Work and Health.

Jacobs, H. E. (1993). *Behavior analysis guidelines and brain injury rehabilitation: People, principles, and programs.* Gaithersburg, MD: Aspen.

Johnson-Laird, P. N. (1995). Deductive reasoning ability. In R. Sternberg (Ed.), *Human abilities: An information-processing approach.* New York: Freeman.

Josselson, R., & Lieblich, A. (Eds.). (1995). *Interpreting experience: The narrative study of lives* (Vol. 3). Thousand Oaks, CA: Sage.

Katz, N. (Ed.). (1992). *Cognitive rehabilitation: Models for intervention in occupational therapy.* Stoneham, MA: Butterworth-Heinemann.

Kielhofner, G. (1977). Temporal adaptation: A conceptual framework for occupational therapy. *American Journal of Occupational Therapy, 31,* 238.

Kielhofner, G. (1982). Qualitative research. Part 2: Methodological approaches and relevance to occupational therapy. *Occupational Therapy Journal of Research, 2,* 150–164.

Kielhofner, G. (1985). *A model of human occupation.* Baltimore: Williams & Wilkins.

Klatzy, K. (1980). *Human memory: Structure and processes.* San Francisco: Freeman.

Kluwe, R. H. (1987). Executive decisions and regulation of problem solving behavior. In F. E. Weinert & R. H. Kluwe (Eds.), *Metacognition, motivation, and understanding.* Hillsdale, NJ: Erlbaum.

Koegel, L. K., Koegle, R. L., & Ingham, J. C. (1986). Programming rapid generalization of correct articulation through self-monitoring procedures. *Journal of Speech and Hearing Disorders, 51,* 24–32.

Krefting, L. M. (1989). Reintegration into the community after head injury: The results of an ethnographic study. *Occupational Therapy Journal of Research, 9,* 67–83.

Krefting, L. M. (1991). Rigor in qualitative research: The assessment of trustworthiness. *American Journal of Occupational Therapy, 45* (3), 214–222.

Krefting, L., & Krefting, D. (1990). Leisure activities after a stroke: An ethnographic approach. *American Journal of Occupational Therapy, 45* (5), 429–436.

Krinsky, R. (1990). The visionary world of Beatriz Abreu. *Advance, 6* (11), 7, 13.

Lampert, J., & Lapolice, D. J. (1995). Functional considerations in evaluation and treatment of the client with low vision. *American Journal of Occupational Therapy, 49,* 885–890.

Lee, W. A. (1989). A control systems framework for understanding normal and abnormal posture. *American Journal of Occupational Therapy, 43,* 291–301.

Lezak, M. D. (1983). *Neuropsychological assessment.* New York: Oxford Unversity Press.

Light, K. E. (1990). Information processing for motor performance in aging adults. *Physical Therapy, 10,* 820–826.

Luria, A. R. (1973). *The working brain.* New York: Basic Books.

Mattingly, C., & Fleming, M. H. (1993). *Clinical reasoning: Forms of inquiry in a therapeutic practice.* Philadelphia: Davis.

McColl, M. A. (1994). Holistic occupational therapy: Historical meaning and contemporary implications. *Canadian Journal of Occupational Therapy, 61* (2), 72–77.

McColl, M. A., Gerein, N., & Valentine, F. (1997). Occupational therapy: Meeting the challenges of disability. In C. Christiansen & C. Baum (Eds.), *Occupational therapy: Enabling function and well-being.* Thorofare, NJ: Slack.

McColl, M. A., Law, M., & Stewart, D. (1993). *Theoretical basis of occupational therapy: An annotated bibliography.* Thorofare, NJ: Slack.

Miller, R. (1992). Introducing holistic education: The historical and pedagogical context of the 1990 Chicago Statement. *Teacher Education Quarterly, 19* (1), 5–13.

Mosey, A. C. (1986). *Psychosocial components of occupational therapy.* New York: Raven Press.

Mosey, A. C. (1989). Editorial: The proper focus of scientific inquiry in occupational therapy: Frames of reference. *Occupational Therapy Journal of Research, 9* (4), 195–201.

Mosey, A. C. (1992). *Applied scientific inquiry in the health professions: An epistemological orientation.* Bethesda, MD: American Occupational Therapy Association.

Mosey, A. C. (1993). Partition of occupational science and occupational therapy: Sorting out some issues. *American Journal of Occupational Therapy, 47* (8), 751–754.

Nachmanovitch, S. (1990). *Free play: The power of improvisation in life and the arts.* New York: Putnam.

Nashner, L. (1982). Adaption of human movement to altered environments. *Trends in Neuroscience, 5,* 358–366.

Neistadt, M. E. (1992). The classroom as clinic: Applications for a method of teaching clinical reasoning. *American Journal of Occupational Therapy, 46,* 814–817.

Nelson, D. L. (1987). Occupational: Form and performance. *American Journal of Occupational Therapy, 42,* 633–641.

Neville, A. (1980). Temporal adaptation: Application with short term psychiatric patients. *American Journal of Occupational Therapy, 34,* 328.

Newton, R. A. (1995). Balance abilities in individuals with moderate and severe traumatic brain injury. *Brain Injury, 9* (5), 445–451.

Norman, D. A. (1969). *Memory and attention: An introduction to human information processing.* New York: Wiley.

Norman, D. A. (1979). Perception, memory and mental processes. In L. Nilsson (Ed.), *Perspectives on memory research.* Hillsdale, NJ: Erbaum.

O'Dell, M. W., Jasin P., Lyons, N., Stivers, M., & Meszaros, F. (1996). Standardized assessment instruments for minimally-responsive, brain-injured patients. *Neurorehabilitation, 6,* 45–55.

O'Dell, M. W., & Riggs, R. V. (1996). Management of the minimally responsive patient. In L. J. Horn & N. D. Zasler (Eds.), *Medical rehabilitation of traumatic brain injury.* Philadelphia: Hanley & Belfus.

Ottenbacher, K., & Christiansen, C. (1997). Occupational performance assessment. In C. Christiansen, & C. Baum (Eds.), *Occupational therapy: Enabling function and well-being.* Thorofare, NJ: Slack.

Paris, S. G., & Winograd, P. (1990). How metacognition can promote academic learning and instruction. In B. F. Jones & L. Idol (Eds.), *Dimensions of thinking and cognitive instruction.* Hillsdale, NJ: Erlbaum.

Parham, L. D. (1987). Toward professionalism: The reflective therapist. *American Journal of Occupational Therapy, 41,* 555–561.

Patterson, J. B., & Marks, C. (1992). The client as customer: Achieving service quality and customer satisfaction in rehabilitation. *Journal of Rehabilitation, 58* (4), 16–20.

Pellegrino, J. W. (1995). Inductive reasoning ability. In R. J. Sternberg (Ed.), *Human abilities: An information-processing approach* (pp. 195–225). New York: W. H. Freeman.

Peloquin, S. M. (1990a). Helping through touch: The embodiment of caring. *Journal of Religion and Health, 28* (4)and also reprinted in *Hakomi Forum,* 299–322.

Peloquin, S. M. (1990b). The patient therapist relationship in occupational therapy: Understanding visions and images. *American Journal of Occupational Therapy, 44,* 13–21.

Peloquin, S. M. (1993a). Beliefs that shape care: Reflections from narratives. *American Journal of Occupational Therapy, 47,* 935–942.

Peloquin, S. M. (1993b). The depersonalization of patients: A profile gleaned from narratives. *American Journal of Occupational Therapy, 47,* 830–837.

Peloquin, S. M. (1995). The fullness of empathy: Reflections and illustrations. *American Journal of Occupational Therapy, 49,* 24–31.

Peloquin, S. M. (1996). Using the arts to enhance confluent learning. *American Journal of Occupational Therapy, 50,* 148–151.

Pierce, D., & Frank, G. (1992). A mother's work: Two levels of feminist analysis of family-centered care. *American Journal of Occupational Therapy, 46,* 972–980.

Polkinghorne, D. E. (1988). *Narrative knowing and the human sciences.* Albany: State University of New York Press.

Pollock, N. (1993). Client-centered assessment. *American Journal of Occupational Therapy, 47,* 298–301.

Posner, M. I. (1988). Introduction: What is it to be an expert? In M. T. H. Chi, R. Glaser, & M. J. Farr (Eds.), The nature of expertise. Hillsdale, NJ: Erlbaum.

Prigatano, G. P., Altman, I. M., & O'Brien, K. P. (1990). Behavioral limitations that traumatic-brain-injured patients tend to underestimate. *Clinical Neuropsychologist, 4* (2), 163–176.

Psathas, G. (1995). *Conversation analysis: The study of talk-in-interaction.* Thousand Oaks, CA: Sage.

Rappaport, M. (1986). Brain evoked potentials in coma and the vegetative state. *Head Trauma Rehabilitation, 1* (1), 15–29.

Reed, E. S. (1982). An outline of a theory of action systems. *Journal of Motor Behavior, 14,* 98–134.

Reed, E. S. (1989a). Neural regulation of adaptive behavior. *Ecological Psychology, 1,* 97–118.

Reed, E. S. (1989b). Changing theories of postural development. In M. H. Wollacott & A. Shumway-Cook (Eds.), *Development of posture and gait across the life span.* Columbia: University of South Carolina Press.

Rehak, A., Kaplan, J. A., Weylman, S. T., Kelly, B., Brownell, H. H., & Gardner, H. (1992). Story processing in right-hemisphere brain-damaged patients. *Brain and Language, 42,* 320–336.

Riessman, C. K. (1993). *Narrative analysis.* (Qualitative Research Methods Series 30). Thousand Oaks, CA: Sage.

Rosenberg, J., & Ashwal, S. (1996). Recent advances in the development of practice parameters: The vegetative state. *NeuroRehabilitation, 6,* 79–87.

Schloss, P. J., & Wood, C. E. (1990). Effect of self-monitoring on maintenance and generalization of conversational skills of persons with mental retardation. *Mental Retardation, 28* (2), 105–113.

Schoenfield, A. H. (1987). What's all the fuss about metacognition? In A. H. Schoenfeld (Ed.), *Cognitive science and mathematics education.* Hillsdale, NJ: Erlbaum.

Schon, D. A. (1987). *Educating the reflective practitioner.* San Francisco: Jossey-Bass.

Schmidt, R. A. (1988). *Motor control and learning: A behavioral emphasis* (2nd ed.). Champaign, IL: Human Kinetics.

Schmidt, R. A., & Bjork, R. A. (1992). New conceptualizations of practice: Common principles in three paradigms suggest new concept for training. *Psychological Science, 3,* 207–217.

Schwartz, R. K. (1985). *Therapy as learning.* Dubuque, IA: Kendall.

Schwartz, R. K. (1991). Education and training strategies: Therapy as learning. In C. Christiansen & C. Braun (Eds.), *Occupational therapy: Overcoming human performance deficits.* Thorofare, NJ: Slack.

Schwartzberg, S. L. (1994). Helping factors in a peer-developed support group for persons with head injury, Part 1: Participant observer perspective. *American Journal of Occupational Therapy, 48,* 297–304.

Segal, M. E., & Schall, R. R. (1995). Assessing handicap of stroke survivors: A validation study of the Craig Handicap assessment and reporting technique. *American Journal of Physical Medicine and Rehabilitation, 74* (4), 276–286.

Shaw, R. (1986). Persistent vegetative state: Principles and techniques for seating and positioning. *Head Trauma Rehabilitation, 1* (1), 31–37.

Shriberg, L. D., & Kwiatkowski, J. (1990). Self-monitoring and generalization in preschool speech-delayed children. *Language, Speech, and Hearing Services in Schools, 21,* 157–170.

Siev, E., Freishtat, B., & Zoltan, B. (1986). *Perceptual and cognitive dysfunction in the adult stroke patient* (rev. ed.). Thorofare, NJ: Slack.

Silver, E. A. (1987). Foundations of cognitive theory and research for mathematics problem-solving instruction. In A. H. Schoenfeld (Ed.), *Cognitive science and mathematics education.* Hillsdale, NJ: Erlbaum.

Sohlberg, M. M., & Mateer, C. A. (1989). Training use of compensatory memory books: A three stage behavioral approach. *Journal of Clinical and Experimental Neuropsychology, 11* (6), 871–891.

Spencer, J., Krefting, L., & Mattingly, C. (1993). Incorporation of ethnographic methods in occupational therapy assessment. *American Journal of Occupational Therapy, 47,* 303–309.

Stein, F. (1989). *Anatomy of clinical research: An introduction to scientific inquiry in medicine, rehabilitation and related health professions.* Thorofare, NJ: Slack.

Stineman, M. G., Hamilton, B. B., Granger, C. G., Goin, J. E., Escarce, J. J., & Williams, S. V. (1994). Four methods for characterizing disability in the formation of function related groups. *Archives of Physical Medicine and Rehabilitation, 75,* 1277–1283.

Strauss, A., & Corbin, J. (1994). Grounded theory methodology: An overview. In N. K. Denzin & Y. S. Lincoln (Eds.), *Handbook of qualitative research.* Thousand Oaks, CA: Sage.

Stuss, D. T. (1992). Biological and psychological development of executive functions. *Brain and Cognition, 20,* 8–23.

Sunderland, A., Harris, J. E., & Gleave, J. (1984). Memory failures in everyday life following severe head injury. *Journal of Clinical Neuropsychology, 6* (2), 127–142.

Swanson, H. L. (1990). Influence of metacognitive knowledge and aptitude on problem solving. *Journal of Educational Psychology, 82* (2), 306–314.

Toglia, J. (1991). Generalization of treatment: A multicontext approach to cognitive perceptual impairment in adults with brain injury. *American Journal of Occupational Therapy, 45,* 505–516.

Toglia, J. (1993). Attention and memory. In C. B. Royeen, *AOTA self-study series: Cognitive rehabilitation.* Bethesda, MD: American Occupational Therapy Association.

Trombly, C. (1993). The issue is anticipating the future: Assessment of occupational function. *American Journal of Occupational Therapy, 47,* 253–257.

Van Zomeren, A. H., & Brouwer, W. H. (1994). *Clinical neuropsychology of attention.* Oxford: Oxford University Press.

VanLehn, K., Jones, R. M., & Chi, M. T. H. (1991). Modeling the self-explanation effects with Cascade 3. *Proceeding of the Thirteenth Annual Conference of the Cognitive Science Society.* Hillsdale, NJ: Erlbaum.

VanLehn, K., Jones, R. M., & Chi, M. T. H. (1992). A model of the self-explanation effects. *Journal of the Learning Sciences, 2* (1), 1–60.

Vygotsky, L. S. (1978). *Mind in society: The development of higher psychological processes.* Cambridge: Harvard University Press.

Warren, M. L. (1993). A hierarchical model for evaluation and treatment of visual perceptual dysfunction in adult acquired brain injury: Parts 1 and 2. *American Journal of Occupational Therapy, 47,* 42–66.

Warren, M. (1995). Providing low vision rehabilitation services with occupational therapy and ophthalmology: A program description. *American Journal of Occupational Therapy, 49,* 877–883.

Webster, J. S., & Scott, R. R. (1983). The effects of self-instructional training on attentional deficits following head injury. *Clinical Neuropsychology, 5* (2), 69–74.

Weitzman, E. A., & Miles, M. B. (1995). *Computer programs for qualitative data analysis.* Thousand Oaks, CA: Sage.

White, J. A. (1996). Temporal adaptation in the intensive care unit. In R. Zemke & F. Clark (Eds.), *Occupational science— The evolving discipline.* Philadelphia, PA: Davis.

Willer, B., Ottenbacher, K. J., & Coad, M. L. (1994). The community integration questionnaire. *American Journal of Physical Medicine and Rehabilitation, 73,* 103–111.

Wilson, B. A. (1987). *Rehabilitation of memory.* New York: Guilford Press.

Winne, P. H. (1995). Inherent details in self-regulated learning. *Educational Psychologist, 30* (4), 173–187.

Wood, W., Abreu, B., Duval, M., & Gerber, D. (1994). Occupational performance and the function approach. In C. B. Royeen (Eds.), *AOTA self-study series: Cognitive rehabilitation.* Bethesda, MD: American Occupational Therapy Association.

World Health Organization (WHO). (1980). *International classification of impairments, disabilities, and handicaps.* Geneva: Author.

Yerxa, E. A. (1992). Foreword. In N. Katz (Ed.), *Cognitive rehabilitation: Models for intervention in occupational therapy.* Stoneham, MA: Butterworth-Heinemann.

Ylvisaker, M., & Szekeres, S. F. (1989). Metacognitive and executive impairments in head-injured children and adults. *Topics in Language Disorders, 9* (2), 34–49.

Zemke, R. (1989). The continua of scientific research designs. *American Journal of Occupational Therapy, 43,* 551–553.

Zemke, R., & Clark, F. (1996a). Preface. In R. Zemke & F. Clark (Eds.), *Occupational science—The evolving discipline.* Philadelphia: Davis.

Zemke, R., & Clark, F. (1996b). Defining and classifying. In R. Zemke & F. Clark (Eds.), *Occupational science—The evolving discipline.* Philadelphia: Davis.

Zimmerman, B. J. (1995). Self-regulation involves more than metacognition: A social cognitive perspective. *Educational Psychologist, 30* (4), 217–221.

CHAPTER 3

Cognitive Rehabilitation:
A Retraining Model for Clients
Following Brain Injuries

Sara Averbuch, MA, OTR, and Noomi Katz, PhD, OTR

A cognitive retraining or remediation approach in occupational therapy was developed by occupational therapists at Loewenstein Rehabilitation Hospital (LRH) and derives originally from clinical experience with clients following traumatic brain injury. The target population consisted of clients following both cerebrovascular accident (CVA) and traumatic brain damage (TBD), as well as clients with other neuropsychological dysfunctions. The approach was also adapted to treat adolescents with learning difficulties or underachieving school students. Clients were treated along the whole process, from the acute phase, until they reached a plateau in their progress. Then the treatment continued within the community, until the client found his or her place as a productive person in society. Treatment focused mainly on cognitive training, because this area is affected the most by brain damage and has direct implications for function. At the beginning phase of treatment, training was mainly remedial, in order to lessen cognitive deficits. In the next phase, our effort was centered on functional treatment and compensations, in order to enable the client to adapt to the community with his or her specific deficits.

This chapter describes the theoretical base, the assessment tools with research findings, and the cognitive treatment goals and applications we used. Case studies are presented from different client populations, and implications for future knowledge development are discussed.

Theoretical Base

In reference to this approach, we based our rationales on neuropsychological and cognitive theories (developmental and information processing). Neuropsychology provides the understanding of brain function, the basis and justification for treatment, whereas cognitive theories provide an understanding of the nature of intellectual processes and developmental sequence. Cognitive theories also influenced the development of the evaluation tools and treatment methods we used. These knowledge bases were then combined with occupational therapy principles of active intervention and philosophical assumptions, regarding the quality of life and the importance of independent coping with daily tasks.

The Neuropsychological Rationale

The cortex is described as a network of fibers, as "wiring diagrams" (Braitenberg, 1978). Each brain region is involved in various functions and interacts with other regions in completing a specific task. Thus, every normal act is a result of a dynamic balance between all brain structures. According to Luria (1973, p. 31), "Mental function . . . cannot be localized in narrow zones of the cortex . . . but must be organized in systems of concretely working zones, each of which performs its role in complex functional system." Luria also states that global function is constant, while the relationships among its components are variable and influenced by specific circumstances under which the function is performed. Thus, the way (or the action) through which the specific task is performed varies according to circumstances. The system, the "network of fibers" of the higher mental processes in the human cortex, constantly changes during the child's development and is influenced by his or her environment (learning and training process). The structures of higher mental processes change, and with them, so do their relationships with each other (i.e., their "intellectual organization") (Vygotsky, 1962). Thus, normal function is the result of a dynamic balance between all brain structures.

Brain injury causes a disturbance in the delicate balance between brain structures, which is not only the result of a localized lesion of one of the brain areas. A lesion in each zone or area may lead to disintegration of the entire functional system (Luria, 1973; 1980). In other words, the functional system as a whole can be disturbed by a lesion affecting a very large number of areas, and it can be disturbed differently by lesions in different localizations.

Brain damage can also cause symptoms that result from disinhibition of an intact area, and not only from the damaged area. Therefore, treatment aims to regain a balance between the brain structures and to create compensatory strategies for improving function. Because there are several ways to perform cognitive functions, these ways offer the rationale for training that creates alternative strategies and achieves the reorganization of impaired intellectual abilities.

In summary, "the multiplicity of functions fulfilled by cortical regions, the variety of ways in which complex cognitive functions can be performed, and the different contingencies of learning tasks on an intact brain offer a substrate for the functional reorganization of impaired intellectual abilities" (Rahmani, 1987, p. 5).

The Cognitive Rationale

Cognitive theories study the information processing of the normal intellect. The information an individual has to process comes from three sources:

(1) his or her environment, (2) his or her memory, where the information is compared to previous experiences, and (3) the feedback he or she receives after the action (Bourne et al., 1979). Information passes through several stages, during which it is received, registered, and encoded. This processed information is then organized as a schemata. Neisser (1976, p. 54) defines schema as "that portion of the entire perceptual cycle which is internal to the perceiver, modifiable by experience, and somehow specific to what is being perceived. The schema accepts information as it becomes available at sensory surfaces and is changed by that information; it directs movements and exploratory activities that make more information available by which it is further modified." Schema enables us to handle a large body of information by allowing us to compare new stimuli with previous experiences and then modify and change the schema. This is similar to Piaget's process of assimilation and accommodation (Ginsburg & Opper, 1979).

The normal individual actively seeks and assimilates information in relation to his or her ability to understand and then remember it. This search is guided by schemata representing the layout of our memories and knowledge. Perception, thinking, and memory are constantly interacting. Comprehension and memory depend on what and how we perceive. Perception is influenced by our ability to

1. Appreciate the relevance of the information
2. Distinguish among hierarchical constellations of attributes characteristic of different information
3. Distinguish among hierarchical constellations of attributes characteristic of different information that is perceived.

These abilities further rely strongly on previous experiences and accumulated knowledge.

For example, visual identification is strongly affected by the ability to analyze the information according to its hierarchical attributes and previous experiences. Identification is much clearer when we deal with incomplete or partial information as presented in embedded figures. Identification is made according to characteristic features, the prototype of the groups to which the specific item belongs (Rahmani, 1982; 1987). As noted in Rosch studies (1975, 1978), the formation and learning of components is based on forming preferential levels of abstraction, selecting prototypes, creating object categories, and determining the degree of category membership. In a similar way, the learning process and memory are strongly affected by the perception process. The various mechanisms of the cognitive functions of perception, thinking operations, and memory provide the procedures for cognitive retraining of the impaired intellectual processes in brain-damaged clients.

Occupational Therapy for Clients with Brain Damage

For a long time, occupational therapists have treated clients with brain damage caused by traumatic injuries, stroke, and other neurological causes. Recently, however, there has been an increased interest in developing knowledge of the relationships between cognitive deficits and functional performance. In almost all occupational therapy models, cognition is considered one of the major performance or competence components determining occupational performance or human occupation (Allen, 1985; Katz, 1985; Kielhofner, 1995; Mosey, 1986; Pedretti, 1985). Moreover, we believe that cognitive components are the major cause of rehabilitation outcomes in clients with brain damage, so we therefore focused on these assets (Bernspang et al., 1989; Katz, 1992; Rahmani, 1982).

Neistadt (1988; 1990) divided the different approaches of cognitive treatment in occupational therapy into two main categories: the adaptive or functional approach, which emphasizes the functional and practical aspects of every day activities, and the remedial approach, which emphasizes the training of the cognitive components and their generalization across all activities. To these two categories dynamic assessment and treatment was added by Toglia (in this book) based on Vygotsky and Feuerstein (Hadas-Lidor & Katz in this book).

Underlying the remedial approach to (or retraining of) cognitive deficits is the assumption that generalization occurs from practice in one modality to adaptation within other modalities and

tasks. The functional approach assumes that brain-damaged clients must practice directly every activity they have to perform, and generalization cannot be taken for granted. However, using a combination of both during the rehabilitation process seems to be the correct approach for adult brain-damaged clients. Practice of only specific tasks would limit the client's adaptation, while training in tabletop or computer tasks without practicing the actual tasks themselves may be inadequate. Our model combines the two approaches in the cognitive rehabilitation program, although the retraining phase is central to the process.

Furthermore, for occupational therapists, the real test of treatment success is performance of purposeful activities in the person's real world environment. Therefore, even though the main part of treatment in this approach is the retraining of cognitive skills, their actual internalization and generalization across tasks must be tested in real life situations similar to the level of transfer developed by Toglia (1992; in this book). Only then is full rehabilitation accomplished (Katz, 1994).

Definition of Main Cognitive Concepts

Cognition

"Cognition is the activity of knowing: the acquisition, organization, and use of knowledge" (Neisser, 1976, p.1). It consists of the intellectual processes that are responsible for function and behavior. Cognition is prerequisite for managing all encounters with the environment. Cognition consists of interrelated processes, including the ability to perceive, organize, assimilate, and manipulate information (Abreu & Toglia, 1987). By the same token, cognition (according to Piaget) is equated with intelligent adaptation to the environment. "Cognition is conceived of as a general term that covers attention, perception, thinking operations, and memory" (Katz et al., 1989, p. 186). Lidz (1987) provides a comprehensive definition, namely the individual's capacity to acquire and use information in order to adapt to environmental demands. This definition incorporates cognitive skills with information processing to functional adaptation.

Perception

Perception is the ability to perceive information and is regarded as the first step and prerequisite to higher function. However, perception relies on the perceiver's experience and previous knowledge. Perception centers on all sensory areas: visual, spatial, auditory, and tactile. In the literature, the study of perception focuses largely on visual identification. Visual identification of objects is based on the perceiver's ability to appreciate objects' characteristic features and their relevance (Neisser, 1976).

Visuomotor Organization

Visuomotor organization, or constructional ability, is the area that combines perceptual activity with motor response. It has a spatial component, including activities such as drawing, copying, building, or assembling. Difficulties in this area are expressed in the performance of ADL and complex activities of any kind (Lezak, 1995).

Thinking Operations

Thinking operations consist of conceptual and learning processes and include the ability to categorize, relate information to a hierarchical order, determine the relevance of the information according to a particular situation, sequence information, and solve problems. Problem solving is a behavior directed toward achieving a goal. It involves breaking the goal down into hierarchical tasks that will result in achieving the goal (Rahmani, 1987).

Memory

Memory refers to the capacity for keeping an amount of information in an active state (short-term memory) or the ability to recall or retrieve from long-term memory. However, information can be used only in an active state, and active modes of processing are needed to remember information. Memory is the output of well-processed information from a proper thinking process. New material can be learned by visual and/or verbal encoding (Paivio, 1975).

Attention and Concentration

Attention and concentration are the basis of any cognitive performance. Attention is a limited mental resource, which can be allocated at the most to a few cognitive processes at a time. Processes that require attention are called controlled processes (Shiffrin & Schneider, 1977). Attention is the ability to focus on specified information at a given time or on different information at a certain point in time. Concentration is the ability to apply attention over a specific time course (Hoofien, 1987).

Target Population

The Cognitive Retraining Approach was originally developed for adults with traumatic brain injuries, but is now used with almost all neuropsychologically impaired clients. It has also been adapted for adolescents with learning problems.

Evaluation and Research

Cognitive rehabilitation theory assumes that most normal adults achieve a basic cognitive task performance. We therefore start by assessing the client's current cognitive task performance. This assessment serves as a baseline for measuring progress, and, together with premorbid information, a sensorimotor evaluation, and a functional status evaluation in daily activities, it forms the basis for treatment planning (Katz, Hefner, & Reuben, 1990).

Assessment of cognition within this model includes the following cognitive batteries: The Loewenstein Occupational Therapy Cognitive Assessment (LOTCA) battery or the LOTCA-Geriatric (Itzkovich, Elazar, Averbuch, & Katz, 1990; Katz, Elazar, & Itzkovich, 1995); the Rivermead Behavioral Memory Test (Wilson, Cockburn, & Baddeley, 1985, Hebrew translation with permission Averbuch & Katz, 1991); the Behavioral Inattention Test for clients post-CVA to assess presence of unilateral-visual neglect (Wilson, Cockburn, & Halligan, 1987a; Hebrew translation with permission Katz, Averbuch, & Itzkovich). In addition, sometimes the Neurobehavioral Cognitive Status Examination (Cognistat, formerly known as NCSE) is used for screening mental status (Cognistat, 1995).

Loewenstein Occupational Therapy Cognitive Assessment (LOTCA)

At the Loewenstein Rehabilitation Hospital (LRH) in Israel, the staff developed the Loewenstein Occupational Therapy Cognitive Assessment (LOTCA) in order to assess basic cognitive abilities of clients following brain injury (Katz, Itzkovich, Averbuch, & Elazar, 1989; Najenson, Rahmani, Elazar, & Averbuch, 1984). Basic cognitive abilities are those "intellectual functions thought to be prerequisite for managing everyday encounters with the environment" (Najenson et al., 1984, p. 315).

The staff derived foundations for the LOTCA battery from clinical experience as well as from Luria's (neuropsychological) and Piaget's (developmental) theories and evaluation procedures (Golden, 1984; Inhelder & Piaget, 1964). As a starting point for occupational therapy intervention and a screening test for further neuropsychological assessment, the battery provides an initial profile of cognitive abilities of the brain-injured client. It consists of 20 subtests and 5 areas of division: orientation, visual and spatial perception, praxis, visuomotor organization, and thinking operations. A 4- or 5- point scale accompanies each subtest, from which the evaluator may obtain a profile of functioning in a specified area. While the entire battery takes 30 to 45 minutes to administer, the evaluator can divide the testing into sessions if necessary. The instructions include procedures for evaluating clients with expressive language deficits.

Also, evaluators used the LOTCA as a measure of the client's status over time (i.e., clinical change). In those cases where deficits were present at initial assessment, evaluators employed the LOTCA as a follow-up in reference to the client's progress. In general, in order to avoid simple memory carry-over, it is best to repeat the assessment after an interval of at least 2 months. However, since clients practice many similar tasks during treatment, and learning is a possible explanation for higher scores, it is an important factor to consider. This learning, if generalized, is precisely the purpose of treatment. Therefore, in contrast to the view of measurement

theory, we should not regard it as a threat to validity (Katz et al., 1990) (see Appendix for current scoring sheet).

Reliability and Validity

Initially, the researchers established the battery's measurement properties in different ways. They determined interrater reliability coefficients of .82 to .97 for the various subtests and, upon using patient groups and a normal control group, found an alpha coefficient of .85 and above in reference to the internal consistency of perception, visuomotor organization, and thinking operations. (Katz et al., 1989). Next, the researchers determined validity in differentiating between known groups. The Wilcoxon two-sample test showed that between the control groups and the client groups of traumatic brain injuries (TBI) and craniovascular accidents (CVA), all subtests differentiated at the $p < .0001$ level of significance. Through the use of an exploratory factor analyses, they examined initial construct validity, which showed a three-factor solution and a total amount of variance explained above 60% (i.e., substantial). This result supported the assumed structure of the LOTCA (Katz et al., 1989) and led to further investigation. In order to test the area of visuomotor organization in reference to the criterion validity within the TBI group, the examiners used the block design subtest of the WAIS (Wechsler, 1981). They found a Pearson correlation coefficient of $r = .68$ between the score on the block design and the mean score of the visuomotor organization subtests of the LOTCA, and an $r = .77$ when the testing did not measure time on the block design. The results were almost identical for a group of adult clients with chronic schizophrenia ($r = .69$ and $r = .78$) (Katz & Hiemann, 1990).

In order to determine the validity of the LOTCA in reference to American subjects, the researchers compared both American and Israeli healthy adults, as well as those among the two countries who experienced a stroke (Annes, Katz, & Cermak, 1996; Cermak, Katz, McGuire, Greenbaum, Peralta, Maser-Flanagan, 1995). Comparison of means and standard deviations of each LOTCA subtest revealed strong similarities between the American and Israeli healthy adult samples. The similarities in ability to perform accurately between the two groups support the use of the LOTCA battery in the United States.

Comparison of clients who experienced a recent stroke showed that on the majority of LOTCA subtests, there were no significant differences between American and Israeli subjects. Thus, the LOTCA is an appropriate tool to assess Americans who have had a stroke. The American healthy data serve as standards of performance. Additionally, in accordance with its design, the study compared the performance of clients post right and left CVA (Cermak et al., 1995). Few differences existed between the two groups in both countries. Only one subtest, the pegboard construction, revealed significant differences among both American and Israeli subjects. Therefore, the conclusions indicated that for the most part the LOTCA subtests are not specific to right or left cerebral hemisphere, and show more integrative cognitive abilities.

However, through the use of one-way ANOVA, comparison of clients following TBI ($n = 25$) and right CVA, both with neglect ($n = 19$) and without neglect ($n = 21$), showed significant F tests for three of the cognitive areas on the LOTCA (i.e., all except orientation). Scheffe post hoc tests showed that the source of difference was the neglect group, which performed lower in all areas. A Wilcoxon analysis, which compared all LOTCA subtests, showed the same results. In other words, clients post TBI performed significantly higher than clients post RCVA with neglect, while the nonneglect RCVA group was not significantly different from the TBI group.

Annes and colleagues compared the performance on the LOTCA between older (40 to 70 years old) and younger American adults (17 to 25 years old) in two ways: accuracy on all subtests and length of time to perform the visuomotor organization subtests. Similarity in accuracy of performance between older and younger adults was significant on almost all subtests and supported the consideration of the group as one. However, although nearly all normal adults achieved maximum performance on the LOTCA subtests, younger adults required significantly less time to complete all the visuomotor organization subtests. Based on these results, it appears that time, at least for the visuomotor organization subtests, can be used as a more sensitive measure for screening among healthy adults or adults with mild cognitive deficits.

Additionally, Katz, Champagne, and Cermak (1997) found similar results regarding the puzzle subtest. Groups of younger and older American adults were tested on three versions of the puzzle construction subtest. On all versions, the younger adults performed faster than the older adults. Older adults performed faster in the simplified version of the LOTCA-Geriatric (LOTCA-G) than in the original LOTCA subtest in both conditions either on top of the design (as required in the test) or in front of it.

Recently, the relationship between cognitive performance and daily functioning in clients following RCVA, with and without neglect, was studied by Katz, Elazar, Itzkovich, Ring, and Soroker (1996). The study comprised 40 clients with RCVA and first stroke as its sample. Based on the Behavioral Inattention Test (BIT) conventional subtests cutoff point (Wilson et al., 1987a), they assigned clients into neglect ($n = 19$) and nonneglect ($n = 21$) groups. Within both groups, the mean age of the subjects was approximately 58 years old. In both groups, the number of men outweighed the number of women. The functional measures included the Functional Independence Measure (FIM) (Granger et al., 1993), an ADL checklist (Hartman-Maeir & Katz, 1995), and the Rabideau Kitchen Evaluation-Revised (RKE-R), which includes drink and sandwich preparation (Neistadt, 1992).

They assessed subjects in three periods: at admission to the rehabilitation program, at the time of discharge, and at a 6 months' follow-up session. Results of Spearman correlation analysis of the four LOTCA areas with the functional measures at these three assessment periods were as follows.

At admission, in the neglect group, perception correlated with the ADL checklist ($r = .47$), visuomotor and thinking operations correlated with the FIM total and motor ($r \sim .50$). In the nonneglect group, all areas correlated with the FIM cognitive ($r = .50$ to $r = .67$); perception and thinking correlated with the ADL checklist ($r \sim .45$).

At discharge, in the neglect group, moderate to high correlations (range $r = .48$ to $r = .80$) revealed a significant relationship between the LOTCA (except orientation), and all performance measures.

The highest correlations were between visuomotor and thinking with drink and sandwich preparation ($r \sim .80$). In general, within the nonneglect group, significant correlations were moderate (range $r = .36$ to $r = .62$). The highest correlation appeared between the visuomotor organization area and the FIM total ($r = .62$).

At follow-up, subjects participated in only three LOTCA visuomotor subtests: colored block design, puzzle, and drawing a clock. In the neglect group, moderate to high correlations (range $r = .40$ to $r = .77$) appeared with the functional measures (except for clock with the FIM total and cognitive, which was $r \sim .30$). The puzzle subtest correlated the highest with all functional measures ($r \sim .70$). When comparing the two groups, the number of significant correlations within the nonneglect group was smaller and lower than in the neglect group. The highest correlation appeared between the puzzle and sandwich preparation ($r = .70$).

In order to explore the predictive validity of the LOTCA to daily function, from the time of admission to follow-up, the researchers computed a multiple regression analysis. In reference to the entire sample of RCVA subjects ($n = 40$), the BIT conventional score explained about 60% of the variance of all functional measures at follow-up. Depending on the measure (FIM, drink or sandwich), the LOTCA area scores of perception, visuomotor or thinking operations explained only an approximate, additional 5% of variance. A separate analysis for the groups revealed that in the nonneglect group, perception explained 57% and the visuomotor an additional 13% of the FIM total; perception explained 62% of the sandwich preparation; thinking explained 44%, and perception an additional 12% of the drink preparation. Thus, these results identified neglect to be the major variable predicting daily functioning in clients post RCVA with neglect. However, for those clients who do not suffer from neglect, cognitive deficits have a major contribution to the level of daily functioning.

Children's Performance

The testing of 240 normal primary school children determined age-level standards among 40 subjects in each age group, between the ages of 6 and 12 years old. In order to determine age norms of the various subtests, as well as to verify the hierarchical order in which the various cognitive competencies included in the battery are acquired, the study assessed the performance of children on the LOTCA. The results showed a clear, developmental sequence in performance along the LOTCA subtests. Performance levels increased steadily with age, while the performance speed of visuomotor tasks decreased concomitant with the increase toward maximal performance (Averbuch & Katz, 1991).

Presently, we are in the process of adapting the LOTCA to assess children aged 6 to 12 in a more dynamic approach, using Toglia's guidelines (Toglia, 1994) and with some item modifications. The research project in progress includes assessment of healthy children and two groups of children: those with learning disabilities and those following traumatic brain injuries.

Geriatric Version of LOTCA (LOTCA-G)

Clinical experience alerted the researchers to the difficulties in administering the battery to elderly clients. For example, some items are too small to see or manipulate, and the battery as a whole is too long. Therefore, an adapted geriatric version of the LOTCA was developed and researched (Katz, Elazar, & Itzkovich, 1995). Based on literature and clinical observations, the geriatric version, LOTCA-G (Elazar, Itzkovich, & Katz, 1996), was changed according to the following criteria: enlargement of items to reduce difficulties with vision and/or motor coordination; reduction of details in some items for lower task complexity; shortening of subtests, and thus the whole battery, in order to reduce general length of time; and addition of three memory subtests.

Through comparing 33 elderly post stroke and 43 healthy, independent elderly subjects, Katz and colleagues determined construct validity for the LOTCA-G. The subjects' mean age of 77 was similar for both groups, and the range of age spanned from 70 to 91 years old. Among both groups, men represented a third of the population sample. With the exception of praxis and colored block design, all subtests differed significantly between the groups and indicated healthy elderly to be performing better. On all perception subtests, both groups performed well. In order of severity, the most noted decline in the stroke group was in visuomotor organization, thinking operations, and orientation.

The mean length of time to perform the whole assessment for both groups on the LOTCA was about 55 minutes, with a range of 30 to 90 minutes, showing a large amount of variance. On the LOTCA, healthy elderly and clients post CVA showed no significant difference, suggesting normal slowness at older age, upon performance of complex tasks. In contrast, the LOTCA-G showed that clients' performance time was 45 minutes, with a range of 20 to 60 minutes, while that of healthy elderly was 31 minutes, with a range of 20 to 45 minutes. Within the stroke group, the LOTCA took a greater amount of time (57 versus 45 minutes), although this was statistically insignificant. In comparison, within the healthy group, the difference in time was very significant (51 versus 31 minutes). A two-way ANOVA showed overall significant statistical differences (F = 11.26, P < .0001). Scheffe's post hoc test showed that the differences are (1) in the healthy group, between both the LOTCA and LOTCA-G versions, and (2) between both of the healthy and client post CVA groups, in reference to the LOTCA-G.

The Rivermead Behavioral Memory Test (RBMT)

In reference to the evaluation of memory deficits, the Rivermead Behavioral Memory Test is a battery that assesses memory abilities in everyday tasks. "It is assessing skills necessary for adequate functioning in normal life and can also be used to help therapists identify areas for treatment" (Wilson et al., 1985, p. 4).

The RBMT consists of 11 subtests that assess verbal and visual recognition and recall, learning and recall of instructions, and recall of a spatial root. Subtests include remembering a name, belonging, appointment, pictures, story (immediate and delayed), faces, route (immediate and delayed), message, orientation, and date. All subtests use simple, everyday items. For example, one of the instructions is to remember to ask when the next appointment is, when the clock rings, or to ask for a personal

belonging at the end of the assessment that had been given to the therapist at the beginning of the session. In order to make it possible to repeat the assessment a few times, the test includes four alternative versions. Each subtest has a screening with a scoring system of pass/fail (maximum 12) and a standardized profile 3-point score (normal, marginal, and deficit, maximum 24).

In differentiating clients following traumatic brain injury or stroke and healthy persons, the test showed validity (Goldberg & Katz, 1994; Wilson, Cockburn, & Baddeley, 1986). Also, it correlated significantly more with functional outcomes than with other formal memory tests. Existence of norms for elderly above age 70 appeared mainly within the profile scores (Cockburn & Smith, 1989). Apparently, without any culture-related difficulties, occupational therapists in Israel use the Hebrew translation of the RBMT (Goldberg & Katz, 1994).

In 1994, in order to increase the difficulty of the test, Wall, Wilson, and Baddeley studied an extended version (ERBMT). The authors combined two parallel versions into one test, which extended the test to include a double amount of material in each subtest. Subjects consisted of 26 healthy middle-aged persons and 22 healthy elderly persons. The findings suggested that the test was more sensitive in detecting small age differences but required further investigation to ascertain its ecological validity.

The Behavioral Inattention Test (BIT)

The design makeup of the Behavioral Inattention Test (BIT) (Halligan, Cockburn, & Wilson, 1991; Wilson, Cockburn, & Halligan, 1987a; Wilson, Cockburn, & Halligan, 1987b), which consists of six conventional subtests and nine behavioral subtests, aims to identify a wide variety of visual neglect behaviors. The conventional subtests include line crossing, letter cancellation, star cancellation, figure and shape copying, line bisection, and representational drawing. They vary in reference to scoring range, and their combined total allows for a maximum of 146 points.

The behavioral subtests evaluate aspects of daily life: scanning three pictures (plate of food, bathroom sink, and a room), telephone dialing, menu reading, article reading, telling time, coin sorting, address and sentence copying, map navigation, and card sorting. Each subtest score allows for a maximum of 9 points, totaling a maximum of 81 points. Scores can provide a functional profile of neglect and a meaningful guide for treatment.

Reliability and Validity

From a sample of 50 non–brain-damaged subjects and 80 CVA clients (i.e., 54 with right-brain damage and 26 with left-brain damage, the researchers collected normative as well as reliability and validity data. They used the scores of the control subjects to establish cutoff points for individual subtests and total scores. Interrater, parallel form, and test–retest reliability were all high ($r = .99 .91 .99$, $P < .001$ respectively). They established validity in two ways: first, by examining the relationship between the conventional and behavioral test scores ($r = .92$, $P < .001$), a measure of concurrent validity; and second, by examining the relationship between the behavioral scores and therapists' observations of the clients' ADL ($r = .67$, $P < .001$) (Wilson et al., 1987a; Halligan et al., 1991). In 1992, Shiel and Wilson found a strong association between neglect, as assessed by the BIT, and ADL as assessed by the Rivermead ADL assessment and Frenchay Activities Index. Their study contributed to the enhancement of the ecological validity of the BIT.

In a 1989 critique of the BIT, Cermak and Hausser suggested performing additional validity studies to determine whether the BIT indeed relates to actual functional performance. Following these suggestions, Hartman-Maeir and Katz (1995) studied 40 Israeli subjects with right cerebrovascular accident (RCVA), from both day center and hospital settings. Three measures were used in the evaluation: the BIT, performance tasks, and a checklist of activities of daily living. Results showed that seven out of nine BIT behavioral subtests differentiated significantly between subjects with visual neglect and those without neglect. Additionally, six out of nine subtests correlated significantly with parallel performance tasks or ADL checklist items. These findings, which support the validity of the BIT in predicting daily function, also suggest that the test is valid for use in Israel. Furthermore, as described above (Katz et al., 1996), the BIT

conventional score explained about 60% of the variance of all functional measures at follow-up, within an additional group of 40 RCVA clients.

The Neurobehavioral Cognitive Status Examination (Cognistat)

The Cognistat (1995), a screening test formerly known as the NCSE, determines the cognitive status of the client. In Israel, occupational therapists use the test in general hospitals, as a screening of cognitive deficits and as a base line in neurosurgical departments (Weiss, 1994). In practice, since the test provides more information for intervention planning than the Mini Mental Status Exam, the Cognistat also functions well as an assessment of elderly clients.

The test assesses five major cognitive areas: language, constructions, memory, calculations, and reasoning. The evaluation process begins with level of consciousness, orientation, and attention, and only then do other areas of assessment follow. All areas of testing occur within a screen and metric paradigm. First, the client receives the screen task, which is the most difficult item. If the client performs well at this point, the assumption is that the involved, cognitive skill represents normal functioning in that area and requires no further testing. If the client fails the screen task, the administration of the metric tasks takes place. The metric part consists of a series of test items of increasing difficulty. Performance in this area determines whether cognitive skill impairment is present, and if so, to what degree. Scores appear on a profile, which is arranged into four performance levels: average, mild, moderate, and severe (Cognistatl, 1995) (see figure 3-1).

Studies in a variety of client populations, where the suspicion of brain dysfunction exists, show that the Cognistat is sensitive in detecting cognitive impairments, differentiating between groups, and measuring changes over time (Lezak, 1995; Logue, Tupler, D'amico, & Schmitt, 1993; Mysiw, Beegan, & Gatens, 1989; Osmon, Smet, Winegarden, & Gandhavadi, 1992; Schwamm, Van Dyke, Kierman, Merrin, & Mueller, 1987).

Using this version, Katz, Elazar, and Itzkovich (1996) compared the performance of 24 Israeli healthy independent elderly and 15 clients post

Figure 3-1

Cognistat profiles of 3 groups:
Healthy elderly (n=47); DAT (n=42);
Neurosurgical patients (n=47)

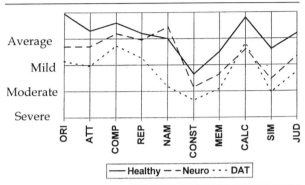

CVA, all above the age of 70. In reference to all subtests, the results showed that healthy elderly scored higher than clients post CVA. The researchers also found significant correlations between compatible subtests of the LOTCA and the Cognistat and low correlations between cognitive skills from different domains. These findings supported the validity of both tests. In an additional study, Katz, Weiss, Armon, and Hartman-Maeir (1997) compared the performance of 47 healthy independent elderly, 47 neurosurgical clients, and 42 persons suffering from dementia. The raw scores of all individual subtests and on four performance levels revealed statistically significant differences among the three groups. All groups produced low scoring on the construction subtest, which seemed to detect the aging process, rather than only disease-related dysfunction. For most subtests, the mean scores and standard deviations of all groups appeared similar or a little lower to those reported in the test manual, which supports the use of the test in Israel. Figure 3-1, taken from Katz, Weiss, Armon, and Hartman-Maeir (1997) presents the profiles of the three groups.

Treatment

The clients' cognitively impaired functions are one of the most important factors influencing their daily lives. Therefore, the aims of cognitive retraining are to enlarge and enhance cognitive ability, by providing the tools and reinforcing the clients' ability to cope with everyday tasks of life.

Cognitive Effects of Brain Damage

Brain damage reduces the individual's ability to process the information needed for identification, thinking operations, and remembering and executing everyday tasks. It limits the individual's ability to organize the information required for planning acts. The brain-damaged person is limited in the number of items he or she can manipulate simultaneously or sequentially. Thus, his or her ability to find various solutions to a given problem is limited. His or her cognitive behavior is concrete and relies strongly on personal experience.

However, brain damage does not affect the various cognitive components equally. The damage always has a predominant effect on one of the cognitive areas. In other words, perception, thinking operations, or memory is not equally impaired. Some sustain more damage, while others, although affected, are less impaired and function better. Cognitive deficits minimize the brain-damaged person's efficiency in every aspect of life: self-care, social behavior, and professional life.

Treatment Goals

The general purpose of retraining the perception processes, thinking operations, and memory is to broaden the client's capacity to handle information and transform it into purposeful activities (Rahmani et al., 1987). Training is expected to lead the client to a systematic search for information, a process that can be generalized to other tasks.

The therapist's first goal in cognitive treatment is to enhance and strengthen the client's remaining or less weakened cognitive abilities. As mentioned earlier, when brain damage is involved, not all cognitive functions are equally impaired. By strengthening the intact areas of cognitive ability, we create the base for new cognitive strategies. Creating new alternative strategies is the second goal of treatment. Alternative strategies are different tools or ways to receive and accumulate information. The therapist uses alternative strategies to train the client to systematically perceive, process, and act according to specific information. The goal is to help the client acquire the strategy to decide which information is the most relevant to him under given circumstances, and accordingly be able to solve problems in different ways. Achieving these goals will lead to the creation of new functional patterns, the result of which will be a different behavioral cognitive structure. In turn, this will improve functional performance.

Treatment Process

The treatment process has two phases. First, the treatment focus is on the cognitively impaired areas. Second, the focus is on adaptation to the environment. The cognitive treatment is based on the results of the different assessments and the premorbid cognitive ability of the client, as it is given by his family in the anamnestic interview. The training is constructed on different levels in every cognitive area: perception, visuomotor organization, thinking operations, and memory. Each level is characterized by the amount of information present to be processed and its complexity. On each level, the client is trained to develop specific strategies adequate to the cognitive area and to the particular level. These strategies are the base for the functional scheme, which will help in developing skills to handle more complex tasks and prerequisite for training at the next, more complex level. On each level, once the client has internalized the given cognitive strategies and can manipulate them on different modalities, he or she will be trained to adjust and adapt them to activities of real life. In other words, at first the client will be trained in specific strategies that strengthen his or her intact cognitive skills, in order to deal with the impaired cognitive areas. The training will be done in the occupational therapy department with specific tools, similar to those in a laboratory environment. After the strategies are learned and, within the laboratory environment, the client can manipulate them on different materials, he or she will be instructed and encouraged to transfer them to real life situations. At first, this application will occur

in the hospital environment in activities of daily living, and later, at home.

The end result of the treatment is that the client integrates the different learned strategies into schematic patterns, and finally, into a new functional behavioral system. For simplicity and clarity, the following description of the treatment process is divided into the different cognitive components. The areas are, of course, interrelated, as are the treatment and its effects.

Training of Visual Perception

The first purpose of visual perception training is to reinforce the identification of concrete objects. In order for the client to be able to identify objects and to understand the consistent combination of their attributes, the therapist shows the client how to search for information. The therapist uses different procedures, and they are given here in a hierarchical order, from simple to complex. The complexity depends on the number of stimuli and the clarity of their representation.

In the beginning of the process, various concrete, daily objects are presented. First, they are presented separately, and later, together. The client has to search for the relevant attributes that create the object (color, shape, material, etc.). Touch and sound are used as additional sources of information. After the client has become acquainted with the strategy, he or she is required to use it to identify objects that are grouped together. This task is more complex because parts of the information are hidden.

Second, the client is trained to identify pictorial and schematic presentations of those objects from the first step. By drawing the client's attention toward the specific features of the objects, as they are represented in pictures, the therapist broadens the strategy.

Third, the client is trained to identify pictures of various degrees of ambiguity. The ambiguity can be pictures of embedded objects, photos of objects taken from unusual angles, or drawings of objects based on their parts. All of these procedures help to develop the client's ability to identify objects in the presence of incomplete information.

Fourth, the client is taught to discriminate subtle differences between objects. This is done by comparing pictures that differ in one or more details or through matching pictures with large number of variables.

Finally, the fifth stage involves the most complex task, which is to identify a pictorial situation. Although this task is not purely visual and combines more than one cognitive area, it can be used for training the specific weak area.

At each level, the client is trained to use specific strategies in real life, such as to identify items according to a list in the supermarket, to find the car in the parking lot, or to identify the needed key.

Training of Spatial Perception

The training consists of developing the client's orientation in personal and extrapersonal space, as well as his or her recognition of spatial reversal.

Personal Space. In this task, the procedures used include identifying body parts, knowing their location, and displaying awareness of the body's midline and its right-left and up-down position. Treatment focuses on helping the client cross the midline smoothly, by using activities that include features that are among all of the self-care tasks (washing, dressing, etc.).

Extrapersonal Space. The treatment purpose is to identify the position of objects near-far from client, above-under, and at his or her left-right: the relations between space and person. Training procedures such as arranging the table for dinner or arranging clothes in the closet are used.

Reversal. In reversal, the purpose is to identify reversed directions in space: first on the trainer's body, while he or she is sitting in front of the client, later in the street, and finally on the map.

Training of Visuomotor Organization

This area combines the abilities of perception and motor action. Constructional activities at any level are the expression of perceptual abilities, praxis abilities, and organization. The client is trained to analyze perceptual models, to plan their reproduction, and finally to construct them. The main purpose of this strategy is the ability to analyze and synthesize given plans. Various procedures are used in order to train and enhance the constructional strategy.

First, the client has to learn to scan a given model to analyze its combination of components. In order to achieve this, he or she must copy simple forms or reproduce designs combined of clearly distinct parts. Then, gradually, through more demanding tasks in terms of components, the schema will be enlarged. The client will have to copy complex forms. He or she will be trained to reproduce models that require counting and accurate part or model location, without clear distinction of the compounding parts. Part of the training includes reproducing three-dimensional models as well as models in perspective. Finally, the client will have to alter his or her learned strategy, by constructing new strategies according to professional plans.

We should comment that not everyone needs all levels of this area in their daily life; not all clients will be able to or need to read and reconstruct a plan. However, almost everyone can learn the simple forms when necessary. What we have described is the extent of our training in occupational therapy. However, when the client needs these elaborate skills for his or her profession, he or she will be further referred for vocational training.

Training of Thinking Operations

The basis of thinking operations is classification skills and simple logical sequence. In order to develop classification skills, the client is trained to make the distinction between relevant and irrelevant features of objects. Then he or she must choose the hierarchical order of the relevant features and create simple categories and subcategories according to the most relevant feature. The features become a criteria for creating a category, and the client must be able to shift from one criteria to another. The ability to shift between criteria is the difference between concrete and flexible thinking. These skills in everyday life can be used with activities that require planning and organization:

shopping, arranging things in drawers or cupboards, preparing ingredients for cooking, etc.

The next step of our training, the logical operations of transitivity and of cause and effect relations, is done with different materials and different modalities. Clients will learn to solve logical problems that involve one, two, or more compounding parts and mathematical problems. Clients will read short stories and answer questions about what they have read, displaying the level of ability to draw conclusions. Each of these tasks demands systematic strategies of thinking. Sequence is another essential thinking operation. In order to solve a problem, operations have to be done in the right order. This order depends on the client's ability to sequence. The tasks we use involve arranging pictorial situations and different series of numbers, forms, etc. In order to solve problems, one must have the ability to draw conclusions from one stage to another. Also, one needs the ability to judge and appreciate the results of his or her solutions. Finally, it is crucial to train these strategies in real problems of everyday life.

Training of Memory

Memory deficits are a major problem for clients with brain damage. Often, they are the only problem the client notices. Brain-damaged clients complain about their lack of memory, even when it, objectively, is not their main problem. Memory seems to be the most concrete difficulty; it is easily understood by others and accepted as a very plausible excuse for many other disabilities. However, memory is affected by many cognitive components, and memory problems are also the result of other impairments. For example, if clients have difficulties in thinking operations, they will ultimately have memory problems. Information that was not systematically perceived will be stored directly, and its retrieval from memory will be incomplete and incoherent. In order to create functional schemes for learning and remembering, the client must use other cognitive components, such as perception skills, association cues, sequencing, and problem-solving strategies. At the same time, the client will be trained to use adaptive tools, such as notebooks or tape recorders.

Orientation. The first purpose of training is to help the client to orient himself or herself to the immediate place and time. The task begins by orienting the client to the immediate environment of the department and hospital. The therapist administers the training through three parallel channels. Through conversation, the client is supplied first with accurate information about his or her physical environment, and then with information in reference to his or her time schedule. Then the client is given the same information in the form of written instructions that are the basis of experiencing everyday tasks. The same bits of information must be given in conversation, writing, and real experience. New information will be added gradually, as soon as the client is able to handle the old information. When training topographic memory of the environment, the therapist instructs the client to create landmarks of perceptual cues along the way. During real experience training, the client has to recite aloud what has been learned through conversation, reading the written instruction, and showing mastery of his or her ability in actions. Gradually, the training will be enlarged to the outside world and home surroundings, using the same procedures.

Short-Term Memory. A common sign indicating a short-term memory deficit is that, when the client cannot recall an immediate item, usually he or she will be surprised that something has already been presented. To reinforce his or her ability, we will use association techniques, the key feature of which is creating familiar associations for the client. In other words, the point of this procedure is to work intensely on the client's perceiving and storing processes. These procedures are very useful for recalling names of people, short events, and short bits of information.

Long-Term Memory. Long-term memory loss is seen through the client's difficulty in learning new material from newspapers or professional materials. The major feature of training at this level is content analysis. This training develops the ability to divide the information into concrete, meaningful parts, as well as to understand and point to the logical sequence of events. As a result, the creation of a framework for arranging and storing information forms. The frame is the anchor, the landmark of recall. Once the information has been systematically stored, it will be much easier to recall if the client is asked general questions about the learning procedures: (What kind of information was it? What was the main topic? What sort of things happened? Was it funny? Was it about people, animals?)

As the client progresses clinically, the questions become increasingly general, and help the client to search for the proper information. As mentioned earlier, the client is trained to use a notebook for recording relevant information, and to use it properly as a reminder, while ignoring what is no longer relevant.

Attention

Often, attention is presented as a major deficit, when discussing cognitive impairment. There are treatment approaches, in which the main effort is made in developing attention. Attention is a major factor of mental function. However, we regard it as inherent in every cognitive process and assume that by training specific cognitive processes, attention will be positively affected. Therefore, we do not train attention as an independent entity but use it as part of the different cognitive areas.

Case Studies

Four case studies are described to illustrate the cognitive retraining approach with adult clients following TBI, right CVA with neglect, left CVA with aphasia, and treatment of an adolescent with learning difficulties.

1. A client following traumatic brain injury

Rachel is 44 years old, married with four children. She works as a family physician. After she suffered from headaches throughout the year, she found out that she had a meningioma on the left frontal lobe of her brain. The meningioma needed to be removed through a bi-frontal craniotomy. Two weeks after the operation, Loewenstein Rehabilitation Hospital admitted her for rehabilitation.

Evaluation results at admission

Motor status. Rachel showed no motor or sensory deficits.

ADL. Rachel was independent in all self-care activities.

Cognitive status—LOTCA results. Orientation, perception, and praxis were intact. The main deficits were in thinking operations and the more complex visuomotor organization subtests (see figure 3-2). She had major difficulties in choosing the right criteria for categorization. When the criteria had been chosen, with the therapist's help, she had fewer problems maintaining categorizing during the sorting phase. Sometimes, during the session, she lost the meaning of categorization and worked in an associative way.

In the beginning, Rachel appeared disheveled and neglected. She could wear the same clothes day after day, without noticing that they were not clean anymore. Her behavior was very passive, and she showed no mimics in her speech and no affect on her face. When speaking of her situation, she expressed feelings of "not being OK" and of feeling helpless. However, she could work for a long period of time, without losing concentration, and with high motivation and will to do anything, in order to progress.

Treatment process

The first goal involved developing basic, logical thinking, through training Rachel to perform simple sorting tasks of concrete categories, and then to sequence. We began by sorting everyday objects according to their attributes, and then proceeded with learning the meaning of categories. First, we addressed concrete and practical categories that people need daily and that differ from each other, such as clothing and food. In each group, we used four or five objects, while focusing on the relevant criteria for sorting. Rachel learned to analyze an object through asking such questions as "What are its attributes?" and "How do they relate in hierarchical order?" and "What is the most meaningful attribute that defines the object?" She

Figure 3-2

Case 1, LOTCA Performance

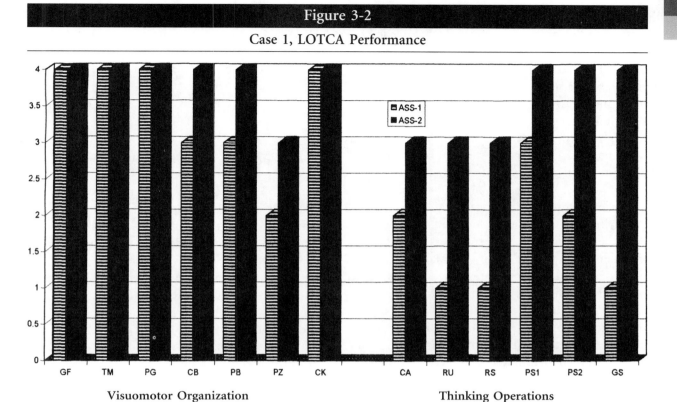

Visuomotor Organization
(Note: see abbreviations in Appendix)

Thinking Operations

learned, for example, that the most meaningful attribute of a pencil is its use for writing. This method of training bases its foundation on the fact that many concrete objects obtain their definition according to their usage. After Rachel developed capability in sorting objects correctly, and it became clear that she learned the way to accomplish the task, the direction of the training aimed at transferring the skill to activities of daily living. Together with her therapist, she began to organize her schedule for the day. At this point, Rachel began treatment in the outpatient clinic and remained at home for half her day. We sorted out the required tasks according to different criteria, such as time of performance, morning tasks or activities of personal ADL, child care tasks (e.g., making her children's breakfast and sandwiches for school), and housekeeping activities. Next, we arranged and recorded each group of activities into a hierarchical and sequential format. Rachel's spending significant time at home necessitated her to follow the schedule. With much effort, we emphasized the goal of improving her appearance.

Upon completion of this aspect of learning, Rachel readily integrated it into her home environment, and her family began to report constant improvement in her duties at home.

As the training sessions continued, we gradually expanded demands for her thinking ability to deal with more abstract categories and began to work on medical study materials. Utilizing the same techniques of investigation in reference to the relevant attributes of the objects, we began to construct a schema of analyzing a text. The schema consisted of finding the main issues and underling the important paragraphs, distinguishing between relevant and irrelevant information, recording them according to their order of importance in relation to the main issue, and finally, drawing conclusions from the given information. At first, Rachel had great difficulty locating important information. She expressed sensing a lack of comprehension, in reference to the meaning of the sentences. As she had been reading medical material previously known to her, she became quite shocked regarding her difficulties. In order to "survive" what seemed to be a nightmare, she needed much support from others. At this stage of training, Rachel needed to confront the demands of the medical material. When she successfully found the main paragraphs, she reached a milestone and turning point within her training. At that moment, she needed to learn the whole procedure of manipulating the schema, through which, as described before, she could learn relevant material from her medical books. On an emotional level, she responded with mixed feelings of joy and fear and asked about her chances of ever returning to her practice.

During this period at home, although she required more time and performed less pedantically, she demonstrated the ability to maintain fulfillment of all of her duties as previously. At this stage, one of the physicians at the hospital volunteered to work with us, in order to assess the extent of her professional abilities. The main problem that appeared was that, after hours of training and learning of certain material, Rachel still could not properly recall it. The physician stated, "she knows everything but can't use it alone properly." Upon request of knowing Rachel's impression, she expressed that she forgets everything. Together, in order to overcome this obstacle, we constructed an empty draft suitable to her material. It consisted of headlines, such as diagnoses, clinical signs, treatments, differential diagnoses, and side effects. We often used this method, by filling the draft with different information, according to what she already learned. The method helped, and she progressed significantly in performance.

Finally, Rachel began to work and assist both her colleague in his clinic and the staff in the hospital emergency room twice a week. In both places, she began to work under the close supervision of her colleagues. The reports of her performance were positive, and the greatest critique of her work came from Rachel herself. Rachel proved to be a very responsible person. When she felt confident enough, she returned to her work, with the knowledge that when she would encounter difficulties, she would need to consult a colleague from the medical profession.

In summary, a year after the craniotomy, Rachel was back at home and at work. She complained only of fatigue and difficulty falling asleep early at nights. Her family agreed with her report but added feeling regret over the loss of a certain quality of Rachel's personality. The profile in figure 3-2 illustrates her improvement on the LOTCA. Through intensive treatment and much effort on the part of Rachel, she gradually achieved marked and significant progress.

2. A client following right CVA with neglect

Joan is 55 years old married with three children. She has a high school education (12 years). As her main role, she functions as a housewife, and she most enjoys playing bridge and painting. She lives in a private house with two flights of stairs. Following a vascular accident at the right middle cerebral artery, the Loewenstein Rehabilitation Hospital diagnosed her as having a right CVA with hemiplegia and accepted her for treatment. Prior to the event, she smoked heavily and suffered from high blood pressure and diabetes.

Evaluation results at admission

Motor status. Joan ambulated through the use of a wheelchair. On the left hemiplegic side, she was flaccid in tone and showed no active movement. She displayed complete deficiency of proprioception and superficial sensitivity.

ADL. While she independently ate and drank, she otherwise required full assistance. Through observation of her behavior and performance, it became clear that her main problem entailed unilateral spatial neglect, which affected the execution of every function.

Cognitive status—LOTCA results. Orientation in time, visual perception, and praxis remained intact. Orientation in place, spatial perception, visuomotor organization, and thinking operations revealed deficits. Detailed functional assessment noted dressing apraxia, as a result of both her spatial problems and her inability to attend efficiently to the left field. Performance in the area of thinking operations was relatively better, as long as she did not need to actually perform the task. While she verbally located criteria for categorization and shifted it mentally, she became lost when she actually had to perform the categorization tasks. Similarly, in the pictorial sequence task, she understood the story properly and described it accurately; however, she mixed up the pictures and "forgot" some, when trying to reorganize them. The LOTCA profile (see figure 3-3) matches the large lesion in the right hemisphere that appeared in the CT scan.

The middle cerebral artery, the location of Joan's vascular accident, is responsible for the blood supply to large portions of the frontal, temporal, and parietal lobes (an area that covers almost the whole hemisphere). Thus, this vascular accident resulted in a basic inability to divide spatial attention properly, especially to the left field, and caused unilateral neglect and dressing and constructional apraxias. Joan's verbal abilities, memory, and verbal problem solving remained intact.

Treatment process

The cognitive training focused on improving Joan's spatial attention, which seemed to be the basic deficit that affected her performance in every domain, as well as spatial orientation, body perception, and visuomotor organization. The treatment sessions, which incorporated parallel training in ADL, motor, and cognitive tasks, maintained the same goal of improving spatial attention. To achieve this goal, tasks included scanning, systematically searching the whole spectrum, attending to different stimuli, and combining and using all sensory and communication-oriented channels (i.e., auditory, visual, tactile, verbal, and motor).

In order to increase Joan's involvement in treatment, higher levels of cognitive functions supported the training by increasing her awareness and understanding of her deficits. Since her verbal thinking abilities were relatively intact, she succeeded in understanding the treatment goals. However, the therapist needed much alertness and energy in order to maintain Joan's attention during treatment sessions. Within each domain, she applied the same strategies and sequence of actions in reference to treatment. For example, in the areas of spatial attention and searching systematically the whole spectrum, she worked with ADL training

through the strategies of searching for clothing, identifying body parts, planning in advance before acting, and verbalizing every step of the activity. As another example, in reference to spatial orientation, she applied the strategies of searching and scanning the hospital surroundings, while verbalizing and learning about it, and in the occupational therapy department, using the same strategies in tabletop visuomotor organization tasks and computer exercises.

She demonstrated application of the following strategies during ADL training:

1. Attending to the left side of the body and to the near space in the room
2. Scanning both sides and crossing the body midline
3. Relating body parts to suitable clothing
4. Verbally planning and organizing specific performance before executing it
5. Training specific techniques for dressing with one hand.

In the next phase, Joan needed to apply the learned strategies to ADL tasks, first before discharge from the hospital, and then upon reintegration into the home and community.

After 3 months of intensive treatment, Joan was reevaluated with the LOTCA, which showed a marked improvement (see Figure 3-3).

Although Joan's orientation of time and place improved within familiar environments, she increasingly experienced difficulty applying it in new places. Her left side neglect remained, but she gained awareness of it, could control her searching strategy, and thus progressed in performance. Specifically, she performed better on tabletop tasks and in defined narrow space. When she was in a large room or outside in new surroundings, accentuation of the neglect appeared. In visuomotor organization tasks using learned techniques, Joan improved and dealt well with analyzing simple tasks but continued to experience difficulties with three-dimensional and perspective models. In ADL, Joan required assistance only for mobility, especially upon encountering certain obstacles. She maneuvered her wheelchair without bumping into walls and doors. She showed marked improvement

Figure 3-3

Case 2, LOTCA Performance

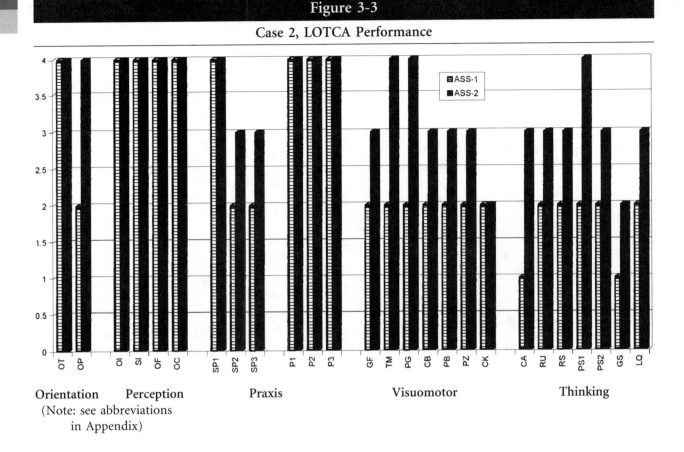

Orientation   Perception   Praxis   Visuomotor   Thinking
(Note: see abbreviations
       in Appendix)

through an increase in concentration, which in no way negatively impacted on her performance.

Following her release from the hospital, Joan received recommendations to continue treatment in the community.

3. A client following Left CVA with aphasia

Tom is 37 years old, married with no children. He has an undergraduate degree in mathematics and computers (15 years of schooling). He worked as a computer programmer in a high-tech company. Prior to the stroke, he was a healthy, nonsmoking individual.

Tom received the diagnosis of severe rheumatic mitral stenosis with an enlarged left atrium with thrombus, chronic atrial fibrilation, left CVA with right hemiplegia, and motor and partially sensory aphasia. The CT scan showed edema of the left hemisphere that pushed aside the midline, as well as a collapse of the third and forth rooms, and

right hydrocephalus. Two months after the stroke, Tom had a heart operation (an open commissurotomy, in order to enlarge the mitral stenosis, and a removal of the thrombus). A month after the operation, Loewenstein Rehabilitation Hospital admitted him for rehabilitation. A second CT scan showed a large fronto-temporal left infarct. The rooms remained functional.

Evaluation results at admission

Tom was an alert, cooperative, and well-oriented individual; his eye fields were intact; he had right facialis with difficulty swallowing liquids.

Motor status. Tom ambulated with right plantar flexion, which was insufficiently stable. In his right hand, distal active movements functioned better than proximal movements. He also lacked sensation, both proprioceptively and superficially.

ADL. In basic self-care functions, such as eating, washing, and dressing, he demonstrated independence in wheelchair mobility, he maneuvered his wheelchair by himself.

Cognitive status—LOTCA results. During the assessment, Tom displayed an accentuation of language problems, which necessitated the distribution of tests adapted to his aphasic condition. Orientation, visual and spatial perception, as well as praxis abilities remained intact. In visuomotor organization tasks, Tom performed better on clearly structured tasks and experienced more difficulties on less structured tasks (such as the clock).

The major problems appeared in thinking operation tasks, in which he showed difficulties in categorizing and concreteness in shifting sets. He related to the simple criteria of color or shape but could not find more complex criteria. Similarly, in reference to pictorial sequencing tasks, he arranged the central part of the sequence but experienced problems with the more detailed pictures (i.e., the ones in between). During the assessment session, he showed slight attention problems. In summary, the main cognitive problems were in thinking operations, which also affected his ability to organize unclear visuomotor tasks. He showed mental slowness with slight performance preservation (see Figure 3-4).

Treatment process

Since Tom was independent in basic ADL tasks, we focused on cognitive training and addressed his language difficulties, as a preliminary to training in IADL and returning to work. The first goal involved strengthening the preserved cognitive abilities, since they consisted of the base for developing alternative schemes for higher mental functions.

According to Rahmani (1987), normal mental functions consist of two main parts: the steadiness of the goal and the flexibility of various ways to achieve it. Thus, training focuses on teaching alternative strategies for achieving the mental goal in the dysfunctional cognitive skills. In this case, while bearing in mind Tom's limited language ability, the intact abilities, such as visual and spatial perception and praxis, constituted the base for improving thinking operations. For example, training in categorization, in order to enhance his ability of problem solving, requires the following steps:

1. Gathering and analyzing data
2. Designing a hierarchy of the data (i.e., deciding what is more important and when)
3. Choosing the criteria (i.e., deciding what, when, and how to work and with which criteria)
4. Changing criteria, according with environmental changes
5. Using feedback at every stage and judging the whole process.

After Tom learned the steps of the strategy, he needed to apply them to different tasks and materials. Upon working on transferring of learned strategy, he worked at first with limited data and clear information, and then he enlarged it, by gradually adding more ambiguous information. He made a special effort to apply the strategies and exercises to mathematics, his domain of interest. It seemed that the general improvement resulted also in improvement of the mental slowness.

For approximately 4 months, Tom remained hospitalized, during which he received daily treatment. He showed marked improvement in both cognitive and language skills but only partially achieved the goals. His language improvement consisted of understanding better oral information, demonstrating an ability to express several words at a time (which made communication with him easier), and showing good ability to use gestures. Tom will need to continue speech therapy for a long time. Additionally, Tom improved in his cognitive skills, especially in thinking operations but still did not reach full ability (see the second LOTCA assessment, Figure 3-4). As expected, this improvement affected his ability in other functional areas and his mental speed. Upon discharge, as Tom was still young and work-eligible, he received an intensive plan for further treatment in the community.

4. An adolescent with learning difficulties

Mary is a 16-year-old high school student. The youngest of two, she has an older brother who

Figure 3-4

Case 3, LOTCA Performance

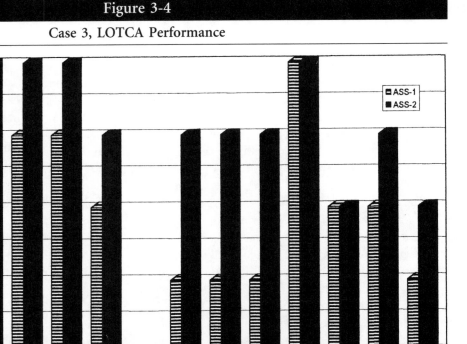

Visuomotor Organization
(Note: see abbreviations in Appendix)

Thinking Operations

is a student in computer engineering. Mary was considered to be a poor learner, and her parents, as well as her teachers, were discussing the possibility of interrupting her studies. To assist in the decision-making process, she received a battery of tests at school, including the Bender, the WISC-R, the WMS-R, perception tests, and specifically didactic tests. The results revealed that she was both functioning below her ability and lacking learning strategies. Overall, her abilities seemed to be average, showing better results on nonverbal tests than on verbal ones.

The school educational psychologist referred Mary for occupational therapy treatment. During the meeting, the psychologist emphasized that Mary showed an average cognitive ability and a poor prognosis for making significant progress at school, but a good prognosis for finishing high school before the age of army service. When discussing the possibility of professional school, Mary expressed no preference and appeared emotionally young in relation to her biological age.

Mary arrived at the first session with her mother. She was a tall, obese girl, who dressed in a plain and old-fashioned manner, and appeared clean but somehow neglected. She seemed shy and spoke only in response to others (i.e., typically, her mother did the talking). Her mother complained of low marks in all school subjects. She stated that the excessive study hours, which Mary spent learning with her parents, minimally affected her grades. The mother expressed feelings of being tired of tutoring, and that the circumstance frustrated the whole family. She seemed angry when discussing Mary's dependence, inability to take responsibility for her studies, and words of accusation against her parents for her failures. Throughout the conversation, Mary remained silent. In response to a direct question, if she agreed with her mother's description of the situation, she stated that her mother was probably correct and that her failures were a fact. When asked to state her favorite school subject, she answered: "I like literature, but only in class. I don't like reading."

With summertime as the deadline for goal completion, so that she would appear better prepared for school, Mary began treatment before the summer. During the first sessions, Mary seemed very passive but very attentive. She worked hard, showing motivation and determination. It quickly became obvious that she had no learning skills, and that she tried to memorize whatever she read, without any insight or comprehension into the material. She could not distinguish between main ideas and details, and she identified everything as consisting of the same level of importance. As for her ability to integrate or understand what she read, she could only tell the subject, in the same way she memorized it, and could not display any thinking process. Similarly, it was beyond her capacity to "read between the lines" or to draw conclusions. As an additional obstacle, her vocabulary was very dull. Her thinking process was on such a concrete level that she often misunderstood a given question or paragraph, and she could not grasp the concept that one word could have more than one meaning.

The first goal aimed at improving her thinking process. We began with the concept of categorization, working on locating the criteria for junking, and changing it according to different properties or needs. At the beginning, Mary experienced many difficulties. She became frustrated that she could not find more than one or two criteria for grouping, and that, through the session, she discovered numerous other possibilities. It was necessary to show her how to create the need for criteria, to analyze the properties of an object, and to make the applications. Frequently, Mary questioned, "Why do I need this? How is it going to help me with my studies?" Her questions revealed not only the need for developing her basic thinking process but the necessity for showing her what the applications include regarding the things we learned.

The treatment followed two parallel systems. The first system, which was remedial, addressed the thinking process in the following ways:

1. Detecting the attributes or properties of an object or group
2. Finding the hierarchical order of the attributes, according to the needs of the situation
3. Changing the criteria, according to different demands.

The second, which was functional, approached the subject of learning to apply the newly developed thinking skills to everyday situations, which in Mary's case entailed learning school material. In other words, the same schema that guided finding the criteria to categorize it should be applicable to any learning material. This method of learning allowed Mary to relate to both a greater amount and a greater level of abstractness, in reference to information.

Below is an example of steps that Mary needed to learn, in order to properly process an article:

1. Learn that the headings indicate the subject matter, and on this basis, develop expectations from the article
2. Form sets of questions and record them, so that the options of expectations are concrete and clear
3. Locate the answers to what was expected, during reading time
4. Determine which questions were irrelevant and which expectations did not fit, and replace them with others from the reading material
5. Write in a table format or as a list of main points, in reference to the important information located in the article, through paraphrasing the main ideas
6. Judge the importance of each main point of information and arrange them in hierarchical order.

This information processing demands from the learner exploratory work, judging and comparing, junking, and leaving details according to the material and need. This form of work maintains the attention and alertness of the learner and deepens the processing level, since, in every phase, the objectives change.

In Mary's case, we first applied the model with short, clear pieces of information (i.e., a sentence). Then we gradually expanded the amount of work to include a paragraph, a short story, and finally, a whole article. As we applied the strategies with different subjects and learning materials, Mary's repertoire of learning strategies gradually increased in both quantity and quality, and she began to work with more difficult and abstract material. With time and experience, she internalized the process and worked more independently. The next step involved guiding her to work with complicated examination questions, to detail them, and to decipher the main questions and determine the supporting information needed. In time, through hard work at home and attempts to apply what she gained in treatment, Mary progressed significantly. When school began, she appeared more relaxed and less frightened, and, finally, she knew what to do. For the first time she realized that she had meaningful things to say and that she knew how to say them, and she began to participate. Her teachers reported good and encouraging feedback. We continued to meet each week, mainly to provide her with support. When the exam period began, Mary expressed feeling excited but capable. She felt that this would be an ultimate and real experience. For the first time, she demonstrated confidence in her ability to cope alone and that she did not need to ask for assistance from her parents. The results on her examinations, including those in mathematics and geography, which we never addressed with her, were significantly better. Finally, we observed ultimate proof that she really internalized the whole process and that she was able to transfer and apply it when needed.

Gradually, we reduced our meetings to once a month or to when Mary felt the need to see me. At the end of the semester, Mary passed all of her exams with B and A marks, and by the end of the year, she earned only As. The process not only affected her learning abilities, although that was our focus in treatment, but also developed a more positive and confident attitude in her. She cut her hair in a more fashionable way and paid more attention to her attire. At school, she began to approach students. Sometimes, when she felt rejected, she raised the issues at our meeting, in order to understand and cope with her stress, thus showing improvement over her previous behavior of running away from the event. When she finished the year, she expressed feeling strong and ready for an upcoming students' trip abroad. Mary is an example of how, through the provision of the right tools and support and encouragement, the cognitive model positively influences one's level of studies as well as all aspects of life.

Implications for Further Knowledge Development

The cognitive approach presented in this chapter centers around clinical practice. The development of it followed a pass of practice to theory to research and back to practice. The starting point was the observation of TBI clients' performance whose major dysfunction appeared in the area of cognitive deficits and their influence on function. Despite the assumption that the retraining approach enlarges the functional schemes and as such may generalize to all functional areas, an adaptive approach accompanies the whole treatment process: applying learned strategies to actual everyday activities.

Further knowledge development through research studies of treatment effectiveness is needed. As reported in the evaluation section, numerous studies have been conducted to determine reliability and validity of the assessment instruments, their cross-cultural applicability, and further development and adaptation to different age populations (e.g., elderly, children). However, we are now at a point where outcome studies and treatment effectiveness are essential.

References

Abreu, B. C., & Toglia, J. P. (1987). Cognitive rehabilitation: A model for occupational therapy. *American Journal of Occupational Therapy, 41,* 439–453.

Allen, C. K. (1985). *Occupational therapy for psychiatric diseases: Measurement and management of cognitive disabilities.* Boston: Little, Brown.

Annes, G., Katz, N., & Cermak, S. A. (1996). Comparison of younger and older healthy adults on the Loewenstein Occupational Therapy Cognitive Assessment. *Occupational Therapy International, 3,* 157–173.

Averbuch, S., & Katz, N. (1991). Age level standards of the Loewenstein Occupational Therapy Cognitive Assessment (LOTCA). *Israeli Journal of Occupational Therapy, 1,* E1–15.

Bernspang, B., Viitanen, M., & Eriksson, S. (1989). Impairments of perceptual and motor functions: Their influence on self-care ability 4 to 6 years after a stroke. *Occupational Therapy Journal of Research, 9,* 27–37.

Bourne, L. E., Dominski, R. L., & Loftus, E. F. (1979). *Cognitive processes.* Englewood Cliffs, NJ: Prentice-Hall.

Braitenberg, V. (1978). Cortical architectonic: General and areal. In M. A. Brazier & H. Petsche (Eds.), *Architectonics of the cerebral cortex*. New York: Raven Press.

Cermak, S. A., & Hausser, J. (1989). The Behavioral Inattention Test for Unilateral Visual Neglect: A critical review. *Physical and Occupational Therapy in Geriatrics, 7* (3), 43–53.

Cermak, S. A., Katz, N., McGuire, E., Greenbaum, S., Peralta, C., & Maser-Flanagan, V. (1995). Performance of Americans and Israelis with cerebrovascular accident on the Loewenstein Occupational Therapy Cognitive Assessment (LOTCA*). American Journal of Occupational Therapy, 49,* 500–506.

Cockburn, J., & Smith, T. P. (1989). *The Rivermead Behavioral Memory Test,* Supplement 3: Elderly people. Titchfield: Thames Valley Test Company.

COGNISTAT, *The Neurobehavioral Cognitive Status Examination Manual* (1995). Fairfax, CA: Northern California Neurobehavioral Group.

Elazar, B., Itzkovich, M., & Katz, N. (1996). *LOTCA-G Manual.* Pequannock, NJ: Maddak.

Giles, G. M., & Clark-Wilson, J. (1988). The use of behavioral techniques in functional skills training after severe brain injury. *American Journal of Occupational Therapy, 42,* 658–665.

Ginsburg, H., & Opper, S. (1979). *Piaget's theory of intellectual development.* Englewood Cliffs, NJ: Prentice-Hall.

Goldberg, S., & Katz, N. (1994). The validity of the Rivermead Behavioral Memory Test for assessing everyday memory of elderly Israeli CVA clients and a normal control group. *Israeli Journal of Occupational Therapy, 3,* H149–168.

Golden, C. J. (1984). Rehabilitation and the Luria-Nebraska Neuropsychological Battery. In B. A. Edelstein & E. T. Couture (Eds.), *Behavioral assessment and rehabilitation of the traumaticaly brain-damaged.* New York: Plenum Press.

Granger, C. V., Cotter, A. C., Hamilton, B. B., & Fiedler, R. C. (1993). Functional assessment scales: A study of persons after stroke. *Archives of Physical Medicine and Rehabilitation, 74,* 133–138.

Halligan, P. W., Cockburn, J., & Wilson, B. A. (1991). The behavioural assessment of visual neglect. *Neuropsychological Rehabilitation, 1,* 5–32.

Hartman-Maeir, A., & Katz, N. (1995). Validity of the Behavioral Inattention Test (BIT): Relationships with functional tasks. *American Journal of Occupational Therapy, 49,* 507–516.

Hooffien, D. (1987). Rehabilitation of Attention. In A. Mazzucchi (Ed.), *Neuropsychological rehabilitation*. Bologna Italy: Il Mulino.

Inhelder, B., & Piaget, J. (1964). *The early growth of logic in the child.* New York: Morton.

Itzkovich, M., Elazar, B. Averbuch, S., & Katz, N. (1990). *LOTCA Manual.* NJ: Maddak.

Katz, N. (1985). Occupational therapy's domain of concern: Reconsidered. *American Journal of Occupational Therapy, 39,* 518–524.

Katz, N. (1992). *Cognitive rehabilitation: Models of intervention in occupational therapy.* Stoneham, MA: Butterworth-Heinemann.

Katz, N. (1994). Cognitive rehabilitation: Models for intervention and research on cognition in occupational therapy. *Occupational Therapy International, 1,* 34–48.

Katz, N., Champagne, D., & Cermak, S. A. (1997). Comparison of younger and older adults on three versions of a puzzle reproduction task. *American Journal of Occupational Therapy, 51,* 562–568.

Katz, N., Elazar, B., & Itzkovich, M. (1995). Construct validity of a geriatric version of the Loewenstein Occupational Therapy Cognitive Assessment (LOTCA) Battery. *Physical & Occupational Therapy in Geriatrics, 13,* 31–45.

Katz, N., Elazar, B., & Itzkovitch, M. (1996). Validity of the Neurobehavioral Cognitive Status Examination (Cognistat) in assessing clients post CVA and healthy elderly in Israel. *Israeli Journal of Occupational Therapy, 5,* E185–198.

Katz, N., Elazar, B., Itzkovitch, M., Ring H., & Soroker, N. (May 1996). Paper presented at the First Mediterranean Congress of Physical Medicine and Rehabilitation, Herziliya, Israel.

Katz, Hartman-Maeir, Weiss, & Armon. (1997). *Neuro-Rehabilitation, 9,* 179–186.

Katz, N., Hefner, D., & Rueben, R. (1990). Measuring clinical change in cognitive rehabilitation of clients with brain damage: Two cases, traumatic brain injury and cerebral vascular accident. *Occupational Therapy in Health Care, 7,* 23–43.

Katz, N., & Heimann, N. (1990). Review of research conducted in Israel on cognitive disability instrumentation. *Occupational Therapy in Mental Health, 10,* 1–15.

Katz, N., Itzkovich, M., Averbuch, S., & Elazar, B. (1989). Loewenstein Occupational Therapy Cognitive Assessment (LOTCA), battery for brain injured clients: Reliability and validity. *American Journal of Occupational Therapy, 43,* 184–192.

Katz, N., Weiss, P., Armon, N., & Hartman-Maeir, A. (1997). Comparison of cognitive status profiles of healthy elderly, persons with dementia and neurosurgical patients using the Neurobehavioral Cognitive Status Examination. *Neuro-Rehabilitation, 9,* 179–186.

Kielhofner, G. (Ed.). (1995). *A model of human occupation* (2nd ed.). Baltimore: Williams & Wilkins.

Lezak, M. (1995). *Neuropsychological assessmen* (3rd ed.). New York: Oxford University Press.

Lidz, C. S. (1987). *Dynamic assessment.* New York: Guilford Press.

Logue, P. E., Tupler, L. A., D'amico, C., & Schmitt, F. A. (1993). The Neurobehavioral Cognitive Status Examination: Psychometric properties in use with psychiatric inclients. *Journal of Clinical Psychology, 49,* 80–89.

Luria, A. R. (1973). *The working brain.* England: Penguin Books.

Luria, A. R. (1980). *Higher cortical functions in man.* New York: Basic Books.

Mosey, A. C. (1986). *Psychosocial components of occupational therapy.* New York: Raven Press.

Mysiw, W. J., Beegan, J. G., & Gatens, P. F. (1989). Prospective cognitive assessment of stroke clients before inpatient rehabilitation. *American Journal of Physical Medicine & Rehabilitation, 68,* 168–171.

Najenson, T., Rahmani, L., Elazar, B., & Averbuch, S. (1984). An elementary cognitive assessment and treatment of the craniocerebrally injured client. In B. A. Edelstein & E. T. Couture (Eds.). *Behavioral assessment and rehabilitation of the traumatically brain-damaged.* New York: Plenum Press.

Neistadt, M. E. (1988). Occupational therapy for adults with perceptual deficits. *American Journal of Occupational Therapy, 42,* 434–440.

Neistadt, M. E. (1990). A critical analysis of occupational therapy approaches for perceptual deficits in adult with brain injury. *American Journal of Occupational Therapy, 44,* 299–304.

Neistadt, M. E. (1992). The Rabideau Kitchen Evaluation-Revised: An assessment of meal preparation skill. *The Occupational Therapy Journal of Research, 12,* 242–253.

Neisser, U. (1976). *Cognition and reality.* New York: W. H. Freeman.

Osmon, D. C., Smet, I. C., Winegarden, B., & Gandhavadi, B. (1992). Neurobehavioral Cognitive Status Examination: Its use with unilateral stroke clients in a rehabilitation setting. *Archives of Physical Medicine, 73,* 414–418.

Paivio, A. (1975). Perceptual comparisons through the mind's eye. *Memory and Cognition, 3,* 635–647.

Pedretti, L. W. (1985). *Occupational therapy practice skills for physical dysfunction* (2nd ed.). St. Louis: Mosby.

Rahmani, L. (1982). The intellectual rehabilitation of brain-damaged clients. *Clinical Neuropsychology, 4,* 44–45.

Rahmani, L. (1987). Neuro-cognitive theory and the intellectual rehabilitation of brain damaged clients: An introduction. Unpublished paper.

Rahmani, L., Geva, N., Rochberg, J., Trope, I., & Bore, B. (1987). Issues in neurocognitive assessment and treatment. In E. Vakil, D. Hoofien, & Z. Groswasser, *Rehabilitation of the brain injured.* London: Freund.

Rosch, E. (1978). Principles of categorization. In E. Rosch & B. Lloyed (Eds). *Cognition and categorization.* Hillsdale, NJ: Erlbaum.

Rosch, E., & Mervis, C.B. (1975). Family resemblances: Studies in the internal structure of categories. *Cognitive Psychology, 7,* 573–605.

Schwamm, L. H., Van Dyke, C., Kierman, R. J., Merrin, E. L., & Mueller, J. (1987). The Neurobehavioral Cognitive Status Examination: Comparison with the cognitive capacity screening examination and the Mini-Mental State Examination in a neurosurgical population. *Annals of International Medicine, 107,* 486–490.

Shiel, A., & Wilson, B. A. (1992). The relationship between unilateral neglect and dependence in activities of daily living. Paper presented at the European Occupational Therapy Conference, Dublin, Ireland.

Shiffrin, R. M., & Schneider, W. (1977). Controlled and automatic human information processing: II-Perceptual learning, automatic attending: A general theory. *Psychological review, 84,* 127–190.

Toglia, J. P. (1992). A dynamic interactional approach to cognitive rehabilitation. In N. Katz, *Cognitive rehabilitation: Models of intervention in occupational therapy.* Stoneham, MA: Butterworth-Hienemann.

Toglia, J. P. (1994). *Toglia Categorization Assessment (TCA).* Pequannock, NJ: Maddak.

Vygotsky, L. S. (1962). *Thought & language.* Cambridge: MIT Press.

Wall, C., Wilson, B. A., & Baddeley, A. D. (1994). The Extended Rivermead Behavioral Memory Test: A measure of everyday memory performance in normal adults. *Memory, 2,* 149–166.

Wechsler, D. (1981). Wechsler Adult Intelligence Scale. New York: Psychological Corporation.

Weiss, P. (1994). The occupational therapist's role in assessment of clients with suspected normal pressure hydrocephalus as predictore of good shunt outcome. *Israeli Journal of Occupational Therapy, 3,* E33–E42.

Wilson, B., Cockburn, J., & Baddeley, A. (1985). *The Rivermead Behavioral Memory Test Manual.* London: Thames Valley.

Wilson, B., Cockburn, J., & Baddeley, A. (1986). *The Rivermead Behavioral Memory Test.* Second supplement. London: Thames Valley.

Wilson, B. A., Cockburn, J., & Halligan, P. W. (1987a). *Behavioural Inattention Test Manual.* Fareham, Hants, England: Thames Valley.

Wilson, B. A., Cockburn, J., & Halligan, P. W. (1987b). Development of a behavioral test of visuospatial neglect. *Archives of Physical Medicine and Rehabilitation, 68,* 98–102.

LOTCA Battery - Revised Scoring sheet
(circle the appropriate number)

SUB-TESTS		SCORE								COMMENTS
		low				high				
ORIENTATION										
Time	OT	1	2	3	4	5	6	7	8	
Place	OP	1	2	3	4	5	6	7	8	
VISUAL PERCEPTION										
Object Identification	OI	1		2		3		4		
Shape Identification	SI	1		2		3		4		
Overlapping Figures	OF	1		2		3		4		
Object Constancy	OC	1		2		3		4		
SPATIAL PERCEPTION										
Directions on Ps' Body	SP1	1		2		3		4		
Spatial Relations	SP2	1		2		3		4		
Spatial Relations on Picture	SP3	1		2		3		4		
PRAXIS										
Motor Imitation	P1	1		2		3		4		
Utilization of Objects	P2	1		2		3		4		
Symbolic Actions	P3	1		2		3		4		
VISUOMOTOR ORGANIZATION										
Copying Geometric Forms	GF	1		2		3		4		
Two-Dimensional Model	TM	1		2		3		4		
Pegboard Construction	PG	1		2		3		4		
Colored Block-Design	CB	1		2		3		4		
Plain Block-Design	PB	1		2		3		4		
Puzzle	PZ	1		2		3		4		
Drawing a Clock	CK	1		2		3		4		
THINKING OPERATIONS										
Categorization	CA	1		2	3		4		5	
ROC Unstructered	RU	1		2	3		4		5	
ROC Structered	RS	1		2	3		4		5	
Pictorial Sequence A	PS1	1		2		3		4		
Pictorial Sequence B	PS2	1		2		3		4		
Geometric Sequence	GS	1		2		3		4		
Logic Questions	LQ	1		2		3		4		
ATTENTION AND CONCENTRATION		1		2		3		4		
Indicate: Length of time:										
Assessment was performed in:		☒ one session					☒ two sessions or more			

CHAPTER 4

A Neurofunctional Approach to Rehabilitation Following Severe Brain Injury

Gordon Muir Giles, MA, DipCot, OTR

This chapter describes a neurofunctional approach to rehabilitation of patients following severe central nervous system trauma (Giles & Clark-Wilson, 1993; Yuen, 1994). The approach was developed to be applicable to persons with acquired neurological impairments that affect cognitive functioning, including individuals with traumatic brain injury (penetrating/nonpenetrating, focal/diffuse), anoxic damage (and other neurochemical imbalances or poisonings causing neurological damage, e.g., carbon monoxide poisoning), infections (e.g., encephalitis, meningitis), some types of vascular events (e.g., aneurysms), and some types of cerebrovascular accidents. The World Health Organization has advanced a tripartite classification of dysfunction, comprising impairment, disability, and handicap; the approach described in this chapter emphasizes the reduction of disability and handicap (WHO, 1980). The neurofunctional approach considers the constraints placed on the person's functioning by the nature of the injury. In addition, the approach considers evidence from cognitive neuroscience and learning theory in the design and implementation of retraining programs. Although the approach addresses cognitive functioning, its focus is not the retraining of cognitive processes (componant areas) but the retraining of real world skills (performance areas).

Rationale

Most people recover following acute neurological damage. The rapid nature of the early improvement implicates a neurophysiological process or processes, other than learning. Although the cause of the recovery is unknown, therapists have attempted to potentiate the process by stimulating the patient. In the early acute period coma stimulation is viewed as an important component of treatment by many therapists (Giles & Clark-Wilson, 1993). In later stages of recovery occupational therapists have attempted to stimulate patients by the use of tasks of graded difficulty. Hierarchies in various cognitive, behavioral, and physical domains have been constructed, and therapists attempt to help patients progress through these (Soderback & Normell, 1986a; 1986b). It has been suggested that the earlier a patient can be exposed to rehabilitation, the greater the recovery (Cope & Hall, 1982). Acute rehabilitation could have an effect both on the rapidity of improvement and on its overall extent. Alternatively, it could alter the slope of recovery but not the ultimate level of outcome. Of course, it could also have neither effect. Accelerated improvement—whether or not it has durable effects—could result in the patient leaving the hospital earlier and suffering fewer medical and psychological complications. There would be considerable cost savings. Animal models of recovery from neurological trauma suggest that there is considerable effect of early physical intervention. In a comparison of early and late motor "rehabilitation" in monkeys, delayed intervention resulted in more rapid improvement, but the ultimate level of recovery of the early rehabilitation group was never achieved (Black, Markowitz, & Cianci, 1975). There have been no animal studies directly supporting a comparable effect for cognitive functions. Attempts to study the benefits of early intervention on human subjects (Cope & Hall, 1982; Mackay, Bernstein, Chapman, Morgan, & Milazzo, 1992) have been so complicated by methodological difficulties that results have been difficult to interpret (Giles & Clark-Wilson, 1993). There are, however, reports of patients removed from nursing homes and admitted to rehabilitation facilities whose rapid improvement suggests that some stimulation is necessary to ensure that patients function up to the level permitted by their neurological recovery (Shaw, Brodsky, & McMahon, 1985; Bell & Tallman, 1995). There is no evidence that one specific form of interaction has a greater effect than another at this early stage on potentiating recovery.

In the postacute recovery period, therapists have also attempted to directly address the cognitive substrata of perception, attention, memory, judgment, reasoning, and so on. The advantage of these basic cognitive interventions, were they to be effective, would be the "trickle down" effect that improvement in basic cognitive skills would have on all aspects of the person's functioning. For example, improved attention would improve the ability to keep track of ongoing events, work performance, etc. The disadvantage of attempting to remediate basic cognitive functioning is that this type of intervention is of unproved efficacy, so that time and effort may be devoted to a pointless task and result in no functional improvement.

Instead of addressing basic cognitive deficits some therapists have attempted to train brain-injured patients in compensatory approaches to specific deficits (Wilson & Moffat, 1984). Unfortunately patients are often taught techniques without adequate consideration being given to whether the likely improvement in quality of life warrants the effort required to learn them. Patients must be able to transfer a compensatory strategy to novel situations encountered in the real world. Brain-injured individuals can often learn strategies but be unable to apply them. Compensatory behaviors that are most successful are those that the individual may overlearn to the point of automaticity. Compensatory techniques that remain effortful despite overlearning (such as visualization strategies in memory retraining) are usually too demanding to be used outside the training sessions.

As an alternative to the above techniques specific task approaches train people to perform a specific functional behavior. In specific task training the therapist attempts to teach an actual functional task. The intervention may or may not involve task-specific compensatory training. (For example, a hemianopic patient who is being taught to cross the street may be trained to overcompensate by turning the head to the left.) Using the terminology of the World Health Organization (WHO, 1980) the intention is to reduce disability or handicap. Task-specific training is the essence of the neurofunctional approach, but it also includes other important features. The intervention must address a behavior of clinical importance and to an extent that makes a real difference. In most cases training must be complete enough to be self-sustaining (i.e., used spontaneously and habitually) by the time the patient is discharged from the treatment setting. Training should be attempted in the same way across domains so that only a limited amount of new learning is required. Patients may then be able to generalize skills learned in one setting to other settings. Events that occur in the environment, which precede a behavior, are recognized as important in affecting the likelihood that a behavior will occur. Therapists should consider the stimulus demands of the environment when developing retraining programs. An emphasis is placed on metacognitive functions so that the individual can use retained executive skills to compensate for basic process deficits. By addressing basic skills we may be able to improve patient insight, mental efficiency, and organization, resulting in continued cognitive improvements. Evidence is reviewed below that suggests that functional improvements may continue in patients provided with functional retraining following the cessation of the program itself. In this sense the neurofunctional approach is a bottom-up rather than a top-down approach.

Theoretical Base

Neurofunctional retraining must consider the person's learning characteristics in the design and implementation of programs. Since memory, attention, and frontal lobe impairments are central to many patients' problems, these areas must be considered in the development of retraining programs.

They are not here considered as areas to be treated directly but only instrumentally in the design of functional skills programs. A theoretical framework for considering these deficits will be discussed before an outline of a system of neurofunctional retraining is described.

Memory

Memory can be conceptualized under the headings declarative and nondeclarative. Declarative memory is available to introspection and may be divided into semantic and episodic subtypes. Episodic memory is information about temporally dated events and the temporal-spatial relations between these events. It refers to "historical" information specific to the individual. Semantic memory is organized knowledge about the world, which is not tied to context (it includes the majority of information learned in institutional education, e.g., scientific facts and historical dates) (Tulving, 1972). Tulving (1983) maintains that the retrieval of information (from the episodic or semantic memory systems) constitutes an episode. One implication of this theory is that the act of remembering is recorded in the episodic memory store, thus changing its overall contents. Episodic memory is the most vulnerable to impairment. Though deficits in acquiring new semantic information probably occur in tandem with episodic memory deficits, semantic memory stores may still be accessed and learning may take place via frequent repetition of to-be-remembered information.

Nondeclarative memory (also called procedural learning) can be thought of as the store of acquired patterns of behavior not necessarily mediated by cognitive learning. Nondeclarative "knowledge" is not available to introspection; information is accessed through performance. Learning may occur without the subject being aware that learning has taken place. Nissen and Bullemer (1987) examined the attentional requirements of procedural learning to determine whether attention is necessary for procedural learning as it is for introspectively available forms of knowledge acquisition. A computerized serial reaction time task was used. A light appeared at one of four locations. Subjects pressed one key out of a set of four located directly below the position of the light. Learning was evaluated

by measuring facilitation of performance on a repeating 10-trial stimulus sequence to which the subjects were naive. In nonneurologically impaired subjects there was considerable improvement in performance when this was the only task. However, when given in a dual-task condition (a condition reducing the subject's ability to attend to the task), learning of the sequence, as assessed by verbal report and performance measures, was minimal. Patients with Korsakoff's syndrome were also able to learn the sequence in the single task condition despite their lack of awareness of the repeating pattern. Nissen and Bullemer (1987) conclude that improved performance in the task, which is dependent on procedural memory, required the subject to attend to it.

There is increasing interest in the role of nondeclarative memory in the acquisition of complex behaviors. Lewicki and coworkers in a series of experiments (Lewicki, Czyzenska, & Hoffman, 1987; Lewicki, Hill, & Bizot, 1988) have examined the ability of individuals to acquire relatively complex nondeclarative knowledge. Results confirmed that nonconsciously acquired knowledge can be utilized to facilitate performance, but of particular note in the reports of Lewicki and colleagues (1987, 1988) is the extreme complexity of the tasks employed. Although the skill acquisition is likely to be via nondeclarative learning, the tasks were far more complex than those normally thought to be subserved by this memory system.

An alternative model of memory functioning that regards memory as a property of systems has been proposed by Fuster (1995). In this theory a memory is a network of neocortical neurons and the connections that link them. The network is formed by experience as a result of the concurrent activation of neuronal ensembles that represent diverse aspects of the internal and external environment and of motor action. Networks are modified by experience. Memory is regarded as a functional property of all areas of the cerebral cortex. Memory is one aspect of perceiving, acting, and representing. Cortical areas have different functions and therefore different types of memory. Also memory has active and inactive states (attention). All memory is seen as essentially associative, with short- and long-term memory having the same underlying mechanism. Memory is global and nonlocalizable. One implication of this view is that memory is not subserved by anatomically discrete systems but that different types of memory functioning are the result of differential involvement of anatomically localized components of the memory process.

One possibility is that the establishment of episodic memories, i.e., memories that have specific temporal and sensory attributes, requires the participation of the hippocampus as well as other neocortical areas in the storage process. In some cases patients with severe memory impairments may by frequent repetition of material access the declarative memory system; that is, the patient can learn and describe their knowledge, if the information is repeated frequently enough. However, this material is without specific temporal or sensory provenance. The frequent repetition of material may allow for the development of cortical connections robust enough to allow "spontaneous" availability without the participation of the hippocampus. For example, the patient described in the Case Example below was taught to wash and dress in a novel way despite amnesia following herpes simplex encephalitis. At 3 months post training the patient continued to use the novel washing and dressing procedure independently and could state the new order of washing and dressing behaviors. However, when questioned about the retraining program, which he had participated in for 20 minutes morning and evening for over 3 months, he had no recollection of it, claiming simply that he had "always washed and dressed this way."

Attention

Increased understanding of attention as a set of complex interrelated processes may help clarify how voluntary control is exerted over more automatic processes. Posner and Peterson (1990) highlight three principles central to the understanding of attention: (1) that the attentional system is separate from the more basic systems to which attention is allocated, (2) that the attentional system depends on the interaction of different anatomical areas, and (3) that the areas involved in attention are specific and distinct from one another and the rest of the brain (i.e., that attention is neither the property of a single center nor a property of the brain as a whole). Posner and Peterson describe three attentional processes with their anatomical locations: orienting, target detection, and tonic arousal. The ability to orient to visual stimuli in space is associated with the posterior parietal lobe, thalamic nuclei, and the superior colliculus. Target detection (and response activation) appears to be associated with midline frontal areas, including the anterior cingulate gyrus and supplementary motor area. Damage to medial prefrontal structures tends to diminish both the speed and the amount of human activity. The medial sagittal areas are also part of a system that includes brain stem structures that are responsible for tonic arousal. Tonic arousal appears to be subserved by pathways originating in the locus coeruleus and terminating in frontal areas with the function lateralized to the right.

The distinction between conscious and automatic processes may reflect the participation of different neural mechanisms subserved by different neuroanatomical systems. The participation of the attentional system in conscious processing may be analogous to the functioning of midline temporal structures in the declarative memory system. Many of the cognitive processes that may be disrupted following brain injury may be attributed to deficits in attention.

Automatic and Controlled Processing

Shiffrin and Schneider (1977) describe attention in terms of attention-dependent controlled processing and attention-independent automatic processing. Controlled processing is capacity limited and is required for new learning to occur. During the learning phase of an activity, the unskilled individual relies heavily on feedback about performance and devotes conscious attention to the activity (controlled processing). This focused attention continues during the practice stage of response acquisition. Once the action is learned, the individual's performance is controlled by a series of "prearranged instruction sequences" that act independently of feedback (automatic processing), leaving the individual free to concentrate on other aspects of the same or different tasks. Automatic processing occurs without conscious control and places only limited demands on the information processing system. Observations of individuals following severe brain injury suggest that activities that were previously automatic are disrupted by brain injury. Levin, Goldstein, High, and Williams (1988) administered free recall and frequency of occurrence tasks to patients with severe brain injury and a control group. In their first experiment, Levin et al. (1988) found that both free recall (an effortful task) and judgment of relative frequency of occurrence (an automatic task) were impaired in 15 brain-injured patients relative to a control group. In a second experiment, the authors corroborated this finding and showed that estimates of frequency were also impaired in a different groups of 16 brain-injured patients. Shiffrin and Schneider (1977) have described two types of attentional system break down: divided attentional deficits and focused attentional deficits.

Divided Attentional Deficit

A divided attentional deficit (DAD) indicates a failure of the capacity limited attentional system to accommodate all the information necessary for optimum task performance (Schneider, Dumais, & Shiffrin, 1984). For example, in gait retraining a patient may be able to ambulate with standby assistance, unless a person walks across his or her visual field or says "good morning," whereupon the patient loses balance. This failure constitutes a divided attentional deficit, because the patient had insufficient attentional capacity to walk and attend to any other information. Stuss, Stethem, Hugenholtz, Picton, Pivik, and Richards (1989) confirmed the existence of DAD among brain-injured patients using a complex reaction time task. Patients are slow in tasks that require consciously controlled information processing and demonstrate an inability to process multiple pieces of information rapidly. Stuss et al. (1989) found this to be so even of mildly injured patients.

Focused Attentional Deficit

A focused attentional deficit (FAD) typically occurs when an unfamiliar response is required to a stimu-

lus, which already has an overlearned response linked to it (Schneider, Dumais, & Shiffrin 1984). Continuous attention from the individual may be required to suppress this automatic behavior. Stuss et al. (1989) developed a series of computer tasks designed to assess focused attentional deficits; the central feature of the FAD to be analyzed was the inability to suppress a previously learned complex level of processing when a simpler level of processing was demanded. A complex reaction time computer program task that required multiple discrimination (shape, internal line orientation, color) was followed by a task, the outward appearance of which was identical to this complex task but which required a far less complex level of discrimination. Although both patients and controls were informed of the change, the patients were less able than the controls to inhibit the processing of redundant information.

Selectivity

Task performance is influenced by the presence of competing attentional demands (Kewman, Yanus, & Kirsch, 1988). The ability to selectively attend depends on discriminating task-relevant information from background stimuli. For example, following traumatic brain injury, individuals have difficulty in filtering out distracting verbal information from relevant verbal information (Kewman, Yanus, & Kirsch, 1988). Part of the difficulty in maintaining selective attention may be due to an inability to suppress responses to novel or irrelevant stimuli. As a task is practiced, novel and irrelevant stimuli become less distracting as the individual habituates to them (Lorch, Anderson, & Well, 1984). In Solokov's view (1963) habituation occurs because repeated presentation allows the individual to construct a mental representation of the irrelevant stimuli as irrelevant. There is no evidence, however, to suggest that generalization of the habituation process occurs.

Alternating Attention

The ability to alternate attention in rapid succession between tasks is an important attentional capacity. The ability to suppress a response tendency and shift sets is an ability that can be disrupted by frontal lobe impairment.

Frontal Lobe Functions

Below we describe some important functions of the frontal lobes that may interact with basic cognitive deficits and that may result in impaired functional skills.

Planning and Initiation

Many individuals with frontal brain damage appear not to prepare responses. Freedman, Bleiberg, and Freedland (1987) examined the ability of persons with brain injury to forward plan, using a conditioning paradigm (a shuttlebox-analog avoidance task). When compared to a group of patients after a cerebrovascular accident, the brain-injured patients demonstrated greater anticipatory behavior deficits despite the fact that the two groups did not differ on escape behavior, and that the closed brain-injured group was equivalent or better on performance of individual tests of the Halstead-Reitan Battery and Wechsler scales. Neither clarification of the instruction, additional trials, nor enhancement of the warning cue appeared to ameliorate the anticipatory behavior deficit. The authors suggested that patients with anticipatory behavior deficits would show deficits in situations where current behavior should be regulated on the basis of expected future consequences. Vilkki (1988), using a task similar to the token test but with more ambiguity, found that patients with frontal lobe deficits fail to identify the appropriate categories for sorting. Cicerone, Lazar, and Shapiro (1983) found that subjects with frontal lobe lesions failed to systematically explore a hypothesis (general concept formation) and failed to discard inappropriate hypotheses. Shallice and Evans (1978) noticed that many of their patients with frontal lobe impairment demonstrated a gross inability to produce adequate cognitive estimates. The authors asked the patients questions that tapped areas of knowledge that most people possess but that require material to be accessed and manipulated in novel ways. Answering such questions adequately involves the selection of an appropriate plan to answer the question and check possible answers mentally for error. Examples of the questions included "On average how many TV programs are shown on one TV channel between 6:00 p.m. and 11:00 p.m.?" and "What is the length of an average man's spine?" In the latter question, one must compare the spontaneous estimate of an average person's height with the percentage of an individual's height accounted for by the spine. The patients with anterior lesions performed considerably worse than either the patients with posterior lesions or the normal controls. The authors interpret this finding as a deficit in planning and checking answers against multiple types of data for bizarreness and inconsistency.

Persons with brain injury may not engage in the internal behaviors necessary for planning and subsequently executing complex dependent action sequences. In order for a person to carry out complex behaviors that require the initiation of novel behaviors through time, it is necessary to develop a plan and then initiate a check act/wait cycle (Reason, 1984). Once the plan is developed, the individual compares plan time with real time in order to determine whether he or she needs to initiate a plan component or to wait. For example, to get to an appointment 45 minutes across town, a person intermittently checks the time throughout the day. Each time the individual looks at the clock he or she decides whether to leave or wait. As the time for leaving approaches, the person looks at the clock with greater frequency and also begins to adjust other activities so as to leave on time. Many patients, particularly whose with marked frontal lobe impairment, appear unable to initiate this type of planning behavior. They do not develop action plans or the "drive" required for the check act/wait cycles. The present author found it particularly instructive to observe some severely injured patients doing their laundry. Many of these patients were unable to check to see if their laundry was dry. The absence of checking could not be accounted for by memory impairment (the patients when questioned were aware that their clothes were in the dryer) nor by lack of knowledge about the laundry procedures involved, nor by lack of motivation. The patients nonetheless required an external cue to enable them to initiate the behavior. Many therapists attempt to have patients practice problem solving and reasoning to overcome these deficits. However, the patient is unable to spontaneously develop and monitor a novel dependent sequence of actions. Rather than have patients attempt to improve their responses to novelty, an alternative approach is to have patients overlearn needed behavioral sequences. Some types of novelty can be accommodated by training patients in metacognitive control strategies such as the use of a diary or other form of external memory aid (Giles & Shore, 1989b; Giles & Clark-Wilson, 1993). However, patients must have adequate self-awareness and adequate metacognitive control. The overlearning of the metacognitive control strategy must also be part of the training.

Self-Awareness

The term anosagnosia was initially used to describe denial of left hemiplegia and has since been extended to include many types of failure to understand current limitations. Various theories have been proposed to explain the clinically observable phenomena but do not capture the full range of patient behaviors, suggesting that they are not completely adequate. The more concrete the limitations, the more likely they are to be recognized by the person. Individuals who are unaware of motor deficits are unaware of cognitive deficits, but the reverse is not the case. Motor deficits are more concrete and have more direct perceptual salience.

Individuals develop a sense of self over time, and it may be this sense of self that remains stable despite the changes produced by the brain injury. A combination of deficits of attention, memory impairment, and impairments in the integration of the new information into a revised view of "self" may result in what we as clinicians experience as denial. It is also probable that the patient may refuse to believe that new information presented about the patient's "new self" is accurate, preferring to utilize more conventional explanations

from his or her previous (nonneurologically impaired) life. Some researchers suggest that there is a distinction between motivated lack of awareness and organic lack of awareness (see, e.g., McGlynn & Schacter, 1989). However, the current author views the two types of denial as overlapping and not mutually exclusive phenomena. A complete description of this theoretically position is to appear elsewhere (Giles, in preparation). Admission of errors in activities that should clearly be within the individual's capability is an embarrassment, and patients may believe that what they are being told about their own performance cannot be true. That this part of the response is a ubiquitous human phenomenon rather than a neurological deficit is demonstrated by this response style being common among a patient's family members.

Metacognitive Functioning

The term metacognition has been used to describe a person's understanding and use of his or her own basic cognitive and perceptual processes. Nelson and Narens (1994) describe a two-level, two-process model of cognitive functioning. The two levels are the basic object level and the metalevel, and the two processes are monitoring in which the flow of information is from the object level to the metalevel and the control in which the flow of information is from the metalevel to the object level. Contained within the metalevel is a model of how the object level works. The model is necessarily imperfect. If, following brain damage, there is no change in the model of object level functioning, then the individual will have no ability to adjust control functions to compensate for the impairment. A readjustment of the model would, however, give the patient the opportunity to engage in new object level regulatory behaviors that could improve performance.

The patient's memory, attentional skills, and frontal lobe functioning constrain the types of interventions the patient can make use of. These limitations can be considered constraints on learning imposed by the injury. The neurofunctional approach considers these contraints in the development of retraining programs.

Intervention

Severe brain injury often results in the loss or disruption of patterns of adaptive behavior. Additionally the individual's ability to reacquire adaptive patterns of behavior is impaired. The frequency of disruption of basic self-care skills has been estimated at 5 to 15% (Jennett & Teasdale, 1981; Jacobs, 1988). Disruption of more complex self-care skills appears to be more common (Jacobs, 1988). The extent and location of brain injury places constraints on human learning, but the ability to acquire new behaviors is retained in all but the most profoundly injured.

Assessment

Neurofunctional assessment may make use of a range of evaluation techniques. Methods include standardized assessments, questionnaires, checklists, rating scales, and observation. The most important of these is observation. Occupational therapists typically assess patients over a wide range of basic areas of functioning that may be divided into sensory, perceptual, motor, cognitive, and affective skills. A nonexhaustive list of factors to be considered on initial assessment is provided in table 4-1. Observation of real life functioning is the primary mode of assessment because there is almost never a one-to-one correspondence between observed cognitive deficits and impaired performance of functional skills. Observational techniques can be described as falling into two categories: naturalistic and structured. In naturalistic observation environmental demands are not specifically manipulated, allowing the therapist to develop an understanding of the patient's overall behavioral repertoire. It is important to establish what the patient does unconstrained by external cues or demands, so the therapist can evaluate whether the patient produces any compensatory behaviors (appropriate or inappropriate). Structured observations fall into two categories. First, specific areas of functioning can be cued and observed, e.g., washing and dressing behavior, street crossing, transfers. Second, specific behaviors can be evaluated for frequency of occurrence and eliciting factors, and for frequency baselining or antecedent/behavior/consequence (ABC) recordings. This second type of recording is often used to describe and measure inadequate behavioral control or social skills deficits (baselining techniques are described in more detail in Giles & Clark-Wilson, 1993). Despite careful observation the origin of some functional skills deficits can remain unclear. In those instances the occupational therapist may use standardized testing to attempt to elicit the true cause of the problem so that an adequate treatment plan can be developed.

The functional skills assessed by occupational therapists are most often low-frequency behaviors (like bathing and eating). For this reason observation needs to be scheduled. It should be remembered that this necessarily affects the patient's behavior. For example, a patient may show adequate performance when prompted to wash and dress but not engage in either behavior spontaneously. Central to the assessment of function is not what the patient can do, but what he or she actually does on a day-to-day basis. As an example of behavioral observation, let us take street crossing. Initially the therapist makes a determination of how safe it is to assess this behavior (i.e., a patient who is delusional, aggressive, or confused and given to impulsive behavior might have this aspect of the assessment deferred). A purposive route (e.g., to the coffee shop) may be selected. The patient is told that the purpose of the trip is to see if he or she can get to the store safely (and find the way back); the patient is not specifically cued to safe street crossing. The therapist then walks with (but a little behind) the patient so as not to give physical cues. The first street to be crossed should be quiet so as to give the therapist an opportunity to estimate performance in a relatively safe environment. The therapist should be ready to stop the patient if they are unsafe. If the patient is safe in crossing quiet streets, he or she may progress to busier streets both with and without crossing lights. The therapist should also assess the patient's ability to maintain safety when distracted by conversation. If the patient is initially unsafe (i.e., does not check for traffic, inadequately checks for traffic, or checks but nonetheless behaves unsafely), the therapist's task is to determined what additional cues are required to elicit safe behavior. For some patients a simple instruction to pay attention to how they

Table 4-1
Initial Screening

Sensation	Motor skill	Affect
Vision	Biomechanical	Depressed (tearful, psychomotor
Acuity	Fractures	retardation)
Visual fields	Contractures	Euphoric
Diplopia	Heterotopic ossification	Labile
Depth perception	Peripheral nerve injuries	Anger/short-temperedness
Color	Strength	Flat or constricted affect
Hearing	Endurance	Insight
Touch	Neuromuscular	
Superficial	Ataxia	
Deep	Tremor	
Sustained pressure	Apraxia	
Temperature	Spasticity	
Pain	Akinesia	
Proprioception	Bradykinesia	
Position sense	Rigidity	
Kinesthetic sense	Cognitive	
	Orientation (person, place, and time)	
Perception	Attention	
Visual	Memory (for current ongoing information)	
Visual neglect	Frontal lobe functioning	
Visual suppression	Planning	
Form discrimination/constancy	Initiation (level of spontaneously occurring behavior)	
Visual agnosia	Self-awareness	
Tactile	Metacognitive functions	
Tactile neglect		
Tactile suppression		
Steriognosis		

cross the street may be adequate. Others may need additional opportunities to practice focusing on safe street crossing behaviors as outlined by the therapist. Where there is a marked deficit or an identifiable perceptual deficit, or where the individual is unable to respond to general street crossing stimulation, a more structured approach should be considered. The therapist should determine the most appropriate techniques, type of prompts, reinforcers, and frequency of practice. Similarly an appropriate measure of task acquisition should be selected. Progress in assessment is the same for all functional domains, from least structured to most structured.

Neurofunctional assessment determines current level of functioning and assists in the determination of optimal forms of retraining. The neuro-functional assessment is central to the selection of goals and target behaviors required for the rehabilitation team's integrated treatment plan. Neuro-functional assessments should be conducted under conditions as close as possible to those the person will experience following rehabilitation. Neuro-functional assessment therefore differs from other types of testing that demand highly standardize conditions. The rigorous control of variables necessary for the pursuit of science is sacrificed in favor of ecological validity. Table 4-2 lists factors to be considered in developing a picture of the individual's behavior in environmental context. There are many variables that influence performance in real world situations, for example, the presence of setting events (Giles & Clark-Wilson, 1993), cues, or environmental conditions.

Table 4-2
The Goals of Neurofunctional Assessment

1. To identify retained functional skills.
2. To identify deficits limiting independent functioning.
3. To identify environmental factors that support independent functioning.
4. To identify the demands placed on the individual by the environment.
5. To identify the strategies used to overcome functional deficits.
6. To identify methods that assist the individual to relearn functional skills.
7. To identify the changes required to enable the individual to function in an environmental context.

Adapted from Giles, G. M., & Clark-Wilson, J. (1993). Rehabilitation of occupational therapy for the brain-injured adult: A neurofunctional approach. London: Chapman and Hall.

Standardized Assessment

In some instances observation alone will not indicate why a person's performance breaks down. Standardized testing may assist in determining the origin of a performance deficit. Recently a number of tests have appeared on the market intended to be ecologically valid. The Test of Everyday Attention (TEA) is the first standardized noncomputerized test of attention available for use by occupational therapists (Robertson, Ward, Ridgeway, & Nimmo-Smith, 1994). The TEA was developed to reflect current theories of attention. The TEA measures selective attention, sustained attention, attentional switching, and the ability to divide attention. The TEA uses relatively familiar everyday materials and is plausible and acceptable to patients.

The second edition of the Rivermead Behavioral Memory Test (RBMT) shows considerable refinement over the first edition and although produced in England contains culturally specific variants for North American users (Wilson, Cockburn, & Baddeley, 1991). Although there are many assessments of memory available, most do not attempt to identify the occurrence of everyday memory problems. The RBMT attempts to assess skills necessary for normal life functioning rather than performance on experimental materials and paradigms. The items involve either remembering to carry out some everyday task or measuring the abilities needed to function in everyday life. There are 11 subtests in the RBMT and four parallel versions so that practice effects that might occur with repeated testing can be avoided.

Retraining

Having discussed some of the factors that lead to the disruption of functional behaviors, it is time to consider how to retrain a cognitively impaired brain-injured person to perform a functional task. Continuing with the example of street crossing, let us consider how an individual with severe memory impairment might be trained to cross the street. During assessment it is determined that the patient has no specific perceptual deficits but that he or she walks across intersections without checking for traffic. Having performed a task analysis the therapist determined that crossing the street safely consists of stopping at the curbside, looking in both directions, and then walking directly across the street, when there are no motor vehicles within a certain distance (depending on the patient's speed of ambulation and so forth). Having performed the task analysis the therapist can develop a program of verbal prompts, the purpose of which is to elicit from the patient safe street crossing and to direct the patient's attention to the factors in the task determining success or failure. The first time the patient practices street crossing is an "episode." It is processed and the specific to-be-learned activity is associated with the specific street intersection, the traffic that is passing, and other incidental information. This episode may not be available later for introspection, but a certain potentiation effect will have occurred. On the second occasion only certain aspects of the situation will have been held constant, for instance, the specific instructions given. As this street crossing routine is repeated, always using the same prompts, the street crossing episodes are not retained. The street crossing memory becomes an abstraction of many specific memory traces, all slightly different, that eventually produce the generalized memory structure of crossing streets. This experience becomes prototypical, and the patient develops a habit of crossing the street in the way that has been practiced. In optimum cases the patient no longer chooses to cross the street in a certain manner; the patient just crosses the street in this way. Initially during treatment there is an attempt to reduce the possibility of failure to a minimum by the cues given. As performance improves, cues may be faded. The task practiced must be ultimately performable given the fixed aspects of the patient's deficits. If the therapist attempts to teach behaviors that are beyond the patient's cognitive ability, the program will fail.

The role of the therapist is to determine the functional skill to be trained, develop methods that allow the patient to perform the task with the minimum amount of new learning, and develop a method that directs the patient's attention to the central components of the task.

Metacognitive Control and Skills Training

Programming may be thought to exist on a behavioral–cognitive behavioral continuum. All treatment centers around modifying the patient's previous responses (Giles & Clark-Wilson, 1988) and replacing them with new and more adaptive ones via practice. Patients who are able to develop a new and more accurate model of their own basic cognitive functioning can learn new metacognitive control strategies. Metacognitive control involves learning a new language or way to think about the postinjury self. Functional skills that require the patient to cope with novelty require a complex set of cognitive abilities. For example, complete functional use of a diary always involves decisions about what information to write down. Practice in how to make entries and what information to enter reduces the difficulty of these tasks, but the patient must nevertheless be able to categorize a particular event as one of the classes of events that should be recorded and then initiate the recording.

Training programs that attempt to address a general behavior such as to reduce a social skills deficit or to develop use of a memory book should include the following three stages. The first stage is a cognitive overlearning element that attempts to focus the patient's attention on the behavior or area of skills deficit and to develop a verbal label for the behavior. The therapist discusses the long-term consequences of the behavior or skill deficit with the patient. The therapist emphases its inconvenience and the benefits likely to accrue to the patient from changing it. If the patient has severe deficits, this cognitive component may need to be reviewed one or more times per day and may continue throughout and/or beyond the other program elements. The second stage is sessional practice of required behaviors. Here the patient practices the behavior for a short period of time in an environment controlled by the therapist. The patient must be able to produce the behavior with only moderate effort in this controlled environment before progressing to stage three, the 24-hour program approach. In this stage there is an attempt to target each instance of the behavior throughout the day. This type of intervention requires an interdisciplinary team and a high level of staff training. Each time the patient exhibits the target behavior, a staff member responds in a predetermined manner usually so as to have the patient attend to the behavior, categorize it as an instance of the target behavior, suppress it and replace it with an alternative or incompatible behavior.

The degree to which a behavior becomes automatic influences its durability. Behaviors that can be developed to a high degree of automaticity such as washing and dressing (and which are practiced repeatedly) are extremely robust. Behaviors that must be consciously initiated by the subject, such as use of a memory book, require more specific and ongoing environmental support.

Interventions

Reinforcement and Skill Building

A reinforcing event is one that increases the likelihood of the behavior that immediately precedes it being repeated. Reinforcers may be primary or secondary. There is some evidence that reinforcement aids learning (Dolan & Norton, 1977; Lashley & Drabman 1974). The reason that reinforcement increases learning is unknown but may be related to the ability of reinforcement to direct attention toward the to-be-learned aspects of the practiced behaviors.

Task Analysis

Task analysis involves a process of dividing tasks into component parts that can be taught. The analysis provides a method of organizing behaviors so as to make them easier to learn. The components of a task analysis may be converted to verbal or visual prompts. When the therapist uses a task analysis to develop a set of verbal cues, the number of cues depends on the patient's ability. For example, in the development of a washing and dressing program some patients require only a few prompts such as "wash your face" to produce complex behavioral chains. Other patients require several prompts, for example, "pick up the washcloth," "put soap on the washcloth," "wash your face," and "rinse the washcloth."

Chaining

Functional tasks can be thought of as complex stimulus-response chains in which the completion of each activity acts as the stimulus for the next step in the chain (Kazdin, 1994). Three chaining options are available for training functional tasks: (1) backward chaining (BC), in which the last step of the task is trained first, followed by the second to last step and the last step and so on progressing backwards through the chain; (2) forward chaining (FC), in which the first step of the chain is trained first, followed by the first and second step and so on, progressing forward through the chain; (3) whole task method (WTM), in which each step of the chain is trained on each presentation. Basic operant researchers have preferred backward chaining on theoretical grounds (Skinner, 1938; Martin, Koop, Turner, & Hanel, 1981), while clinicians have focused on the practical advantages of the whole task method. Contemporary studies have found WTM to be equivalent or superior to BC (Spooner, 1981; Spooner, 1984; Martin et al., 1981; McDonnell & Laughlin, 1989).

Prompts

Events that facilitate the production of a behavior are called prompts (or cues). In many instances prompts are available in the environment but they are no longer sufficient to guide behavior or they have lost their meaning entirely (e.g., arriving at a busy junction no longer cues safe street crossing routines). The therapist adds additional prompts to those already available in the environment. Therapists can facilitate the learning of skills with a range of differing types of prompts. Two types of prompting systems have been evaluated in teaching chained tasks: the system of least prompts (SLP) and time delay procedures. The system of least prompts (sometimes referred to as the increasing assistance procedure) involves the presentation of a prompt hierarchy that is arranged from most general to most specific. The individual is cued progressively through the hierarchy of prompts available for each step in the chain until a correct response is produced. The time delay cueing system typically involves two training stages. (1) A cue designed to elicit the next step in the chain is delivered so as to coincide with the stimulus (i.e., the completion of the previous step in the chain). (2) A defined interval is inserted between the occurrence of the stimulus and the response eliciting cue. Two types of time delay procedures are described in the literature: progressive time delay (PTD) where longer and longer intervals are inserted between the occurrence of the stimulus and the cue, and constant time delay (CTD) where a fixed response interval is inserted between stimulus and cue (Wolery, Griffen, Ault, Gast, & Doyle, 1990). Although the system of least prompts has been used with individuals with brain damage (O'Reilly & Cuvo, 1989; McMillan, Papadopoulos, Cornall, & Greenwood, 1990), the majority of reports of functional interventions using chained tasks have used CTD (Giles & Clark-Wilson, 1988; Giles & Clark-Wilson, 1993; Katzman & Mix, 1994). No studies comparing SLP with time delay methods has been conducted with people with brain injury. However, in studies comparing these methods in persons with mental retardation both CTD and PTD have been shown to be superior to SLP (Wolery et al., 1990; McDonnell, 1987). In most circumstances CTD procedures may be preferred because they require less attention from the therapist to the cueing itself (Wolery et al., 1990). Some therapists may prefer to begin with CTD and utilize PTD as a fading technique. However, PTD should be used only when the patient has already developed the skill to the point where they can be 80 to 90% correct, because otherwise they are likely to "practice" the propagation of incorrect responses—a situation to be avoided. Questions like "What's next?" or instructions telling the individual to "go ahead" can also help the individual initiate the activity and decrease dependence on prompts.

Practice

Repetition of a behavior increases the probability of the behavior being further repeated (Giles & Clark-Wilson, 1993). This is known as response practice and is the most important aspect of successful behavioral training. As practice is continued, the behaviors can become automatic. Overlearning refers to the practice of a skill well beyond the point where mastery has been achieved. Overlearning increases the chances that a skill is consolidated in the individual's repertoire of skills and reduces the effort required for performance of the skill (Giles & Clark-Wilson, 1993).

Shaping

Shaping refers to the reinforcement of closer and closer approximations to the desired behavior. Tasks are graded in difficulty so they are achievable. As competency is demonstrated, the task requirements are increased (see the Case Example below).

Control of a Behavior by Antecedents

The antecedents to a behavior may be altered in an attempt to change the likelihood of occurrence of a behavior. This is a method of setting the environmental conditions—the stimulus events so as to increase the possibility that the patient will emit the desired behavior. The control of specific antecedents may be particularly useful in working with patients with profound memory impairment. Zencius, Wesolowski, Burke, and McQuade (1989) compared the effect of altering antecedents with the effect of varying consequences in three patients with marked memory disorder. Zencius and co-workers (1989) found that for one patient posting a sign regarding breaktimes at the work station drastically reduced the number of unauthorized breaks. In another patient the most effective way to increase cane usage, a goal of the rehabilitation team, was to provide her with a cane to use during her morning activities of daily living. This technique was found to be more effective than social praise, a contract for money, or someone to escort her to get her cane when she was found without it. In a third patient the authors found that a map and a written daily schedule were more powerful than a contract for money in increasing therapy attendance. In each case, alteration of the antecedent produced behavioral improvement following attempts to alter behavior by consequences that had proved to be only marginally successful (for a fuller discussion see Clark-Wilson & Giles, 1993).

Overlearning

Overlearning refers to the practice of a skill well beyond the point where the patient is able to produce the behavior. Overlearning increases the chances that the skill is consolidated—becomes automatic—and reduces the amount of effort required for performance. When a skill becomes automatic, it becomes the easiest behavior to initiate from an array of possible behaviors (i.e., the possibility of an interference error is reduced). The goal of rehabilitation can often best be met by having the individual engage in overlearning. For example, a street crossing program should not be terminated on meeting the functional criteria but on meeting criteria plus a certain number of practice sessions designed to make the behavior automatic. The number of additional sessions required to develop automaticity is unclear. Automaticity is assessed by ongoing monitoring of the patient's behavior in conjunction with distractions.

Encore Procedure

When an individual demonstrates an infrequently displayed skill without prompting, he or she can be prompted to produce several more correct responses. For example, a patient was learning to attract attention appropriately before asking questions or making requests in social skill groups. On any occasion when she asked appropriately, such as by saying the person's name, or saying "excuse me" (rather than screaming or banging objects) and then asking a question, she was given social, and occasionally tangible, reinforcement and asked to repeat the sequence of behaviors again, whereupon she was reinforced again.

Highlighting

Many individuals after brain injury have problems in distinguishing the central aspects of a task. Highlighting refers to a strategy that promotes the discrimination of the crucial elements of an activity by exaggerating the salience of some stimulus features. Prompts are progressively faded once the patient is consistently making correct discriminations. Highlighting might be achieved by emphasizing phrases, pointing, touching, or providing specific reinforcement.

Intervention Using Metacognitive Control Strategies

Metacognitively oriented intervention should involve consideration of the foregoing factors but in addition should maximize use of the patient's own retained learning ability. The therapist's role becomes to supervise the patient in setting his or her own goals and developing his or her own strategies to perform functional tasks based on knowledge of his or her own limitations. For example, a patient who has been working on improving community mobility might set a goal of finding the way to a specific novel location. The patient would then have to develop, with the assistance of the therapist,

a knowledge of the parameters involved in the task, e.g., available means of transportation, time requirements, cost, and route finding methods. As the patient shows increasing competencies, longer periods of time and more complex tasks can be set for the patient. Eventually long periods of the treatment day should be devoted to the patient pursuing her own goals, periodically checking in with the therapist who can ensure that she remains critically self-aware. The therapist's goal is to set tasks and direct the patient's attention on how current experience can be used to improve future task performance. The patient is encouraged to learn about his or her own cognitive abilities and to develop effective metacognitive control strategies.

Goal Statements

The incorporation of goal statements in each session has a number of advantages. It may increase participation, help the patient attend to the to-be-learned aspect of activities (this discriminatory aspect may need to be repeated throughout the session); and it communicates respect from therapist to patient. For patients with lack of insight it orients them to their deficits and cues them as to how the to-be-undertaken therapeutic activity will help them achieve their own goals. Therapists may wish to present the session as a scientific endeavor, in which either the therapist or the patient is allowed to have incorrect notions, but in which an empirical question is examined. With some patients, however, active agreement with the therapeutic intervention is not attainable, and the therapist seeking agreement will only derail the therapeutic endeavor. The therapist is not advised to abandon the goal of developing functional skills by waiting until the patient knows that he or she has deficits. Goal-directing statements, for example, for 5 minutes at the beginning of each session and interspersed statements throughout, orienting patients to these issues is frequently indicated. For example, "As you know as a result of your severe brain injury you have needed some help in washing and dressing yourself. We are working with you every morning so that you can develop a system to be independent. You can now perform all but three of the activities of washing and dressing completely independently."

Debriefing

Regular debriefing about performance (knowledge of results) is indicated in producing positive behavioral change. Telling the patient that he or she has done well is encouraging, but nonspecific and damaging if untrue. Feedback about results should be concrete and accurate; written materials that the patient can refer to such as graphs or logs should be used where possible.

Management of Denial

Awareness of deficits improves with spontaneous recovery. Physical problems are likely to be recognized before psychological problems, and the implications of the problems for future plans and life goals are often recognized last. The process of adjustment can be seen as falling into three stages: active denial, ambivalence, and engagement. In active denial the patient rejects any information relating to deficit and states that there is nothing wrong. The patient is often actively hostile to the treatment staff and denies any similarity between himself or herself and other patients. In the stage of ambivalence the patient begins to come to terms with some brain-injury–related changes and begins to develop a new self-concept. A typical statement at this stage might be "I can't believe that this is so difficult for me." In the engagement stage the patient recognizes the problems and actively engages with the problem and with treatment staff about developing an effective and tolerable way of "being in the world." The therapist assists the patient in changing the patient's frame of reference or the explanatory stance in order to assist the patient in understanding how to best cope with a current situation. In one sense the patient is taught a new language of brain injury. The importance of emotional support and a positive frame of reference cannot be overstated. The desire to confront the patient into accepting the disability should be resisted.

Case Example

During the final year of an undergraduate course in electrical engineering patient 1 developed herpes simplex encephalitis. The patient's acute illness is reported by Greenwood, Bhalla, Gordon, and Roberts (1983); for a full discussion of his early recovery the interested reader is referred there. Following recovery from the acute illness patient 1 was found to be hyperoral, sullenly uncooperative, and aggressive. Patient 1 was also amnestic with an inability to remember new material for more than 30 seconds following presentation. Remote memory was impoverished in content and sequential organization. Patient 1 also had a category-specific knowledge deficit about food and food-related items (he was unable to distinguish food from nonfood items). One year post-onset patient 1 was living at home with his mother who was providing extensive supervision. Early in patient 1's recovery it had been suggested that he keep a diary. Unfortunately this had become a focus for obsessional behavior such that patient 1 was obsessed by recording everything that happened "before I forget." The recording had no functional value because patient 1 was unable to select relevant aspects of his environment (recording largely irrelevant, idiosyncratic, and repetitive themes) and because he only wrote in his diary, and never referred to it. Increasing resistance to basic activities of daily living and escalating physical aggression led to psychiatric hospital admission where his behavior was managed with large doses of major tranquilizers. Following a 1-month trial period, admission was arranged to a specialized behavior disorder program (Eames and Wood, 1985) where the treatment described here took place.

On admission to the unit patient 1 was constantly angry. He paced the unit corridors incessantly with pen and diary in hand. Any frustration was construed as persecutory and frequently resulted in serious aggressive outbursts (patient 1 had been an Olympic-class swimmer and was 6 feet 3 inches tall). Patient 1 maintained a constant stream of repetitive questions particularly related to his stated desire to die—stating "all I need is a driver's license" and asking for "suicide pills." Patient 1 would approach staff, standing 6 inches away, glaring down at them and ask "How long does it take for a pointless place to admit they can't help your illness?" Patient 1 rarely bathed and smelled continuously of sweat and stale soap. He was constantly hungry and believed that staff were trying to stave him to death. However, he remembered that he was given medications and referred to his "constant pill diet."

Initial observation revealed that patient 1 would attempt to use environmental cues and to verbally regulate his behavior; unfortunately his attempts were mostly inappropriate. For example, patient 1 would not wash under his arms because "it is cold outside so I cannot have been sweating." It was also realized that although amnestic patient 1 could learn new information by constant repetition. Patient 1 had some insight into his circumstances and a paranoid and negative attitude toward himself, his environment, and those around him (particularly staff). It was recognized that if intervention were to be effective, changes meaningful to patient 1 would have to take place. The interdisciplinary team established the following goals: elimination of physical aggression, elimination of the "diary," improved personal hygiene, increased positive social interaction, and independence in preparing one meal per day.

The unit on which this treatment program occurred utilized a "extinction approach" to aggression with time-out in a time-out room for 5 minutes for any instance of physical aggression. On admission patient 1 was averaging five instances of physical aggression per week.

Following 2 weeks' evaluation it was clear to staff that treatment could not be effective as long as patient 1 retained his diary. Staff were unable to engage patient 1 in any meaningful therapy because he was constantly recording in his notebook his paranoid interpretation of the "ridiculous" events occurring around him. The decision to remove the diary was made reluctantly because the "diary" was seen by staff as patient 1's attempt to bring order and stability into his life and because it was reasonable to expect that removal of the diary would provoke an escalation of his behavior disorder. Following a period of additional staff training patient 1 had all his writing equipment and notebooks taken from him. During this first day patient 1 was physically aggressive eight times. Figure 4-1 shows the patients' gradual reduction of physical aggression over the next 5

months. Patient 1 was being treated concurrently with carbamazapine.

Removal of the diary allowed staff to engage in other therapeutic interventions. Personal hygiene was selected because patient 1's unpleasant odor significantly affected his social acceptability. Baseline observations indicated that patient 1 could manage functions such as washing his face or brushing his teeth but that he could not put these units together nonrepetitively into a coherent sequence. For example, he might wash his face, brush his teeth four times, and then stop. A behavioral program utilizing verbal mediation was selected because patient 1 spontaneously attempted to verbally regulate his own behavior. Staff performing the program timed-out on-the-spot (ignored) any inappropriate verbalizations. The program is described in detail elsewhere (Giles & Morgan, 1989). Patient 1 was told a phrase that linked the act performed to one that immediately followed it, e.g., "Teeth cleaned now shave. Say after me. . . ." He was rewarded (with chocolate) and praised for repeating the link phrase and then again for initiating the behavior. Eight mediating phrases were used to link the nine activities of the program together. Failure to perform the activity—which was surprisingly rare—lead to a 30-second time-out on-the-spot followed by reprompting by the therapist. The program was carried out twice per day 5 days a week. As learning occurred, reinforcement was made increasingly intermittent. It was hoped that patient 1 would learn to verbally mediate his own behavior in the sequence that he was being taught. Figure 4-2 shows his progress over the 14 weeks of treatment. There was an unexpected reduction in "acts of washing verbally mediated" toward the end of the program because patient 1 consolidated part of the sequence into "wash the body from top to bottom." At 3 months' follow-up the patient continued to be independent in basic activities of daily living and continued to use the same behavioral sequence.

Social interaction was addressed using a shaping procedure. When not escorted to a specific location, patient 1 would pace around the unit in an agitated state. The goal of the intervention was to encourage him to sit with others and engage in appropriate conversations. Initially a staff member would stand by the doorway to the patient lounge

Figure 4-1

The response of patient 1 to a program of 5 minutes time-out
in a time-out room for physical aggression.

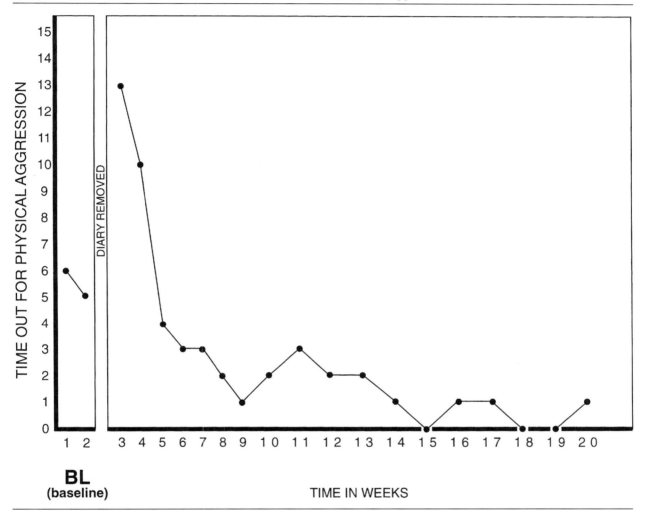

and give patient 1 praise and a cookie for approaching the doorway. Later patient 1 was rewarded for entering the room and provided with additional reinforcement for each 30 seconds he stayed in the room. Later he was only reinforced when he was sitting down, and still later only for sitting quietly or when engaged in socially appropriate conversation. Inappropriate behaviors were timed-out on-the-spot (ignored). The program was rapidly effective with patient 1 attending the patient lounge independently during scheduled breaks.

Despite the ongoing success of the programs described above patient 1 remained preoccupied by the idea that staff were attempting to starve him and keeping him on "a pointless pill diet." Physical confrontations with staff were often about access to food (e.g., taking food from others). Staff hypothesized that if patient 1 could be taught to prepare a meal for himself he would be less likely to believe that he was being starved. Teaching patient 1 to prepare a meal was complicated by a number of factors. Patient 1 was amnestic and had a category-specific loss of information for food and objects in the kitchen. Patient 1 could not distinguish food from nonfood items, did not know what color toast should be when it was done,

Figure 4-2

The response of patient 1 to a washing and dressing training program.
WVM = Acts of washing verbally mediated. WPS = Acts of washing performed in sequence.
WPI = Acts of washing performed independently.

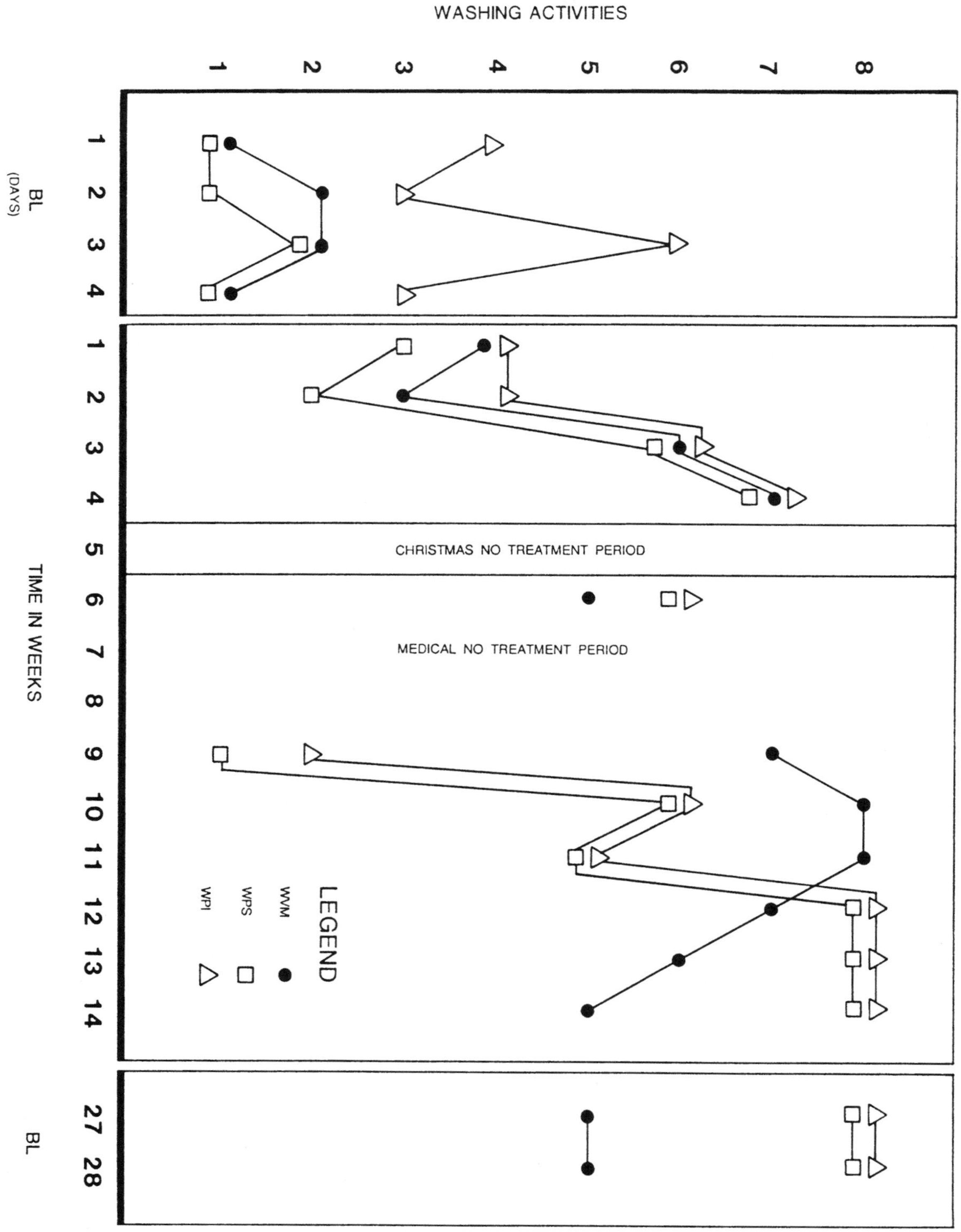

WASHING ACTIVITIES

did not know what "boiling" meant, and could not recognize an oven, a grill, or basic kitchen implements. Patient 1 was observed for 1 week attempting to make a breakfast consisting of two slices of toast with a can of baked beans and sausages (his selection). A program of written instructions was developed and modified in response to difficulties patient 1 experienced in carrying them out. Patient 1 was prompted with "check instructions" on entering the kitchen. All the food items to make breakfast were set out with a copy of the instructions and a pen for patient 1 to check off each item as it was completed. For the first 2 weeks patient 1 continued to require verbal instructions as well as the written instructions, but by the end of the third week he was independent with the instruction sheet and supervision was withdrawn. After performing the program every morning for 6 weeks the instruction sheet was withdrawn and food was left in the cupboard and patient 1 continued to make his breakfast independently. Nonetheless for a further 6 weeks patient 1 had to be escorted to the kitchen each morning despite his protests that he could not cook. On a day approximately 14 weeks after the beginning of the program patient 1 greeted every person who entered the unit with a broad smile of excitement and the statement "I can make my own break-

Figure 4-3

The response of patient 1 to a cooking program. A = Food and instruction sheet on counter and with additional verbal prompts when necessary (primarily "check instructions"). B = Food and instruction sheet on counter. C = Food left in cupboards, no instruction sheet.

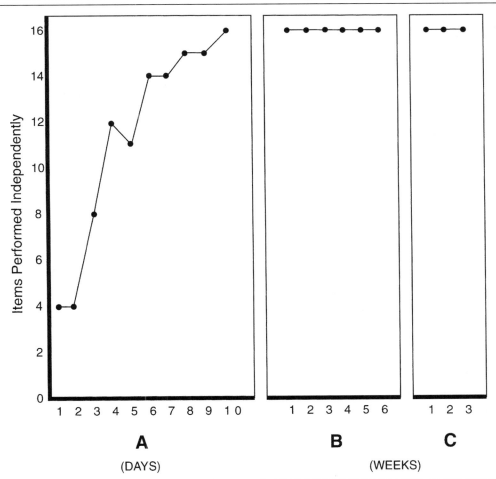

fast!" Patient 1 ceased protesting that he was being starved.

Patient 1's ability to explore the environment for information that could guide his behavior was used later to train him to go into town and do his shopping, do his laundry, and eventually hold a job.

The foregoing case example indicates how strengths and weaknesses are assessed, why specific areas were targeted for intervention, how an understanding of strengths and weaknesses was incorporated into a retraining program. This case example highlights the principal features of the neurofunctional approach.

Outcome Studies

Single-case or small-group studies have demonstrated the efficacy of functional task training with brain-injured adults in the areas of continence (Cohen, 1986), self-feeding (Hooper-Row, 1988), transfers (Goodman-Smith & Turnball, 1983), personal hygiene (Giles & Clark-Wilson, 1988; Giles & Shore, 1989a; Giles, Ridley, Dill, & Frye, 1997), mobility and community skills (Giles & Clark-Wilson, 1993), and social skills (Gajar, Schloss, Schloss, & Thompson, 1984; Brotherton, Thomas, Wisotzek, & Milan, 1988; Giles, Fussey, & Burgess, 1988). Single-case and small-group designs allow treatment to be specifically tailored to the patient's needs while maintaining the controls necessary for determining the effects of treatment (Giles, 1989; 1994). Lloyd and Cuvo (1994) reviewed results of behavioral interventions concluding that treatment effects are robust and enduring. A number of follow-up studies have examined the effectiveness of post-acute brain-injury programs. Even when cognitive skills are directly addressed it is often functional skills that improve (Mills, Nesbeda, Katz, & Alexander, 1992). Follow-up of 42 patients treated at an outpatient post-acute cognitive rehabilitation found that cognitive measures were not significantly affected by treatment but that there was significant improvement in patients' functional performance and that this was maintained at 18 months' follow-up (Mills, Nesbeda, Katz, & Alexander, 1992). Johnston and Lewis (1991) assessed the one-year outcome of 82 pa-

tients treated at post-acute community reentry programs and found that there were enduring improvements in independent living and productive activities with patients requirements for supervision showing substantial decline. Although improved independent living and household skills were the most frequent dimension of actual benefit they were seldom documented as goals (Johnston, 1991). An outcome study of 21 persons treated at a transitional living program found that improvements in independence documented at one year had remained stable or had improved at three years' follow-up (Harrick, Krefting, Johnston, Carlson, & Minnes, 1994). Bell and Tallman (1995) describe significant functional improvement in five patients admitted for rehabilitation from a skilled nursing facility. All patients were at least one year post injury. Mean treatment duration was 51 days. Following rehabilitation all patients were discharged to the community (e.g., a board and care home). The greatest improvements occurred in functional skills with inconsistent improvement in the areas of language and cognition, which, the authors conclude, were less crucial to their functioning in a structured community setting (Bell and Tallman, 1995). Other workers have found that functional performance may continue to improve following the end of a program of functional retraining even in patients who are significantly post injury (Fryer and Haffey, 1987). Elsewhere I have argued that it is important to learn from the history of brain-injury rehabilitation and to focus on where we can have the most positive impact on patient outcomes (Giles, 1994). Evidence is mounting that individuals after brain injury can be assisted to redevelop independent living skills that significantly reduce their need for supervision and institutional care.

Conclusion

Occupational therapy must be judged as a discipline on whether patients demonstrate improved functioning. Interventions should be tailored to the individual patient. Attention should be paid to what the patients need to learn to be independent in their environment. In addition treatment methods should consider the constraints placed on the patients' learning by the injury itself. This chapter has outlined an approach to assessment and intervention. Emphasis has been placed on the variables of practice, attention, memory, and frontal lobe functioning. Rather than attempt to address the elusive "underlying cause" of a functional impairment this chapter highlights the advantages of a more direct approach. Evidence is growing that functionally oriented rehabilitation can produce meaningful changes in functional outcomes for patients following brain injury.

Acknowledgments

Thanks are due to the *Journal of Clinical and Experimental Neuropsychology* for permission to reprint material previously published, vol. 11, 311–318, 1989.

References

Bell, K. R., & Tallman, C. A. (1995). Community re-entry of long-term institutionalized brain-injured patient. *Brain Injury, 9*, 315–320.

Black, P., Markowitz, R. S., & Cianci, S. N. (1975). Recovery of motor function after lesions in the motor cortex of monkey. In CIBA Foundation Symposium 34. New Series. *Outcome of severe damage to the central nervous system.* Amsterdam: Elsevier.

Brotherton, F. A., Thomas, L. L., Wisotzek, I. E., & Milan, M. A. (1988). Social skills training in the rehabilitation of patients with traumatic head injury. *Archives of Physical Medicine and Rehabilitation, 69*, 827–832.

Cicerone, K. D., Lazar, R. M., & Shapiro, W. R. (1983). Effects of frontal lobe lesions on hypothesis sampling during concept formation. *Neuropsychologia, 21*, 513–524.

Cohen, R. E. (1986). Behavioral treatment of incontinence in a profoundly neurologically impaired adult. *Archives of Physical Medicine and Rehabilitation, 67*, 833–834.

Cope, D. N., & Hall, K. (1982). Head injury rehabilitation: Benefits of early intervention. *Archives of Physical Medicine and Rehabilitation, 63*, 433–437.

Dolan, M. P., & Norton, J. C. (1977). A programmed training technique that uses reinforcement to facilitate acquisition and retention in brain damaged patients. *Journal of Clinical Psychology, 33*, 496–501.

Eames, P., & Wood, R. (1985). Rehabilitation after severe brain injury: A follow-up study of a behaviour modification approach. *Journal of Neurology, Neuro, surgery, and Psychiatry, 48*, 613–619.

Freedman, P. E., Bleiberg, J., & Freedland K. (1987). Anticipatory behaviour deficits in closed head injury. *Journal of Neurology, Neurosurgery, and Psychiatry, 50*, 398–401.

Fryer, L. J., & Haffey, W. J. (1987). Cognitive rehabilitation and community readaptation: Outcomes from two program models. *Journal of Head Trauma Rehabilitation, 21*, 51–63.

Fuster, J. M. (1995). *Memory in the cerebral cortex.* Cambridge: MIT Press.

Gajar, A., Schloss, P. J., Schloss, C., & Thompson, C. K. (1984). Effects of feedback and self-monitoring on brain trauma youth's conversational skills. *Journal of Applied Behavior Analysis, 17*, 353–358.

Giles, G. M. (1989). Demonstrating the effectiveness of occupational therapy after severe brain trauma. *American Journal of Occupational Therapy, 43*, 613–615.

Giles, G. M. (1994). The status of brain injury rehabilitation. *American Journal of Occupational Therapy, 48*, 199–205.

Giles, G. M., & Clark-Wilson, J. (1988). The use of behavioral techniques in functional skills training after severe brain injury. *American Journal of Occupational Therapy, 42*, 658–665.

Giles, G. M., & Clark-Wilson, J. (1993). *Brain injury rehabilitation: A neurofunctional approach.* San Diego: Singular.

Giles, G. M., Fussey, I., & Burgess, P. (1989). The behavioral treatment of verbal interaction skills following severe head injury: A single case study. *Brain Injury, 2*, 75–81.

Giles, G. M., & Morgan, J. H. (1989). Training functional skills following herpes simplex encephalitis: A single case study. *Journal of Clinical and Experimental Neuropsychology, 11*, 311–318.

Giles, G. M., Ridley, J., Dill, A., & Frye, S. (1997). A consecutive series of brain injured adults treated with a washing and dressing retraining program. *American Journal of Occupational Therapy, 51*, 256–266.

Giles, G. M., & Shore, M. (1989a). A rapid method for teaching severely brain-injured adults to wash and dress. *Archives of Physical Medicine and Rehabilitation, 70*, 156–158.

Giles, G. M., & Shore, M. (1989b). The effectiveness of an electronic memory aid for a memory-impaired adult of normal intelligence. *American Journal of Occupational Therapy, 43*, 409–411.

Goodman-Smith, A., & Turnbull, J. (1983). A behavioral approach to the rehabilitation of severely brain injured adults: An illustrated case history. *Physiotherapy, 69*, 393–396.

Greenwood, R., Bhalla, A., Gordon, A., & Roberts, J. (1983). Behavioral disturbance during recovery from herpes simplex encephalitis. *Journal of Neurology, Neurosurgery, and Psychiatry, 46*, 809–817.

Harrick, L., Krefting, L., Johnston, J., Carlson, P., & Minnes, P. (1994). Stability of functional outcomes following transitional living programme participation: 3 year follow up. *Brain Injury, 8*, 439–447.

Hooper-Row, J. (1988). Rehabilitation of physical deficits in the post-acute brain-injured: Four case studies. In I. Fussey

& G. M. Giles (Eds.), *Rehabilitation of the severely brain-injury adult: A practical approach.* London: Croom Helm.

Jacobs, H. E. (1988). The Los Angeles head injury survey: Procedures and initial findings. *Archives of Physical Medicine and Rehabilitation, 69,* 425–431.

Jennett, B., & Teasdale, G. (1981). *Management of head injuries.* Philadelphia: Davis.

Johnston, M. V. (1991). Outcomes of community re-entry programmes for brain injury survivors. Part 2: Further investigations. *Brain Injury, 5,* 155–168.

Johnston, M. V., & Lewis, F. D. (1991). Outcomes of community re-entry programmes for brain injury survivors. Part 1: Independent living and productive activities. *Brain Injury, 5,* 141–154.

Katzman, S., & Mix, C. (1994). Improving functional independence in a patient with encephalitis through behavior modification shaping techniques. *American Journal of Occupational Therapy, 48,* 259–269.

Kazdin A. (1994). *Behavior modification in applied settings* (5th ed.) Pacific Grove, CA Brooks/Cole.

Kewman, D. G., Yanus, B., & Kirsch, N. (1988). Assessment of distractibility in auditory comprehension after traumatic brain injury. *Brain Injury, 2,* 131–137.

Lashley, B., & Drabman, R. (1974). Facilitation of the acquisition and retention of sight-word vocabulary through token reinforcement. *Journal of Applied Behavioral Analysis, 7,* 307–312.

Levin, H. S., Goldstein, F. C., High W. M., & Williams, D. (1988). Automatic and effortful processing after severe closed head injury. *Brain and Cognition, 7,* 283–297.

Lewicki, P., Czyzenska, M., & Hoffman, H. (1987). Unconscious acquisition of complex procedural knowledge. *Journal of Experimental Psychology: Learning, Memory and Cognition, 13,* 523–530.

Lewicki, P., Hill, T., & Bizot, E. (1988). Acquisition of procedural knowledge about a pattern of stimuli that cannot be articulated. *Cognitive Psychology, 20,* 24–37.

Lloyd, L. F., & Cuvo, A. J. (1994). Maintenance and generalization of behaviors after treatment of persons with traumatic brain injury. *Brain Injury, 8,* 529–540.

Lorch, E. P., Anderson, D. R., & Well, A. D. (1984). Effects of irrelevant information on speeded classification tasks: Interference is reduced by habituation. *Journal of Experimental Psychology: Human Perception and Performance, 10,* 850–864.

Mackay, L. E., Bernstein, B. A., Chapman, P. E., Morgan, A. S., & Milazzo, L. S. (1992). Early intervention in severe head injury: Long-term benefits of a formalized program. *Archives of Physical Medicine and Rehabilitation, 73,* 635–641.

Martin, G. L., Koop, S., Turner, G., & Hanel, F. (1981). Backward chaining versus total task presentation to teach assembly tasks to severely retarded persons. *Behavior Research of Severe Developmental Disabilities, 2,* 117–136.

McDonnell, J. (1987). The effect of time delay and increasing prompt hierarchy strategies on the acquisition of purchasing skills by students with severe handicaps. *Journal of the Association for the Severely Handicapped, 12,* 227–236.

McDonnell, J., & Laughlin, B. (1989). A comparison of backward and concurrent chaining strategies in teaching community skills. *Education and Training in Mental Retardation, 24,* 230–238.

McGlynn, S. M., & Schacter, D. L. (1989). Unawareness of deficits in neuropsychological syndromes. *Journal of Clinical and Experimental Neuropsychology, 11,* 143–205.

McMillan, T. M., Papadopoulos, H., Cornall, C., & Greenwood, R. J. (1990). Modification of severe behavior problems following herpes simplex encephalitis. *Brain Injury, 4,* 399–406.

Mills, J. M., Nesbeda, T., Katz, D. I., & Alexander, M. P. (1992). Outcomes for traumatically brain-injured patients following post-acute rehabilitation programmes. *Brain Injury, 6,* 219–228.

Nelson, T. O., & Narens, L. (1994). Why investigate metacognition. In J. Metcalf & P. Shimamura (Eds.), *Metacognition: Knowing about knowing.* Cambridge: MIT Press.

Nissen, M. J., & Bullemer, P. (1987). Attentional requirements of learning: Evidence from performance measures. *Cognitive Psychology, 19,* 1–32.

O'Reilly, M. F., & Cuvo, A. J. (1989). Teaching self-treatment of cold symptoms to an anoxic brain injured adult. *Behavioral Residential Treatment, 4,* 359–375.

Posner, M. I., & Peterson, S. E. (1990). The attentional system of the human brain. *Annual Review of Neuroscience, 13,* 25–42.

Reason, J. (1984). Absent-mindedness and cognitive control. In J. E. Harris & P. E. Morris, *Everyday memory actions and absent-mindedness.* London: Academic Press.

Robertson, I. H., Ward, T., Ridgeway, V., & Nimmo-Smith, I. (1994). *The Test of Everyday Attention.* Bury St. Edmund's, England: Thames Valley Test.

Schneider, W., Dumais, S. T., & Shiffrin, R. M. (1984). Automatic and control processing and attention. In R. Parasuraman, & D. R. Davis (Eds.), *Varieties of attention.* London: Academic Press.

Shallice, T., & Evans, M. E. (1978). The involvement of the frontal lobes in cognitive estimation. *Cortex, 14,* 294–303.

Shaw, L., Brodsky, L., & McMahon, B. T. (1985). Neuropsychiatric intervention in the rehabilitation of head injured patients. *Psychiatric Journal of the University of Ottawa, 10,* 237–240.

Shiffrin, R. M., & Schneider, W. (1977). Controlled and automatic information processing: II. Perceptual learning, automatic attending, and a general theory. *Psychological Review, 84,* 127–190.

Skinner, B. F. (1938). *The behavior of organisms: An experimental analysis.* New York: Appelton-Century-Crofts.

Soderback, I., & Normell, L. A. (1986a). Intellectual function training in adults with acquired brain damage: An occupational therapy method. *Scandinavian Journal of Rehabilitation Medicine, 18,* 139–146.

Soderback, I., & Normell, L. A. (1986b). Intellectual function training in adults with acquired brain damage: Evaluation. *Scandinavian Journal of Rehabilitation Medicine, 18,* 147–153.

Solokov, E. N. (1963). *Perception and the conditioned reflex.* Oxford: Pergamon Press.

Spooner, F. (1981). An operant analysis of the effects of backward chaining and total task presentation. *Dissertation Abstracts International, 41* (3), 992A.

Spooner, F. (1984). Comparison of backward chaining and total task presentation in training severely handicapped persons. *Education and Training of the Mentally Retarded, 19,* 15–22.

Stuss, D. T., Stethem, L. L., Hugenholtz, H., Picton, T., Pivik, J., & Richards, M. T. (1989). Reaction time after head injury: Fatigue, divided attention and consistency of performance. *Journal of Neurology, Neurosurgery, and Psychiatry, 52,* 742–748.

Tulving, E. (1972). Episodic and semantic memory. In E. Tulving & W. Donaldson (Eds.), *Organization of memory.* New York: Academic Press.

Tulving, E. (1983). *Elements of episodic memory.* Oxford: Clarendon Press.

Vilkki, J. (1988). Problem solving after focal cerebral lesions. *Cortex, 24,* 119–127.

Wilson, B. A., Cockburn, J., & Baddeley, A. (1991). *The Rivermead Behavioral Memory Test* (2nd ed.). Bury St. Edmund's, England: Thames Valley Test.

Wilson, B. A., & Moffat, N. (1984). *Clinical management of memory problems.* London: Croom Helm.

Wolery, M., Griffen, A. K., Ault, M. J., Gast, D. L., & Doyle, P. M. (1990). Comparison of constant time delay and the system of least prompts in teaching chained tasks. *Education and Training in Mental Retardation, 25,* 243–257.

World Health Organization. (1980). *International classification of impairment disabilities and handicaps.* Geneva: World Health Organization.

Yuen, H. K. (1994). Neurofunctional approach to improve self-care skills in adults with brain damage. *Occupational Therapy in Mental Health, 12,* 31–45.

Zencius, A. H., Wesolowski, M. D., Burke, W. H., & McQuade, P. (1989). Antecedent control in the treatment of brain injured clients. *Brain Injury, 3,* 199–205.

Mental Health

CHAPTER 5

The Dynamic Interactional Model in Schizophrenia

Naomi Josman, PhD, OTR

There exists a traditional distinction in medicine between mental disorders and physical disorders. Mental disorders refers to those diseases and conditions with manifestations that seem mostly to affect a person's behavior: how a person feels, how a person thinks, how he remembers, and how those victims perceive and view the world around them (Levy, 1982). In the past, psychiatric conditions were attributed to environmental factors or to psychosocial influences (Andreasen, 1989; Donohue, 1993). Since the introduction of neuroleptic drugs in the 1950s and 1960s, a plethora of drug studies have contributed significantly to revealing, at least partially, the underlying biological bases of mental disorders. Simultaneously, neuroscientific findings of the past 2 decades and the burgeoning interdisciplinary interest in the interaction between central nervous system development, the environment, and illness have raised hopes for stimulating more effective treatment methods (Fine, 1993).

In considering similar problems among the mentally ill, more recently developed conceptualizations and interventions, which address the cognitive difficulties experienced by clients following brain-injuries, appear to be a most valuable resource. Cognitive methods for the rehabilitation of mentally-ill clients were initially introduced in the 1980s (Anthony, 1980), and Allen (1985) was the first to propose a cognitive intervention model for occupational therapy with mentally ill clients.

In this chapter I propose adopting the Dynamic Interactional Model for evaluating and treating mentally ill clients, an approach initially developed by Toglia for use with clients following brain injuries (Toglia, 1992). Although the cognitive disorders that will be described are characteristic of many psychiatric disorders, including both schizophrenia and primary affective disorders, the focus is on schizophrenia and cognitive disorders. Moreover, while it may be assumed that the Dynamic Interactional Approach is highly appropriate for interventions with several mental health disorders, this chapter concentrates specifically on the cognitive/neuropsychological disorders of schizophrenia.

This chapter initially provides an overview of the theoretical base for schizophrenia and cognitive disorders: memory disorders, frontal lobe disorders, and awareness disorders in schizophrenia. Thereafter, the Dynamic Interactional Model and its adaptation to clients suffering from schizophrenia is discussed, with special reference to evaluation and treatment methods for intervention and implications for the study of relevant instruments. Two case studies are presented to illustrate the intervention. The chapter concludes with the description of three research studies, using the Dynamic Interactional Assessment (DIA) instruments and recommendations for adopting this model to other mental health disorders, and proposes further research into the utility and efficacy of the DIA model for evaluation, treatment, and rehabilitation of mentally ill clients.

Neuropsychological/Neuroscientific Evidence of Cognitive Deficits in Schizophrenia

Growing evidence in psychiatry proposes biological explanations for clients' functional disorders, as manifest in schizophrenia and primary affective disorders. The cognitive symptoms of schizophrenia have been well established and include thought disorder, hallucinations, and delusions. For a long time, these symptoms also have been the targets of various therapeutic approaches and interventions. Cognitive or neuropsychological deficits in schizophrenia include problems of attention, concentration, and memory, as well as impairment in abstraction and concept formation abilities, and have only comparatively recently become targets of research and treatment (Stuve, Erickson, & Spaulding, 1991). An abundant literature documents the presence of significant neuropsychological impairments in schizophrenia (David & Cutting, 1994).

The contemporary diagnostic trends in schizophrenia consider the inclusion of two conditions classified according to the symptomatology of functional and relational abilities. These two conditions are termed positive and negative symptoms (Andreasen, 1989). Positive symptom schizophrenia is characterized by highly visible psychotic symptoms, such as blatant auditory hallucinations, bizarre delusions of persecution or outside control, and disorders of thought and association. Negative symptom schizophrenia is characterized by marked deficits, such as poverty of speech, poor judgment, social withdrawal, and lack of emotional responsiveness (Andreasen, 1989; Crow, 1985). According to Cornblatt, Lenzenweger, Dworkin, and Erlenmeyer-Kimling (1985), positive symptoms appear to be specifically associated with distractibility, whereas negative symptoms appear to be related only to more complex cognitive deficits.

Psychiatric clients experience everyday difficulties that are characteristic of cognitive disability (Allen, 1992). Their difficulties are similar to those found in people with other diagnoses, including people following brain injuries. Moreover, these people share common learning difficulties, which can be divided into component parts of brain function, such as apraxia and impairment of perception, attention, memory, and orientation.

According to Weinberger, Aloia, Goldberg, and Berman (1994), many persons with schizophrenia show clinical signs of frontal lobe dysfunction, including blunted affect, difficulty with problem solving, and impoverished thinking.

Anthony and Liberman (1986) describe a conceptual model for psychiatric rehabilitation. They theorize that the conceptual model introduced to physical medicine and rehabilitation was integrated later into the mental health disciplines. The rehabilitation process of both populations begins when the pathology and impairments of the acute stage stabilize. Three major cognitive areas are described in the following section.

Memory Disorders

Memory impairments in schizophrenia have been well documented (Clare, McKenna, Mortimer, & Baddeley, 1993). According to Calev and Edelist (1993), these impairments represent the most significant neuropsychological problems in schizophrenia. Several investigators have found that the memory deficit observed in schizophrenia may not be attributable to poor cooperation, lack of motivation, overall intellectual impairment, distraction by symptoms, or medication (Clare, McKenna, Mortimer, & Baddley, 1993; Duffy & O'Carroll, 1994).

More recently, a number of studies have found that the memory deficit in schizophrenia, unlike the classical amnestic syndrome observed after brain injury, involves both episodic and semantic memory. Therefore, schizophrenic individuals exhibit impairment in general knowledge of concepts, categories, and meanings (Chen, Wilkins, & McKenna, 1994; Clare, McKenna, Mortimer, & Baddeley, 1993; Duffy & O'Carroll, 1994).

Encoding is a major memory process, defined as a mental activity or a type of strategy that the learner employs when studying material to be remembered. A number of studies link memory recall deficits in schizophrenic clients to ineffective encoding of to-be-remembered verbal materials (Calev, Venables, & Monk, 1983; Harvey, Earle-Boyer, Wielgus, & Levinson, 1986). In a study by Larsen and Fromholt (1976), schizophrenic participants required more trials than normal participants to organize a set of words consistently on a sorting task. However, after accomplishing the task, their recall was comparable to the recall of normal participants in terms of number of words and categorical order. Thus, it is evident that induced affective or semantic encoding strategies attenuate the encoding deficit in schizophrenia. Further studies have found the process of making meaningful sentences out of to-be-remembered words (Koh, Marusarz, & Rosen, 1980), and an increase in the level of semantic processing (Koh, Grinker, Marusarz, & Forman, 1981) to have similar normalizing effects in recall of schizophrenic clients.

There are, however, some noncorroboratory findings, wherein schizophrenic subjects have exhibited a recall deficit, even after inducing effective encoding and mnemonic organization (Calev, Venables, & Monk, 1983). They interpret these discrepant findings in terms of the specific samples studied: their schizophrenic sample included chronic, severely disturbed, individuals, who had at least 2 years of cumulative hospitalization before their present admission, in distinct contrast to Koh and his colleagues' (1981) sample of young schizophrenic clients who were mildly disturbed, nonchronic, and well conditioned.

There is evidence that the memory deficits in encoding that remanifest by schizophrenic subjects may be related to inefficient use of mnemonic strategies, rather than to irreversible structural defects (Koh & Peterson, 1978). While these clients demonstrate the potential to use mnemonic organizational properties, they may fail to do so at the encoding stage (Calev, Venables, & Monk, 1983).

A number of different hypotheses have been proposed to account for the difficulties in using efficient encoding strategies, which schizophrenic individuals seem to experience. Recent findings have led some investigators to propose that the lack of efficient organizational strategies observed during encoding may be related to a disorder of semantic category structure, or to abnormalities in the network of semantic relations. Chen, Wilkins, and McKenna (1994) found that schizophrenic individuals needed to overextend the boundaries of categories, taking the longest time to respond to semantically related items not belonging within the category.

The impaired capacity to form meaningful and efficient associations that constitute the founda-

tions of memory may be attributable to overinclusive thinking. Gray, Feldon, Rawlins, Hemsley, and Smith (1991) proposed that the basic problem in schizophrenia may be a weakening of the ability to utilize and incorporate past experiences in current learning. Duffy and O'Carroll (1994) have further hypothesized that the cognitive mechanisms involved in the formation and retention of association networks in general may be dysfunctional in schizophrenia. Alternatively, Schwartz, Rosse, and Deutsch (1993) have suggested that schizophrenic clients may have difficulty in using conceptual or organizational processes in performing tasks that require explicit retrieval of contextual information.

Frontal Lobe Disorders

There is accumulating evidence that clients with schizophrenia are unable to fully activate their frontal lobes during cognitive tasks, requiring sustained frontal lobe activation (Melzer, 1994). Many clients with schizophrenia show clinical signs of frontal lobe dysfunction, including blunted affect, difficulty with problem solving, and impoverished thinking (Weinberger, Aloia, Goldberg, & Berman, 1994).

One of the critical cognitive difficulties that characterizes many clients with schizophrenia is demonstrated on the Wisconsin Card Sorting Test (WCST) (Heaton, Chelune, Talley, Kay, & Curtiss, 1993). The performance of schizophrenic clients on the WCST, a test that is sensitive to frontal lobe dysfunction, was inferior to that of normal controls; in addition, neuroleptic treatment did not correct the deficit (Melzer, 1994).

Weinberger's (1987) controlled studies of postmortem brain tissue have yielded nonspecific, but objective evidence of anatomical pathology in schizophrenia in the periventricular limbic and diencephalic areas, and in the prefrontal cortex. These studies, however, have not demonstrated, a characteristic lesion, or even a consistent pathological picture, in part because of differing methods of tissue examination. Weinberger (1987) concluded that in a generic sense, these studies suggest that pathology of the limbic system is a replaceable phenomenon in schizophrenia. More recently, Weinberger et al. (1994) have suggested that the failure of intracortical connectivity of the prefrontal cortex may account for both cognitive and psychotic manifestations of this illness.

Cutting, David and Murphy (1987) compared two groups of adults diagnosed with schizophrenia and a control group of individuals diagnosed as neurotic on four tests of categorical thinking, in an attempt to discover the nature of overinclusive thinking. Results showed that schizophrenics were poorer on nonverbal than on verbal categories, with more conceptual loosening and a tendency toward overcategorization. Schizophrenic individuals adopted a piecemeal strategy, suggesting a deficit in their ability to form a Gestalt of the task.

Heinrichs (1990) examined the WCST performance of 56 neuropsychiatric clients referred for neuropsychological assessment. Using descriptive statistics, he showed a high degree of impairment of the sample as a whole on the WCST. Point-biserial correlations between WCST variables and frontal cerebral involvement were significant, but relatively modest. No relationship between schizophrenia or mood disorder and the WCST indices was found. Hospitalization was also related to WCST variables: outpatients demonstrated less impairment than inpatients. Heinrichs interpreted the results in terms of the validity of the WCST as a predictor of neurological, psychiatric, and functional statuses in different clinical populations.

Green, Ganzell, Satz, and Vaclav (1990), commenting on a study by Goldberg, Weinberger, Pliskin, Berman, and Podd (1989), suggested that schizophrenic clients were unable to learn the WCST due to suboptimal behavioral contingencies needed for learning. They therefore conducted a new pilot study with 10 schizophrenic individuals and examined their performance on the WCST under four conditions. Data showed a learner–nonlearner distinction, possibly representative of separate etiological subtypes, which might identify those clients who would benefit from rehabilitation and training.

Awareness Disorders

A lack of awareness of existing deficits has been documented for a broad range of neuropsychological syndromes. In addition, this phenomenon has significant implications for treatment and management. Clients who are unaware of their problems are unlikely to cooperate with treatment plans or accept help from concerned family members (McGlynn & Kaszniak, 1986). Furthermore, these clients may attempt to perform activities that are entirely unrealistic, considering their given disabilities.

Schizophrenic clients who lack awareness of their deficits may also pose serious problems for family members and other caretakers. Several studies have indicated that persons suffering from schizophrenia are largely unaware of their abnormal involuntary movements. The motor disturbance in schizophrenia generally has been attributed to the effect of long-term treatment with neuroleptic drugs and is referred to as tardive dyskinesia. However, these movement disorders in schizophrenia were observed and documented long before the advent of neuroleptic medication (Crow, Cross, Johnstone, et al., 1982). Greenfield (1985) claimed that clients who lack awareness of their mental illness, insisting that they have no illness or symptoms requiring treatment, are virtually inaccessible to treatment.

Delusions have been considered, by definition, to be outside the realm of patients' awareness. Kihlstrom and Hoyt (1988) viewed delusions as part product of disordered perceptual and attentional processes. According to this view, schizophrenic clients are entirely unaware of their most fundamental psychological deficit: a perceptual-attentional disorder. As a consequence, they search for some explanation for their anomalous experiences, not realizing their own role in constructing the bizarre experiences. Schizophrenia with negative symptoms, however, provides evidence that brain dysfunction is restricted primarily to subcortical structures and the frontal lobes. Stuss and Benson (1986) discussed the possible contribution of frontal lobe damage to the pathogenesis of anosognosia. The role of frontal damage in unawareness of deficits is further indicated by the extensive literature on people following head injuries, who often exhibit symptoms of frontal lobe damage with unawareness of deficits (McGlynn & Kaszniak, 1986).

Amador, Flaum, Andreasen, et al. (1994) conducted a study to assess insight into multiple aspects of mental disorder using a standardized measure. Their sample of 412 patients included clients with psychotic and mood disorders. Their results indicate that poor insight is a prevalent feature of schizophrenia. Moreover, a variety of self-awareness deficits were found to be more severe and pervasive in subjects with schizophrenia than in clients with schizoaffective or major depressive disorders, with or without psychosis.

In summary, persons diagnosed as suffering from schizophrenia have a disorder that encompasses multiple aspects of psychopathology. Efforts of contemporary researchers, theorists, and practitioners focus currently on the neuropsychological/cognitive aspects of the schizophrenic disorder. The focal question that arises is: Do we have a direction or method for helping and treating these people? In the following section, I propose using the DIA to further our understanding and enhance our ability to intervene with such clients.

The Dynamic Interactional Model

Toglia's model (1992) uses a broad definition of cognition that encompasses information processing skills, learning, and generalization. Moreover, cognition is not merely divided into distinct entities but rather cognitive abilities and deficiencies are analyzed according to underlying processes, strategies, and potential for learning. In essence, cognition is viewed as an ongoing product of the dynamic interaction between the individual, the task, and the environment (see chapter 1). Clinical application of this model will provide essential information about individuals' potential for change, and will also help to answer the following questions: How promptly does an individual learn new material? How well do they retain it? How do they go about organizing new information? How do they proceed with decisions in response to environmental demands? How orderly and comprehensive are their problem-solving strategies (Erickson & Binder, 1986)?

The Dynamic Interactional Model addresses learning potential, analyzes individual processing strategies and style, and provides important guidelines for treatment. Implementing this elaborate method with clients suffering from schizophrenia may significantly advance our understanding of the disorder and enhance the capacity for effective therapeutic intervention.

Intervention, including Evaluation Procedures, Assessment Instruments, and Treatment Methods

The initial step in evaluating schizophrenic clients should be based on the use of static assessments, such as standardized cognitive screening instruments. The results of such an evaluation will define a client's "here and now" performance baseline. The objectives of the static assessment are the identification and quantification of cognitive deficits, which is essential information for diagnosing, progress monitoring, discharge planning, and client or caregiver education regarding expected behaviors (Toglia, 1989). At the following more elaborative step of evaluation, the therapist should use the Dynamic Interactional Assessment (DIA) and instruments developed and studied by Toglia (see chapter 1).

In Figure 1-3 Toglia analyzes the differences between static, qualitative, and dynamic assessment methods. The main contribution of the DIA is that, at the conclusion of the evaluation process, a therapist is able to provide answers to three questions: Can performance be facilitated or changed? What conditions increase or decrease client symptoms? What is the client's potential for learning? The DIA consists of three components that are integrated during assessment: awareness questions, cueing and task grading, and strategy investigation.

The following three paragraphs briefly describe instruments developed by Toglia: Contextual Memory Test (CMT), Toglia Category Assessment (TCA), and Deductive Reasoning Test. All three instruments are in practical use with schizophrenic clients. Full details of the instruments can be found in their manual and in chapter 1 of this book. The Contextual Memory Test (CMT) was designed to objectively investigate awareness and the use of strategy, as well as to screen memory deficits. The CMT provides a measure of three related aspects of memory:

- awareness of memory capacity—general questioning, prediction of memory capacity prior to task performance, and estimation of memory capacity following task performance

- recall of line-drawn objects—both immediate and delayed recall
- strategy use—the ability to describe the use of strategy, and the ability to benefit from a strategy provided by the examiner (Toglia, 1993).

The Toglia Category Assessment (TCA) was designed to examine the ability of adults to establish categories and to switch conceptual sets. An objective investigation of awareness is included both before and after task performance. The evaluator investigates the relationship between subject estimation and his or her actual TCA score. The test uses plastic utensils that can be sorted according to size, color, and type. The test objectively examines the client's ability to profit from cues and/or task modification (Toglia, 1994).

The Deductive Reasoning Test, which is a continuation of the TCA, employs the same plastic utensils, and should be administered as the next step immediately after the TCA. A questioning game is introduced, wherein the client is instructed to guess which utensil the examiner is thinking of. The client can respond only with questions having yes or no answers, in trying to guess the correct utensil. The examiner does not actually think of an item but answers "no" uniformly to all questions until only one possibility remains. The correct answer should be attained within five questions (Toglia, 1994). A person can have difficulty with this task for a number of reasons, including failure to keep track of previous questions or answers, failure to utilize feedback, failure to discard an inappropriate hypothesis, decreased ability to attend to the relevant attribute, impulsivity (Toglia, 1994).

Treatment

Treatment planning in general is dependent not only on the occupational therapist but on the decisions of a multidisciplinary team. The occupational therapist needs to be aware of the clinical work setting and context, the overall purposes of the setting, his or her specific professional role, goals and objectives, and his or her contribution as a staff member best serving the clients' needs. In light of the contemporary practice policy of many health services, most schizophrenic clients are admitted to psychiatric hospitals in an acute stage, where efforts are aimed at stabilizing psychotic symptoms and expediting the transfer of clients to a rehabilitation center. In light of this situation, the main purpose of occupational therapy interventions is assessment, treatment goal-setting, and production of a clear and coherent report. As previously mentioned, initial static standardized assessment tools should be employed to uniformly evaluate all clients. Most frequently, the client is discharged before having a chance to undergo a DIA. However, for those occupational therapists working in a long-term rehabilitation setting, it is recommended that both the DIA and the treatment methods derived from this evaluation process be used.

If the DIA reveals that a client's performance cannot be facilitated through cueing or task modification, then a functional or skill-training approach may be appropriate (Neistadt, 1990). The various treatment methods are fully detailed by Allen (1985) and Fleming Cottrell (1993), but lie outside the scope of this chapter. If, however, the assessment reveals that a client's performance may be facilitated by any kind of mediation, the therapist should then employ a multicontextual treatment approach to facilitate the client's ability to process information and implement it flexibly across task conditions.

The following list states the main multicontextual treatment principles for clients suffering from schizophrenia. A full description of this method is presented in Chapter 1 as well as in other sources (Toglia, 1989; 1991; 1992).

- The sequence of treatment is not predetermined, but is rather developed step by step, according to the client's achievements.
- During all treatment sessions, the therapist analyzes the processing strategies employed by the client, and determines whether the task may be performed in a more efficient way.
- Determining client motivation is crucial for this kind of treatment. When planning and selecting

treatment activities, the therapist needs to consider learner characteristics, including motivation and individual personality characteristics.

■ Treatment usually begins at the level where performance breaks down, or the point at which the client is able to successfully complete the task with the aid of only one to three cues.

■ Treatment needs to use activities that meet the abilities of the individual.

■ Task complexity is not increased until evidence of generalization is observed at all levels of transfer.

■ The underlying strategy or conceptual characteristics remain the same in all treatment tasks, whereas the surface characteristics of the task change gradually as treatment moves from near transfer to far transfer (Toglia, 1991).

■ The therapist needs to define the goals of each activity in clear and concrete terms that are comprehensible to the client.

■ The therapist uses a variety of computer, gross motor, table-top, and functional tasks in treatment; the therapist avoids the use of one exclusive type of activity in order to ensure that, while the instruction may have been embedded in one context, the learned skills may still be accessible in relation to that specific context (Toglia, 1991).

■ Metacognitive training to promote awareness and self-monitoring skills should be incorporated into each treatment session, as well as in different situations.

■ In order to help the client adapt to different environments, both individual and group activities should be employed.

Case Report 1

Nancy is an 18-year-old female with a diagnosis of schizophrenia with negative symptoms. She recently showed improvement after medication with Clozapine. On her initial evaluation using the Allen Cognitive Level (ACL) test, she scored at level 4—goal-directed actions, defined by Allen (1992) as the level where the subject "sequences the self through a series of steps to match a concrete sample or known standard of how the finished product should appear" (p. 5). Nancy's occupational thera-

pist observed marked task impairment and reported that she was inattentive to the task requirements. For example, she did not wait or ask for assistance and would continue performing a task obviously incorrectly, unaware of her poor results. She either ignored or omitted many aspects of the task and the social environment. A DIA was administered to provide insight into Nancy's underlying cognitive strengths and deficits.

Awareness   Prior to performing the TCA, Nancy denied changes in her thinking skills, yet overestimated the difficulty of the task. Immediately following task performance, Nancy claimed that her thinking was "not as sharp as it used to be." She then admitted to sometimes missing the point of a conversation or joke. She accurately rated the sorting task as difficult.

Task Performance   Nancy had no difficulty sorting the utensils according to type, but needed five to six cues to sort them according to color. She demonstrated a tendency to perseverate on the utensil-type category. However, when the therapist pointed out the difference between the utensils, she then immediately rearranged the utensils into the correct category. On the third round of sorting Nancy needed only two cues to accurately categorize the utensils according to size. She appeared to have learned from the previous trial and actively sought to identify further differences between the utensils.

While using the CMT, Nancy showed very similar problems on the awareness part of the test. She first denied changes in her memory performance and overestimated her ability to recall items. She estimated that she would remember 15 out of the 20 items to be presented to her. In fact, she was able to recall only eight items in the immediate recall and seven in the delayed recall. Following task performance, she claimed that her memory was not as good as it had been prior to her hospitalization, and she was able to estimate accurately, having recalled eight items in the immediate recall and seven in the delayed recall.

Strategy Use   When asked to describe how she studied the items, Nancy responded, "I just looked at them." Her order of recall did not reveal any clustering or grouping of associated items. In part II however, when she was given cues to use the contextual information, both her immediate and delayed recall increased by three or four points. In addition, the order of recall revealed smaller clustering of related items. This seems to indicate that although Nancy did not appear to initiate the use of efficient strategies, she was quite able to implement strategies when prompted to do so.

Summary   Nancy evidenced recall deficits, and demonstrated a decrease in ability to estimate her quality of performance, as well as an impaired use of strategies. However, performance in all three areas can be improved. Nancy's performance demonstrated a learning curve on both tests, as well as a "carry over" generalization effect in the use of strategies. She thus appears to be a suitable candidate for metamemory training and cognitive training in other areas.

Treatment Objectives

- Nancy will demonstrate the ability to estimate the amount of information to be correctly recalled within three to five points.
- Nancy will demonstrate the ability to estimate the level of difficulty of a sorting task.
- Nancy will demonstrate the ability to initiate use of a grouping strategy three out of five times in tasks where items are closely related.
- Nancy will demonstrate the ability to apply use of an organizing strategy to two different tasks without prompting.

Case Report 2

Rena is a 45-year-old female with a diagnosis of schizophrenia with both positive and negative symptoms. Rena is a highly intelligent woman but is functionally impaired. She has become increasingly preoccupied with her slowness and her difficulties with self-care and home management activities. Her high anxiety and demoralization in response to these problems became partially linked to the earlier loss of her house and furniture, during

a prolonged psychotic episode. The stress provoked by these memories appeared to limit her already compromised problem-solving capacities. Different treatment techniques had previously been used, practiced, and mastered—in both individual and group settings. However, these methods failed at home, where she was unable to transfer what she had learned in treatment and when she was having the greatest need for intervention.

Evaluation   Rena's personality and emotional problems were already well known to the therapist. Task and environment variables were reviewed through observation and analysis in her home. The main question was: Why was Rena unable to generalize acquired skills and transfer them specifically to her home situation?

A DIA was introduced. A battery of assessments including the CMT and the TCA was chosen to identify deficits and conditions that maximize performance. Surprisingly, most of Rena's difficulties were primarily those of style rather than capacity. Both short-term and long-term memory as well as basic organizational capacities were sufficiently intact but not always accessible, because of inefficient employment, such as overattentiveness to details during the sorting of items or difficulty in disengaging from a task. Inadequate self-monitoring skills were also observed.

During assessment sessions, Rena was responsive to cueing, and was able to retain information and apply it to other assessment tasks that appeared different, as well as to improve the efficiency of her cognitive operations.

Treatment Plan   As a result of the assessment data, efforts to engage her potential were shifted from the skills-training group to individual session training self-management techniques, aimed at enhancing her ability to self-monitor her tendencies to overfocus on details, making necessary work for herself, and displaying sluggishness in completing tasks. Rena was given written guidelines to help her organize her thoughts before initiating any task. The same techniques were applied to a succession of other meaningful activities, such as cooking tasks requiring recipe selection, shopping, and budgeting. In each task, the behaviors that Rena seeks to monitor are identified, and manageable goals, questionnaires, and guidelines are developed with the therapist. Rena's responsiveness to this approach has been notable, and she was able to transfer the same strategies to other activities. As mentioned earlier, Rena is an intelligent woman and highly motivated toward her treatment; this kind of treatment strategy was therefore reasonable and productive.

Research

Using the tools developed in the DIA, three different studies will be reported in this section: (1) A study using the TCA with both schizophrenic and brain-injured participants (Toglia & Josman, 1994); (2) Study of differences in metamemory in chronic schizophrenic participants and controls, using the CMT (Josman, unpublished); and (3) Study of memory functions in chronic schizophrenic participants using the CMT (So, Toglia, & Donohue, 1997).

Josman's (1993) study was designed to examine categorization skills in schizophrenic and brain-injured participants, and compare the performance of these two populations. A total of 70 hospitalized adult subjects were examined, including 35 schizophrenic and 35 brain-injured subjects. The schizophrenic population included participants with paranoid schizophrenia, simple-type schizophrenia, residual schizophrenia, and schizo-affective disorders. Participants with active hallucinations or delusions were excluded from the study. The mean age for the schizophrenic subjects was 39 (SD = 12), while the mean age for the brain-injured subjects was 54 (SD = 19). The age difference between the two groups reflected differences between the two populations. In general the average age at onset of schizophrenia is in the mid-20s, while cerebral vascular accidents are more commonly seen in the elderly population.

In this study the brain-injured population was generally more educated than the schizophrenic population. A positive correlation of r =.59 (p < .001) between level of education and the TCA was found. The higher educational level of the brain-injured population may partially account for the higher scores obtained by this population as compared to the schizophrenic population. It should be noted that the brain-injured population constituted an acute population, whereas the schizophrenic population had been in treatment for an average of 12.48 years, with a standard deviation of 9.5 (Toglia & Josman, 1994).

Description of performance

The mean performance score of the schizophrenic subjects on the TCA was 23.08 (SD = 7.60), while the score of the brain injured subjects on the TCA was 25.17 (SD = 6.3). Overall, the brain-injured population scored slightly higher than the schizophrenic population, but the difference was not significant. This indicated that the TCA should not be used to discriminate between schizophrenic and brain-injured adults. This finding is not surprising, because there is evidence that chronic schizophrenic participants show decline in cognition and are assumed to have structural neurological changes located in the frontal lobe (Weinberger, Aloia, Goldberg, & Berman, 1994). Most neuropsychological tests are unable to differentiate between chronic schizophrenic and brain-injured subjects (Lezak, 1995). The TCA was not designed with the purpose of differential diagnosis or discrimination between organic and psychiatric illnesses, but rather to provide information that may be helpful for treatment planning.

Awareness Performance

In this study, questions pertaining to awareness were included immediately following task performance. There were significant differences between the mean awareness scores: the brain-injured subjects obtained poorer estimation scores than their schizophrenic counterparts. In addition, there was a significant correlation between the total TCA score and the awareness score for the schizophrenic subjects (r = .40), but not for the brain injured subjects. Brain-injured subjects, however, demonstrated an interesting crossover pattern: those who estimated the task to be easy tended to have more difficulty than those who estimated the task to be difficult whereas participants who estimated the task to be difficult, tended to perform better than they had estimated.

This finding is consistent with other studies, which have found that a similar failure to recognize the difficulty of a task in relation to one's own abilities results in impaired performance (McGlynn & Kaszniak, 1986). Results also indicate that questions pertaining to awareness may be sensitive in differentiating between schizophrenic and brain-injured populations.

Using the CMT

In a recent study, Josman (unpublished) compared the performance of chronic schizophrenic participants to healthy controls. A total of 89 subjects were examined including 30 chronic schizophrenic clients hospitalized within three different psychiatric hospitals in Israel and 59 healthy controls. The mean age for the chronic schizophrenic subjects was 35.6 (SD = 8.94), and for the control subjects was 37.3 (SD = 14.3). All other demographic variables were very similar for both groups and showed no significant differences.

The CMT (Toglia, 1993) was used to measure three aspects of memory: (1) awareness (general, prediction, and estimation), (2) recall (immediate and delayed), and (3) strategy use. The test was administered uniformly to all participants without the provision of any interventions or cues during administration. The restaurant version was administered to half the subjects, and the morning version was administered to the remainder of the subjects.

Memory performance

Significant differences were obtained on both immediate and delayed recall between schizophrenic subjects and healthy controls. The mean score of recall performance of the healthy subjects (immediate = 14.6; delayed = 14.3) fell within normal limits, according to the CMT manual (Toglia, 1993), while that of the schizophrenic subjects (immediate = 10.1; delayed = 8.6) fell into the mild category of memory ability.

The mean scores of the schizophrenic subjects ($\bar{x}$ = 22.3; SD = 5.3) were significantly lower (t = 3.85 p <.001) than the scores of the healthy subjects ($\bar{x}$ = 25.8; SD = 3.2).

The prediction scores before immediate recall were very similar for both healthy ($\bar{x}$ = 11.9) and schizophrenic subjects ($\bar{x}$ = 11.3). However, the schizophrenic subjects overestimated the number of pictures to be remembered, while the healthy subjects underestimated them. The mean estimation scores directly following the immediate recall of both the schizophrenic ($\bar{x}$ = 10.8) and the healthy ($\bar{x}$ = 14) subjects were more reflective of their true recall scores: only the mean estimation scores of the healthy subjects were statistically significant with the true recall score obtained, but not for the schizophrenic subjects. The estimation scores after the delayed recall for both groups were more reflective of actual recall scores and statistically significant. This finding indicates that the schizophrenic participants' awareness of their memory ability differed from the awareness of the healthy subjects. It should be noted that the schizophrenic participants overestimated their recall ability before task performance, but their estimation was more accurate immediately after recall performance.

Strategy Use

A significant difference between the schizophrenic and healthy participants was found in reference to their strategy use. The healthy participants used higher order strategies such as restaurant or association/group, whereas a third of the schizophrenic participants used a visualization strategy. Most of the schizophrenic participants did not report the use of any strategy.

In response to this finding, So, Toglia, & Donohue (1997) studied the memory performance of chronic adult schizophrenic participants in terms of (1) awareness of memory capacity, (2) immediate and delayed recall, and (3) strategy use and ability to use contextual information using the CMT (Toglia, 1993).

Twenty-three chronic schizophrenic participants with a mean age of 38.3 (SD = 6.5), residing in a state psychiatric hospital in New Jersey, were included in the study. The study consisted of 18 males and five females with the mean number of years of education of 11.7 (SD = 2). The mean duration of inpatient stay was 38.6 months (SD = 54.1). The mean number of years since either the onset of illness or the participants' first admission was 15.87 (SD = 7.4). The primary diagnosis of the participants included 11 (47.8%) chronic paranoid schizophrenic and 12 (52.2%) chronic undifferentiated schizophrenic individuals. Among the 23 subjects, 14 (60.9%) indicated a history of alcohol abuse, drug abuse, or both. All subjects were being treated with neuroleptic medication.

In part I of the test, each participant was assessed without the aid of any cueing. In part II, each subject was provided with cueing through being told the theme prior to viewing the objects. This is the usual sequence of directions for the CMT. Part II was administered at least 3 days after the presentation of part I to minimize the learning effect. This study investigated whether the cue of providing the theme or context facilitated recall.

The Brief Psychiatric Rating Scale-Anchored (BPRS-A, Woerner, Mannuzza, & Kane, 1988) and the Scale for the Assessment of Negative Symptoms (SANS; Andreasen, 1989) were used and scored based on the information derived from the interview with the investigator, from chart review of nursing notes, and from consultation with other medical staff.

A quasi-experimental design using a one-group, pretest posttest design format was employed. In part I but not in part II, the participant had to estimate his or her own memory capacity.

Immediate and Delayed Recall

In part II (with cue providing the theme), the participants achieved higher mean scores in both immediate (10.7) and delayed (9.2) recall than in part I (without cue) immediate (8.5) and delayed (7.5) recall. The differences between the two mean scores in immediate recall was 2.08 (SD = 2.72), ($t = -3.67$, $p < .001$). The differences between the two mean scores for delayed recall was 1.65 (SD = 3.11), ($t = -2.55$, $p < .05$).

Recall and Positive and Negative Symptoms

All participants manifested negative-symptom schizophrenia as classified by Andreasen (1982, 1985, 1989). Participants showed varying degrees of severity of negative symptoms, indicating a range of chronicity. The mean score of the BPRS-A was 31.21 (SD = 8.1). Pearson correlations were computed between the scores of BPRS-A and immediate and delayed recall in both parts of the CMT.

The results reveal significant inverse correlations between the scores of the BPRS-A and the scores of recall (r ranging from $-.65$ to $-.83$, $p < .01$). The mean scores of the SANS items was 61.6 (SD = 29.9). Pearson correlations were computed between the sum scores of the SANS and the scores of recall on CMT (r ranging from $-.64$ to $-.77$, $p < .01$).

An analysis of variance was performed between the global rating of each individual category of the SANS and the CMT recall scores. The categories of alogia and attentional impairment showed a significant correlation with the recall scores, while the other three categories showed no consistent significant correlations.

Recall and Strategy Use

The sum of the scores on questions 15 and 16 was calculated. These two questions asked the participants what they did to recall the item (Toglia, 1993). Pearson correlations were then computed between the scores of strategy use and the scores of recall. The correlation coefficient of immediate recall increased from $r = .61$ in part I to $r = .63$ ($p < .01$) in part II. The correlation coefficient of delayed recall increased from $r = .60$ in part I to $r = .69$ ($p < .01$) in part II.

Recall and Awareness of Memory Capacity

The participants were only asked to estimate their own memory capacity on part I of the CMT. Of these participants, 65.2% rated their memory capacity in the 51 to 100% range in reference to their performance before illness, while 30.43% of the participants rated themselves within a 0 to 50% range. One participant was unsure about his memory capacity. Participants reported experiencing a lower frequency of forgetting things.

The participants were required to estimate how many items out of 20 they could remember, and following the recall task, to estimate how many items they did remember. Correlations between prediction and recall ranged from $r = .08$ to $r = .32$ and those between recall and estimation ranged from $r = .31$ to $r = .75$ ($p < .01$).

A posthoc question was raised as to whether a difference could be observed between paranoid and undifferentiated schizophrenic participants in their CMT performance. In three out of the four memory tests, paranoid participants achieved mean scores 40% higher than the undifferentiated schizophrenic participants.

Summary and Implications for Further Knowledge Development and Directions for Future Research

In this chapter, I have proposed adopting the Dynamic Interactional Approach for evaluating and treating mentally ill clients focusing on schizophrenia and cognitive disorders, an approach initially developed by Toglia for use with clients following brain injuries (Toglia, 1992). While it may be assumed that the DIA be highly appropriate for interventions with several mental health disorders, such as schizoaffective and affective disorders, the DIA requires further exploration with these populations before advocating its clinical adoption and use. Further studies comparing the performance of chronic clients following brain injury and schizophrenia, as well as at the stage of acute brain injury and acute schizophrenia should be conducted using the DIA instruments. Reliability and validity studies with adolescent schizophrenic clients should be done to broaden the use of the DIA instruments. The effectiveness of the multicontextual treatment with clients suffering from schizophrenia should be investigated.

As Toglia stated in her chapter, in the absence of research evidence demonstrating the therapeutic efficacy of one cognitive approach over the other, occupational therapists should employ the approach that best fits the individual client and his or her specific disability.

Acknowledgment

I thank Mrs. Yaara Harary, Mrs. Ayelet Rabinowitz, and Mrs. Yael Yaron, senior occupational therapy students at Haifa University, for their assistance with testing.

References

Allen, C. K. (1985). *Occupational therapy for psychiatric diseases: Measurement and management of cognitive disabilities.* Boston: Little, Brown.

Allen, C. K. (1992). Cognitive Disabilities. In N. Katz (Ed.), *Cognitive rehabilitation models for intervention in occupational therapy.* Stoneham, MA: Butterworth-Heinemann.

Amador, X. F., Flaum, M., Andreasen, N. C., Strauss, D. H., Yale, S. A., Clark, S. C., & Gorman, J. M. (1994). Awareness of illness in schizophrenia and schizoaffective and mood disorders. *Archives of General Psychiatry, 11,* 826–836.

Andreasen, N. C. (1982). Negative symptoms in schizophrenia: Definition and reliability. *Archives of General Psychiatry, 39,* 784–788.

Andreasen, N. C. (1985). Positive and negative schizophrenia: A critical evaluation. *Schizophrenia Bulletin, 3,* 380–389.

Andreasen, N. C. (1989). The scale for the assessment of negative symptoms (SANS): Conceptual and theoretical foundations. *British Journal of Psychiatry, 155,* 49–52.

Anthony, W. A. (1980). A rehabilitation model for rehabilitating the psychiatrically sidabled. *Rehabilitation Counseling Bulletin, 24,* 6–21.

Anthony, W. A., & Liberman, R. P. (1986). The practice of psychiatric rehabilitation: Historical, conceptual, and research base. *Schizophrenia Bulletin, 4,* 542–559.

Calev, A., & Edelist, S. (1993). Affect and memory in schizophrenia: Negative emotion words are forgotten less rapidly than other words by long-hospitalized schizophrenics. *Psychopatology, 26,* 229–235.

Calev, A., Venables, P. H., & Monk, A. F. (1983). Evidence for distinct verbal memory pathologies in severely and mildly disturbed schizophrenics. *Schizophrenia Bulletin, 9,* 247–264.

Chen, E. Y. H., Wilkins, A. J., & McKenna, P. J. (1994). Semantic memory is both impaired and anomalous in schizophrenia. *Psychological Medicine, 24,* 193–202.

Clare, L., McKenna, P. J., Mortimer, A. M., & Baddeley, A. D. (1993). Memory in schizophrenia: What is impaired and what is preserved? *Neuropsychologia, 31,* 1225–1241.

Crow, T. J. (1985). The two-syndrome concept: Origins and current status. *Schizophrenia Bulletin, 11,* 475–485.

Cornblatt, B. A., Lenzenweger, M. F., & Dworkin, R. H., & Erlenmeyer-Kimling, L. (1985). Positive and negative schizophrenic symptoms, attention, and information processing. *Schizophrenia Bulletin, 11,* 397–407.

Crow, T. J., Cross, A. J., Johnstone, E. C., Owen, F., Owens, D. G. C., & Waddington, J. L. (1982). Abnormal involuntary movement in schizophrenia: Are they related to the disease process or its treatment? Are they associated with changes in dopamine receptors? *Clinical Psychopharmacology, 2,* 336–340.

Cutting, J., David, A. S., & Murphy, D. (1987). The nature of overinclusive thinking in schizophrenia. *Psychology, 24,* 213–219.

David, A. S., & Cutting, J. C. (Eds.). (1994). *The neuropsychology of schizophrenia.* Hillsdale, NJ: Erlbaum.

Donohue, M. V. (1993). Abnormal emotional conditions. In H. Cohen (Ed.), *Neuroscience for rehabilitation.* Philadelphia: Lippincott.

Duffy, L., & O'Carroll, R. (1994). Memory impairment in schizophrenia: A comparison with that observed in the Alcoholic Korsakoff Syndrome. *Psychological Medicine, 24,* 155–165.

Erickson, R. C., & Binder, L. M. (1986). Cognitive deficit among functionally psychotic patients: A rehabilitative perspective. *Journal of Clinical Experimental Neuropsychology, 3,* 257–274.

Fine, S. (1993). Neurobehavioral perspectives on schizophrenia. In J. Van Deusen (Ed.), *Body image and perceptual dysfunction in adults.* Philadelphia: Saunders.

Fleming Cottrell, R. P. (Ed.). (1993). *Psychosocial occupational therapy proactive approaches.* Bethesda, MD: American Occupational Therapy Association.

Goldberg, T. E., Weinberger, D. R., Pliskin, N. H., Berman, K. F., & Podd, M. H. (1989). Recall memory deficit in schizophrenia: A possible manifestation of prefrontal dysfunction. *Schizophrenia Research, 2,* 251–257.

Gray, J. A., Feldon, J., Rawlins, J. N. P., Hemsley, D. R., & Smith, A. D. (1991). The neuropsychology of schizophrenia. *Behavioral and Brain Science, 14,* 1–14.

Green, M. F., Ganzell, S., Satz, P., & Vaclav, J. F. (1990). Teaching the Wisconsin Card Sorting Test to schizophrenic patients. *Archives of General Psychiatry, 47,* 91–92.

Greenfeld, D. (1985). *The psychotic patient.* New York: Free Press.

Harvey, P. D., Earle-Boyer, E. A., Wielgus, M. S., & Levinson, J. C. (1986). Encoding, memory and thought disorders in schizophrenia and mania. *Schizophrenia Bulletin, 12,* 252–261.

Heaton, R. K., Chelune, G. J., Talley, J. L., Kay, G. G., & Curtiss, G. (1993). *Wisconsin Card Sorting Test Manual.* Odessa, FL: Psychological Assessment Resources.

Heinrichs, R. W. (1990). Variables associated with Wisconsin Card Sorting Test performance in neuropsychiatric patients referred for assessment. *Neuropsychiatry, Neuropsychology, and Behavioral Neurology, 3,* 107–112.

Josman, N. (1993). *Assessment of categorization skills in brain injured and schizophrenic persons: Validation of the Toglia Category Assessment (TCA).* Doctoral Dissertation, New York University.

Josman, N. (unpublished). Study of differences in metamemory in chronic schizophrenic participants and controls, using the CMT.

Kihlstrom, J. F., & Hoyt, I. P. (1988). Hypnosis and the psychology of delusions. In T. F. Oltmanns and B. A. Maher (Eds.), *Delusional beliefs.* New York: Wiley.

Koh, S. D., Grinker, R. R., Marusarz, T. Z., & Forman, P. L. (1981). Affective memory and schizophrenic anhedonia. *Schizophrenia Bulletin, 7,* 292–307.

Koh, S. D., Marusarz, T. Z., & Rosen, A. J. (1980). Remembering of sentences by schizophrenic young adults. *Journal of Abnormal Psychology, 87,* 303–313.

Koh, S. D., & Peterson, R. A. (1978). Encoding orientation and the remembering of schizophrenic young adults. *Journal of Abnormal Psychology, 89,* 291–294.

Larsen, S. F., & Fromholt, P. (1976). Mnemonic organization and free recall in schizophrenia. *Journal of Abnormal Psychology, 85,* 61–65.

Levy, R. (1982). *The new language of psychiatry.* Boston: Little, Brown.

Lezak, M. D. (1995). *Neuropsychological assessment* (3rd ed.). New York: Oxford University.

McGlynn, S. M., & Kaszniak, A. W. (1986). Unawareness of deficits in dementia and schizophrenia. In G. P. Prigatano (Ed.), *Neuropsychological rehabilitation after brain injury.* Baltimore: Johns Hopkins University Press.

Meltzer, H. Y. (1994). Frontal and non-frontal lobe neuropsychological test performance and clinical symptomatology in schizophrenia. In J. A. Talbott (Ed.), *The year book of psychiatry and applied mental health.* St. Louis: Mosby.

Neistadt, M. (1990). A critical analysis of occupational therapy approaches for perceptual deficits in adults with brain injury. *American Journal of Occupational Therapy, 44,* 299–304.

Schwartz, B. L., Rosse, R. B., & Deutsch, S. I. (1993). Limits of the processing view in accounting for dissociation among memory measures in clinical population. *Memory and Cognition, 21,* 63–72.

So, Y. P., Toglia, J., & Donohue, M. V. (1997). A study of memory functioning in chronic schizophrenic patients. *Occupational Therapy in Mental Health., 13,* 1–23.

Stuss, D. T., & Benson, D. F. (1986). *The frontal lobes.* New York: Raven Press.

Stuve, P., Erickson, R. C., & Spaulding, W. (1991). Cognitive rehabilitation: The next step in psychiatric rehabilitation. *Psychosocial Rehabilitation Journal, 1,* 9–26.

Toglia, J. P. (1989). Approaches to cognitive assessment of the brain-injured adult: Traditional methods and dynamic investigation. *Occupational Therapy Practice*, 1, 36–55.

Toglia, J. P. (1991). Generalization of treatment: A multicontext approach to cognitive perceptual impairment in adults with brain injury. *American Journal of Occupational Therapy*, 45, 505–516.

Toglia, J. P. (1992). A Dynamic Interactional Approach to cognitive rehabilitation. In N. Katz (Ed.), *Cognitive rehabilitation models for intervention in occupational therapy*. Stoneham, MA: Butterworth-Heinemann.

Toglia, J. P. (1993). *The Contextual Memory Test Manual*. Tucson: Therapy Skill Builders.

Toglia, J. P. (1994). *Dynamic assessment of categorization: TCA—The Toglia Category Assessment*. Pequannock, NJ: Maddak.

Toglia, J. P., & Josman, N. (1994). Preliminary reliability and validity studies on the TCA. In J. P. Toglia, *Dynamic assessment of categorization: TCA—The Toglia Category Assessment*. Pequannock, NJ: Maddak.

Weinberger, D. R. (1987). Implications of normal brain development for the pathogenesis of schizophrenia. *Archives of General Psychiatry*, 44, 660–669.

Weinberger, D. R., Aloia, M. S., Goldberg, T. E., & Berman, K. F. (1994). The frontal lobes and schizophrenia. *Journal of Neuropsychiatry and Clinical Neurosciences*, 6, 419–427.

Woerner, M. G., Mannuzza, S., & Kane, J. M. (1988). Anchoring the BPRS: An aid to improved reliability. *Psychopharmacology Bulletin*, 24, 112–117.

CHAPTER 6

The Cognitive-Behavioral Model in Mental Health

Linda Duncombe, MSc, OTR

The cognitive-behavioral model is perhaps most frequently practiced in occupational therapy in the form of psychoeducational groups. Additionally, some of the many cognitive-behavioral techniques are incorporated into individual treatment sessions or when working on individual goals within a group context.

To aid in understanding the theoretical background of the cognitive-behavioral frame of reference, the development of cognitive therapy, the beginnings of behavior therapy, and their synthesis will be presented. Next, the relevance of this model to occupational therapy will be discussed. A section on intervention will include a discussion of appropriate assessments and ways in which occupational therapy practitioners have used cognitive-behavioral concepts in treatment. Psychoeducational groups, specifically, will be highlighted. Three cases will exemplify intervention strategies: one describes a patient in an acute in-patient unit who is discharged to day treatment, one is a resident in a group home where the occupational therapist is a consultant, and one is from a wellness program. Finally, research, especially the use of outcome measures, and implications for use of this model in the context of trends in health care will be discussed.

Development of Cognitive-Behavioral Therapy

Cognitive Therapy

Departing from the psychoanalytic traditions in which they had been trained, early cognitive therapists proposed that behavior could be changed through alterations in an individual's thoughts (Beck, 1970; Ellis, 1985; Frankl, 1985; Glasser, 1965). In fact, some historians write, cognitive therapy really began in 1911 when Sigmund Freud and Alfred Adler agreed to disagree and parted ways (Werner, 1982). Adler had difficulty accepting Freud's belief that all psychological problems were the result of intrapsychic conflict. It was Adler's belief, instead, that each individual's personality functioned as a unified whole and that conflicts in people resulted from distorted thinking about the world around them and their place (competency/function) within that world. Thinking, not unconscious drives, shapes behavior. Adler's Law of Compensation, which suggests that an organism can and does change its behavior to compensate for personal deficits that interfere with *adaptation to the environment,*[1] provided the rationale for his later addition of cognition to his earlier theoretical constructs about feelings of inferiority and the striving for mastery (Shulman, 1985).

Adler had many followers in the 1920s and 1930s, but after his death in 1937 interest in his work declined until about 1956 when excerpts of his writings were republished (Werner, 1982). Since then, interest in his partially cognitive approach and in other forms of cognitive therapy has been steadily increasing. The Adlerian therapist, however, does not think of himself or herself entirely as a cognitive therapist. The goal of therapy, in large part, is to change the way one thinks about the world and reacts to it; in

---

1. *denotes relevance to occupational therapy philosophy.*

addition, the individual is asked to use his or her insights to make changes in emotions and behavior as well.

There is at least one other aspect of Adler's theory that relates to cognitive therapy. Adler placed great importance on the *uniqueness of each person*. This leads to the individuality of each treatment plan for each client. A variety of techniques is used, depending on the individual's needs and capacities. These include the "as if" method (instructing the client to act "as if" he or she could), "creating images" of what one wants to happen, "the push-button technique" in which the client pushes the happy or sad button to indicate his or her emotional tone, the "paradoxical technique . . . to create cognitive dissonance," and "confrontation" (Shulman, 1985, p. 254).

Albert Ellis, whose work also derives from the psychoanalytic tradition, suggested that insight alone was not enough to change the behaviors of his clients. He believed that we say sentences to ourselves that affect our behavior. We can control the content of those sentences cognitively and thus change, in a positive direction, both emotion and behavior (Ellis, 1958). A mentally healthy person has accurate perceptions of himself or herself, his or her environment, and his or her behavior in relation to that environment. He or she then is acting on an accurate understanding of reality. If an individual does not have a realistic view of his or her world and his or her place in the world, it is the therapist's role to clarify reality.

Ellis attempted to do this by systematically convincing clients of the fallacy of their internalized assumptions, distorted perceptions, and illogical thinking. The goal was "cognitive restructuring." The client had to accept what the therapist considered to be rational in an effort to change emotions and behaviors (Hoffman, 1984). In Ellis's own words, which build on the work of Adler, one of the tenets of rational-emotive therapy is that "humans are purposeful, or goal-seeking creatures and . . . they bring to A (activating events or activating experiences) general and specific goals (G)" (Ellis, 1985). Rational or irrational beliefs (rBs or iBs) help or get in the way of these goals. A × B = C (cognitive, emotional, or behavioral consequences). This is quite simplistic, as Ellis explains, but can serve as a starting place for understanding the relationship between one's thinking, emotions, and behaviors (Ellis, 1985, p. 314).

Therefore, in addition to being a framework for treatment of dysfunctional individuals, it "also is a personality theory that shows how people largely create their own normal or healthy (positive and negative) feelings and how they can change them if they wish to and work at doing so" (Ellis, 1985). One final note about rational-emotive therapy is the use of homework. Clients are asked to continue the work of therapy during the week, between appointments. For some situations, standard homework sheets are given. At other times, individuals are given specific tasks, for example, participating in a feared social event. This is part of altering one's consciousness about how one is currently thinking, acting, and feeling. The use of homework in today's psychoeducational groups may stem from this aspect of Ellis's theory.

William Glasser published *Reality Therapy: A New Approach to Psychiatry* in 1965. This approach was quite different from the approaches discussed above. Proposed was a way of changing thinking and emotions by first changing behavior. The major tenet of reality therapy was that one has the responsibility to meet one's own needs without infringing on the rights of others to meet their needs. The first question asked by a reality therapist is not "How are you feeling?" but rather "What are you doing?" Next, the therapist points out that what the client is doing is obviously not helping if he or she is feeling bad enough about himself or herself that he or she has sought counseling. Therapy then proceeds through the arrangement of a daily schedule of client activities chosen for their success potential. Emphasis is placed on taking small steps over short periods of time. When there is success in small things, it is hypothesized, the client then can progress toward success in larger things. As the success experiences increase in number, self-esteem improves and thinking and feeling have been changed in a positive direction through doing. Glasser's approach may be considered a cognitive therapy in that there is no time spent on the search for insight or on an analysis of intrapsychic conflict.

A theorist whose name has become almost synonymous with cognitive therapy is Aaron Beck. He added to Adler's belief that *thinking shapes behavior* in noting that thinking shapes behavior and emotion. "In a broad sense, any technique whose major mode of action is the modification of faulty patterns of thinking can be regarded as cognitive therapy. "However, cognitive therapy may be defined more narrowly as a set of operations focused on a patient's cognitions (verbal or pictorial) and on the premises, assumptions, and attitudes underlying these cognitions" (Beck, 1970, p. 187). The basic concepts of cognitive therapy include the underlying theory of cognitive therapy, strategies for working in the cognitive sphere, and specific techniques for use in the therapy process. More specifically, Beck identified the central processing abilities of individuals as necessary for survival. That processing includes receiving information from the environment, synthesizing it with what has already been processed, and planning and acting on the results of the processing (Beck & Weishaar, 1994). Based on his belief that one's thinking about events leads to emotional reactions, the goal of therapy is to "reshape the erroneous beliefs which produce inappropriate emotions and behavior" (Werner, 1982, pp. 19-20). The strategies used to produce this *cognitive shift* are *collaborative empiricism*, in which the patient and therapist work together to use the exploratory principles of scientific thinking to determine "dysfunctional interpretations" (Beck & Weishaar, 1994, p. 286), and *guided discovery*, in which misperceptions of the past are identified as being similar to those in the present. Clients are asked to take note of the experiences in their lives and identify what they believe to be the associated dysfunctional thought processes (Vallis, 1991). Although this sounds like Ellis's rational-emotive therapy, the techniques of Beck's form of cognitive therapy are less teacherlike (no homework sheets; homework is more experientially based) and involve more discussion about questions raised by the therapist. These interventions are considered less forceful; greater emphasis is placed on learning while doing. Beck's cognitive therapy focuses on empowering the individual to change thought processes from dysfunctional to functional, enhancing one's ability to cope (Beck & Weishaar, 1994).

Aspects of cognition that are emphasized in cognitive therapies are automatic thoughts, underlying assumptions, and cognitive distortions (Freeman, Pretzer, Fleming & Simon, 1990). *Automatic thoughts* are immediate interpretations of events. Everyone has automatic thoughts but in psychopathology these may be distorted, mistaken, or unrealistic. *Underlying assumptions* are the beliefs of an individual that shape his or her perceptions and interpretations of events. Similar beliefs or beliefs entrenched over a period of time are frequently called *schemas.* These are usually unspoken and may not be in the immediate awareness of the individual until discovered in diagnostic interviews or during empirical data gathering. *Cognitive distortions* are also referred to as *errors in logic* (Beck, 1970). Distortions in thinking can increase the effect of underlying assumptions.

Treatment in the cognitive model is aimed at changing any and all of the above aspects of the cognitive process. A feedback loop is envisioned in which beliefs and assumptions (internally generated), external events, responses of others to one's interpersonal behavior, and emotional reactions based on perception and memory all contribute to the automatic thoughts that direct future behavior. Therapy, then, is focused on breaking the cycle described above, so that automatic thoughts can be modified. This should improve one's mood and change behavior. As emotions and behavior change, so will the feedback to the system, diminishing the negative impact of the cycle (Freeman, Pretzer, Fleming, & Simon, 1990).

The *goal* in cognitive therapy is "to achieve greater self-esteem, improved functioning at work and school and more satisfying personal relationships" (Burns, 1989a, p. ix).

In the 1970s there was a burgeoning of literature from behaviorists who were beginning to wonder if the positive results they were attributing to behavior therapy were actually due to cognitive aspects of therapy, such as a client's expectation of positive results (Hoffman, 1984). As the basis of behavior in learning theory was further examined, some began to identify various cognitive processes as being responsible for the changes effected by behavioral therapy (Hoffman, 1984; Seiler, 1984).

Behavior Therapy

The *classical conditioning* techniques of Pavlov, with contributions by Watson, Cover-Jones, Dunlap, Mowrer, and later, Wolpe, Lazarus, Reyna, Salter, and Eysenck, provided the foundation from which behavior therapy emerged (Mahoney, 1984). As interest in *operant conditioning* of Skinner (1953) and other pioneers grew stronger, in the 1950s and 1960s, behaviorists began to employ behavior modification strategies such as *token economies* and *shaping*. During this time, two developments are identified (Mahoney, 1984) as historical antecedents for the movement toward a combined cognitive-behavioral approach. These are Skinner's reference to behavioral self-control (1953) and the description by Homme and Cautela of "coverants: the operants of the mind" (Mahoney, 1984). Self-control refers to the ability of the individual to have some influence in the direction his or her life will take (Bruce & Borg, 1993). Coverants refer to thoughts and thought processes that follow the principles of operant conditioning. For example, a therapist might instruct a client to picture himself or herself performing a desired behavior and then have him or her imagine a pleasant event as the result (coverant reinforcer) of that behavior (Hoffman, 1984). Bandura (1985) later elaborated upon these notions of self-control and coverant thought in describing the importance of the central nervous system processes in behavior modification in 1969.

By the 1970s, there were two behaviorist schools of thought: the cognitive and the noncognitive. Beck is an example of a cognitive therapist who, although taking behavior therapy techniques into account, did not attempt to integrate the tenets of behavior therapy with cognitive therapy (Semmer & Frese, 1984). Seiler (1984), however, documented the appearance of cognitive interpretations for what had been the domain of behavioristic research. Positive results from behavior therapy techniques were potentially explained in cognitive therapy terms. Skinner and his followers, conversely, rejected any attempt at explaining behavior therapy through cognitive descriptions, for example with references to "the inner man" (Hoffman, 1984, p. 54). There were, however, enough behaviorists who were interested in the cognitive components of behavior to form a special interest group for cognitive-behavioral research within both the Association for the Advancement of Behavioral Therapy and the Association for Behavioral Analysis. These groups studied the inner person within the confines of behavior therapy and the result of this was what is now known as cognitive-behavioral psychology (Bruce & Borg, 1993).

Contemporary Cognitive-Behavioral Therapy

cognitive-behavioral interventions . . . (include) . . . behavior therapists' increasing concern with mediational (mental/cognitive) therapeutic approaches and cognitive therapists' growing recognition of methodological behaviorism. (Kendall & Hollon, 1979, p. 2)

Thus, as contemporary cognitive-behavioral therapy has evolved, practitioners acknowledge both the mediating impact of thoughts on behavior and the importance of behavioral methodology in changing how one thinks and feels about oneself. In addition, when cognitive and behavioral treatment methods are combined, they must include both verbal intervention procedures for cognitive change and environmental/activity manipulations to encourage behavioral change (Hollon & Kendall, 1979).

Much of current cognitive therapy has been influenced by behavior analysis and therapy. For example, Dobson's (1988) covert conditioning models included the covert conditioning of Cautela (1967) and the thought-stopping techniques of Wolpe (1958). Bandura's social learning theory (1985) incorporated observational learning as well as other nonbehavioral techniques such as *self-efficacy*. Meichenbaum developed self-instructional training, D'Zurilla and Goldfried wrote about problem-solving treatment using cognitive restructuring, and Rehm developed self-control therapy (Vallis, 1991). These forms of cognitive therapy were highly structured, didactic, and educational; little attention was paid to the development of a therapeutic relationship.

In considering the intertwining of cognitive and behavioral therapy, it is important to trace theoretical underpinnings of each. Beck (1976) described behavior therapy as being a subset of cognitive therapy, but articulated how similar they are in comparison to psychoanalytic theory. Commonalities are a structured therapeutic interview, description of the presenting problem in cognitive or behavioral terms, and determination of an intervention plan, including identification by the therapist of the expected response or expected goal of treatment (Beck, 1976). Four threads, or influences, also have been identified (Kendall & Hollon, 1979). The first is that thoughts are subject to the same laws of learning as are overt behaviors. Second, "attitudes, beliefs, expectancies, attributions, and other cognitive activities are central to producing, predicting, and understanding psychopathological behavior and the effects of therapeutic intervention" (Kendall & Hollon, 1979, p. 5). The third influence comes from the social learning theorists like Kanfer and Bandura, who used behavioral paradigms to look at self-efficacy and self-regulation. The last thread refers to the combination of cognitive interventions with behavioral management so that the result is an expected and meaningful outcome.

The *principles of traditional cognitive therapy* that must be reflected in a cognitive-behavioral approach are phenomenology, collaboration, activity, empiricism, and generalization. The following set of descriptors relies on the work of Vallis (1991).

Principle 1: *Phenomenology* is a critical aspect of cognitive therapy in that information about the individual, and how important that background information is to the individual, must be gathered from the client himself or herself. A series of diagnostic interviews is conducted in order to obtain a detailed description of their subjective experience. This forms the basis for the treatment plan. How this information is used, i.e., how the treatment plan is established or how much emphasis is placed on various aspects of cognition (content, process, structure, etc.), varies with the conceptual model. As first identified by Adler, the individual is the unique piece in the puzzle.

Principle 2: *Collaboration* is another cornerstone of cognitive therapy. The therapist and the client decide together on the path to take, then work together toward their goals. The knowledge that one is participating in the planning and the working through of the treatment plan should be beneficial

to the patient. Within a frame of reference in which cognition is thought to be responsible for action and feeling, this reaffirms the ability of the individual to shape his or her own destiny. There is a better chance that the client will carry out the treatment plan if he or she participates in the planning. Collaboration also decreases resistance and opposition.

Principle 3: *Activity*, not just verbal interactions between therapist and client, is necessary to change behavior. Attention is paid to the ways in which different behaviors affect mood and to how thinking can set the stage for satisfying interpersonal interactions. The strategic use of activity in the therapeutic context clearly differentiates the cognitive therapists from the psychoanalysts.

Principle 4: *Empiricism* is the process that enables the therapist and the client to look at cognition, behavior, and emotion as through a magnifying glass. In some cases, the client is asked to collect data that the therapist and the client can look at together as part of understanding where to go next with the treatment plan. When the client and the therapist participate in guided discovery, the client does not feel that the therapist is imposing professional ideas.

Principle 5: *Generalization* refers to guaranteeing that therapeutic changes will benefit the individual beyond as well as within the therapy sessions. The homework given to clients is one way of ensuring that some activity takes place in the intended environment.

The *principles of behavior therapy* that must be included in a cognitive-behavioral model are: the use of a behavioral assessment, treatment aimed at specific behaviors or components of behaviors, and specific treatment strategies that are individualized to attend to the specific behaviors in the unique environment of that person (Wilson, 1994). These principles are based on a learning theory model in which behavior (response) is believed to be the result of an event (stimulus). In addition, "behavior is learned when it is immediately reinforced" (Stein, 1982, p. 36).

There is agreement about the importance of the scientific method (empiricism) within the principles of cognitive and behavioral therapy. The other principles are combined throughout treatment and in specific techniques.

Techniques on Cognitive-Behavioral Therapy

There are many more techniques used in cognitive-behavioral therapy than can be presented here, but some examples have been selected to illustrate what this form of treatment might look like. Freeman, Pretzer, Fleming, and Simon (1990) have provided a structure for identifying these techniques, which could actually be placed along a continuum from primarily cognitive to primarily behavioral (see Table 6-1).

Cognitive techniques can be described in the following six categories:

1. Techniques for challenging automatic thoughts. An example of this would be *challenging absolutes*. In this technique the therapist asks questions that help the patient discover the lack of logic in his thinking. The Socratic method of questioning, frequently used with this technique, is a hallmark of Beck's cognitive therapy (Beck & Weishaar, 1994).

2. Techniques for eliminating cognitive distortions. *Decatastrophizing*, also referred to as the "what if" technique (Beck & Weishaar, 1994,

p. 309), is an example of this. The therapist requests that the patient think of the opposite of what he or she fears, attacking head on, the cognitive distortion of "catastrophizing . . . (which is the) . . . extreme exaggeration of impending doom" (McMullin, 1986, p. 14).

3. Techniques for challenging underlying assumptions. Assumptions tend to surface as underlying themes in the automatic thoughts that guide one's behavior. One way to challenge them is to have the patient *write an alternative assumption* (McMullin, 1986, p. 11). This is frequently done through the medium of a journal. First, the patient is asked to write down his or her worst emotions and what he or she thought instigated the feelings. Next, the patient is to record his or her interpretation of the situation. For example, a neighbor does not say hello as he walks by. The patient might feel rejected and the interpretation might be that "I am not liked/unlovable." The next assignment is for the patient to think of three or four additional interpretations for why the neighbor might not have spoken. Each interpretation is examined for how plausible it might be, being as objective as

---

Table 6-1

Cognitive and Behavioral Techniques

Primarily Cognitive Techniques	Primarily Behavioral Techniques
For Challenging Automatic Thoughts ■ Challenging Absolutes	For Behavioral Change ■ Graded Task Assignments ■ Activity Scheduling ■ Social Skills Training ■ Assertiveness Training ■ Behavioral Rehearsal
For Eliminating Cognitive Distortions ■ Decatastrophizing	
For Challenging Underlying Assumptions ■ Write an Alternate Assumption	To Achieve Cognitive Change ■ Behavioral Experiments ■ Role Playing ■ Role Reversal
Mental Imagery ■ Replacement Imagery ■ Flooding Imagery ■ Cognitive Rehearsal	
For Controlling Recurrent Thoughts ■ Thought Stopping ■ Refocusing	
For Changing and Controlling Behavior ■ Self-Instructional Training	

possible. Finally, one is selected as being the most probable. In the example, the patient might decide that the neighbor was deeply engrossed in thought and did not see him or her standing there. The patient and therapist can continue examining other underlying assumptions until the process becomes automatic for the patient.

4. Mental imagery techniques. *Replacement imagery* and *flooding imagery* are two ways to enable patients to alter the mental scenes they have conjured up in response to events or perceived events. Patients frequently report visual images associated with anxiety or fears (Beck & Weishaar, 1994). When one is instructed to visualize something in place of the feared event, replacement imagery is being used. Flooding imagery is an example of desensitization in which the patient imagines the feared scene and identifies the concurrent irrational thoughts. As the image becomes more and more real, the patient's feelings build and build until they eventually go away (McMullin, 1986). Another example in this category of techniques is *cognitive rehearsal* in which patients rehearse, in their thoughts only, what they need to say before it has to be done in real life.

5. Techniques for controlling recurrent thoughts. *Thought stopping* is a method in which, in a relaxed state, the therapist yells "Stop," at the point at which the patient identifies the beginning of an obsessional thought (Salkovskis & Kirk, 1989). The patient is taught to do this for himself or herself eventually. A less immediate approach is *refocusing* in which the therapist first asks the patient to focus on the troublesome emotion and the event that triggered that emotion. Then the patient is asked to identify similar situations to the antecedent event that did not result in the negative emotion and to practice replacing or refocusing on the more positive feelings.

6. Techniques for changing and controlling behavior. *Self-instructional training* results in a series of instructions the individual uses as self-talk to carry out a task or perform an activity that would otherwise be difficult or impossible. For example, an individual might learn to say "Relax and take a deep breath" prior to a situation that is seen as anxiety-provoking (Meichenbaum & Asarnow, 1979).

Behavioral techniques are described as follows:

1. Techniques for behavioral change. *Graded task assignments* are simply sequenced tasks and subtasks, which an individual must perform, to increase the probability for success. Generally, they are organized from simple to complex or "least demanding to most demanding" (Hollon & Beck, 1979, p. 185). Glasser (1965) explains the use of this technique in *Reality Therapy*. Occupational therapists use graded activities throughout treatment, frequently in a growth-facilitating environment (Mosey, 1972). Outcomes of treatment can be determined from graded task assignments because of the specificity of the task definition. *Activity scheduling* is a continuation of graded task assignments in that the patient's entire day is scheduled, hour by hour. This has been noted as especially helpful with depressed patients (Hollon & Beck, 1979). *Social skills training* and *assertiveness training* are also examples of techniques for behavioral change. In both of these techniques, specific skills are taught to patients using tangible and nontangible/social reinforcers, usually in a group setting so that patients can learn the specific skills necessary to function in their expected environments. Both techniques require practice of the skills being learned. The practicing is a form of *behavioral rehearsal*. However, any skill or interaction can be rehearsed before the actual event happens.

2. Techniques to achieve cognitive change. *Behavioral experiments*, or trying different ways of acting in a particular situation, provide information which the patient can think about in terms of each behavior's effectiveness and the emotional response connected to it. Both *role playing* and *role reversal* are used to give the patient insight into both how he or she might act and how he or she is perceived. These techniques provide behavioral information that can be explored cognitively. In some cases, the patient is asked to take a role opposite one he or she usually plays and convince the therapist, who is playing the role of the patient, that his or her thoughts are irrational (McMullin, 1986).

One other category of techniques has been identified. These are *educational techniques* (Vallis, 1991). Many of the techniques identified above can be provided in an educational setting. Thus, rather than educational techniques being different in content, they differ in the way in which they are presented to the client. For example, in stress management groups, the techniques of mental imagery, cognitive rehearsal, and self-instructional training may be combined with graded task assignments and role playing to educate individuals about stress and stress management as well as to modify stress producing thoughts and behaviors. When this type of group is offered in a mental health setting, it is frequently referred to as a psychoeducational group.

Given the many techniques available to the cognitive-behavioral therapist, one might wonder how one selects the appropriate strategy. There are two guiding principles (Freeman et al., 1990): the more verbal the client, the more cognitive the strategy; and the more anxious the client, the more behavioral the strategy. In addition, each of the different techniques, with emphasis on education, cognition, and behavior, plays a different role in working on changing one's thinking, feeling, and behavior. If one wants to change an individual's thinking through knowledge, then an educational approach might be the strategy of choice. If one wants to attack the distorted thinking directly, a more cognitive approach might be best. For techniques that focus on behavior, the goal is to change the individual's cognitions and affect through the feedback from the activity.

Occupational therapy practice literature identifies the use of the educational, cognitive and behavioral techniques described above. Therefore, cognitive-behavioral therapy will be presented in terms of its congruence with the philosophy and models of current occupational therapy practice.

Cognitive-Behavioral Treatment and the Philosophy of Occupational Therapy

In the first stated philosophy of occupational therapy, Meyer (1922) spoke of *habits*, which he described as organized patterns of behavior *and* thinking. Meyer believed that people with mental illness could be helped through altering their milieu and modifying their habits of thinking (Lidz, 1985). *Ergasia* (from the Greek, meaning work) was a term created by Meyer that referred to "mentally integrated activity" (Lidz, 1985, p. 44). Meyer believed that, in order to help a patient solve or resolve a problem, one needed to focus on those personal/environmental aspects of the individual to which one had access. The available options for doing this are changing the environment and altering habit patterns (behaviors) and ways of thinking (cognition). These are also the underlying tenets of the cognitive-behavioral therapists.

The most recently stated philosophy of occupational therapy includes the statement, "Purposeful activity facilitates the adaptive process" (Representative Assembly, 1979a, p. 785). In cognitive-behavioral therapy, purposeful activities are explored. Then environmental feedback is given and intrinsic feedback occurs to help the individual effect changes in thinking and future behaviors so he or she will be better able to function in his or her environment. Since there is theoretical compatibility between occupational and cognitive-behavioral therapies, occupational therapy practitioners can appropriately incorporate cognitive behavioral strategies into their practice. One cognitive-behavioral therapist defined the goal of cognitive-behavioral therapy as achieving "greater self-esteem, improved functioning at work and school and more satisfying personal relationships" (Burns, 1989a). This is also an appropriate goal of occupational therapy.

Cognitive-Behavioral Therapy in Occupational Therapy

Behavior therapy has been described as consistent with occupational therapy philosophy and theory base (Diasio, 1968; Levy, 1993; Sieg, 1974; Stein, 1982) and demonstrated as effective in occupational therapy treatment (Jodrell & Sanson-Fisher, 1975; Sieg, 1974; Smith & Tempone, 1968; Zschokke, Freeberg, & Erickson, 1975). Some have felt, however, that the reliance on external reinforcement in behavior therapy is incompatible with the occupational therapy practitioner's belief in the inherent motivation of activity (Barris, Kielhofner, & Watts, 1983; Bruce & Borg, 1993).

The principles of cognitive therapy—phenomenology, collaboration, activity, empiricism, and generalization—are more than compatible with the beliefs of occupational therapy. Both place emphasis on

1. The phenomenologic experience of the individual
2. The collaborative interaction between client and therapist regarding goals and treatment
3. The use of rational thinking to solve problems and increase cognitive awareness of behavior
4. The importance of ensuring the generalizing of therapy to an individual's functioning in his or her environment.

More specifically, the therapeutic use of purposeful activity, one of the hallmarks of occupational therapy, is also what is said to set cognitive therapists apart from psychoanalytic (verbal) therapists. Just as the cognitive-behavioral therapist believes that a change in one's thinking can change behavior and that a positive experience can change one's thinking about oneself, occupational therapy practitioners have long believed that "Man is an active being whose development is influenced by the use of purposeful activity" (Representative Assembly, 1979a, p. 785). Fidler(1969) stated it well in relation to task-oriented groups:

The intent of the task-oriented group is to provide a shared working experience wherein the relationship between feeling, thinking and behavior, their impact on others and task-accomplishment and productivity can be viewed and explored. (Fidler, 1969, p.45)

The biopsychosocial model (Mosey, 1974) was suggested to the occupational therapy community as an alternative to either the medical model with its focus on pathology or a health model, which primarily emphasizes an individual's assets. More recently, in discussing schizophrenia, Fine (1993) referred to the relevance of the biopsychosocial theory for all disabilities. The cognitive-behavioral model is similar to the biopsychosocial model in that the latter "directs attention to the body, mind, and environment of the client" (Mosey, 1974, p. 138). As in most other occupational therapy models, the biopsychosocial model focuses on the teaching and learning process that takes place during an occupational therapist-planned activity, on the goal of adaptive functioning in an individual's environment and on the use of specific behavioral objectives.

The role of the occupational therapy practitioner when using the cognitive-behavioral model has been identified as being that of an educator-facilitator, modeling a scientific attitude, questioning generalizations, a participant-observer, forming a collaborative relationship, and using activities to assess knowledge and skill level (Bruce & Borg, 1993). Cole (1993) describes how cognitive-behaviorism may be used by occupational therapy practitioners in psychoeducational groups, such as stress management, time management, leisure planning, and health education. Further, she refers to the role of the occupational therapist as educator-facilitator, helping patients to change their distorted thinking. "We can teach our group members to challenge each other and to encourage their use of rational thinking to solve problems" (Cole, 1993, p. 132). This is accomplished most realistically with patients who function at Level 5 or 6 on the Allen Diagnostic Battery (Allen, Earhart, & Blue, 1992; Earhart, Allen, & Blue, 1993). In addition, Cole incorporates the principles of cognitive behavior therapy into her seven-step format for activity groups (individualizing the treatment for each member, working together through an activity, problem-solving, and generalizing).

Cognitive-behavior therapy, which combines activity with the cognitive awareness necessary for change, provides an appropriate theoretical model for use with patients who have a psychosocial dysfunction as well as in prevention (DeMars, 1992; Johnson, 1987; Taylor, 1988). Although the cognitive-behavioral model of treatment is not an occupational therapy model, its use by occupational therapy practitioners can be recommended.

A number of similarities between occupational therapy and cognitive-behavioral therapy have been identified. As one looks at the differences, it is important to consider the two types of change that take place: peripheral and deep (Bruce & Borg, 1993). Occupational therapy practitioners' methods have an immediate effect on peripheral change. Only additional insight and more intensive cognitive therapy can be responsible for the deep change in which core beliefs and cognitive structures are altered to change one's identity (Bruce & Borg, 1993). Peripheral change should not be considered unimportant. It may be the first step, in a series of small steps, toward deep change, or it may be the change in thinking about the current reality that enables an individual, in the midst of an acute crisis, to be able to face the demands of his or her life. Role playing, social skills training, assertiveness training (Bruce & Borg, 1993) and stress management are examples of techniques that might result in peripheral change. It is also possible that, in longer-term treatment settings, daily practice of functional skills with increased cognitive awareness will result in deep change.

An extensive literature review revealed that many occupational therapy practitioners have used the principles of cognitive behavior therapy in their practice with a variety of populations, and still others have led psychoeducational groups that are based on the principles of cognitive behavior therapy (Crist, 1986; Goldstein, Gershaw, & Sprafkin, 1979; Greenberg, et al., 1988). Criteria for including articles as cognitive-behavioral were the presence of the five cognitive principles of phenomenology, collaboration, activity, empiricism, and generalization and the presence of behavioral methodology. Some psychoeducational programs were identified as being based on behavioral/learning theory principles. However, if in the presentations of these programs a discussion was described in which patients were expected to think about their behavior and identify feelings connected with the behaviors or skills being learned or practiced, that discussion was considered to be a cognitive component to what had been described as a behavioral approach. It should be noted that the use of a cognitive-behavioral technique or referring to treatment as psychoeducational does not mean that the therapy has been carefully designed as cognitive-behavioral therapy. This will be discussed further in the intervention section below. We will first look at the types of assessments used by occupational therapists, then the different cognitive-behavioral interventions will be described and the populations/diagnoses treated will be identified.

Evaluation

One of the purposes of an initial evaluation is to identify the current functioning of an individual and how it compares with what the individual should and could be doing. To determine if the cognitive-behavioral model of treatment is appropriate for a patient, one also must determine the ability of the patient to participate in, and benefit from, therapy using cognitive-behavioral strategies and techniques. Some believe that only patients who score at level 5 or level 6 in the Allen Diagnostic Battery, which consists of the Allen Cognitive Level Scale (ACLS-90), the Allen Diagnostic Module (ADM), and the Routine Task Inventory (RTI) (Allen & Reyner, 1996), are appropriate for cognitive-behavioral treatment (Cole, 1993). While it is clear that patients who are functioning at fairly high cognitive levels will benefit from cognitive-behavioral therapy, the flexibility is there to adjust the techniques so that the more highly cognitive the patient, the more cognitive the therapy and the less cognitively capable the patient, the more behavioral the treatment. In all cases, one certainly needs to ascertain the cognitive abilities of patients as well as to consider information relevant to the other strategic aspects of cognitive therapy (phenomenology, collaboration, activity, empiricism, and generalization). Appropriate types of reinforcers, preferred methods of feedback, and relevant aspects of the expected environment are important to know for the behavioral aspect of the therapy. Finally, in order to determine outcome goals, the current functional behavior of the individual must be identified.

Nineteen articles referring to psychoeducation or cognitive-behavioral treatment in occupational therapy were reviewed for assessment techniques. Five of those articles did not mention assessment (Eilenberg, 1986; Friedlob, Janis, & Deets-Aron, 1986; Goldstein, et al., 1979; Johnson, 1986; Nickel, 1988). The remaining 14 articles yielded 17 different evaluations. Two categories of evaluations emerged: those that yielded information about the cognitive abilities of patients and those that identified the presence or absence of skills and behaviors necessary to function in one's environment. While some assessments incorporated aspects of both categories, the motivation and goals of patients could be elicited in any of them. Most practitioners who described the evaluation process identified more than one method to provide relevant information.

Formal But Nonspecific Assessments

An *interview* was mentioned most frequently (Courtney & Escobedo, 1990; DeMars, 1992; Giles & Allen, 1986; Maslen, 1982; Taylor, 1988). During the interview, the therapist attempted to elicit an individual's cognitive abilities, such as memory, attention, concentration, and judgment, as well as motivation to participate and identification of the goals/needs from the patient's perspective. This addresses the *phenomenological* perspective of the individual, required in a cognitive-behavioral approach, as well as initiating shared *collaboration* around treatment goals. Several articles mentioned the use of *questionnaires* that may have been given in interview format as well (Crist, 1986; Maslen, 1982). One article referred to the use of a self-assessment (Greenberg, et al., 1988).

Observations of patients in structured and unstructured *activities* were helpful in identifying skills and problem-solving strategies (Fine, 1993). More specifically, a collage activity was suggested to provide information about knowledge and feelings of self and self-esteem (Lindsay, 1983). Two authors referred to the need to evaluate the cognitive levels/abilities of patients, but did not describe how this was, or should be, done (Courtney & Escobedo, 1990; Kaseman, 1980).

Standardized Assessments Yielding Information about Cognitive Abilities

Two occupational therapy evaluations provide valuable information about cognitive abilities. Since one can determine levels of cognitive abilities by giving the Allen Diagnostic Battery, it has been suggested as an instrument of choice for this frame of reference (Cole, 1993). The Allen Diagnostic Battery is presented in chapter 8 in this book. The Bay Area Functional Performance Evaluation (BaFPE) (Bloomer & Williams, 1982) evaluates the cognitive components of memory for written/verbal instructions, organization of time and materials, attention span, evidence of thought disorder, and ability to abstract. In addition, there are opportunities for the therapist to observe qualitative signs that might indicate organic involvement, interfering with functional activities. The BaFPE requires 30 to 45 minutes to administer and must be given individually. Those working in an acute care setting might have difficulty using it as a basic screening for all patients.

Although developed for use with adults with brain injury, a dynamic investigative approach to assessment of cognition must be mentioned (Toglia, 1992). This occupational therapy assessment provides opportunities for problem-solving, then changes the task and/or the environment and provides cueing in order to determine learning potential. This assessment is presented in depth in chapter 1 in this book.

The Woodcock Johnson Psycho-Educational Battery (Woodcock & Johnson, 1977; Christiansen & Baum, 1991), although not specific to occupational therapy, also yields cognitive abilities.

Formal/Standardized Assessments That Focus on Functional Living Skills

1. Basic Living Skills Battery (Skolaski & Broekema, 1986)
2. Kohlman Evaluation of Living Skills (McGourty, in Hemphill, 1988; Crist, 1986; Lillie & Armstrong, 1982)
3. Living Skills Evaluation (Ogren, 1983)
4. Phillip's Social Skills Criterion Scale (Phillips, 1978; Crist, 1986)
5. Scorable Self-Care Evaluation (Clark & Peters, 1984; Crist, 1986)
6. Stress Management Questionnaire (Stein & Nikolic, 1989)
7. Task Check List (Lillie & Armstrong, 1982)

These suggested assessments are useful in initial data gathering, but evaluation is an ongoing process (Bruce & Borg, 1993; Giles, 1985) and provides the opportunity to scientifically examine the cognitive, affective, and behavioral barriers to functioning. This is part of the *empirical focus* of this frame of reference.

Finally, one needs to ascertain the patient's view of his or her environment and current and expected environmental demands (Bruce & Borg, 1993). This provides information about *generalization*, without which treatment is merely an exercise.

To summarize, when performing an evaluation in the cognitive-behavioral frame of reference, one needs to identify the following:

- Cognitive components:

    - ability to think and process information (concrete, abstract, metacognition)
    - ability to communicate thinking through words
    - attention span/concentration
    - memory
    - problem solving/judgment
    - learning style

- Behavioral components:

    - appropriate reinforcement (tangible/intangible)
    - feedback—patient's preferred form
    - specific adaptive/maladaptive behaviors

- Cognitive and behavioral components combined:

    - motivation to participate in treatment
    - goals/identified needs.

The evaluation process should include an interview, observation of the patient performing an activity, and a standardized/formal assessment that can be the basis for showing that change has taken place after treatment has concluded. "Clearly, the art of assessment requires the capacity to narrow the focus and magnify particular components of performance without losing sight of the bigger psychosocial picture." (Fine, 1993, p. 94).

The results of the evaluation must be shared with the patient. Then collaborative, specific, functional outcomes should be agreed to. These goals should be based on the patient's cognitive abilities and current adaptive and maladaptive functional behaviors/living skills. The intervention phase, during which there is ongoing evaluation and collaboration, then commences.

Intervention

A good intervention plan starts with specific behavioral objectives. There are four target areas for change: the environment, thoughts/attitudes, knowledge, and skills (Bruce & Borg, 1993). Just as one has to include both the cognitive and behavioral aspects of the evaluation procedure, the same is true for treatment. In this process it is useful to keep in mind that the more cognitively capable the individual, the more cognitive the approach can be, and the less cognitively capable the person, the more behavioral the approach may need to be. Flexibility in adapting techniques to changes in a patient's level of function is also important. Cognitive-behavioral strategies must be carefully selected to effect change in relevant cognitive and behavioral aspects of the individual (Johnson, 1987).

The ultimate goal of all occupational therapy treatment, regardless of the theoretical model or techniques being used, is to increase the functioning of an individual in his or her environment of choice. In the cognitive-behavioral frame of reference, the general goal is self-regulation through improved cognitive function (Bruce & Borg, 1993). Cognitive behaviorists believe that one's thoughts/feelings/beliefs can, and do, affect one's behavior or ability to function in his or her environment. Also feedback about how one acts, from both the nonhuman and human environment, can alter one's thinking/beliefs/feelings about one's capabilities; this, in turn, will affect behavior. As occupational therapy practitioners work toward functional goals, they use their role as teacher/collaborator, in role modeling, problem-solving, and other activities to build skills and to provide feedback and cognitive awareness necessary for a change in one's cognitive beliefs.

Occupational therapy practitioners employ a variety of cognitive-behavioral strategies and techniques to achieve functional occupational therapy goals with patients. Bruce and Borg (1993) listed a number of strategies and techniques, including homework tasks, bibliotherapy, process task groups such as assertiveness and social skills groups, films, modeling and role-play, physical guidance during tasks (graded activities), identifying cognitive distortions, testing cognitions (reality testing), and providing knowledge in an educational format. Social skills/life skills groups and stress management/relaxation groups are examples of psychoeducational groups that have been successful in helping patients meet their goals. These groups will be described below.

Since cognitive-behavior therapy requires some ability to reflect on one's thinking and on the feedback from one's behavior, it is not surprising that occupational therapy practitioners have reported success using cognitive-behavioral techniques with patients whose diagnoses have not affected their basic cognitive structures and/or cognitive abilities. More specifically, occupational therapists have identified cognitive-behavioral therapy as effective in working with alcoholism (Lindsay, 1983; Moyers, 1988; Stoffel, 1994), eating disorders (Giles, 1985; Giles & Allen, 1986), depression (Eilenberg, 1986; Johnson, 1986; Stein & Smith, 1989) and chronic pain (Engel, 1991; Engel & Rapoff, 1990). In addition, specific techniques and programs have been identified for schizophrenic patients (Stein & Nikolic, 1989) in both acute settings (Bradlee, 1984; Fine & Schwimmer 1986; Greenberg, et al., Ogren, 1983) and long-term settings (Campbell & McCreadie, 1988; Drouet, 1986; Friedlob, et al., 1986; Nickel, 1988). For many of these patients, the techniques need to be more behavioral because of limited ability to take advantage of the cognitive aspects of the therapy.

Various psychoeducational groups and programs for specific populations will be described in more detail. Three case studies will be presented to provide a view of treatment in a variety of settings, with different populations and with different roles for the occupational therapist. The first case study will explain and exemplify the more traditional role of working in an acute in-patient psychiatric unit and a partial hospital treatment program. The patient described has a diagnosis of depression with suicidal ideation. Next, cognitive-behavioral therapy will be described for the occupational therapist who is functioning as a consultant to a group home. Social skills training for the patient with chronic schizophrenia will be highlighted in this case. Finally, coping skills groups will be presented in the context of the role of the occupational therapist working with a well population. A couples communication group provides an example for this type of group.

Cognitive-Behavioral Techniques in a Traditional Psychiatric Setting

Occupational therapists use cognitive-behavioral techniques while working with patients on a short- or long-term basis, even when the patients are engaged in groups that would not fall into the category of psychoeducational. Cognitive-behavioral therapy is as much a philosophy as a set of guiding principles. Because the philosophy of cognitive-behavioral therapy dovetails with the philosophy of occupational therapy, the techniques are logical to include. This has been illustrated in numerous descriptions of programs for in-patients (Bradlee, 1984; Courtney & Escobedo, 1990; Fine & Schwimmer, 1986; Giles, 1985; Giles & Allen, 1986; Greenberg, et al., 1988; Heine, 1975; Klein, 1988; Ogren, 1983; Stein & Smith, 1989) and in day-treatment (Campbell & McCreadie, 1988; Courtney & Escobedo, 1990; Crist, 1986; Johnson, 1986; Kaseman, 1980; Nickel, 1988; Stein & Nikolic, 1989). This case presentation will highlight a patient in an acute in-patient setting who is then discharged to day-treatment where occupational therapy is continued.

Case 1: Treatment in an Acute In-patient Unit and Partial Hospital Treatment Setting (Case Contributed by Deane B. McCraith, MS, OTR/L)

Setting: The setting for this case study is a community mental health center that provides a range of mental health services designed to meet a variety of consumer needs along the continuum of care. The center has a 20-bed acute in-patient unit with 4 to 7 days as the average length of stay. The partial hospital program meets 9 am-3 pm. Participants in this program are required to attend full time for a minimum of 2 weeks. The partial hospital program offers a variety of daytime groups and vocational/educational services and supported work programs for persons requiring longer term care and follow-up. The out-patient program offers day and evening counseling for individuals and groups. All programs use a cognitive-behavioral model that emphasizes a goal-oriented, problem-focused, and usually, a here-and-now perspective.

The overall philosophy is that changes in thoughts, attitudes, and behavior can significantly impact moods and feelings, leading to changes in overall quality of life satisfaction and performance effectiveness. The ultimate goal is to help clients take control of their own recovery process by learning new or modified ways of thinking and doing that are most effective for satisfying their own needs as well as meeting the expectations of their chosen environment. Within this context, additional therapeutic approaches and techniques are used as appropriate for an individual client. The occupational therapy program uses the Allen Cognitive Disability Levels to identify cognitive level of function so that cognitive-behavioral interventions can be graded to meet the patient's cognitive and related performance abilities, as well as to optimize motivation, self-control, successful learning, generalization to discharge environment, and return of higher level cognitive abilities where this potential exists. The occupational therapy program emphasizes choice-making, problem-solving, and participation in success-oriented activities.

Background Chart Information: Edna is a 57-year-old, widowed mother of two grown daughters. She was admitted to the acute in-patient psychiatric unit following a suicide attempt. Prior to her husband's death in an automobile accident 4 months ago, Edna worked as a postal clerk and enjoyed a modest lifestyle raising her children with her husband of 40 years. One month after her husband's death Edna attempted to return to work. Usually a conscientious, cheerful employee, her supervisor reported to Edna's daughter that she frequently called in sick. On the job, she was distracted, short-tempered with frequent tearful outbursts, and slow in completing routine tasks. After 2 months, Edna was given a 3-month medical leave of absence. Edna's daughter reported that Edna continued to do poorly. Usually active in her church and community, Edna canceled or forgot appointments and avoided doing things with friends and family. Never a TV watcher, she spent hours sitting in front of the television, frequently sleeping or staring vacantly at the screen. Once a meticulous homemaker, she let dust accumulate and mail pile up. Although she maintained her

personal hygiene, she lost interest in her appearance and stopped wearing makeup and having her hair professionally styled. Approximately 1 month after going on medical leave from work, Edna called her daughter and tearfully told her that she had ingested an overdose of pills because she felt useless, saw no hope for the future without her husband, and wanted to relieve her family and friends of the burden she had become. At this point, Edna's daughter brought Edna to the hospital.

On admission, Edna complained of severe depression with frequent suicidal ideation. She reported lack of energy, anxiety and irritability, and difficulty concentrating. She expressed a pervasive sense of hopelessness and helplessness about her future without her husband and about her inability to "pull herself together, get back to work, and be a decent person." She also expressed the certainty that she would be fired from her job. The nursing staff described Edna as compliant, withdrawn, agitated, lethargic, and tearful.

Psychiatric diagnosis, treatment plan, and goals: Edna was diagnosed with Major Depression (DSM-IV, Axis I, 1994) related to the unexpected, traumatic loss of her spouse of 40 years. The long-term in-patient goal (6 to 7 days) was to discharge Edna home with follow-up partial hospital or outpatient care, as appropriate. The short-term inpatient goals were:

1. Stabilize Edna's mood with continued antidepressant medication and supportive milieu
2. Assess safety and suicidal risk
3. Provide education on grief, loss and depression
4. Provide opportunities for examining/modifying thought distortions regarding her current life circumstances and the future
5. Plan for discharge including continued support and structure for recovery.

Occupational therapy evaluation: The occupational therapy evaluation included a modified Occupational Performance History Interview

(OPHI)[2] (Kielhofner, Henry & Walens, 1989) and the Allen Battery[3] consisting of the ACLS-90, RTI-2, ADM (Allen & Reyner, 1996; Allen, 1996; Allen, Earhart, & Blue, 1992; Earhart, Allen, & Blue, 1993). Edna was cooperative but did not independently initiate any conversation or task behavior during the evaluation sessions.

In the OPHI interview, Edna identified her husband's death as the major downhill turning point in her mood and performance abilities. Prior to that she described herself as a "good wife, mother and grandmother," a caring person active in church and community, and a hardworking postal clerk who had recently been honored for her 30 years of competent service. She reported that she used to be a creative and fun-loving person, enjoying quilting, crafts, gardening, and bowling. Edna tearfully described travel plans that she and her late husband had been making for their retirement years. However, she told the occupational therapist that "now my life is over. I can't do anything anymore. I'm useless and it would be best for everyone if I were gone, too." When pushed to identify possible distortions in this self assessment of her abilities and worth to herself and others, she was able to do so.

---

2. The Occupational Performance History Interview (OPHI) is an historical interview designed to collect information about an individual's occupational performance in the areas of organization of daily living routines; life roles, interest, values and goals; perception of ability and assumption of responsibility; and environmental influences.

3. The Allen Battery consists of three assessment tools. The Allen Cognitive Level Screen (ACLS): 1990 is a standardized screening tool and performance test designed to measure a person's ability to function and learn. It provides an indication of global cognitive performance deficit and/or performance ability based on a leather lacing activity. The Allen Diagnostic Module (ADM) is also a standardized screening tool designed to verify the ACLS-90 score. It involves the completion of a craft project standardized to control the new information presented to the individual being evaluated. It also yields indication of global cognitive performance deficit and/or performance ability based on completion of a meaningful, novel task. The Routine Task Inventory (RTI-2) is an observational or interview guide for assessing functional ability on 40 routine, familiar tasks that are apt to be affected by a cognitive disability (e.g., activities of daily living (ADL) and Instrumental ADL (IADL), occupational and social role skills).

On the Allen Cognitive Level Screen (ACLS-90), Edna scored a 5.2. This indicated that Edna was able to be goal directed, to initiate new procedures, and to remember and complete several steps at a time. However, she had difficulty planning ahead and used trial and error to problem-solve, giving up easily when frustrated. This typical Level 5 behavior was also very apparent in the Occupational Therapy Task Evaluation Group using the Allen Diagnostic Module (ADM). With encouragement, Edna reluctantly selected a wooden tile trivet project stating, "I used to like to do this kind of thing, but now I'll probably make a mess of it." In beginning the project, she scanned written directions and precautions but used trial and error problem-solving to complete the project. She was impatient in sanding and staining. Thus, the stain was uneven and darker where the inadequately stained wood absorbed too much stain. She worked very slowly, giving the tiles some attempt at even spacing. She did not have time to grout the tiles.

The Routine Task Inventory Rating (RTI-2), based on information in the chart from Edna's daughter and employer and on Edna's OPHI self-report, indicated that Edna's basic living skill performance (grooming, dressing, toileting, bathing, and feeding) were adequate, but that her performance problems at work, her isolating behaviors, her neglect of homemaking interests and chores, and her apparent difficulty adjusting to changes since her husband's death were clear evidence of both occupational and social role disability typical of Cognitive level 5 performance.

In summary, the occupational therapist noted that Edna's 5.2 level of function was consistent with moderate depression. However, given the information on her highest level of function prior to her husband's death, including her competence at work, her social and community involvement, and her interests, she probably could be capable of 5.8 or 6.0 functioning. This suggested, that with medication and cognitive-behavioral intervention related to her depression, loss, and future performance potential, Edna should be able to return to a fulfilling and satisfying lifestyle in her major life roles as worker, mother and grandmother, and community service provider.

Occupational Therapy Treatment: Edna and the occupational therapist collaboratively decided that Edna's occupational therapy goals while in the hospital would focus on modifying her negative self-assessment, particularly as it related to her role performance as worker and valued family member and on planning her time use routines and coping skills after discharge. Her goals were:

1. Engage in activities in which she could experience success and positive feedback about her performance
2. Gain knowledge about grief, loss, and depression, and their impact on work and interpersonal performance
3. Learn several relaxation and stress reduction techniques to decrease anxiety and negative self-talk/suicidal ideation
4. Practice techniques for decreasing or modifying her negative thoughts so that she could more realistically assess her abilities, deficits, and future goals as worker and family member
5. Identify new daily routine and leisure activities to replace time use patterns established with husband.

Edna agreed to attend the following groups:

1. Daily morning exercise group that included education about the positive effects of exercise for health, stress reduction, and for relieving symptoms of depression (led by a certified occupational therapy assistant),
2. Stress reduction/relaxation group that met daily and included education and skill practice as well as discussion on use of techniques after leaving the hospital (led by a certified occupational therapy assistant and a nurse),
3. Daily occupational therapy task group for social interaction and successful task performance experience, for work on concentration and planned actions, as well as for further task performance evaluation (co-led by an occupational therapist and an occupational therapy student)
4. Coping skills group that met 3 times per week and included cognitive behavioral education and skill practice using techniques like thought stopping, role-playing, identifying and correcting thought distortions, and assertiveness skills.

As an occupational therapy group, much of the focus was on decreasing thoughts/behaviors that interfered with role and task performance and on increasing thoughts/behaviors that encourage role and task performance (co-led by an occupational therapist and psychologist).

The last three groups were specifically designed for persons with ACL of 5.0 or above so that the tasks, teaching-learning methods, and discussions could be graded to fit the members cognitive abilities, thus enhancing potential for successful learning and performance, self-control, and generalizing to discharge environment.

Progress: After 6 days, the treatment team noted that Edna seemed less anxious and withdrawn. She was attending all scheduled groups and activities without needing to be reminded. In occupational therapy task group, Edna completed three projects and acknowledged praise for the quality of her work. She demonstrated modest improvement in her ability to concentrate, problem-solve, and follow directions, although she continued to have difficulty initiating conversation, asking for help when needed, and planning ahead. She was still easily discouraged and frustrated. Frequently, she needed encouragement and support to keep from slipping into negative self-talk. Although she attended exercise and stress reduction/relaxation groups, she usually chose to watch, stating that she did not have the energy for anything physical or meditative. In the coping skills group, Edna completed the learning assignments but expressed doubts about them working for her. While still expressing depressed and negative thoughts with frequent tearful episodes, her mood was noted to be improved. She was able to verbally relate these thoughts and moods to the traumatic loss of her husband and her concerns about losing her job and the respect of her daughters. She also indicated that she would try to recognize her all or nothing thinking and catastrophizing, and that she would call her daughter if she felt like acting on her suicidal thoughts. Edna concurred with her treatment team's perception that she was sufficiently safe and in control of her thoughts and actions to be discharged to her daughter's home. She also agreed to attend the partial hospital program for 2 weeks for further cognitive-behavioral training to cope with her loss and depression, for evaluation and structuring of her home routine and leisure time use, and for evaluation of her potential to return to work.

Day Hospital OT Treatment: In the partial hospital program, Edna continued with the occupational therapy goals established while an inpatient with the addition of a sixth goal: to evaluate potential and to suggest a time frame for return to work. She attended the daily occupational therapy task group with a similar focus to the inpatient group, a leisure activity group, and a 10-session structured learning group. This group was led by a nurse, a social worker, and an occupational therapy practitioner. Sessions were run like classes and covered the following topics: coping with mental illness, medication side effects, community resources, communication skills, assertiveness skills, anger management, time management, vocational readiness, techniques for managing negative self-talk, and relapse prevention.

A fourth group, called Like Choices and Options Group, focused on the process of changing one's attitude from seeing oneself as a victim of life's circumstances to seeing oneself as a person with choices and options. In this group, co-led by an occupational therapist and a social worker, patients were expected to write an autobiography with a positive outcome for the ending. Group members helped each other work on identifying choices and options for solving problems related to major life roles that had been impacted by their mental illness. Members gave each other feedback on their thoughts, behavior, and feelings and used role playing, modeling, and problem solving to modify distorted thoughts and maladaptive behaviors and to practice alternative performance and attitudinal options. In this group, Edna focused on reality testing and modifying her perceptions that her life was over, that she was a burden to everyone, and that she would be fired from her job. She worked on planning a new daily routine without her husband and on a plan for her time use until she returned to work.

After 14 days in the partial hospital program, Edna was reassessed on the ACLS-90. She achieved a score of 5.8 that indicated that her psycho-

pharmacologic treatment along with a supportive milieu and a collaborative role in her cognitive-behavioral treatment with the occupational therapy practitioners and other team members had been successful. Through these interventions, Edna was able to decide to ask for an additional month leave of absence from her work so that she could continue with her recovery before taking on the pressures of work. In preparation, she practiced role playing if her boss said no. She also worked out a structured schedule to keep from having too much free time at home and selected three leisure pursuits: gardening, rubber stamp art, and counted cross stitch. She decided to try walking with a neighbor for exercise, to return to her volunteer work at church, and to do some daytime baby-sitting for her grandchildren.

At the point of discharge, Edna reported feeling less discouraged and expressed a willingness to try to be more patient with herself, allowing time to grieve the loss of her husband and to adjust to her changed lifestyle. Edna collaborated with her treatment team in deciding to attend the outpatient service for monthly medication follow-up and weekly supportive cognitive-behavioral therapy. She also chose to attend a weekly grief and loss support group.

Social or Life Skills

Many descriptions of social or life skills groups include behavior therapy as their underlying theoretical base, but in reality there is the expectation of cognitive awareness and of the individual participating in the activities for the intrinsic value of the activity, not merely for an external reinforcement (Drouet, 1986; Liberman, Massel, Mosk, & Wong, 1985).

When one examines the procedure utilized in a social skills approach (Hayes, 1989; Hewitt, Wishart, & Lambert, 1981; Kaseman, 1980), it includes the five principles of cognitive therapy (individualization, collaboration, activity, problem solving, and generalization). One occupational therapist described a group, clearly utilizing cognitive-behavioral techniques, without identifying it as such (Heine, 1975). Another practitioner created a social skills game that incorporated cognition, behavioral skills, and self-awareness (Love, 1988).

Although some programs used tangible reinforcements (Drouet, 1986; Hayes, 1989), all other requirements of cognitive-behavior therapy were met.

Since these groups are based on cognitive-behavioral therapy principles, the groups must be organized around the needs/behavioral goals of the individuals in the groups. The following case will provide an example of the treatment process using cognitive-behavioral therapy with social/life skills groups.

Case 2: A Group Home with an Occupational Therapist Consultant

Bob is a resident in a group home. He is 70 years old. His diagnosis is chronic schizophrenia. He was hospitalized in a state hospital until the facility was closed 5 years ago. He was selected for inclusion in a group home because he was well maintained on his medication, had no history of violence, and currently had no active hallucinations. Because he had been hospitalized for most of his life, he is very dependent on staff to take care of all his daily needs. He is mostly independent in activities of daily living, needing reminders about shaving and not wearing dirty clothes. He is dependent on staff for the maintenance of his clothes (laundry) and for shopping, preparing, and cleaning up after his meals. He can read but does not chose to. He mostly sits, head down, and waits for something to do. He participates in a group activity but never suggests one. He greets staff but does not talk to fellow residents unless it is in the context of a group activity, or he is asked by a staff member to elicit information from another resident.

The occupational therapist is a consultant to his group home and routinely evaluates group members and identifies programs run by the staff which are appropriate for selected members to attend. The occupational therapist also participates in staff training and supervision in leading a variety of groups, including leisure skills, gardening, cooking, exercise, reminiscence, and others which incorporate interests of the staff or are suggested by residents.

Bob was given two formal assessments, the Bay area Functional Performance Evaluation (BaFPE) (Bloomer & Williams, 1982) and the Kohlman Evaluation of Living Skills (KELS) (McGourty, 1988).

The BaFPE was administered on March 18. This standardized assessment consists of five tasks that differ in degree of complexity and structure and yield scores in three component areas: cognitive, performance, and affective, as well as qualitative indicators of possible organic involvement. Bob scored one standard deviation (s.d.) below the norm in 7 out of 12 function areas. Cognitive Component: Bob scored more than one s.d. below the norm in memory for written/verbal instructions, organization of time and materials, and attention span. Primarily because of these three areas, he also performed below the norm in the total cognitive score. He scored within normal limits (WNL) in ability to abstract and there was no evidence of thought disorder. Performance Component: Bob's scores were WNL for two of the three areas tested: task completion and efficiency. He scored one s.d. below the norm in errors. Affective Component: He scored more than one s.d. below the norm in frustration tolerance, self-confidence, and general affective impression. His scores were WNL for motivation. In reference to Structure/Complexity, Bob scored more than one s.d. below the norm in money and marketing, a cognitively-oriented task involving several steps, in a home drawing in which there was some structure and some choice, and in the block design—a visual memory task. In both the money and marketing and the home drawing tasks, although he was able to give some idea of what he was expected to do before he began, he appeared to not know what was expected during the actual task. It is unclear whether he forgot the instructions, had intervening thoughts or preoccupations that interfered with his remembering, never really comprehended what he was to do, or was not able to act on what he heard and could verbalize having heard. He scored WNL for the structured task of sorting shells and for the least structured task, the kinetic person drawing. His total score for this task-oriented assessment was more than one s.d. below the norm for the sample group with which he was compared. (This client's scores were compared to norms from a population of people with chronic mental illness whose demographics resemble those of this particular client.)

The Kohlman Evaluation of Living Skills (KELS) is a currently nonstandardized assessment. Although research on validity and reliability has been conducted, more is needed (McGourty, 1988). Scores are available in 18 living skills. In addition, "Throughout the KELS, there are many opportunities to assess the patient's cognitive abilities such as memory, attention span, and comprehension" (McGourty, 1988, p. 138). On March 25, Bob was given nine areas that were considered relevant to his living situation. Under Self-Care, he needed assistance in appearance, specifically in hair care and shaving. He was dressed appropriately in street clothes, but the cleanliness of the clothes was questionable. He reported daily performance of some activities, like tooth brushing, but not of washing and shaving. In the Safety and Health category, he was aware of dangerous household situations, but not what to do about them. He had some idea of appropriate action for sickness, but not for accidents. He had no knowledge of emergency phone numbers or of availability of medical and dental facilities. He reported being totally dependent in the area of Money Management. He bought coffee regularly and always got the same change back, but in using real money and store items he was unable to determine how much change he should receive from a one dollar bill. Likewise, he was dependent on others for his Transportation needs and had no knowledge of the transit system. Although he said he knew how to use the telephone book, he said he had no need to do so. Finally, for Work and Leisure, he had no plans to seek employment and listed only three activities that he liked to do in his spare time: go on trips (especially out to eat), watch television, and read the newspaper.

General Observations: Bob was compliant throughout. He slowly attempted every task presented. He spoke in a low, monotone voice, and displayed no affect toward the examiner or to anything she did or said. When it was time to end each session, the examiner said "Thank you for your cooperation." To which he replied, without emotion "It was a pleasure." Throughout all tests and tasks, he seemed to have the most difficulty following directions. In some cases, he thought he understood the directions when he did not. In other cases, he began to work before the examiner finished giving the directions. In still other situations, directions needed to be repeated for every item in the category. Finally, psychomotor retardation and lack of initiative were apparent throughout the evaluation sessions.

Based on the results of these assessments, social/life skills training in the cognitive-behavioral frame of reference seemed appropriate. Bob's motivation was high, and the presence of the cognitive ability to abstract indicated the potential for self-awareness. His other cognitive abilities, although low, seemed adequate to work on the skills suggested as lacking in the KELS: Activities of Daily Living (ADL), safety, money management, and leisure.

The results of the evaluation were explained to Bob with some ideas of areas in which he might be able to function better in his structured living situation. He was asked what he would like to be able to do better. He said he had concern about what he would do if his roommate started choking. (When asked why he was concerned about this, he responded that his roommate often ate in their room, even though this was not allowed, and he, Bob had never learned any first aid.) He would like to manage his money better. He is frustrated with the staff at the group home in the lack of activities and feels the members need to take more charge of this. He enjoys going out on trips and realizes that, to be more acceptable to people he meets, he needs to be more consistent about his physical appearance.

With this in mind, Bob and the therapist created the following goals:

1. In a safety skills group, Bob will:
   a. show evidence of being able to dial 911 and of what to say to the person on the other end of the line
   b. make a card that indicates the information to give a 911 operator and place it at the phone near his room
   c. demonstrate the Heimlich maneuver

   d. make a card with personal emergency infor-
      mation and carry it in his wallet
   e. during a fire drill in his home, successfully
      exit within 1 minute.
2. During a 3-week money management course,
   Bob will:
   a. demonstrate ability to count change for one
      dollar, five dollars, ten dollars, and twenty
      dollars
   b. problem-solve and role-play with others
      what to say if he believes the change is in-
      correct
   c. list weekly items he would like to buy and
      activities in which he would like to partici-
      pate that cost money, compare this with his
      weekly allowance, and create a personal
      budget.
3. In an ongoing leisure skills group, Bob will:
   a. give at least one suggestion at every discus-
      sion for possible activities
   b. participate in either preparation or cleanup
      of the activity once every other week
   c. start a conversation once each group with at
      least one other member of the group
   d. participate in making weekly schedule post-
      ers for the house members.
4. Bob and his resident advisor will make a chart
   of ADL tasks to be done and when they should
   be done. Bob will check off when he has done
   the listed activities and after 2 weeks, the chart
   can be modified or the frequency of Bob's
   checked responses on the chart can be changed
   as Bob and his resident advisor see progress.
   After all morning ADL activities are completed,
   Bob will be asked how he thinks he looks, and
   he will write that in the appropriate space on
   the chart.

Bob participated in three groups/classes, one on
safety, one on money management, and one on
leisure activities. They were all psychoeducational
groups with homework, practical activities built
into the groups, role playing, printed information,
and instructional videotapes. At the end of each
group, the group leader elicited from each participant his or her thoughts and feelings about the
content of the group and how he or she might
change his or her behavior as a result of the group.
The occupational therapist met weekly with staff

concerning supervision of the groups. Bob also
worked with his resident advisor on activities of
daily living. This latter endeavor was mostly behavioral with a slight cognitive component built in.

Does this fit for the cognitive-behavioral frame
of reference? In terms of *phenomenology*, the interview included Bob's concerns and goals and what
he thought some of the problems were. Both the
goals and the intervention plan were created *collaboratively* with Bob. All interventions included *activity*. In terms of *empiricism*, Bob was asked to help
problem-solve why he felt anxious about safety
situations and his identification of a lack of knowledge of safety led to a group for all interested
members in his house. This procedure was carried
out for all goals. Since Bob's goals and activities
were being carried out in the environment in which
they were expected to occur, *generalization* was
expected to take place. The *reinforcement* schedule
for his ADL needed to be changed so that Bob was
aware that he had made these changes and so that
his involvement in them would become self-rein-
forcing.

Three months later: In a follow-up session with
Bob, the occupational therapist asked how things
were going. He was well-dressed, clean-shaven, and
sat upright. He reported that he was pleased with
his "courses." He was no longer worried about the
safety of his room-mate. The "class" on safety/first
aid had decided to do follow-up safety drills, like
fire drills, once in a while to keep people "on their
toes." He felt more competent with his money,
and the food servers where he occasionally bought
coffee had complimented him on his appearance
during a money transaction. The one area he was
still concerned about was leisure activities. There
had been recent turnover of weekend staff, and he
did not yet feel comfortable enough with the new
people to voice his opinions. After problem-solving
around this concern, he decided to suggest the idea
of a planning group at a group home meeting.

Stress Management and Relaxation Training

These groups have been documented for schizophrenia (Stein & Nikolic, 1989), depression (Stein
& Smith, 1989), alcoholism (Moyers, 1988; Stoffel,
1994), eating disorders (Giles, 1985), and with a

well population (Burns, 1989b). There is generally an educational component to these groups in which the "students" learn about stress and then are asked to identify how they know when they are feeling stress, how they feel stress in their body, and how they act when they are feeling under stress. Homework sheets usually help group members begin to identify stress and their own coping or noncoping strategies on a daily basis. Once the stress factors have been identified, individuals are asked to problem-solve and identify stress management or relaxation techniques that might be helpful. Next they practice the techniques, first in the group and then as homework, and give feedback to themselves and the group about the effectiveness of the techniques. Generalization, making sure that the group members continue to use the stress management techniques after they leave the treatment facility, is probably the most difficult part in the strategy. Examples of other coping skills groups are anger management and communication skills.

Case 3: A Wellness Group

This is a couples communication group offered by a health maintenance organization. It is advertised as a health and wellness group for people who want to improve their communication skills with a significant other. (No singles are permitted to attend the group.) The group meets for 6 weeks, one evening a week. An occupational therapist is the group leader. She identifies herself as an occupational therapist and defines her goal: that everyone in the group will function optimally in his or her environment, specifically in the area of communication with another person. Although they have arrived as couples, each individual in the group introduces himself or herself and identifies his or her goals and why he or she has chosen to attend this group. Because this is not a treatment situation, there are no clinical evaluations. Instead, each person is asked to take a pretest, identifying areas of concern or potential conflict, such as competition, workload, cultural backgrounds, relationships with partner's family, need for emotional space, and willingness to change the current communication style (Cohen-Kaplan, 1991). Then, in psychoeducational format, a lecture/discussion

about communication styles/skills starts the classes. Each participant receives his or her own booklet of handouts that includes a bibliography of layman's books of the subject, and several are recommended as "texts" for the course. During the 6 weeks, couples learn about their own communication style and practice different styles. A homework log, in which they record when they use different styles and what the results are, is brought back to class and discussed. Assertiveness is defined, discussed, practiced, and discussed again. The participants are taught, and learn through role playing, how to listen and respond in a nondefensive way to their partner as they learn about conflict resolution. The group explores anger and how to handle it. They write their life scripts and share them with their partner. To focus on the real issues for each couple, much of the time is devoted to role playing actual conversations which the couples have chosen as a focus. The group gives the couple feedback and they are encouraged to change their behavior. There is no follow-up after the couples' communication group is over, but several groups of couples have spontaneously organized support groups to carry on the work of the group.

This is the story of Peter and Valerie. Peter and Valerie had been married for a little over 2 years. They both worked and had no children. They were saving for a house and had been spending much time on house-hunting in the recent past. They felt they had a healthy relationship in that they had maintained their own interests and friends as well as doing things together. However, something was wrong. They both recognized it. Valerie would go out on a Friday evening with her friends from work. Peter felt that he was okay with that and found ways to occupy his time. Then on Saturday mornings, Peter would frequently play golf with his brother and/or his father. He could not understand why Valerie would be so upset when he got home from these activities. It was identified, during the communication style exercise, that Peter tended to be compliant (passive) in his communication style and that Valerie tended to be passive-aggressive. Thus, Peter had responded to this situation by saying nothing, yet silently wondering and worrying about what was wrong. Valerie, in a passive-aggressive style, had been unpleasant and sarcastic until her mood wore off. Each person was committed to identifying the problem and had been reading the texts and doing the homework faithfully. They participated in the role-play, accepting feedback and discussing the group's reaction to their styles. They also provided excellent feedback to other members. The night arrived for them to role-play a real situation in their lives. Each had selected a different scenario to role-play and had received permission from the other person to share that with the group. Peter went first and described the interaction after his return from a golf game with his father. When Valerie appeared passive-aggressive, the group identified that for her and she tried to be more assertive. Peter was admonished for being passive. The reenactment of their role-play progressed, but seemed like acting, not like genuine change. Neither described any difference in thinking or feeling after their role-play. Valerie gave the background for the communication she wanted to examine. It took place at the home of her in-laws. During this description and role-play it was evident that Valerie had a lot of feeling about her relationship with her husband when he was with his family. Valerie explained what she had observed, how she felt about it, and what she desired. Peter listened. When his turn came to report on what he had heard, an amazing thing happened. He had truly heard Valerie for the first time on this issue. Maybe she had communicated clearly about it for the first time, however, he realized that rather than her being jealous of the time he spent with his family, she was reacting to the way he acted toward her when they were together with his family. She felt ignored and not respected as an individual. They both responded positively to their new found knowledge about each other and the way in which they communicated their important concerns. They agreed to continue communicating in this style and reported in later sessions that this particular interaction was a major breakthrough for them. They had changed their thinking about themselves, about each other, and about how to communicate.

The cognitive-behavioral aspects of this group are more clearly seen, perhaps, because this group has more of the cognitive components in it than behavioral. Activities are used throughout to identify the thoughts and feelings that group members have that are interfering with the ability to communicate with each other. The uniqueness of each person in the group is emphasized and nothing is done without collaborating and problem-solving with the person involved. Many cognitive-behavioral techniques are used including bibliotherapy, role playing, homework, role modeling, cognitive rehearsal, identifying cognitive distortions, feedback from group members, and the use of an educational format.

Three cases have been presented that illustrate the use of cognitive-behavioral therapy within the context and philosophy of occupational therapy. Although the philosophy is stable, the context of occupational therapy is ever changing. For that reason, the cases were described in four different settings. The role of the occupational therapy practitioner in direct treatment, both in- and out-patient, consultation, and community education was meant to reflect the changes in health care.

Research

The value of any treatment method based on one or many theoretical rationales must be determined through research. One of the differences between cognitive therapy and psychoanalytic therapy has been identified as the researchability of cognitive therapy: "outcome studies are easily conducted because the principles of cognitive therapy can be systematized within a relatively uniform set of therapeutic procedures" (Beck, 1976, p. 318). "Cognitive therapy has been extensively tested since the first outcome study was published in 1977" (Beck, 1995, p. 2). (For references on treatment efficacy for depression, anxiety, panic disorders, phobias, substance abuse, eating disorders, and couples' problems, see Beck, 1995.) Although descriptions abound of occupational therapy practitioners using cognitive-behavioral techniques, the research on the efficacy of these techniques is sparse.

In reviewing the literature for effectiveness of treatment with schizophrenia, Hayes (1989) found four treatment methods most often mentioned. Two of these, social skills training and living skills training, have a cognitive component even though they are considered more behavioral than cognitive. This places them in the realm of cognitive-behavioral therapy. However, because of methodological flaws, one cannot infer that the treatment described would have the same effect in other settings and with other patients (Hayes, 1989). Non–occupational therapy literature has indicated that social skills training increased patients' skills, but this has yet to be documented in occupational therapy. One study did document that social skills training was effective in increasing social behavior of schizophrenic patients but not in transferring those skills to their community settings (Hayes, Halford, & Varghese, 1991).

The presence of patients' money management skills was identified before and after they were included in a life skills program (Kaseman, 1980). Although only raw data were presented, the results indicated an increase of skills. Two other descriptions of outcomes were of a living skills group for psychiatric patients in an acute setting (Ogren, 1983) and in a well population (DeMars, 1992). Again, no statistics were available to present data more scientifically. Two outcome studies did add statistical support to the use of social skills training with psychiatric patients (Campbell & McCreadie, 1983; Friedlob et al., 1986). They were limited, however, to small numbers of patients.

From the research thus far, it seems that several factors would facilitate our ability to document outcomes in the area of mental health. First, the number of patients we have assigned to groups and on whom we collect data has been limited. We need to find ways to combine data to increase our members rather than being isolative in our research efforts. Since the wide variety of diagnoses and medication may impact on the treatment and provide uncontrollable variables (Hayes, 1989), the combining of data across clinics would help with increasing numbers in similar groups. Additionally, occupational therapy practitioners are not using standardized measures for pre- and post-testing.

Thien (1987) suggested that occupational therapy practitioners could provide outcome data on patients by assessing their progress toward goals, utilizing patient satisfaction questionnaires, and using behavior rating scales. These suggestions are appropriate in the cognitive-behavioral frame of reference. Behavioral rating scales could provide pre and post data for the specific behaviors identified in behavioral objectives as was done in a documentation review system that was set up to look

at outcomes (Thien, 1987). Because of the emphasis in cognitive-behavioral therapy on the individual taking responsibility for himself or herself through cognitive awareness, the use of patient satisfaction questionnaires is also appropriate. This is an excellent way to determine if the coping skills taught have generalized to the environment in which the individual needs to use them (Thien, 1987).

The use of standardized measures for determining progress has been quite limited in occupational therapy outcome research. Several studies have used standardized measures outside of, but related to, occupational therapy such as the Simple Rathus Assertiveness Schedule (McCormick, 1985) and the Tennessee Self-Concept Scale (Stoffel, 1993). Several assessments mentioned earlier in the chapter are standardized and could be used for research purposes to show efficacy of treatment. Clearly we also need more standardized assessments, but work is currently progressing on providing data for several (KELS, ACLS-90). The Stress Management Questionnaire (Stein & Smith, 1989) has recently been standardized (Stein, in preparation). Its use as an assessment tool has been recommended for occupational therapy practitioners leading stress management groups or working with a depressed population.

There is promise in these attempts to develop standardized assessments and to document outcomes. To further demonstrate the value of occupational therapy and of the use of specific methods in occupational therapy practice, we need to "clarify which patients respond to what particular forms of treatment, what behaviors and symptoms can be changed and whether specifically trained skills generalize to the home, and to the community" (Hayes, 1989, p. 151).

The Challenge of the Future

The changes in health care toward cost-containment through managed care have had a profound effect on how and where we function as occupational therapy practitioners. Just as a car mechanic is expected to diagnose the problem, provide an estimate of costs, estimate the amount of time necessary to fix the vehicle, and determine the expected performance of the vehicle after repair, so are health care providers expected to inform patients regarding specific functional goals, the time needed to achieve these goals, and the effectiveness of the treatment they will receive. As reported above, our outcome measures are sorely lacking. An emotional belief that what we do is beneficial is not sufficient. Before we can validate our presence in *any* context, we need to document the effectiveness of what we do.

Also, in the era of cost-containment, management is determining who does what best and in the least expensive way. We need to ask the question, what can occupational therapy add to a mental health team that is unique; then we need to capitalize on that uniqueness. I propose that one of the unique aspects of occupational therapy is not the use of cognitive-behavioral techniques, but the ability to identify the combination of a patient's cognitive abilities coupled with the identification of functional skills needed for survival in his or her community. When this information is synthesized with contributions of other team members, the foundation for a holistic intervention plan is in place.

Our goal must be to document what we are doing and provide the measures of effectiveness necessary for validation of our unique skills. Further, we are challenged to change (Fidler, 1991) the arena in which we have been working for so long and move to where managed care is placing our patients.

The basic tenets of cognitive-behavioral therapy and the philosophy of occupational therapy have many commonalities. Occupational therapy practitioners have adopted many cognitive-behavioral strategies and techniques in conjunction with other occupational therapy frames of reference. The intent of this chapter has been to define the relationship of a cognitive-behavioral approach to occupational therapy and to provide an understanding of the theoretical antecedents of the cognitive-behavioral components of occupational therapy practice. Understanding the background of these cognitive-behavioral techniques should prove useful to the occupational therapist as he or she creates an eclectic approach for an individual patient. "It is necessary to combine several schools of thought and draw from many resources when working with populations whose illness reflects biopsychosocial phenomena. Neither the patient, nor the course of a given illness, are unidimensional. Different treatment models can augment or jointly stimulate desired effects, and changing needs certainly may require different approaches" (Fine, 1991, p. vii).

Finally, when occupational therapy practitioners apply techniques to meet occupational therapy treatment goals, it does not mean that they are cognitive-behavioral therapists. Furthermore, the technique is not the goal of treatment. We are not specialists in stress management or coping or rational thinking. Our uniqueness as occupational therapy practitioners lies in our professional judgment and ability to identify patients' global cognitive assets and limitations and how they affect functional behavior. We use a variety of techniques and strategies, graded to the patients' cognitive abilities to enable them to learn the functional skills and behaviors necessary for meaningful lives in their environment of choice.

Acknowledgment

The author would like to thank Deane McCraith, Frank Stein, Virginia Stoffel, Hilda Versluys, and Deborah Youngman for support through providing related material, for valuable suggestions, and for reviewing earlier drafts of this manuscript.

References

Allen, C. (1996). *Allen Cognitive Level Screen, 1996 test manual*. Colchester, CT: S & S Worldwide.

Allen, C. Earhart, C., & Blue, T. (1992). *Occupational therapy treatment goals for the physically and cognitively disabled*. Bethesda, MD: American Occupational Therapy Association.

Allen, C. & Reyner, A. (1996). *How to start using the Allen Diagnostic Module* (2nd ed.). Colchester, CT: S & S Worldwide.

American Psychiatric Association. (1994). *Diagnostic and statistical manual of mental disorders* (4th ed.). Washington, DC: Author.

Bandura, A. (1985). Model of causality in social learning theory. In M. Mahoney & A. Freeman (Eds.), *Cognition and psychotherapy*. New York: Plenum Press.

Barris, R., Kielhofner, G., & Watts, J. (1983). *Psychosocial occupational therapy*. Laurel, MD: Ramsco.

Beck, A. (1970). Cognitive therapy: Nature and relation to behavior therapy. *Behavior Therapy, 1,* 184–200.

Beck, A. (1976). *Cognitive therapy and emotional disorders.* New York: International University Press.

Beck, A., & Weishaar, M. (1994). Cognitive therapy. In R. Corsini & D. Wedding (Eds.), *Current psychotherapies* (4th ed.). Itasca, IL: Peacock.

Beck, J. (1995). *Cognitive therapy: Basics and beyond.* New York: Guilford Press.

Bloomer, J., & Williams, S. (1982). The Bay Area Functional Performance Evaluation. In B. Hemphill (Ed.), *The evaluative process in psychiatric occupational therapy.* Thorofare, NJ: Slack.

Bradlee, L. (1984). The use of groups in short-term psychiatric settings. *Occupational Therapy in Mental Health, 4* (3), 47–57.

Bruce, B., & Borg, B. (1993*). Psychosocial occupational therapy: Frames of reference for intervention* (2nd ed.). Thorofare, NJ: Slack.

Burns, D. (1989a). Foreword. In J. Persons, *Cognitive therapy in practice: A case formulation approach.* New York: Norton.

Campbell, A., & McCreadie, R. (1988). Occupational therapy is effective for chronic schizophrenic day patients. *British Journal of Occupational Therapy, 46,* 327–328.

Cautela, J. (1967). Covert sensitization. *Psychological Reports, 20,* 459–468.

Christiansen, C., & Baum, C. (1991). *Occupational therapy: Overcoming human performance deficits.* Thorofare, NJ: Slack.

Clarck, E., & Peters, M. (1984). *Scorable self-care evaluation.* Thorofare, NJ: Slack.

Cohen-Kaplan, E. (1991). *Couples communication skills course.* Boston: Harvard Community Health Plan.

Cole, M. (1993). *Group dynamics in occupational therapy.* Thorofare, NJ: Slack.

Courtney, C., & Escobedo, B. (1990). A stress-management program: Inpatient-to-outpatient continuity. *American Journal of Occupational Therapy, 44,* 306–310.

Crist, P. (1986). Community living skills: A psychoeducational community-based program. *Occupational Therapy in Mental Health, 6* (2), 51–64.

DeMars, P. (1992). An occupational therapy life skills curriculum model for a native American tribe: A health promotion program based on ethnographic field research. *American Journal of Occupational Therapy, 46,* 727–736.

Diasio, K. (1968). Psychiatric occupational therapy: Search for a conceptual framework in light of psychoanalytic ego psychology and learning theory. *American Journal of Occupational Therapy, 22,* 400–406.

Dobson, K. (1988). *Handbook of cognitive-behavioral therapies.* New York: Guilford Press.

Drouet, V. (1986). Individual behavioral programme planning with long-stay patients. Part 1: Programmes planned and followed in an occupational therapy department. Part 2: Social skills training. *British Journal of Occupational Therapy, 49,* 227–232.

Earhart, C., Allen, C., & Blue, T. (1993). *Allen Diagnostic Module: Instruction manual.* Colchester, CT: S & S Worldwide.

Eilenberg, A. (1986). An expanded community role for occupational therapy: Preventing depression. *Physical and Occupational Therapy in Geriatrics, 5* (1), 47–57.

Ellis, A. (1958). Rational psychotherapy. *Journal of General Psychology, 59,* 35–49.

Ellis, A. (1985). Expanding the ABC's of rational-emotive therapy. In M. Mahoney & A. Freeman (Eds.), *Cognition and psychotherapy.* New York: Plenum Press.

Engel, J. (1991). Social validation of relaxation training in pediatric headache control. *Occupational Therapy in Mental Health, 11* (4), 77–90.

Engel, J., & Rapoff, M. (1990). Biofeedback-assisted relaxation training for adult and pediatric headache disorders. *Occupational Therapy Journal of Research, 10,* 283–299.

Fidler, G. (1969). The task-oriented group as a context for treatment. *American Journal of Occupational Therapy, 11,* 43–48.

Fidler, G. (1991). The challenge to change occupational therapy practice. *Occupational Therapy in Mental Health, 11* (1), 1–11.

Fine, S. (1991). Letter to Author, July 1989. In M. Ross, *Integrative group therapy: The structured five-stage approach* (2nd ed.). Thorofare, NJ: Slack.

Fine, S. (1993). Neurobehavioral perspectives on schizophrenia. In J. Van Deusen (Ed.), *Body image and perceptual dysfunction in adults.* Philadelphia: Saunders.

Fine, S., & Schwimmer, P. (1986). The effects of occupational therapy on independent living skills, *Mental Health Special Interest Section Newsletter, 9* (4), 2–3.

Frankl, V. E. (1985). Logos, paradox, and the search for meaning. In M. Mahoney & A. Freeman (Eds.), *Cognition and psychotherapy.* New York: Plenum Press.

Freeman, A., Pretzer, J., Fleming, B., & Simon, K. (1990). *Clinical applications of cognitive therapy.* New York: Plenum Press.

Friedlob, S., Janis, G., & Deets-Aron, C. (1986). A hospital connected half-way house program for individuals with long-term neuropsychiatric disabilities. *American Journal of Occupational Therapy, 40,* 271–277.

Giles, G. (1985). Anorexia nervosa and bulimia: An activity-oriented approach. *American Journal of Occupational Therapy, 39,* 510–517.

Giles, G., & Allen, M. (1986). Occupational therapy in the rehabilitation of the patient with Anorexia nervosa. *Occupational Therapy in Mental Health, 6* (1), 47–66.

Glasser, W. (1965). *Reality therapy: A new approach to psychiatry.* New York: Harper & Row.

Goldstein, A., Gershaw, N., & Sprafkin, R. (1979). Structured learning therapy: Development and evaluation. *American Journal of Occupational Therapy, 33,* 635–639.

Greenberg, L., Fine, S., Cohen, C., Larson, K., Michaelson-Bailey, A., Rubinton, P., & Glick, I. (1988). An interdisciplinary psychoeducational program for schizophrenic patients and their families in an acute care setting. *Hospital and Community Psychiatry, 39,* 277–282.

Hayes, R. (1989). Occupational therapy in the treatment of schizophrenia. *Occupational Therapy in Mental Health, 9* (3), 51–68.

Hayes, R., Halford, W., & Varghese, F. (1991). Generalization of the effects of activity therapy and social skills training on the social behavior of low functioning schizophrenic patients. *Occupational Therapy in Mental Health, 11* (4), 3–20.

Heine, D. (1975). Daily living group: Focus on transition from hospital to community. *American Journal of Occupational Therapy, 29,* 628–630.

Hewitt, K., Wishart, C., & Lambert, R. (1981). Social skills training with chronic psychiatric patients. *British Journal of Occupational Therapy, 44,* 284–285.

Hoffman, N. (Ed.). (1984). *Foundations of cognitive therapy: Theoretical methods and practical approaches.* New York: Plenum Press.

Hollon, S., & Beck, A. (1979). Cognitive theory of depression. In P. Kendall & S. Hollon (Eds.), *Cognitive behavioral interventions.* New York: Academic Press.

Hollon, S., & Kendall, P. (1979). Cognitive-behavioral interventions: Theory and procedure. In P. Kendall & S. Hollon (Eds.), *Cognitive-behavioral interventions.* New York: Academic Press.

Jodrell, R., & Sanson-Fisher, R. (1975). Basic concepts of behavior therapy: An experiment involving disturbed adolescent girls. *American Journal of Occupational Therapy, 29,* 620–624.

Johnson, M. (1986). Use of cognitive-behavioral techniques with depressed adults in day treatment. *Depression: Assessment and treatment update: Proceedings.* Bethesda, MD: American Occupational Therapy Association.

Johnson, M. (1987). Occupational therapists and the teaching of cognitive behavioral skills. *Occupational Therapy in Mental Health, 7* (3), 69–81.

Kaseman, B. (1980). Teaching money management skills to psychiatric outpatients. *Occupational Therapy in Mental Health, 1* (3), 59–71.

Kendall, P., & Hollon, S. (1979). Cognitive-behavioral interventions: Overview and current status. In P. Kendall & S. Hollon (Eds.), *Cognitive behavioral interventions.* New York: Academic Press.

Kielhofner, G., Henry, A., & Walens, D. (1989). *A user's guide to the occupational performance history interview.* Bethesda, MD: American Occupational Therapy Association.

Klein, J. (1988). Abstinence-oriented inpatient treatment of the substance abuser. *Occupational Therapy in Mental Health, 8,* 46–49.

Levy, L. (1993). Behavioral frame of reference. In H. Hopkins & H. Smith (Eds.), *Willard and Spackman's occupational therapy* (8th ed.) Philadelphia: Lippincott.

Liberman, R., Massel, H., Mosk, M., & Wong, S. (1985). Social skills training for chronic mental patients. *Hospital and Community Psychiatry, 36,* 396–403.

Lidz, T. (1985). Adolf Meyer and the development of American psychiatry, *Occupational Therapy in Mental Health, 5* (3), 33–53.

Lillie, M., & Armstrong Jr., H. (1982). Contributions to the development of psychoeducational approaches to mental health service. *American Journal of Occupational Therapy, 36,* 438–443.

Lindsay, W. (1983). The role of the occupational therapist in the treatment of alcoholism. *American Journal of Occupational Therapy, 37,* 36–43.

Love, H. (1988). Concept and use of the social skills game to facilitate group interaction: A case study. *Occupational Therapy in Mental Health, 8* (3), 119–133.

Mahoney, M. (1984). Behaviorism, cognitivism, and human change processes. In M. Reda & M. Mahoney (Eds.), *Cognitive psychotherapies.* New York: Plenum Press.

Maslen, D. (1982). Rehabilitation training for community living skills: Concepts and techniques. *Occupational Therapy in Mental Health, 2* (1), 33–49.

McCormick, I. A. (1985). A simple version of the Rathus Assertiveness Schedule. *Behavioral Assessment, 7,* 95–99.

McGourty, L. (1988). Kohlman evaluation of living skills (KELS). In B. Hemphill (Ed.), *Mental health assessment in occupational therapy.* Thorofare, NJ: Slack.

McMullin, R. (1986). *Handbook of cognitive therapy techniques.* New York: Norton.

Meichenbaum, D., & Asarnow, J. (1979). Cognitive-behavioral modification and metacognitive development: Implications for the classroom. In P. Kendall & S. Hollon, *Cognitive behavioral interventions.* New York: Academic Press.

Meyer, A. (1922). The philosophy of occupation therapy. *Archives of Occupational Therapy, 1,* 1–10.

Mosey, A. (1972). *Three frames of reference for occupational therapy.* Thorofare, NJ: Slack.

Mosey, A. (1974). An alternative: The biopsychosocial model. *American Journal of Occupational Therapy, 28,* 137–140.

Moyers, P. (1988). An organizational framework for occupational therapy in the treatment of alcoholism. *Occupational Therapy in Mental Health, 8* (2), 27–46.

Nickel, I. (1988). Adapting structured learning therapy for use in a psychiatric adult day hospital. *Canadian Journal of Occupational Therapy, 55,* 21–25.

Ogren, K. (1983). A living skills program in an acute psychiatric setting. *Mental Health Special Interest Section Newsletter, 6* (4), 1–2.

Phillips, E. (1978). *The social skills bases of psychopathology.* New York: Grune & Stratton.

Representative Assembly. (1979). Resolution 531-79. *American Journal of Occupational Therapy, 33,* 785.

Salkovskis, P., & Kirk, J. (1989). Obsessional disorders. In K. Hawton, P. Salkovskis, J. Kirk, & D. Clark (Eds.), *Cognitive behaviour therapy for psychiatric problems: A practical guide.* New York: Oxford University Press.

Seiler, T. B. (1984). Developmental cognitive theory, personality, and therapy. In N. Hoffman (Ed.), *Foundations of cognitive therapy.* New York: Plenum Press.

Semmer, N., & Frese, M. (1984). Implications of action theory for cognitive therapy. In N. Hoffman (Ed.), *Foundations of cognitive therapy.* New York: Plenum Press.

Shulman, B. (1985). Cognitive therapy and the individual psychology of Alfred Adler. In M. Mahoney & A. Freeman (Eds.), *Cognition and psychotherapy.* New York: Plenum Press.

Sieg, K. W. (1974). Applying the behavioral model to the occupational therapy model. *American Occupational Therapy Association, 28,* 421–428.

Skinner, B. (1953). *Science and human behavior.* New York: Macmillan.

Skolaski, T., & Broekema, M. (1975). *The basic living skills battery.* Madison, WI: Dane Mental Health Center.

Smith, N., & Tempone, B. (1968). Psychiatric occupational therapy within a learning theory context. *American Journal of Occupational Therapy, 22,* 415–420.

Stein, F. (1982). A current review of the behavioral frame of reference and its application to occupational therapy. *Occupational Therapy in Mental Health, 2* (4), 35–62.

Stein, F., & Nikolic, S. (1989). Teaching stress management techniques to a schizophrenic patient. *American Journal of Occupational Therapy, 43,* 162–169.

Stein, F., & Smith, J. (1989). Short-term stress management programme with acutely depressed in-patients. *Canadian Journal of Occupational Therapy, 56,* 185–191.

Stein, F., & Smith, J. (in preparation). The stress management questionnaire.

Stoffel, V. (1994). Occupational therapists' roles in treating substance abuse. *Hospital and Community Psychiatric, 45,* 21–22.

Taylor, E. (1988). Anger intervention. *American Journal of Occupational Therapy, 42,* 127–155.

Thien, M. (1987). Demonstrating treatment outcomes in mental health. *Mental Health Special Interest Section Newsletter, 10* (4), 2–3.

Toglia, J. (1992). A dynamic interactional approach to cognitive rehabilitation. In N. Katz (Ed.), *Cognitive rehabilitation: Models for intervention in occupational therapy.* Boston: Andover Medical Publishers.

Vallis, T. M. (1991). Theoretical and conceptual bases of cognitive therapy. In T. Vallis, J. Howe, & P. Miller (Eds.), *The challenge of cognitive: Applications to nontraditional populations.* New York: Plenum Press.

Werner, H. D. (1982). *Cognitive therapy: A humanistic approach.* New York: Free Press.

Wilson, G. (1994). Behavior therapy. In R. Corsini & D. Wedding (Eds.), *Current psychotherapies* (4th ed.) Itasca, IL: Peacock.

Wolpe, J. (1958). *Psychotherapy by reciprocal inhibition.* Stanford: Stanford University Press.

Woodcock, R., & Johnson, M. (1977). *Woodcock Johnson psycho-educational battery.* Hingham, MS: Teaching Resources.

Zschokke, J., Freeberg, M., & Erickson, E. (1975). Influencing behavior to improve attendance at occupational therapy in a psychiatric setting. *American Journal of Occupational Therapy, 29,* 625–627.

SECTION 3

Elderly with Dementia

The Cognitive Disabilities Model in Rehabilitation of Older Adults with Dementia

Linda L. Levy, MA, OTR/L, FAOTA

Cognitive impairment, better known as the "cognitive decline of dementia," increases substantially as people age. Current estimates of the prevalence of cognitive impairment vary from 5% to 10% among those over the age of 65; among those over 85, estimates of cognitive impairment range from 25% to 48% (Morris, 1994; U.S. Senate, 1991; Evans et al., 1989). Although different epidemiological studies report variations in prevalence rates, there is overall agreement that the prevalence of cognitive impairment increases significantly with age, and that in the oldest range cognitive impairment is seen in at least one in four older adults. Thus, it is estimated that some 2 million—and possibly as many as 4 million—residents of the United States are suffering from the cognitive impairment of dementia (Advisory Panel on Alzheimer's Disease, 1993; Evans, et al., 1990). These numbers are projected to climb to 7.5 million to 14.3 million by the year 2040 (Evans et al., 1990). Concurrently, the major disorders causing cognitive impairment become increasingly prevalent in later life. Although the leading cause of cognitive impairment in older adults is Alzheimer's disease (NCHS, 1995), brain disorders such as cerebrovascular disease (leading to stroke and vascular dementia) and Parkinson's disease (leading to Parkinson's dementia) also account for the high rates of cognitive impairment seen in the older population (Friedman, 1995; NCHS, 1995). It is clear that occupational therapists who work with older adults will encounter ever-increasing numbers of patients with cognitive impairment regardless of the setting in which they practice, whether in hospitals, rehabilitation units, mental health settings, long-term care facilities, community agencies, adult day care, and/or home care settings; at the same time, therapists must be prepared to assess and treat the functional disabilities arising from cognitive impairment in older adults.

Emergence of a New Approach to Rehabilitation

Until recently, rehabilitation services were considered more appropriate for individuals with disorders resulting in chronic physical impairments, such as heart disease, arthritis, or stroke, than those with disorders resulting in chronic cognitive impairments (Reifler & Teri, 1986). Cognitive impairment was frequently cited as a cause for denial of eligibility for rehabilitation. The rationale was that rehabilitation was essentially a relearning process, and since patients with cognitive impairment have difficult time learning new material, they would be unable to benefit from rehabilitation services. This rationale gained support from a number of studies demonstrating an association between cognitive impairment and rehabilitation failure (Beals, 1972; Klingbeil, 1982; Kotila et al., 1984; Novack et al., 1987; Miller, 1978; Schuman et al., 1981). Yet successful, albeit "reconceptualized," rehabilitation programs for the functional disabilities of cognitively impaired older adults were at the same time beginning to be described in the literature (Levy, 1986a, 1989; Kemp, 1988; Chiu & Smith, 1990; Gottlieb, 1990). These programs demonstrated that environmental modification, prevention of secondary disabilities, and caregiver education and training are essential components of any rehabilitation program, and that rehabilitation needs to be conceptualized as much more than a relearning process.

In 1987, Congress passed the federal Nursing Home Reform Act (NHRA) as part of the Omnibus Budget Reconciliation Act (OBRA) (P.L. 100-203, 1987), which took effect October 1, 1990. The NHRA was the result of intensive study by the Institute of Medicine and a strong advocacy effort for major reform in the long-term care (LTC) industry. This legislation mandates that an LTC facility "provide services and activities to attain or maintain the highest practicable physical, mental, and psychosocial well-being of each resident . . ." (P.L. 100-203, 1987). Here, a rehabilitative philosophy was mandated for *all* disabled older adults. The overall goals of rehabilitation were reframed from whether the older adult could make measured gains in ambulation and self-care independence (P.L. 89-97, 1965) to whether the older adult's quality of life could be improved upon, despite the presence of chronic, progressive, or multiple disabilities. At the same time, the individual's ability to maintain or improve function assumed highest priority, in lieu of an orientation toward medically oriented regimens and disease processes. Concurrently, older adults with cognitive impairments were explicitly included in rehabilitative considerations for the first time since rehabilitative services were made available to older adults (P.L. 89-97, 1965).

Clearly, occupational therapy is well placed to lead rehabilitation efforts on behalf of cognitively disabled older adults in the now reframed tradition of rehabilitation. The recent "reconceptualization" of rehabilitation has been known to occupational therapists for some time, even though it has only recently been accessible to older adults with cognitive impairment. Indeed, this conceptualization is rooted in the tenets of moral treatment practiced by occupational therapists in psychiatric hospitals 100 years ago (Hopkins & Smith, 1993). In addi-

tion, occupational therapy is unique among current rehabilitation professions in its long-standing investment in efforts to develop foundations for rehabilitative intervention with cognitively impaired individuals. To the profession's credit, the oldest and most established cognitive theoretical approach in occupational therapy, Allen's Cognitive Disabilities Model (1985), has already made groundbreaking contributions to this rapidly developing area of rehabilitation (Allen et al., 1989; Chiu & Smith, 1990; HCFA, 1989; Levy, 1986a; Levy, 1989).

This chapter discusses the application of Allen's Cognitive Disabilities Model for rehabilitating cognitively impaired older adults as a benchmark treatment strategy for this now recognized population. Allen's model is particularly useful for occupational therapists because it has been adopted by Medicare to document the functional consequences of cognitive impairment in older adults (Allen et al., 1989; HCFA, 1989). While the cognitive disability model is conceptualized to address the functional consequences of cognitive impairments experienced by individuals from a variety of neurocognitive disorders, this discussion will emphasize the application of Allen's model to the cognitive limitations presented by dementia, the single most common and well-defined cause of cognitive impairment in older adults (NCHS, 1993; U.S. Senate, 1991). The chapter begins with a synthesis of existing knowledge and research on the effects of dementia on cognition, function, and behavior to provide groundwork for discussion of Allen's model as a pioneering intervention strategy in the now reconceptualized tradition of rehabilitation for the cognitively impaired older adult.

Dementia: Overview

To review, dementia is an acquired organic syndrome in which there is progressive deterioration in global cognitive function of such severity that it interferes with the individual's occupational and social performance (APA, 1994). The primary degenerative process remains untreatable. Symptoms include a gradual loss of memory and eventual failure of all body functions directed by the brain, resulting in death. As has been indicated, it is all too common in the aging population. Survey data report an overall prevalence of 5 to 10% among persons aged 65 and older (Jorm, 1990; Morris, 1994); the prevalence roughly doubles with every 5 years of age reaching a level of at least 16% in persons aged 80 and over (Breteler et al., 1992; Katzman & Kawas, 1994), and there is evidence that it can reach 47% among those 85 and older (Evans et al., 1989). The lifetime risk of Alzheimer's disease ranges between 14 and 26% (Terry et al., 1994). In long-term care settings, dementias remain the most frequently diagnosed clinical problem, affecting 50 to 65% of all residents (NCHS, 1993; U.S. Senate, 1991).

Alzheimer's disease is the most common cause of dementia, accounting for 60% or more of dementing illnesses. There are two other types of dementing illnesses. Multi-infarct dementia, now called "vascular dementia" in DSM-IV, accounts for approximately 20% of all dementias. Mixed dementia (Alzheimer's and multi-infarct/"vascular") accounts for another 10 to 15% of all cases and 25% of older adults who have a stroke eventually develop dementia (Katzman & Kawas, 1994). Recent findings (Snowdon, Greiner, Mortimer, Riley, & Markesbery, 1997) suggest a direct link between Alzheimer's and cerebrovascular diseases. Parkinson's dementia afflicts about 30% of older adults with Parkinson's disease (Friedman, 1995). Other dementia syndromes occur with Pick's disease, Creutzfeldt-Jacob disease, Huntington's disease, hydrocephalus, alcohol abuse, schizophrenia, and various medical illnesses (Schneider, 1995). Symptoms in the latter dementias are similar to those of Alzheimer's disease, although they tend to be more variable, with "spotty" rather than complete losses of intellectual abilities (Tatemichi et al., 1994). For example, in Parkinson's dementia, the memory deficit is one of impaired recall with relative sparing of recognition, and language, except for verbal fluency, remains intact. The course of dementia, while inexorably deteriorating, is unpredictable, lasting an average of 10 years.

Characteristics of Dementia

Dementia encompasses a number of conditions characterized by irreversible and progressive deterioration in all cognitive and functional abilities (Eisdorfer et al., 1994). Clinical characteristics of dementia are common to all types. In general, they can be collapsed into three categories: cognitive impairment, functional impairment, and behavioral impairment.

Cognitive Impairment

The most common cognitive impairment seen in dementia is progressively worsening memory impairment. However, over time, all cognitive subcomponents are affected. To review, memory is an exceedingly complex yet basic cognitive function. It builds upon attention (information needs to be attended to before it can be remembered). When impaired, as in dementia, it compromises all higher-order cognitive functions (i.e., learning, reasoning, planning, problem solving, judgment, abstraction, social awareness).

Information processing theorists (Best, 1989; Cerella, 1990) conceptualize memory in terms of three information processing stages: the ability to attend and take in new information through the senses (encoding), retain it for variable periods of time (storage), and then to access the information when needed (retrieval). Even from the earliest stages of dementia, individuals experience difficulty in all three information processing stages. Significant impairment is demonstrated early on in learning (encoding), retaining (storing), and retrieving information, especially with regard to new information that must be remembered for more than a very brief period of time (Bondi & Kaszniak, 1991; Duchek et al., 1991; Peterson, 1994; Welsh et al., 1991). One of the most reliable differential criteria for the disease is the much greater difficulty in recall experienced by patients in the earliest stages (Welsh et al., 1992). Failure to remember recent conversations and/or repeated conversations is a typical consequence of this difficulty.

The most influential structural theory of memory, developed by Atkinson and Shiffrin (1968), proposes that memory involves the processing of information in three distinct types of memory storage systems: sensory memory, primary (short-term) memory, and secondary (long-term) memory. Sensory memory retains raw uninterpreted sensory information for up to 3 seconds. Primary (short-term) memory retains knowledge currently in use for up to 30 seconds. It is closely related to attentional capacity (Nissen, 1986) and is limited to seven (plus or minus two) chunks of information (Miller, 1956). In dementia, deficits are clear in both primary memory and attentional capacity (Botwinick et al., 1986; Storandt et al., 1984). Secondary (long-term) memory is vast and complex. It has an unlimited capacity, retains information permanently, and requires elaboration to better understand how it is affected by dementia.

Tulving (1972, 1983) proposed a framework to help define the nature of secondary memory. First, he conceptualized secondary memory as "declarative," which he proceeded to subdivide into "episodic" and "semantic" memories. Later, he added a second form of secondary memory, which he termed "procedural" (Squire, 1986; Squire, 1987; Tulving, 1985). In Tulving's view, declarative memory includes memories of facts. Further, episodic memory involves the ability to recall information and personally experienced events to a specific time and place. Semantic memory is more conceptual and involves what is learned as general knowledge about the meanings of words, numbers, symbols, and their interrelationships irrespective of time, place, and personal experience. In contrast, procedural memory involves recall of the necessary skills, rules, plans, and/or procedures to perform an activity. Hence, declarative memory (episodic and/or semantic) involves remembering who, what, where, when, or why; procedural memory involves remembering how. Kausler and Lichty (1988) hypothesize that procedural memories are encoded relatively automatically and do not require the deliberate organizational strategies needed by declarative memories.

Research demonstrates that even in the earliest stages of dementia, both episodic and semantic memory are severely affected (Bondi & Kaszniak, 1991; Nebes, 1989, 1992). Yet procedural memory does not appear to be as affected to the same extent as declarative memory by the disease. Just as the most basic sensory and motor abilities are preserved by the disease process (at least until the later stages), it appears that remembering *how* to perform familiar motor behavior is likewise pre-

served (Eslinger & Damasio, 1986; Levy, 1986a, 1989, 1992; Knopman & Nissen, 1987; Knopman, 1991; Grafman et al., 1990; LaBarge et al., 1992; Dick, 1992: Dick et al., 1988; Dick et al., 1996). In addition, research is beginning to demonstrate that even severely impaired Alzheimer's patients can learn and retain tasks involving fine and gross motor skills for at least 1 month (Eslinger & Damasio, 1986: Heindel et al., 1988; Heindal et al., 1989; Grafman et al., 1990; Knopman, 1991; Dick et al., 1996). Hence, the literature is beginning to document that motor-based retraining programs are worthwhile and have the potential to produce lasting changes (Josephsson et al., 1993). Although yet to be carried out by occupational therapists, this research provides occupational therapy with empirical support for intervention strategies that have long been utilized to enable cognitively impaired older adults to relearn and/or retain basic motor skills and activities of daily living (e.g., eating, bathing, dressing) (Allen, 1982, 1985; Allen, Earhart, & Blue, 1992; Levy, 1974, 1986a, 1989). Indeed, what Tulving (1985) described as procedural memory was recognized much earlier in the occupational therapy literature (Allen, 1982, 1985; Levy, 1974); it remains an important source of cognitive capacity that is capitalized upon in rehabilitation for the elderly with cognitive limitations. This will be discussed more fully later.

Although progressively worsening memory deficits are the hallmark cognitive impairments of dementia, higher-order cognitive functions (e.g., reasoning, problem solving, judgment, abstraction) have already been significantly affected (Baum & Edwards, 1993: Mayer et al., 1986; Sullivan et al., 1989). Lower order cognitive components are affected as well. Early in the course of the disease, individuals can experience aphasia, anomia, and language difficulties (Faber-Langendoen, et al., 1988; Herlitz & Backman, 1990). Aphasia appears to be associated with a more rapid course of deterioration (Yasavage, et al., 1993). Word finding and word fluency difficulties are especially common and are generally considered to be secondary to memory deficits. Yet auditory comprehension appears to be retained at least until later stages of the disease (Keane et al., 1994). Agnosia presents as difficulties in the individual's ability to recognize objects and/or people (Mendez et al., 1990, Yasavage et al., 1993); it is particularly difficult for caregivers to cope with.

Apraxia is well documented in the advanced stages of the disease (Edwards et al., 1991; Geschwind & Damasio, 1985; Yasavage et al., 1993), and there is evidence that it can also be present in earlier stages (Foster et al., 1986). Other visuospatial difficulties are common; for example, one of the most frequent first-reported manifestations of the disease is becoming lost in a familiar neighborhood. Although visuospatial difficulties are most often considered to be secondary to memory impairment, lesions in the visual association cortex in some patients have also been reported (Hof et al., 1990). These lesions produce visuospatial impairments in figure ground discrimination, visual recognition and synthesis, and spatial localization (Mendez et al., 1990; Steffes & Thralow, 1987).

By the end stage of the disease, all cognitive components (i.e., judgment, reasoning, planning, problem solving, learning, memory, visuomotor organization, praxis, perception, orientation, and attention) are profoundly impaired. Concurrently, motor control has been severely affected, resulting in incontinence, ataxia, altered proprioception, gait changes, myoclonus, and Parkinsonism (Bucher & Larson, 1987; Visser, 1983). Coma and death follow.

To date, the only FDA-approved treatments for the cognitive symptoms of dementia are Tacrine (approved in 1994) and Aricept (approved in December 1996). Both are cholinesterase inhibitors that increase the concentrations of the neurotransmitter acetylcholine by inhibiting its breakdown. This mechanism is consistent with what neuroscientists have long identified as the "cholinergic hypothesis" (McEntee & Crook, 1992), which proposes that the longer acetylcholine stays in the brain, the longer neurons can call up memories. The therapeutic effects of both of these medications are modest at best. Neuropsychological testing reveals that Mini-Mental State Exam (MMSE) (Folstein et al., 1975) scores may show improvement by two points, which is deemed roughly equivalent to a delay in the progression of the disease by approximately 6 months. For the MMSE, a change of four points a year is expected in

persons with Alzheimer's dementia. Improvements in activities for daily living have not been reported. Between 25 and 50% of patients have shown benefit from Tachrine (Schneider, 1995); however, high rates of side effects such as liver toxicity, nausea, and vomiting are significant risks with these medications. In addition, there is preliminary evidence that nonsteroidal anti-inflammatory drugs (NSAIDs) can slow the rate of cognitive decline (Rogers, 1993). There are also encouraging, albeit preliminary, findings that estrogen supplemention is associated with significant improvements in memory and attention in elderly women with later stage dementia (n = 12) (Henderson, 1994). Researchers at the National Institutes of Health confirmed that exposure to estrogen enriched the complexity of neural synapses that transmit information between neurons in these women's brains (reported at the November 1996 Annual Conference of the Society of Neuroscience in Washington, D.C.). Clearly, this finding bears watching.

Functional Impairment

A hallmark feature in the diagnosis of dementia is evidence of impairment in complex tasks of daily living (APA, 1994). This criterion was designed to distinguish between cognitive impairment of normal aging and that of dementia. As such, functional information is particularly important in detecting early stages of the disease (AHCPR, 1996; Morris et al., 1991). Functional assessment emerged in the 1960s (Katz et al., 1963; Lawton & Brody, 1969; Lawton et al., 1982), and several questionnaire and observational measures have since been developed. For diagnostic and statistical purposes, functional impairment is defined in terms of the ability to manage one's affairs and property, represented by the ability to perform instrumental activities of daily living (IADL), and the ability to care for oneself, represented by the ability to perform basic activities of daily living (ADL) (Dawson et al., 1987; Manton et al., 1993). IADLs typically include six (or seven) home management activities: preparing meals, shopping for personal items, managing finances, using the telephone, doing heavy housework, doing light housework, and less often, managing one's medications (Fillenbaum, 1985; Lawton & Brody, 1969). ADL include six (or seven) personal care activities: dressing, bathing, toileting, grooming, eating, transfers, and occasionally, ambulation (Katz et al., 1963; Lawton & Brody, 1969). The mild to moderate range of functional impairment is tapped by IADL instruments. The severe range is tapped by ADL instruments. In dementia, the most common first manifestation of the disease is difficulty in performing IADL, which progresses over time to the inability to manage any ADL functions (Hughes et al., 1982; Levy, 1986a; Reisberg et al., 1982, 1985). Decline in functional abilities is reported as one of the most difficult aspects of dementia for both patients (Cotrell & Schultz, 1993) and their caregivers (Green et al., 1993).

Although there is an implicit relationship between functional capacity and the extent of cognitive impairment (Bassett & Folstein, 1991; Reisberg et al., 1982, 1985; Zanetti et al., 1993), the precise nature of this relationship has not been determined. To date, attention and memory deficits have been implicated in predicting functional disability and decline (Vitaliano et al., 1984; Vitaliano et al., 1986; Zanetti et al., 1993; Josephsson et al., 1993). However, Wolinsky and colleagues (Wolinsky & Johnson, 1991; Wolinsky et al., 1992) have found that what they now identify as the "advanced ADL"(i.e., those related to competence in the use of the telephone, managing money, preparing meals, and taking medication appropriately) are more directly related to standard assessments of cognitive function than are the more basic household and self-care ADL. This finding is consistent with this author's perspective, as will be discussed in a later section.

At the same time, other researchers (Eisdorfer et al., 1992; Loewenstein et al., 1992; Loewenstein et al., 1995; Paveza et al., 1995) are beginning to question whether functional and cognitive capacities as assessed by traditional neuropsychological instruments are as interdependent as have traditionally been assumed. The Global Deterioration Scale (GDS) (Reisberg et al., 1982), the Functional Assessment Staging Instrument (FAST) (Scalen & Reisberg 1992; Reisberg et al., 1985), and the Clinical Dementia Rating Scale (CDR) (Berg, 1988;

Hughes et al., 1982) are the most highly respected and frequently cited instruments for staging the progression of the disease, and yet each reflect untested assumptions about the interdependence of functional impairment and cognitive losses. In these staging instruments, functional impairment is generally assessed by global ADL-IADL scales (Katz et al., 1963; Lawton & Brody, 1969; Lawton et al., 1982); cognitive loss is assessed by traditional neuropsychological mental status measures such as the Mini-Mental State Exam (MMSE) (Folstein et al., 1975), the Blessed Orientation-Memory-Concentration (BOMC) test (Katzman et al., 1983), the Blessed Information-Memory-Concentration (BIMC) test (Katzman et al, 1983), the Short Portable Mental Status Questionnaire (SP-MSQ) (Pfeiffer, 1975), or other measures of memory and neuropsychological functions. (For discussion of items included in these instruments, see "Cognitive Changes in Later Life," chapter 10 of this volume. Note also that the limitations inherent in using these measures to predict functional potential will be discussed in a section to follow.) Paveza et al. (1995) and Eisdorfer et al. (1992) have challenged the accuracy of GDS and CDR staging instruments to predict cognitive and functional decline in dementia. Both researchers found that functional impairments occur earlier than predicted by the GDS and that they do not demonstrate progressive decline; functional and cognitive deterioration also occurred at different rates (Eisdorfer et al., 1992; Paveza et al., 1995). Such findings point to a pressing need to provide an alternative to staging instruments such as the GDS, FAST, and CDR, which combine functional capacity and cognitive impairment constructs into a single measure that may not accurately reflect the individual's level of impairment. Further development and testing of instruments that derive separate impairment scores for functional capacity and cognitive impairment is needed.

A number of instruments have been developed to stage deficits in functional skills independent of deficits in cognitive abilities. The original and most frequently utilized measures are relatively global; they include the Index of Activities of Daily Living (Katz et al., 1963), the Physical Self-Maintenance Scale (PSMS), and the Lawton-Brody Instrumental Activities of Daily Living Scale (Lawton & Brody,

1969). More recently, instruments have been developed to measure the cognitive dimension of functional performance. The most common include the Functional Activities Questionnaire (FAQ) (Pfeffer et al., 1982; Pfeffer, 1995), the Structured Assessment of Independent Living Skills (SAILS) (Mahurin et al., 1991), the Direct Assessment of Functional Status (DAFS) (Loewenstein et al., 1989; Loewenstein & Rupert, 1995), the Functional Life Scale (FLS) (Sarno et al., 1973), the Dependance Scale (DS) (Stern et al., 1994), the Functional Performance Measure (FPM) (Carswell et al., 1995), the Functional Behavior Profile (FBP) (Baum, Edwards, & Morrow-Howell, 1993), the Daily Activities Questionnaire (DAQ) (Oakley et al., 1991), and the Kitchen Task Assessment (KTA) (Baum & Edwards, 1993). (The Functional Activities Questionnaire (FAQ) is detailed in chapter 10 of this volume.) In addition, there are a number of functional performance instruments based on the Cognitive Disabilities Model such as the Cognitive Performance Test (CPT) (Burns et al., 1994), the Routine Task Inventory II (RTI II) (Allen, Earhart, & Blue, 1992), the Allen Cognitive Level Test (ACL) (Allen, 1985, 1992), and the Enlarged Allen Cognitive Level Test (ACL-E) (Allen, Earhart, and Blue, 1992; Kehrberg et al., 1992; Kehrberg, 1993). These will be discussed more fully in a later section.

With the exception of the informant-based Functional Activities Questionnaire (FAQ), the nonglobal functional instruments listed above are particularly noteworthy because they offer objective, behaviorally based scales that directly assess functional performance on specific functional tasks. These instruments also limit the well-documented reporter biases inherent in self or informant reports of functioning characteristic of most other functional performance measures (Magaziner et al., 1988; Weinberger et al., 1992; Zimmerman & Magaziner, 1994). However, it needs also to be recognized that the majority of these instruments (i.e., FAQ, DAQ, SAILS, DAFS, FLS, DS, GDS, CDR, and FAST) are designed to assess the prevalence and to stage the functional impairment of dementia. They do not purport to be instruments useful for remediation, rehabilitation, and/or management of the functional performance impairments they document. Table 7-1 provides an outline of the most valid, reliable, and widely used instruments used to assess functional impairment in this population.

Allen's Cognitive Disabilities Model approach to the problem of assessing functional impairment differs markedly from that employed by other researchers. In lieu of strategies aimed toward isolating previously conceptualized neuropsychological functions, or developing generalized task lists, to predict extent of functional impairment, the Cognitive Disabilities Model seeks to discover the unique nature of previously unidentified information processing components underlying functional performance.

Further, Allen's approach is clinically driven. The primary focus is the degree to which specifically defined deficits in information processing capabilities compromise performance of IADL-ADL functional activities (Burns et al., 1994). Hence, the manner in which the individual responds to functional task demands of varying complexity is the primary concern. This strategy differs markedly from functional assessment strategies most visible in the literature. Traditionally, the severity of functional disability is assessed by determining the absolute ability versus inability to perform specific IADL-ADL tasks. The resultant number of IADL-ADL deficits are then summed (Lawton & Brody, 1969; Katz et al., 1963; Fillenbaum, 1985; Leon & Lair, 1990); the nonglobal functional status instruments listed above, albeit employed infrequently, are notable exceptions. Occupational therapists have long recognized the limitations of global and numerical ADL assessments of functional performance. These measures are insufficiently sensitive to reflecting changes over time and nonpredictive of how the individual performs in other functional situations, and they provide no basis to generate practical strategies for intervention. Clearly, Allen's model offers considerable assistance in the assessment, staging, and remediation of cognitive and functional impairments, as will be discussed more fully later.

Behavioral Impairment

Unlike cognitive and functional impairments, there is considerable variability in the extent to

Table 7-1
Functional Assessment Instruments

Global Functional Status Measures
Index of Activities of Daily Living (Katz ADL) (Katz et al., 1963)
Physical Self-Maintenance Scale (PSMS) (Lawton & Brody, 1969)
Instrumental Activities of Daily Living Scale (IADL) (Lawton & Brody, 1969)

Functional Performance Measures emphasizing Cognition
Functional Activities Questionnaire (FAQ) (Pfeffer, 1995)
Structured Assessment of Daily Living Skills (SAILS) (Mahurin, DeBettignies, & Pirozzolo, 1991)
Direct Assessment of Functional Status (DAFS) (Loewenstein et al., 1989)
Functional Life Scale (FLS) (Sarno, Sarno, & Levita, 1973)
Dependence Scale (DS) (Stern, Albert, & Sano, 1994)
Functional Behavior Profile (FBP) (Baum, Edwards, & Morrow-Howell, 1993)
Daily Activities Questionnaire (DAQ) (Oakley et al., 1991)

Occupational Therapy Functional Performance Measures emphasizing Cognition
Kitchen Task Assessment (KTA) (Baum & Edwards, 1993)
Functional Performance Measure (FPM) (Carswell et al., 1995)
Cognitive Performance Test (CPT) (Burns, Mortimer, & Merchek, 1994)
Routine Task Inventory II (RTI II) (Allen, Earhart, & Blue, 1992)
Allen Cognitive Level Test (ACL-90) (Allen, 1992)
Enlarged Allen Cognitive Level Test (LACL) (Allen, Earhart, & Blue, 1992)

Cognitive/Functional Staging Instruments
Global Deterioration Scale (GDS) (Reisberg et al., 1982)
Clinical Dementia Rating Scale (CDR) (Hughes et al., 1982)
Functional Assessment Staging Instrument (FAST) (Reisberg, Ferris, & Franssen, 1985)

which individuals experience behavioral problems (Schneider, 1995). In general, behavioral problems occur in response to cognitive impairments, especially the steadily worsening memory impairments. Individuals with progressive memory loss will become increasingly disoriented. They will first forget what time it is, then where they are and where they have placed their belongings. As the dementia worsens, they will even forget their own names. As would be expected, this leads to increasing agitation and confusion. Not knowing what time it is (or even the right decade) nor where they are, they tend to wander (it appears in search of familiar cues) and often get lost. Because they cannot remember where they have put their belongings, caregivers may be accused of stealing and paranoid features may emerge. Significant relationships between the presence and severity of behavioral problems and the severity of the disease have been demonstrated (Rovner et al., 1986; Swearer et al.,

1988). Relationships have also been demonstrated between the severity of behavioral problems and the severity of functional impairment (Teri et al., 1989).

Agitation is the most frequently documented behavioral problem experienced in persons with dementia (experienced by 100%), and it usually presents in the middle to late stages of the disease (Cohen-Mansfield et al., 1990). Agitated behaviors are categorized as verbally "nonaggressive" (constant requests for attention, complaining or whining, negativism), verbally aggressive (cursing, temper tantrums, screaming), physically "nonaggressive" (general restlessness, wandering, repetitious mannerisms), and/or physically aggressive (hitting, pushing, scratching, kicking). "Nonaggressive" agitated behaviors are the more frequent responses to the dementing disease (Cohen-Mansfield et al., 1990; Deutch & Rovner, 1991). When it occurs, physical aggression is more frequent in institutions than in home care settings (Rovner et al., 1986). It is important to recognize that falls, associated with substantial morbidity and mortality, are common in agitated elderly individuals (Cohen-Mansfield et al., 1990).

It is now recognized that agitated behaviors are derived from a variety of causes and have diverse meanings. Agitated behaviors are considered to reflect ineffective attempts to communicate feelings of pain, discomfort, fear, boredom, distress, loneliness, boredom, and/or other basic needs that must be disentangled by responsive caregivers. In addition, such behaviors are often triggered or exacerbated by environmental stimuli, typically sensory overload. Sensory overload is related to the frequency, intensity, and quantity of unpredictable stimuli and can cause markedly increased agitation and "catastrophic reactions" (the overreactions or excessive upsets precipitated by situations that overwhelm the limited thinking capacity of the brain). Moreover, activities such as bathing and changing clothes are commonly cited by caregivers as circumstances that trigger agitation (Mace & Rabins, 1991; Webster et al., 1988). Caregivers need help in identifying alternative approaches. In all cases, agitated behaviors are most effectively addressed in light of their underlying causes or meanings, before the use of behavioral or pharmacologic treatments (Burgener et al., 1992; Cohen-Mansfield & Billig, 1986; Cohen-Mansfield et al., 1993; Feil, 1993; Leibovici & Tariot, 1988). It should also be noted that there is evidence that agitated behaviors in both home and institutional settings decrease when therapeutic activity programs are available (Baum et al., 1993; Rabinovich & Cohen-Mansfield, 1992; Rovner & Katz, 1992; Rovner, 1994).

Behavioral symptoms can also involve mood disturbances. These include depression (both major depression and other less severe depressive states), affective lability, manic or hypomanic states, and what is broadly described as personality changes. (It is ironic that although personality changes are among the most common behavioral symptoms reported in patients with dementia, they have been the least intensively investigated.) In the early to mild stages of the disease, the most frequently reported behavioral symptoms are minor depression and personality changes (Rubin &

Kinscherf, 1989). The prevalence of major depression in dementia is reported to be between 10 and 30% (Burns, 1991; Teri and Wagner, 1992), although there are also studies that suggest prevalence rates as high as 40% (Lazarus et al., 1987) and 86% (Merriam et al., 1988). (Available data vary depending upon the assessment methods used and the nature of the depression being considered.) The evidence is clear that depression should be treated (Teri & Wagner, 1992). Cognitively impaired depressed patients respond to antidepressant therapy as well as those without cognitive impairment. However, they require a longer and more aggressive course of treatment (Reifler et al., 1986; Reynolds et al., 1987). Note also that relationships have been demonstrated to exist between activity involvement and lowered incidence of depression (Rabinovich & Cohen-Mansfield, 1992; Teri & Logsdon, 1991). An institutional focus on individually meaningful and purposeful occupation is a primary method for preventing depression (Langer & Rodin, 1976).

Behavioral symptoms may also include overtly psychotic phenomena such as delusions and hallucinations, although these are rarely seen until the late stages of the disease (Rubin et al., 1988; Rubin & Kinscherf, 1989). When experienced by patients, psychotic symptoms appear to be more important determinants of behavioral problems than severity of cognitive impairment (Rovner et al., 1986). This finding suggests that psychiatric interventions aimed at ameliorating psychotic symptoms should be carefully considered to reduce behavioral problems and to improve function for those patients with hallucinations and delusions.

Caregivers consistently identify the behavioral disturbances of dementia as the most significant sources of caregiver stress, exceeding the level of cognitive impairment (Deimling & Bass, 1986; Swearer et al., 1988; Teri et al., 1989; Zarit et al., 1980). Clearly, the need for around the clock supervision because of wandering and/or impaired judgment can exhaust even the most stable and caring of caregivers. Ultimately, long-term stress places caregivers at high risk for clinical depression (Teri et al., 1994; Teri & Wagner, 1992). There is evidence that it depresses immune system functioning and the caregiver's overall physical health as well (Kiecolt-Glaser et al., 1987). As will be seen, rehabilitation and care for the individual with cognitive impairment requires active participation of the caregiver. For this reason, preservation of the overall health of the caregiver is essential, with particular attention to the treatment and/or prevention of depression.

It is not the cognitive, functional, or behavioral problems associated with dementia per se that cause caregivers to become severely stressed, depressed, or physically ill, but rather the caregivers's inability to cope with them. (Chiu & Smith, 1990; Kemp, 1988; Zarit et al., 1980). Recent studies indicate that family members who cope better with the problems associated with dementia have higher levels of self-efficacy, the belief that one is capable of addressing a problematic behavior because one has the requisite skills, knowledge, and physical capacity (Cummings, 1987; Gallagher et al., 1987; Teri & Logsdon, 1991). Hence, there is a need for strategies to help caregivers develop a sense of self-efficacy to cope with the cognitive, functional, and behavioral problems they encounter. This too is a primary objective of the cognitive disabilities approach to intervention.

Factors Specific to Rehabilitation for Dementia

A number of factors are specific to rehabilitation for dementia:

1. As of now, there is no medical treatment for dementia. However, there is compelling evidence that although the biological aspects of the disease are not currently treatable, some of the cognitive, functional, and behavioral problems are amenable to intervention (Kahn, 1975; Levy, 1986b, 1992; Larson et al., 1984; Kamholz & Gottlieb, 1992; Kemp, 1988; Gottlieb, 1990; Chiu & Smith, 1990; Teri et al., 1992). Interventions are designed to maximize the remaining functional capacity of the impaired older adult. It is not reasonable to assume that intervention will restore cognitive functioning or reverse the organic brain damage that has already occurred (Chiu & Smith, 1990; Gottlieb, 1990; Levy, 1986b).

2. The major tenet of gerontological rehabilitation, i.e., to help the disabled elder to reach his or her highest attainable level of function, is no less applicable to the care of persons with dementia (Chiu & Smith, 1990; Gottlieb, 1990; Reifler & Teri, 1986). In 1987, this position was codified in the Omnibus Budget Reconciliation Act (OBRA) (P.L. 100–203, 1987), federal legislation that mandated a comprehensive rehabilitative and restorative philosophy for all in geriatric health care. In the rehabilitation model, function is emphasized over cure. The overall goals of intervention are to maintain or restore functional capacity, to promote participation in activities that maximize physical and mental health, and to ease the burdens of caregiving activities (Rovner, 1994). Prior to 1990 (when OBRA took effect), older adults with dementia were not viewed as viable rehabilitation candidates.

3. From the earliest stage of the disease process, elders with dementia suffer such severe cognitive and functional impairments that they are only minimally able to participate in the formulation and implementation of the rehabilitation plan. As a result, an adaptive approach (Mosey, 1994) to rehabilitation must be employed (Levy, 1989, 1992). An adaptive approach places emphasis on changing the task, level of cueing, and/or aspects of the environment to compensate for the effects of cognitive deficits on areas of occupational performance, when no change in impairment can be expected. It requires active participation of the caregiver to implement recommended intervention strategies (Chiu & Smith, 1990; Levy, 1986a, 1989, 1992). In this role, the caregiver needs guidance, support, and assistance from knowledgeable and supportive health professionals (Baum, 1991; Edwards & Baum, 1990; Zarit et al., 1985).

4. Dementias are dynamic diseases. They produce progressive declines in function, and different functional issues arise in different stages of the disease. Caregivers must be educated about the trajectory of disability imposed by the disease in order to maximize the capabilities that remain, to recognize and address potentially remediable "excess disabilities" that may emerge (i.e., depression, deconditioning, agitation, dysphagia), and to prepare themselves for the changes to

come (Levy, 1989; Edwards & Baum, 1990; Chiu & Smith, 1990; Gottlieb, 1990). Hence, it is important that functional performance be regularly assessed and monitored over time.

5. Dementia affects not just the older adult, but also the spouse and/or caregiver of that individual (Zarit et al., 1985). While caregivers are a crucial resource in the rehabilitation process, the progressive nature of the disease over many years can create conditions of unrelenting stress that are compounded by numerous practical problems that often overwhelm the coping capacities of affected families. Indeed, there is a breaking point beyond which the burdens of care become overwhelming, and families are no longer able to provide care without jeopardizing their own health and well-being. At all times, rehabilitative goals have a dual focus: to maximize the affected individual's level of functioning and quality of life and to minimize the burden of the caregiver(s) (Mace & Rabins, 1991; Pearlin et al., 1990; Zarit et al., 1985).

6. The concept of rehabilitation of patients with cognitive impairments is relatively new, and the few strategies that have been reported have yet to be evaluated systematically (Chiu & Smith, 1990; Rentz, 1991). Allen was the first to propose a comprehensive rehabilitation theory to address the functional problems experienced the elders with dementia (Levy, 1986a), and her approach has already made benchmark contributions to this rapidly developing area of rehabilitation (Levy, 1986a, 1989; Kemp, 1988; Allen et al., 1989; HCFA, 1989; Chiu & Smith, 1990; Rentz, 1991; Burns et al., 1994). As will be seen, her approach provides practitioners with a conceptual framework that (1) identifies the causes of the functional impairments of dementia, (2) provides guidelines for assessing the specific nature of the cognitive, functional, and behavioral difficulties experienced by the individual, (3) describes viable intervention strategies to assist individuals and their families or caregivers in coping with the wide range of physical, psychological, and social problems that occur as the disease progresses, (4) provides guidance on how best to enable the individual to lead as normal a life as possible given the disability that exists throughout the course of the disease, and

(5) proposes a comprehensive and humanistic approach to care.

The discussion that follows presents an overview of the cognitive disability approach to rehabilitation of the cognitive, behavioral, and functional impairments experienced by the elderly with dementia. For a more comprehensive discussion the reader is referred to Levy (1986a, 1989, 1992); Allen (1985), Allen, Earhart, & Blue (1992), and Allen and Robertson (1993).

Cognitive Disabilities Model

Neuropsychologists approach the problem of cognitive impairment and functional disability in dementing diseases by analyzing the difficulties in terms of specific cognitive components (i.e., attention, memory, orientation, perception, language functions, praxis, abstract reasoning, executive functions) that deviate from test norms. Although relationships between impairments and functional performance have been reported (Vitaliano et al., 1984; Vitaliano et al., 1986; McCue et al., 1990; Camp & McKitrick, 1992; Backman et al., 1991; Zanetti et al., 1993), findings have not led to useful intervention strategies. It should also be noted that dementias are characterized by severe memory deficits early in the course of the disease. This renders neuropsychological tests that are in large part memory driven less useful in assessing and/or staging the severity of the disease (Welsh et al., 1992).

The cognitive disability approach considers the problem of cognitive impairment and functional disability from a global or multicomponent perspective that is specifically addressed to the functional and behavioral consequences of cognitive impairment. It proposes an information processing model of the etiology of the functional impairment that identifies different information processing patterns revealed by different patterns of functional performance. Critical cognitive components such as attention, praxis, and memory are incorporated into the model; however, they are more broadly conceptualized as components of information processing patterns that vary significantly throughout a hierarchy of functional levels.

The primary intent of cognitive disability theory is to identify information processing capacities that determine whether an individual can perform a functional activity safely and successfully, and the specific nature of the cognitive impairments that need to be compensated for in the event of cognitive limitations. To this end, Allen (1985, 1987) has proposed a hierarchy of six cognitive levels that describe the dimensions of information processed in pursuing normal life activities, as well as qualitative differences in functional capacities and limitations. Given the focus on task performance and/or activity, the six levels are considered to represent information processing that is regulated by sensorimotor associations in the brain (Allen, Earhart, & Blue, 1992; Miller, 1981). Allen views three dimensions of cognition as stages of a sensorimotor information processing model that are considered at each of the six hierarchical cognitive levels. They are:

1. *Attention to sensory cues.* All information processing begins with the ability to attend to sensory input from the environment. Allen orders sensory cues that capture and sustain attention from internal cues (subliminal and proprioceptive), to external concrete cues (tactile, visual, and verbal), to increasingly complex abstract cues (related visual cues, verbal hypothetical, symbols or ideas). At lower cognitive levels, attention is limited to internal cues, such as musculoskeletal and proprioceptive sensations. At more advanced cognitive levels, individuals can respond to progressively wider ranges of cues, including tactile, visual, auditory, and eventually complex symbolic cues from the environment. At each succeeding cognitive level, the sensory cues used in performance are more complex, and behavior appears more organized. In order to maximize functional capacities, therapists must adapt activities both to capitalize on the cues that the individual is able to attend to and to limit exposure to activities that require attention to cues that are beyond the individual's range of comprehension.

2. *Sensorimotor associations.* Sensorimotor associations are the interpretive (i.e., learning/encoding) memory processes that follow from attention to sensory cues, and reflect the capacity to translate sensory cues into functional performance. They have also been conceptualized as the comprehendible goals implicit in initiating an action response. Levy (1974) and Allen (1982) were the first to recognize that the implicit goal of the individual performing an action may not be consistent with the more conventional explicit goals in performing an action. Individuals pursue activities with varying goals in mind, ranging, for example, from the simple pleasure of moving, to an interest in the effects of actions, to an investment in producing a high-quality end product. The problem to be recognized is that at lower cognitive levels an individual may only be able to comprehend the procedural memory (i.e., movement-based learning and memory) attributes involved in a desired activity, e.g., the familiar sensory sensations elicited by the motion of pushing a vacuum back and forth, and would not be able to comprehend the more conventional goal—or the result—that would be expected from an individual with higher memory (e.g., declarative) cognitive capacities, namely, a clean rug. Consequently, at lower cognitive levels, unintentional results become commonplace. It is important to recognize that the inability to comply with the traditional goals and expectations of an activity reflects a specific cognitive (i.e., attention and declarative memory) impairment that is outside of the individual's control. Caregivers can compensate for this impairment by adjusting conventional norms and expectations for activity performance.

3. *Motor actions.* Actions are elicited by attention to sensory cues (input), guided by sensorimotor associations (throughput), and can be observed in activity performance (output). They are the final stage of Allen's information processing model. There are two types: spontaneous (self-initiated from available memory stores) and imitated (cued through visual and motor channels by nonverbal, nonlanguage dependent demonstration from another person). At lower cognitive levels, individuals are only able to initiate and imitate motor actions that are near reflexive and/or already very familiar behavioral actions (neuropsychologists now describe this as the capacity to initiate and imitate procedural

memory responses). At more advanced cognitive levels, self-initiated motor actions extend beyond the well rehearsed and familiar, to planned actions that reflect attention to visual and then to abstract cues. Here, individuals use conceptual information (including declarative memory) to produce solutions to everyday problems and are able to participate freely in a broad range of activities.

Consistent with all occupational therapy models, the Cognitive Disabilities Model relies upon activity analysis as a primary means of intervention. Cognitive disability theory provides a means for analyzing the relative difficulty of any desired activity in terms of requisite information processing demands. From this analysis, environmental factors can be identified that facilitate or constrain the production of each cognitive dimension. Rehabilitation strategies are derived from conceptualizing how the environmental elements associated with each cognitive dimension might best be adapted or modified within the structure of a desired activity to capitalize on remaining cognitive capacities and to compensate for cognitive limitations. The intent is to place desired activities within an individual's range of comprehension and control. Specifically, therapists modify the structure of a desired activity to capitalize on and to compensate for (1) the "sensory cues" that the individual is able to attend to while doing an activity at any given cognitive level; (2) the quality of "sensorimotor association" that the individual is able to learn and remember, and/or the goal that the individual is able to act on, at any given level; and (3) the degree of assistance and/or cues required to enable the individual to complete a desired "motor action" at any given level, i.e., whether the desired motor action can be productively self-initiated, verbally or nonverbally cued, or must be directly imitated from the therapist to elicit a productive motor response.

Cognitive Levels in Rehabilitation

Regardless of the level of cognitive function, cognitive processes are maximized and behavioral responses become more effectively organized when environmental stimuli are presented to the impaired individual in a manner that matches his or her level of cognitive functioning (Levy, 1986a). In order to conceptualize rehabilitative intervention, the therapist must identify first the individual's cognitive capacities and limitations, and then must identify the environmental factors that can be modified to enable successful participation in desired activities.

The discussion that follows will provide a brief overview of the three information processing dimensions as they are revealed at each level and the environmental factors associated with each dimension. Guidelines are presented for conceptualizing environmental modification strategies that capitalize on cognitive capacities and compensate for limitations at each of the cognitive levels (Levy, 1989, 1992); intervention priorities appropriate for individuals functioning at each level are also provided. It should be noted that at any given cognitive level individual differences in treatment planning strategies are less nuanced given this disease than occurs within most other disease, because of the severe and progressive nature of memory deficits that characterize the disease. Yet it needs also to be recognized that individual differences are dependent upon personal characteristics that have defined and given meaning to individuals' lives, i.e., hobbies, professional accomplishments, preferred activities, family ties, expressions of faith. It is essential that such knowledge be sought from others familiar with the individual prior to the disease to ensure that the individual's interests, values, and wishes are respected, even when he or she can no longer express preferences.

Finally, Medicare assistance codes for each level (Allen et al., 1989; HCFA, 1989) will be identified. These codes provide therapists with means to document levels of cognitive assistance required to maximize functional performance capabilities throughout the debilitating course of the disease.

Cognitive Level 6: Planned Actions
(Medicare assistance code: Independent)

Attention is captured by abstract and symbolic cues. The *goal* is to use abstract reasoning to plan action sequences and to anticipate errors. *Motor actions* are those that have been planned in advance. Individuals can use complex information to carry out activities with accuracy and safety. Problems are anticipated, errors are avoided, and consequences of actions are considered. Theoretically, this level represents the absence of cognitive disability. Interventions to compensate for cognitive limitations are not required. Note that this is the only level where planning, problem solving, and learning and memory do not depend on overt visuomotor activity or direct external cues, or both.

Cognitive Level 5: Exploratory Actions
(Medicare assistance code: Stand-by/supervision cognitive assistance)

At this level, *attention* is captured and sustained by external cues, specifically the interesting properties of concrete objects. The *goal* of action is to explore the effects of self-initiated motor actions on physical objects and to investigate these effects through the use of planning and overt trial and error problem solving. (Covert problem solving requires conceptual or symbolic declarative memory. It is absent.) *Motor actions* are exploratory to produce interesting effects on material objects, and extend through visual memory to the ability to follow through on a concrete four- or five-step process. The individual is able to learn through direct concrete, visible, and meaningful stimuli.

Many activities can be accomplished successfully at this level because in concrete activities (i.e., those involving familiar four- to five-step motor actions with visibly perceivable results), individuals function relatively independently. However, the cognitive limitations experienced by individuals at this level become apparent when they attempt activities that require attention to abstract and symbolic cues, such as those that involve verbal and written instructions, diagrams, or drawings. Activities requiring attention to these cues (i.e., balancing a checkbook, following a new recipe, planning a multiple-course meal) will accentuate the disability and should be avoided.

Caregivers find that individuals can complete grooming, dressing, bathing, and eating activities without assistance. Household tasks are carried out relatively independently, although the individual

may require assistance in the abstract reasoning required to establish safety procedures and to anticipate hazardous situations. Difficulties are observed with memory (episodic and then semantic), judgment, reasoning, and planning ahead, as well as with the performance of complex daily activities (i.e., reading, writing, job performance, managing finances, shopping, driving). The individual is more repetitive, has more difficulty remembering recent conversations, events, and appointments, and more frequently misplaces objects.

This level parallels stage 4 (the "late confusional"–predementia stage) of the Global Deterioration Scale for the assessment of primary degenerative dementia (Reisberg et al., 1982), one of the most frequently used scales for staging the progression of the disease. Although there are significant differences in the rate of progression through the various stages of the disease (Goldman & Lazarus, 1988), duration in this stage has been estimated to be 2 years.

Cognitive Level 4: Goal-directed Activity
(Medicare assistance code: Minimum cognitive assistance)

Attention at this level is directed to visible as well as tactile cues, and it is sustained throughout familiar short-term activities to their completion. The *goal* in performing a motor action is to perceive a concrete cause and effect relationship between a visible cue and a desired outcome. Problem solving abilities are absent. *Motor actions* are limited to the ability to follow a two- to three-step, highly familiar, motor process that leads to the accomplishment of visible predictable goals. Individuals can learn two- to three-step procedures that have visible and predictable results.

Activities that can be accomplished successfully at this level are those that are adapted to capitalize on the capacity to use two- to three-step familiar motor actions that have predictable visible results, and activities that compensate for the individual's inability to comprehend novelty or unpredictable results, or notice mistakes when they occur. Individuals use what they see in the environment for cues as to what to do. Decisions are made based upon limited, visual information. Assistance is required with the abstract components of concrete tasks, i.e., procuring and setting-up supplies, scheduling activities. At this level, individuals should be provided with opportunities to engage in simple, relatively error-proof, concrete activities that support desired social roles. This goal is best accomplished by incorporating into the individual's daily routine yard work, household chores (e.g., laundry, simple meal preparation, shopping for a few familiar purchases), familiar sports and dance activities, simple board games and puzzles, typing, and walks to familiar destinations.

Despite significant cognitive impairment, the individual appears to be less confused at this level than at the succeeding level because activities are pursued with specific outcomes in mind. Therapists and caregivers should encourage individuals to engage in comprehensible concrete activities that will protect personal dignity and enable social role retention. However, they should not expect the individual to notice mistakes or solve problems when they occur, to retain directions out of context, to plan beyond the immediate situation, to generalize learning to new situations, or to anticipate safety hazards. Recently, vendors have begun to market a variety of crafts, puzzles, videos, and games (both solo and interactive) specifically designed for the needs of the cognitively disabled. These provide caregivers with exceptional opportunities for engaging cognitively impaired individuals in meaningful and productive activity. (Resources include Cross Creek Recreational Products, Millbrook, New York 12545; Geriatric Resources Inc., Winter Park, Florida 32792; S&S Worldwide, Colchester, Connecticut 06415; Potentials, Amherst, New York 14228; Gold Timers, Pecheco, California 94553; and Eldergames, Rockville, Maryland 20852.)

At this stage, most patients are unaware of their symptoms and may deny them, since their reasoning and judgment have become significantly impaired. Declarative memory (both semantic and episodic) is also significantly impaired. Instructions cannot be remembered, and patients are disoriented to time and sometimes to place. Clocks with the date, day, and year may assist orientation. Calendars, notes, labels, or pictures may serve as reminders of daily activities and locations of objects. However, memories of distant (past) events are retained longer and more powerfully than more recent memories, which only adds to the individual's confusion and lack of understanding about current situations. Environmental consistency is particularly important. Predictable routines allow individuals to perceive a greater sense of control.

Ensuring safety is another important concern at this level. Many accidents can be avoided by preventive measures, and the home environment should be carefully scrutinized for potential safety hazards. Particular attention should be paid to clutter, loose rugs, lighting, door locks, electrical appliances, oven knobs (hidden), hot water pipes, outlets (covered), cigarettes, matches, smoke alarms, firearms, power tools, knives, detergents, polishes, household chemicals, medications, and the tub and shower (grab bars, tub seating, skidproof mats, water temperature adjustment to avoid burns, tap water overflow alarms. Should the individual wander and become lost, caregivers should consider purchasing an identification bracelet and should ensure that identifying photographs are available.

It is important to be especially sensitive to the fear and frustration that accompanies the confusion of dementia. At this stage of the disease, individuals are beginning to recognize that their environments are less manageable and understandable in light of their significant memory impairments. Depression, aggression, and anxiety are frequent and reasonable reactions. Therapists must guide individuals to unvarying surroundings or success-oriented (movement-based) activities when they become agitated. At the same time, it is essential to recognize that caring for individuals with this disease exacts a tremendous physical and emotional toll on the caregiver. Seemingly unlimited patience and self-control are needed to cope with common responses of individuals stricken with this disease, such as repetitive and/or unintelligible conversation, complete silence, extreme agitation, or sudden aggression. At the same time, the individual rarely recognizes the extent of caregiving demanded by the disease, and is rarely able to give thanks to the caregiver. It is essential that mechanisms are specifically designed to provide care for the caregiver and to access respite.

Caregivers find that individuals can complete familiar grooming activities, although they may need to be reminded to do so and provided with supplies. Frequently, they neglect areas that are not completely visible. For example, the back of the body may remain unwashed, shampoo may not be rinsed from the back of the head, and the individual may neglect to shave under the chin, unless redirected. Dressing can be accomplished relatively independently, especially when clothing is preselected and placed in full view, and unnecessary clothing is kept from view; otherwise, inappropriate clothing is likely to be selected. The individual can eat independently but may require assistance to season foods, share a limited quantity of food, open unfamiliar containers, or avoid burns. Again, individuals should be protected from invisible hazards from sources such as heat, chemicals, and electricity. Twenty-four-hour supervision is recommended to ensure safety.

This level parallels stage 5 (the "early dementia" stage) of the Global Deterioration Scale (Reisberg et al., 1982). As indicated, there are significant differences in the rate of progression through the various stages of the disease, although the duration of this stage has been estimated at approximately 18 months.

※ *Cognitive Level 3: Manual Actions* (Medicare assistance code: Moderate cognitive assistance)

At this cognitive level, *attention* is directed to tactile cues that can be acted on, and to familiar objects that can be manipulated. The *goal* in performing a motor action is limited to tactile exploration of the kinds of effects one's actions have on the environment. These actions are typically repeated to verify that similar results occur. *Motor actions* are limited to the ability to follow a one-step, highly familiar, action-oriented direction that has been demonstrated for the individual to follow. It is unrealistic to expect the individual to learn new behavior.

Level three functional activities are caregiver intensive. Activities that can be successfully accomplished are those that are adapted to capitalize on the individual's capacity to be cued to imitate one-step, familiar, repetitive, actions that provide predictable tactile effects, and that compensate for the inability to follow multistep directions or to initiate actions required to achieve a goal (i.e., to conceptu-

alize a predictable result). The individual should be provided with opportunities to participate in adapted activities that reinforce the relationship between one's actions and predictable tactile effects on the environment. Some possibilities include sports activities (such as swimming, biking, and playing "catch"); household maintenance activities (such as washing the car, mowing lawns, cultivating gardens, hand washing laundry); kitchen activities (such as washing and drying the dishes, peeling and chopping vegetables, and cleaning countertops); instrumental ADL activities demonstrated one step at a time, and the adapted craft and game activities mentioned above. As in the previous level, functional performance can be maximized by teaching the caregivers how to present activities to the individual in a manner that will best promote productive motor actions. To this end, caregivers must initiate, sustain, and guide the individual through the steps of a functional activity to its completion.

Spontaneous motor actions include such unproductive behaviors as clicking dials on and off, using keys indiscriminately in locks, and pouring soup in the coffee maker. The individual will be drawn to anything that can be touched and manipulated. Hence, potentially dangerous appliances like toasters, blenders, and coffee makers should be hidden from view; if possible, stove knobs should be removed, or push buttons on the stove covered, and lawn and garden tools and chemicals should be hidden. It is no less critical at this level for the caregiver to provide the individual with opportunities for more productive "face saving" and acceptable uses of familiar tactile movement patterns to enable a sense of competence, dignity, and role investment within his or her social environment. To reiterate, however, the goal of an activity is *not* related to a specific outcome or end product but rather to the relationship between actions and their predictable effects. Consequently therapists and caregivers need to appreciate the need for the individual to do the same thing over and over again, even though by traditional standards this behavior might appear to be perseverative or apraxic. Opportunities to engage in activities that appear by conventional standards (i.e., assuming intact declarative memory) to have no specific outcome, such as vacuuming the same spot over and over again and polishing the same spot on the car door, should be encouraged. Such activities are comprehensible to the individual and need also to be deemed acceptable.

It is important to keep the environment as routine and predictable as possible. Since these individuals can respond to the environment in terms of procedural memories only, adjusting to novelty is difficult. Changes in the environment must be accompanied by reassurance and increased emotional support. Relocation is particularly detrimental and is likely to result in a precipitous decline in function.

Make available a sanctioned, easy means of escape from jarring stimuli. Individuals can no longer separate out unnecessary internal or external stimuli. The plethora of impinging stimulation can easily overwhelm the individual who is already struggling to make sense out of an incomprehensible world. Decreasing unnecessary sources of stimulation can help the individual cope more effectively (eliminating unnecessary activities around individuals and turning off TV or radio when not being actively attuned to). Sensory overload is related to the frequency, intensity, and quantity of unpredictable stimuli, and causes increased agitation and often "catastrophic reactions" (the overreactions or excessive upsets precipitated by situations that overwhelm the limited thinking capacity of the brain). Comprehensible routine stimulation is an important factor in avoiding catastrophic reactions.

Caregivers find that individuals are able to brush teeth, wash hands and face, and use familiar table utensils independently, although they need to be reminded to do these activities. In the absence of a concomitant physical disability, they are also able to manage dressing. However, if the caregiver does not select clothing and hand items to the individual one at a time, errors are frequent. For example, underwear may be placed over trousers, clothes may be donned inside out or backwards, and nightclothes may be selected for daytime wear. Most self-maintenance activities must be broken down into one-step motor actions, and supplies for activities such as tooth brushing, shaving, bathing, and hair washing should be presented one at a time. Twenty-four-hour supervision is necessary to ensure safety.

This level parallels stage 6 (the "middle dementia" stage) of the Global Deterioration Scale (Reisberg et al., 1982). The duration of this stage is estimated to be 2½ years.

Cognitive Level 2: Postural Actions (Medicare assistance code: Maximum cognitive assistance)

At this level, *attention* has shifted from external cues to reliance on internal cues. It is now limited to proprioceptive cues from muscles and joints that are elicited by one's own highly familiar body movements. The *goal* in performing a motor action is to repeat the one-step motor action component of the activity for the pleasure of its effect on the body alone (i.e., on one's sense of position and balance, or on sensory input to muscles and joints). *Motor actions* are limited to the ability to imitate, albeit inexactly, a one-step direction only if it involves the use of a highly familiar near-reflexive gross motor pattern. The individual is severely apraxic, agnosiac, and no longer attends to objects (other than eating utensils) in the task environment. Memory is severely impaired such that the individual no longer remembers how to eat, dress, use the toilet, or perhaps even to speak.

Activities that can be successfully accomplished at this level are those that are adapted to capitalize on the capacity to imitate one-step familiar repetitive gross motor actions, and that compensate for the inability to comprehend a purpose beyond the sensation of movement. Therapists and caregivers will find that providing opportunities to imitate simple movement, calisthenics, and modified sports activities are most often useful, but one-step activities (such as folding laundry, chopping vegetables, and polishing furniture) can be imitated if these activities were near habitual prior to the onset of the disease. Similarly, most IADL can be accomplished provided the individual is provided with a model to follow. For instance, to enable the individual to wash his arms, the caregiver should take a washcloth and demonstrate washing his own arms (the washcloth can be dry). Spontaneous behaviors are largely unproductive or bizarre (e.g., sitting backward on the toilet and "driving" it like a car—flushing to "shift gears," constantly disrobing and redressing, reapplying the same lipstick over and over again). It appears as though individuals are searching for opportunities to apply very familiar gross motor patterns (i.e., "procedural memories") to the environment regardless of the context. Hence it is critical that therapists and caregivers provide individuals with opportunities to imitate actions that are appropriate to the environmental context to encourage functional performance and to enable the retention of dignity within the task environment.

It is nonetheless important to remember that dementing diseases affect the cognitive structures most directly yet leave the emotions largely intact. Caregivers should not expect individuals to participate in complex conversations but should not exclude them from family communications either, for they will understand the emotional overtones. When addressing the individual, use simple sentences as well as simple questions, one at a time, repeated, as necessary. One needs to try to communicate with the individual on an emotional level and to be especially sensitive to the emotional tones that words and actions are communicating. When verbal abilities further deteriorate, individuals often substitute familiar and somewhat related words for names of objects or people they can no longer remember. For instance, the word "mom" may substitute for the name of a close female friend, daughter, or sister. Later, when they are no longer able to respond with words, nonverbal communication and gestures such as familiar body movements become the essential modes of communication.

Feil (1993) has recently developed validation therapy, a viable approach to communicating with individuals struggling with the confusion and rampant emotion characteristic of this stage of the disease. Validation therapy is an approach that seeks to connect to the individual's basic needs by sensitively mirroring his or her behavior or words. The caregiver rephrases words with empathy, and matches the nonverbal gestures in order to establish a connection when words are no longer a viable communication option. Case reports indicate a high degree of success in helping individuals reduce agitation and the need for medication. The central concept of this approach is that building trust and connection is far more important than communicating to "make sense."

Therapists and caregivers find that with demonstration, individuals at this level may cooperate by moving body parts to assist in activities such as grooming, dressing, and feeding but that maximal assistance and direct supervision are still essential. Requests related to actions (i.e., raise your arm, sit, stand) may be followed but may require repetition and demonstration of the movement. Awareness is largely limited to movement within the environment as well as items that directly contact the individual's body (i.e., washcloths, clothing, hand lotion). Resisting touch is not uncommon. With supervision individuals may be able to eat unassisted with foods that can be eaten with fingers, and this should be encouraged for those who no longer recognize or use eating utensils. Others may be able to use spoons and nonslip scoop-edged plates or bowls, although other utensils are used incorrectly. Note that is helpful to serve all food in bowls at this level, which are easier to manage with one-step motor actions. It is also important to recognize that individuals are not able to determine what is edible and what is not. Hence, anything that could be mistaken for food should be removed, such as decorative artificial fruit and poisonous house plants. Aimless pacing is common, but the individual will walk in directions guided by companions. However, the environment should be structured to provide a safe space for wandering, with two- to three-step push-button or combination locks on the doors and an unobstructed walkway within the living environment. To prevent voiding in unacceptable locations (and/or to manage incontinence), individuals should be escorted to the bathroom every 2 hours while they are awake and provided with physical assistance and tactile cues; in addition, wastebaskets or any other receptacles that could be mistaken for a toilet should be removed. Individuals at this level are easily confused when essential objects are hidden by doors, drawers, or closets. Whenever possible it is helpful to leave bathroom and bedroom doors open and to place frequently used objects or treasured possessions on furniture surfaces or hangers where they can be seen easily. Twenty-four-hour supervision is required.

This level parallels stages 6 to 7 (the "middle/late dementia" stage) of the Global Deterioration Scale (Reisberg et al., 1982). Depending upon factors such as health status and age at the onset of the disease, the duration of this stage can extend to 6 years.

Cognitive Level 1: Automatic Actions (Medicare assistance code: Total cognitive assistance)

At the first cognitive level, *attention* is limited to subliminal internal cues, such as hunger, taste, and smell. Individuals, while conscious, appear to stare and are largely unresponsive to external stimuli. There is no *goal*, reason, or memory for performing motor actions, hence few motor actions are being performed. *Motor actions* are limited to the potential to follow near-reflexive one-word directives, such as "sip" or "turn." With little (if any) purpose and few (if any) motor actions available, the individual has few cognitive capabilities to capitalize on. It is unrealistic to attempt to modify activities, although the environment can be modified to elicit orienting responses.

Therapists and caregivers find that an orienting response can be elicited by familiar gustatory and olfactory stimuli (e.g., favorite foods and spices fragrant plants, hand lotion, after-shave), gentle touch, massage, or a family pet. They will find that the individual either actively resists or is at best uncooperative in efforts to provide required maximal assistance in grooming, bathing, and feeding. The individual may need to be fed or allowed to eat with the fingers. Walking and transfers from bed to wheelchair may be achieved with physical guidance, provided muscle control has not yet become severely impaired. Assisted ambulation and, later, regular turning and passive, active, and assistive ranges of motion are necessary in order to forestall the secondary complications of the disease (i.e., pressure sores, contractures, osteoporosis, and infection).

This level parallels stage 7 (the "late dementia" stage) of the Global Deterioration Scale (Reisberg et al., 1982). Although it marks the terminal phase of the disease, medical comorbidities and secondary complications of dementia (i.e., aspiration pneumonia, malnutrition, sepsis from pressure ulcers, urinary tract infections, trauma) frequently cause death prior to this stage.

In summary, rehabilitation for the cognitively impaired older adult requires familiarity with information processing dimensions of functional activity conceptualized in Allen's Cognitive Disabilities Model. Environmental elements associated with information processing dimensions are identified for each of the cognitive levels, including:

1. The sensory cues that should be provided by the therapist or caregiver
2. What is comprehended and/or interpreted (i.e., learning and memory capability) based on those cues
3. The type and complexity of cues, assistance, and directions to be given to elicit productive motor actions.

To maximize functional performance throughout the deteriorating the course of the disease, therapists provide caregivers with guidance on how to capitalize on cognitive capabilities of the individual and compensate for specific cognitive limitations by modifying both the demands and the structure of IADL-ADL and desired life activities.

Evaluation and Assessment

Therapists use a variety of methods to assess cognitive-functional capacities and limitations, defined in this model in terms of the three dimensions of cognition processed in the course of pursuing functional activities:

1. Attention to sensory cues
2. Goal-directed learning and memory behavior
3. Capacity for self-initiated and/or imitated productive motor actions.

The most frequently used assessment method is informal and involves "guided observation" of the individual engaged in any desired task, using the concepts and profiles described above to determine level of cognitive function. More comprehensive profiles of the quality of functional tasks associated with each cognitive level are also available (Allen, 1985; Allen, Earhart, & Blue, 1992; Levy, 1992).

Formal assessments include the Allen Cognitive Level Test (ACL) (Allen, 1985; Allen, Earhart, &

Blue, 1992) which is a standardized leather lacing task used as a screening tool. Scoring is based on the complexity of the lacing stitch that the elder is able to imitate, and a numerical score is assigned which represents the elder's cognitive level. An "enlarged" ACL (Allen, Earhart, & Blue, 1992; Kehrberg et al., 1992; Kehrberg, 1993) is available that compensates for the visual and fine motor demands of this task. Heying (1985) demonstrated a significant correlation between the ACL score of patients with dementia and the caregiver's ratings of ADL performance.

Perhaps the most useful tool to assess levels of cognitive capacities and limitations in the elderly is the Routine Task Inventory (RTI I–Allen, 1985; RTI II–Allen, Earhart, & Blue, 1992). The RTI was designed as a practical observational measure of performance within Allen's framework for describing cognitive disabilities, and serves to identify qualitative differences in functional performance. It also provides therapists and caregivers with a comprehensive listing of behaviors indicative of function and dysfunction to be observed in the performance of physical (ADL) and instrumental daily living tasks (IADL) that are specific to each of the cognitive levels.

This assessment methodology has been developed further in the Cognitive Performance Test (CPT), a new instrument for assessing cognitive functional capacities and limitations in patients with dementia (Allen, Earhart, & Blue, 1992; Burns et al., 1994; Thralow & Rueter, 1993). The CPT comprises six tasks, including to dress, shop, make toast, phone, wash, and travel. Because the CPT is administered directly to the patient, reporter bias is not an issue, as is frequent in functional status instruments that rely on self-report or caregiver information (Weinberger et al., 1992; Zimmerman & Magaziner, 1994; Magaziner et al., 1988). It has demonstrated high interrater and test–retest reliabilities for both normal and demented older adults. Concurrent validity was established by correlating the CPT score to scores on the MMSE, the Lawton and Brody (1969) IADL-ADL scales, and, consistent with Allen's theoretical approach, the deficits observed in the CPT predicted functional capabilities on a wide variety of daily life activities. Scores on the CPT also strongly predicted rate of institutionalization over a

four-year follow-up period. The manual for the CPT can be obtained by contacting T. Burns, Geriatric Research, Education, and Clinical Center, Minneapolis Veterans Administration Medical Center, Minneapolis, Minnesota 55455.

The CPT holds enormous promise for future research in this rapidly evolving area of rehabilitation. It provides a single standardized performance-based index to measure functional status at a single point in time and to stage levels of functional impairment across the deteriorating course of the disease and thereby may address a well-recognized need within the health care system. In contrast to the Direct Assessment of Functional Status (DAFS) (Loewenstein et al., 1989; Loewenstein & Rupert, 1995), this measure is provided in the context of a theoretically sound and viable framework to educate caregivers about the effects of the disease on functional abilities of the older adults, about what to expect from the trajectory of disability exacted by the disease, about cognitive assets and deficits that exist, and about viable strategies to optimize functional capabilities that remain throughout the deteriorating course of the disease. In addition, the CPT provides means to evaluate the effects of rehabilitative intervention on caregiver burden/depression and to predict long-term risks of institutional placement and/or disease progression. It may prove of enormous assistance in legal determinations of functional competence for competency or guardianship proceedings. Finally, the CPT may provide a much needed outcome measure for short-term and longer-term pharmacological trials.

Assessment of Rehabilitation Potential

Clinicians have long acknowledged that deciding which older adults would benefit from rehabilitation services is often difficult, especially when cognitive status is impaired (Becker & Kaufman, 1988). To further complicate the issue, it should by now be recognized that rehabilitation goals for the cognitively impaired require modification from those expected of more intact older adults. With the cognitively impaired, goals are more circumscribed and limited; the primary focus is to optimize self-care skills and to minimize caregiver burden with caregiver education. Therapists using the Cognitive Disabilities Model find that rehabilitation success in such goals is possible if the older adult possesses only the most rudimentary of cognitive capacities: attention, procedural memory, and the capacity to imitate or follow nonverbal directions.

The problem is that currently the most frequently used instruments to assess rehabilitation potential are neuropsychological instruments such as the Mini-Mental State Exam (MMSE) (Folstein et al., 1975), the Blessed Orientation-Memory-Concentration Test (BMOC) (Katzman et al., 1983), the Blessed Information-Memory-Concentration (BIMC) test (Katzman et al., 1983), and the Short Portable Mental Status Questionnaire (SPMSQ) (Pfeiffer, 1975). Yet these are screening and tracking instruments that assess higher-order cognitive components (i.e., language, visuoperception, and declarative memory processing) that are predictive of advanced IADL alone (i.e., managing money and taking medications appropriately) (Fitzgerald et al., 1993; Barberger-Gateau et al., 1992). (See chapter 10 for specific cognitive components assessed by these instruments.) As such, they fail to elicit lower-order cognitive functions relevant for rehabilitation of the more basic (ADL) functional deficits of the cognitively impaired. And yet, as a consequence, cognitively impaired older adults are too often eliminated by other screening professionals from consideration for rehabilitation (Rentz, 1991). Occupational therapists need now to press for revision in traditional mental status instruments used by physicians and neuropsychologists to assess rehabilitation potential in the cognitively impaired.

Conclusion

At present, the progressive course of decline caused by dementia is inevitable. However, Allen's Cognitive Disabilities Model presents a sound rehabilitative framework that helps the cognitively impaired older adult attain his or her highest level of function and maintain active participation in as many preferred activities as possible throughout the trajectory of the disease. Using principles derived from Allen's model, therapists assess functional

deficits and teach caregivers how to modify the information processing demands of functional activities to enable the older adult with cognitive impairments to still meet activity demands, despite the significant deficits that exist. By teaching home and institutional caregivers how to modify daily life activities, occupational therapists help to optimize the afflicted individual's remaining capacities and help both individuals and their caregivers to retain a sense of competence, comprehension, and control throughout the deteriorating course of the disease. This emerging concept of rehabilitation holds high promise for interventions to improve functioning and the quality of life for our aging population.

References

Advisory Panel on Alzheimer's Disease. (1993). *Fourth report of the Advisory Panel on Alzheimer's Disease.* Washington, DC: U.S. Government Printing Office, NIH Pub. No. 93-3520, February 1993.

Agency for Health Care Policy and Research (AHCPR) (November 1996). *Recognition and initial assessment of Alzheimer's disease and related dementias: Clinical practice guideline No. 19.* Rockville, MD: U.S. Department of Health and Human Services, Public Health Service, Agency for Health Care Policy and Research. AHCPR Pub. No. 97-0702.

Allen, C. K. (1982). Independence through activity: The practice of occupational therapy. *American Journal of Occupational Therapy, 36,* 731–739.

Allen, C. K. (1985). *Occupational therapy for psychiatric diseases: Measurement and management of cognitive disabilities.* Boston: Little, Brown.

Allen, C. K. (1987). Activity: Occupational therapy's treatment method. *American Journal of Occupational Therapy, 41,* 563–575.

Allen, C. K. (1992). Cognitive disabilities. In N. Katz (Ed.), *Cognitive rehabilitation: Models for intervention in occupational therapy.* Stoneham, MA: Butterworth-Heinemann.

Allen, C. K., Earhart, C. A., & Blue, T. (1992). *Occupational therapy treatment goals for the physically and cognitively disabled.* Bethesda, MD: American Occupational Therapy Association.

Allen, C. K, Foto, M., Moon-Sperling, T., & Wilson, D. (1989). A medical review approach to Medicare outpatient documentation. *American Journal of Occupational Therapy, 43,* 793–800.

Allen, C. K. And Robertson, S. (1993). *Study guide for Occupational therapy treatment goals for the physically and cognitively disabled.* Bethesda, MD: American Occupational Therapy Association.

American Psychiatric Association (APA). (1994). *Diagnostic and Statistical Manual of Mental Disorders* 4th ed. (DSM-IV). Washington, DC: American Psychiatric Association.

Atkinson, R. C., & Shiffrin, R. M. (1968). Human memory: A proposed system and its control processes. In K. Spence & J. Spence (Eds.), *The psychology of learning and motivation*, vol. 2. New York: Academic Press.

Backman, L., Josephsson, S., Herlitz, A., Stigsdotter, A., & Vitanen, M. (1991). The generalizability of training gains in dementia: Effects of imagery-based mnemonic on face-name retention duration. *Psychology and Aging, 6*, 489–492.

Barberger-Gateau, P. Commenges, D., Gagnon, M., Letenneur, L., Sauvel, C., & Dartigues, J. (1992). Instrumental activities of daily living as a screening tool for cognitive impairment and dementia in elderly community dwellers. *Journal of the American Geriatrics Society, 40*, 1129–1134.

Baum, C. M. (1991). Addressing the needs of the cognitively impaired elderly from a family policy perspective. *American Journal of Occupational Therapy, 45*, 594–606.

Baum, C., & Edwards, D. (1993). Cognitive performance in senile dementia of the Alzheimer's type: The kitchen task assessment. *American Journal of Occupational Therapy, 47*, 431–536.

Baum, C. M., Edwards, D., & Morrow-Howell, N. (1993). Identification and management of productive behaviors in senile dementia of the Alzheimer's type. *Gerontologist, 33*, 403–408.

Beals, R. (1972). Survival following hip fracture. *Journal of Chronic Diseases, 25*, 235–244.

Becker, G., & Kaufman, S. (1988). Age, rehabilitation, and research: Review of the issues. *Gerontologist, 28*, 459–468.

Berg, L. (1988). Clinical dementia rating. *Psychopharmacology Bulletin, 24*, 637–639.

Best, J. B. (1989). *Cognitive psychology*. St. Paul, MN: West.

Bondi, M., & Kaszniak, A. (1991). Implicit and explicit memory in Alzheimer's disease and Parkinson's disease. *Journal of Clinical and Experimental Neuropsychology, 13*, 339–358.

Botwinick, J., Storandt, M., & Berg, L. (1986). A longitudinal, behavioral study of senile dementia of the Alzheimer's type. *Archives of Neurology, 43*, 1124–1127.

Breteler M. M. B., Claus J. J., Van Duijn C. M., Launer L. J., & Hofman A. (1992). Epidemiology of Alzheimer's disease. *Epidemiology Review, 14*, 59–82.

Bucher, D. M. & Larson, E. B. (1987). Falls and fractures in patients with Alzheimer's type dementia. *Journal of the American Medical Association, 257*, 1492–1495.

Burgener, S., Jirovec, M., Murrell, L., Barton, D. (1992). Caregiver and environmental variables related to difficult behaviors in institutionalized, demented elderly persons. *Journal of Gerontology, 47*, 242–249.

Burns, A.(1991). Affective symptoms in Alzheimer's disease. *International Journal of Geriatric Psychiatry, 6*, 371–376.

Burns, T., Mortimer, J., & Merchek, P.(1994). Cognitive performance test: A new approach to functional assessment in Alzheimer's disease. *Journal of Geriatric Psychiatry and Neurology, 7*, 46–54.

Camp. C., & McKitrick, L. (1992). Memory interventions in Alzheimer's-type dementia populations: Methodological and theoretical issues. In R. West & J. Sinnot (Eds.), *Everyday memory and aging: Current research and methodology.* New York: Springer.

Carswell, A., Dulberg, C., Carson, K., & Zgola, J. (1995). The functional performance measure for persons with Alzheimer's disease: Reliability and validity. *Canadian Journal of Occupational Therapy, 62*, 62–69.

Cerella, J. (1990). Aging and information-processing rate. In J. E. Birren & K. W. Schaie (Eds.), *Handbook of the psychology of aging* (3rd ed.). New York: Academic Press.

Chiu, H. C. & Smith, B. A. (1990). Rehabilitation of persons with dementia. In B. Kemp, K. Brummel-Smith, & J. Ramsdell (Eds.), *Geriatric rehabilitation*. Boston: Little, Brown.

Cohen-Mansfield, J., & Billig, N. (1986). Agitated behaviors in the elderly I: A conceptual review. *Journal of the American Geriatrics Society, 34* (10), 711–721.

Cohen-Mansfield, J., Marx, M. S., & Rosenthal, A. S. (1990). Dementia and agitation in nursing home residents: How are they related? *Psychology and Aging, 5*, 3–8.

Cohen-Mansfield, J., Werner, P., Marx, M., & Lipson, S. (1993). In L. A. Rubinstein & D. Wieland (Eds.), *Improving care in the nursing home: Comprehensive reviews of clinical research*. Newbury Park, CA: Sage.

Cotrell, V., & Schultz, R. (1993). The perspective of the patient with Alzheimer's disease: A neglected dimension of dementia research. *Gerontologist, 33*, 205–211.

Cummings, J. L.(1987). Neuropsychiatric aspects of multi-infarct dementia and dementia of the Alzheimer type. *Archives of Neurology, 44*, 389–394.

Dawson, O., Hendershot, G., & Fulton, J. (1987). National Center for Health Statistics: Functional limitations of individuals age 65 and over. *Advance data, vital and health statistics, 133*. Hyattsville, MD: US Public Health Service.

Deimling, G. T. & Bass, D. M. (1986). Symptoms of mental impairment among elderly adults and their effects on family caregivers. *Journal of Gerontology, 41*, 778–784.

Deutch, L. H. & Rovner, B. W. (1991). Agitation and other noncognitive abnormalities in Alzheimer's disease. *Psychiatric Clinics of North America, 14*, 341–351.

Dick, M. B. (1992). Motor and procedural memory in Alzheimer's disease. In L. Backman (Ed.), *Memory functioning in dementia*. Amsterdam: North Holland.

Dick, M. B., Kean, M. L., & Sands, D. (1988) The preselection effect on recall facilitation of motor movements in Alzheimer-type dementia. *Journal of Gerontology, 43*, 127–135.

Dick, M., Shankle, R., Bet, R., Dick-Muehlke, C., Cotman, C, & Kean, M. (1996). Acquisition and long-term retention of a gross motor skill in Alzheimer's disease patients under constant and varied practice conditions. *Journal of Gerontology, 51B,* 103–111.

Duchek, J. M., Cheney, M., Ferraro F. R., & Storandt, M. (1991). Paired associate learning in senile dementia of the Alzheimer type. *Archives of Neurology, 48,* 1038–1040.

Edwards, D., & Baum, C. (1990). Caregiver burden across stages of dementia. *Occupational Therapy Practice, 2,* 17–31.

Edwards, D. F., Deuel, R. K., & Baum, M. C. (1991). Constructional apraxia in senile dementia: Contributions to functional loss. *Physical and Occupational Therapy in Geriatrics, 9,* 53–59.

Eisdorfer, C., Cohen, D., Paveza, G., Ashford, J., Luchins, D., Gorelick, P., Hirschman, R., Freels, S., et al. (1992). An empirical evaluation of the global deterioration scale for staging Alzheimer's disease. *American Journal of Psychiatry, 149,* 190–194.

Eisdorfer, C., Sevush, S., Barry, P., Kumar, V., & Loewenstein, D. (1994). Neuropsychological assessment in Alzheimer's disease. In C. Eisdorfer & E. Olson (Eds.), *Medical clinics of North America: Management of patients with Alzheimer's and related dementia.* Philadelphia: Saunders.

Eslinger, P. J., & Damasio, A. R. (1986). Preserved motor learning in Alzheimer's disease: Implications for anatomy and behavior. *Journal of Neuroscience, 6,* 3006–3009.

Evans, D. A., Funkenstein H. H., Albert M. S., Scherr P. A., & Cook, N. R. (1989). Prevalence of Alzheimer's disease in a community population of older persons. *Journal of the American Medical Association, 262,* 2551–2556.

Evans, D. A., Scherr, P. A., Cook, N. R., Albert, M. S., Funkenstein, H. H., Smith, L. A., Hebert, L .E., Wetle, T. T., Branch, L. G., Chown, M., et al.(1990). Estimated prevalence of Alzheimer's disease in the United States. *Millbank Quarterly, 68,* 267–289.

Faber-Langendoen, K., Morris, J. C., Knesevich, J. W., La-Barge, E., Miller J. P., & Berg, L.(1988). Aphasia in senile dementia of the Alzheimer type. *Annals of Neurology, 23,* 465–370.

Feil, N. (1993). *The validation breakthrough.* Baltimore: Health Professions Press.

Fillenbaum, G. G. (1985). Screening the elderly: A brief instrumental activities of daily living measure. *Journal of the American Geriatrics Society, 33,* 698–706.

Fitzgerald, J., Smith, D., Martin, D., Freedman, J., & Wolinsky, F. (1993). Replications of the multidimensionality of activities of daily living. *Journal of Gerontology, 48,* 28–31.

Folstein, M. F., Folstein, S. E., & McHugh, P. R. (1975). Minimental state: A practical method for grading the cognitive state of patients for the clinician. *Journal of Psychiatric Research, 12,* 189–198.

Foster N. L., Chase, T., Patronas, N., Gillespie, M., & Fedio, P. (1986). Cerebral mapping of apraxia in Alzheimer's disease by position emission tomography. *Annals of Neurology, 19,* 139–143.

Friedman, J. (1995). Neurologic diseases in the elderly. In W. Reichel, W. (Ed.), *Care of the elderly: Clinical aspects of aging.* Baltimore: Williams & Wilkins.

Gallagher, D., Lovett, S., & Zeiss, A. (1987). *Interventions with caregivers of frail elderly persons.* Palo Alto, CA: Caregiver Research Program.

Geschwind, N., & Damasio, A. (1985). Apraxia. In J. Frederick (Ed.), *Handbook of clinical neurology,* vol. 45. New York: Wiley.

Goldman, L., & Lazarus, L. (1988). Assessment and management of dementia in the nursing home. *Clinics in Geriatric Medicine, 4,* 589–600.

Gottlieb, G. (1990). Rehabilitation and dementia of the Alzheimer's type. In S. Brody & L. G. Paulson (Eds.), *Aging and rehabilitation II: The state of the practice.* New York: Springer.

Grafman, J., Weingartner, H., Newhouse, P., Thompson, K., Lalonde, F., Litvan, I., Molchan, S., & Sunderland, T. (1990). Implicit learning in patients with Alzheimer's disease. *Pharmacopsychiatry, 23,* 94–101.

Green, C. R., Mohs, R. C., Schmeidler, J., Aryan, M., & Davis, K. L. (1993). Functional decline in Alzheimer's disease: A longitudinal study. *Journal of the American Geriatrics Society, 41,* 654–661.

Health Care Financing Administration (HCFA). (1989). Outpatient occupational therapy Medicare part B guidelines (DHHS Transmittal No. 55). In *Health Insurance Manual.* Baltimore: HCFA.

Heindel, W., Butters, N., & Salmon, D. (1988). Impaired learning of a motor skill in patients with Huntington's disease. *Behavioral Neuroscience, 102,* 141–147.

Heindel, W., Salmon, D., Shults, C., Walicke, P., & Butters, N. (1989). Neuropsychological evidence for multiple implicit memory systems: A comparison of Alzheimer's, Huntington's, and Parkinson's disease patients. *Journal of Neuroscience, 9,* 582–587.

Henderson, V. (1994). Estrogen replacement therapy in older women: Comparisons between Alzheimer's disease cases and nondementia control subjects. *Archives of Neurology, 51,* 896–900.

Herlitz, A., & Backman, L. (1990). Recall of object names and colors of objects in normal aging and Alzheimer's disease. *Archives of Gerontology and Geriatrics, 11,* 147–154.

Heying, L. M. (1985). Research with subjects having senile dementia. In C. K. Allen (Ed.), *Occupational therapy for psychiatric diseases: Measurement and management of cognitive disabilities.* Boston: Little, Brown.

Hof, P. R., Bouras, C., Constantinidis, J., & Morrison, J. H. (1990). Selective disconnection of specific visual association pathways in cases of Alzheimer's disease presenting with Balint's syndrome. *Journal Neuropathology and Experimental Neurology, 49,* 168–184.

Hopkins, H., & Smith, H. (1993). *Willard and Spackman's Occupational Therapy* (8th ed.). Philadelphia: Lippincott.

Hughes, C., Berg, L., Danzinger, W., Coben, L., & Martin, R. (1982). A new clinical scale for the staging of dementia. *British Journal of Psychiatry, 140,* 566–572.

Jorm, A. F. (1990). *The epidemiology of Alzheimer's disease and related disorders. London:* Chapman & Hall.

Josephsson, S., Backman, L., Borell, L., Brenspang, B., Nygard, L., & Ronnberg, L. (1993). Supporting everyday activities in dementia: An intervention study. *International Journal of Geriatric Psychiatry, 8,* 395–400.

Kahn, R. (1975). The mental health system and the future aged. The *Gerontologist, 15* (1, pt. 2), 24–31.

Kamholz, B. & Gottlieb, G. (1992). The nature and efficacy of interventions for depression and dementia. In B. S. Fogel, A. Furino & G. Gottlieb (Eds.), *Access and financing of neuropsychiatric care for the elderly American.* Washington, DC: American Psychiatric Association. Press.

Katz, S., Ford, A., Moskowitz, R., Jackson, B., Jaffe, M., & Cleveland, M. (1963). The index of ADL: A standardized measure of biological and psychosocial function. *Journal of the American Medical Association, 185,* 914–191.

Katzman, R., Brown, T., Fuld, P., Peck, A., Schecter, R., & Schimmel, H. (1983). Validation of a short orientation-memory-concentration test of cognitive impairment. *American Journal of Psychiatry, 140,* 734–739.

Katzman, R., & Kawas, C. (1994). The epidemiology of dementia and Alzheimer's disease. In R. D. Terry, R. Katzman, & K. L. Blick (Eds.), *Alzheimer Disease.* New York: Raven Press.

Kausler, D., & Lichty, W. (1988). Memory for activities: Rehearsal-independence and aging. In M. L. Howe & C. J. Brainerd (Eds.), *Cognitive development in adulthood: Progress in cognitive developmental research.* New York: Springer.

Keane, M., Gabrieli, J., Growdon, J., & Corkin, S. (1994). Priming in perceptual identification of pseudowords is normal in Alzheimer's disease. *Neuropsychologia, 32,* 343–356.

Kehrberg, K. (1993). *The larger Allen Cognitive Level Test. Test kit and instructions.* Colchester, CT: S & S.

Kehrberg, K., Kuskowski, M., Mortimer, J., & Shoberg, T. (1992). Validating the use of an enlarged easier to see Allen Cognitive Level Tin geriatrics. *Physical and Occupational Therapy in Geriatrics, 10* (3), 1–14.

Kemp, B. (1988). Eight methods family members can use to manage behavioral problems in dementia. *Topics in Geriatric Rehabilitation, 4,* 50–59.

Kiecolt-Glaser, J., Glaser. R, Shuttleworth, E., Dyer, C., Ogrocki, P., & Speicher, C. (1987). Chronic stress and immunity in family caregivers of Alzheimer's disease victims. *Psychosomatic Medicine, 49,* 523–535.

Klingbeil, G. (1982) The assessment of rehabilitation potential in the elderly. *Wisconsin Medical Journal, 81,* 25–27.

Knopman, D. (1991). Long term retention of implicitly acquired learning in patient's with Alzheimer's disease. *Journal of Clinical and Experimental Psychology, 13,* 880–894.

Knopman, D. S., & Nissen, M. J. (1987) . Implicit learning in patients with probable Alzheimer's disease. *Neurology, 37,* 784–788.

Kotila, M., Waltimo, M., & Niemi, M. (1984). The profile of recovery from stroke and factors influencing outcome. *Stroke, 15,* 1039–1044.

LaBarge, E., Smith D. S., Dick, L., & Storandt, M. (1992). Agraphia in dementia of the Alzheimer type. *Archives of Neurology, 49,* 1151–1156.

Langer, E., & Rodin, J. (1976). The effects of choice and enhanced personal responsibility for the aged: A field experiment in an institutional setting. *Journal of Personality and Social Psychology, 34,* 191–198.

Larson, E. B., Reifler. B. V., Featherstone, H. J. & English, D. J. (1984). Dementia in elderly outpatients: A prospective study. *Annals of Internal Medicine, 100,* 417–423.

Lawton, M. P. & Brody, E. M. (1969). Assessment of older people: Self-maintaining and instrumental activities of daily living. *Gerontologist, 9,* 179–186.

Lawton, M., Moss, M., Fulcomer, M., & Kleban, M. (1982). The research and service-oriented multi-level assessment instrument. *Journal of Gerontology, 37,* 91–99.

Lazarus, L. W., Newton, N., Cohler, B., Lesser, J., & Schweon, C. (1987). Frequency and presentation of depressive symptoms in patients with primary degenerative dementia. *American Journal of Psychiatry, 144,* 41–45.

Leibovici, A., & Tariot, P. (1988). Agitation associated with dementia: A systematic approach to treatment. *Psychopharmacology Bulletin, 24,* 49–53.

Leon, J., & Lair, T. (1990). *Functional status of the noninstitutionalized elderly: Estimates of ADL and IADL difficulties.* DHHS Pub. No. (PHS) 90–3462. Rockville, MD: Public Health Service.

Levy, L. L. (1974). Movement therapy for psychiatric patients. *American Journal of Occupational Therapy, 28,* 354–357.

Levy, L. L. (1986a). A practical guide to the care of the Alzheimer's disease victim. *Topics in Geriatric Rehabilitation, 1,* 16–26.

Levy, L. L. (1986b). Cognitive treatment. In L. J. Davis and M. Kirkland (Eds.), *Role of occupational therapy with the elderly.* Bethesda, MD: American Occupational Therapy Association.

Levy, L. L. (1989). Activity adaptation in rehabilitation of the physically and cognitively disabled aged. *Topics in Geriatric Rehabilitation, 4* (4), 53–66.

Levy, L. L. (1992). The use of the cognitive disability frame of reference in rehabilitation of cognitively disabled older adults. In N. Katz (Ed.), *Cognitive rehabilitation: Models for intervention in occupational therapy.* Stoneham, MA: Butterworth-Heinemann.

Loewenstein, D. & Rupert, M. (1995). Staging functional impairment in dementia using performance-based measures: A preliminary analysis. *Journal of Mental Health and Aging, 1,* 47–56.

Loewenstein, D., Amigo, E., Duara, R., Guterman, A., Hurwitz, D., Berkowitz, N., Wilkie, F., Weinberg, G., Black, B., Gittleman, B., & Eisdorfer, C. (1989). A new scale for the assessment of functional status in Alzheimer's disease and related disorders. *Journal of Gerontology, 4,* 114–121.

Loewenstein, D., Rupert, M., Arguelles, T., & Duara, R. (1995). Neuropsychological test performance and prediction of functional capacities among Spanish-speaking and English-speaking patients with dementia. *Archives of Clinical Neuropsychology, 10,* 7–15

Loewenstein, D., Rupert, M., Zimmer, N., Guterman, A., Morgan, R., & Hayden, S. (1992). Neuropsychological test performance and prediction of functional capacities in dementia. *Behavior, Health, and Aging, 3,* 149–158.

Mace, N. L. & Rabins, P. V. (1991). *The thirty-six hour day: A family guide to caring for persons with Alzheimer's disease, related dementing illnesses, and memory loss in later life* (rev. ed.). Baltimore: Johns Hopkins University Press.

Magaziner, J., Simonsick, E., Kashner, T., & Hebel, J. (1988). Patient-proxy response comparability on measures of patient health and functional status. *Journal of Clinical Epidemiology, 4,* 1065–1074.

Mahurin, R., DeBettignies, B., & Pirozzolo, F. (1991). Structured assessment of independent living skills: Preliminary report of a performance measure of functional abilities in dementia. *Journal of Gerontology, 46,* 58–66.

McCue, M., Rogers, J., & Goldstein, G. (1990). Relationship between neuropsychological and functional assessment in elderly neuropsychiatric patients. *Rehabilitation Psychology, 35,* 91–99.

McEntee, W., & Crook, T. (1992). Cholinergic function in the aged brain: Implications for the treatment of memory impairments associated with aging. *Behavioral Pharmacology, 3,* 327–336.

Manton, K., Corder, L., & Stallard, E. (1993). Estimates of change in chronic disability and institutional incidence and prevalence rates in the U.S. elderly population from the 1982, 1984, and 1989: National Long Term Care Survey. *Journal of Gerontology, 48,* 153–166.

Mayer, N., Keating, D., & Rapp, D. (1986). Skills, routines, and activity patterns of daily living: A functional nested approach. In B. Uzzell & Y. Gross (Eds.), *Clinical neuropsychology of intervention.* Boston: Martinus Nijoff.

Mendez, M. F., Mendez M. A.., Martin, R, Smyth, K. A., & Whitehouse P. J. (1990). Complex visual disturbances in Alzheimer's disease. *Neurology, 40,* 439–443.

Merriam, A. E., Aronson, M. K., Gaston, P., Wey, S., & Katz, I. (1988). The psychiatric symptoms of Alzheimer's disease. *Journal of the American Geriatrics Society, 36,* 7–12.

Miller, C. (1978). Survival and ambulation after hip fracture. *Journal of Bone and Joint Surgery, 60A,* 930–933.

Miller, G. A. (1956). The magical number seven, plus or minus two: Some limits on our capacity for processing information. *Psychological Review, 63,* 81–97.

Miller, R. (1981). *Meaning and purpose in the intact brain: A philosophical, psychological, and biological account of conscious processes.* New York: Clarendon Press.

Morris, J. C. (1994) Differential diagnosis of Alzheimer's disease. *Clinics in Geriatric Medicine, 10,* 257–276.

Morris, J. C., McKeel, D. W., Storandt, M., Rubin, E., Price, J., Grant, E., Ball, M., & Berg, L. (1991). Very mild Alzheimer's disease: Informant-based clinical, psychometric, and pathologic distinction from normal aging. *Neurology, 41,* 469–478.

Mosey, A. (1994). Working taxonomies. In C. B. Royeen (Ed.), *AOTA Self-Study Series: Cognitive rehabilitation.* Bethesda, MD: American Occupational Therapy Association.

National Center for Health Statistics (NCHS). (1995). *Trends in the Health of Older Americans, 1994.* Washington, DC: U.S. Government Printing Office, DHHS Pub. No. (PHS) 95–1414.

Nebes, R. D. (1989). Semantic memory in Alzheimer's disease. *Psychological Bulletin, 106,* 377–394.

Nebes, R. D. (1992). Cognitive dysfunction in Alzheimer's disease. In F. Craik & T. Salthouse (Eds.), *The handbook of aging and cognition.* Hillsdale, NJ: Erlbaum.

Nissen, M. J. (1986). Neuropsychology of attention and memory. *Journal of Head Trauma Rehabilitation, 1,* 13–21.

Novack, T., Haban, K., & Graham (1987). Prediction of stroke outcome from a psychological screening. *Archives of Physical Medicine and Rehabilitation, 68,* 729–734.

Oakley, F., Sunderland, T., Hill, J., Phillips, S., Makahon, R., & Ebner, J. (1991). The daily activities questionnaire: A functional assessment for people with Alzheimer's disease. *Physical and Occupational Therapy in Geriatrics, 10* (2), 67–81.

Paveza, G., Cohen, D., Jankowski, L., & Freels, S. (1995). An analysis of the global deterioration scale in older persons applying for community services. *Journal of Mental health and Aging, 1,* 35–43.

Pearlin, L., Mullan, J., Semple, S., & Skaff, M. (1990). Caregiving and the stress process: An overview of concepts and their measures. *Gerontologist, 30,* 583–594.

Peterson, R. C. (1994). Memory function in very early Alzheimer's disease. *Neurology, 44,* 867–872.

Pfeffer, R. (1995). A social function measure in the staging and study of dementia. In M. Bergener, J. Brocklehurst, & S. Finkel (Eds.), *Aging, health, and healing.* New York: Springer.

Pfeffer, R., Kurosaki, T., Harrah, C., Chance, J., & Filos, S. (1982). Measurement of functional activities in older adults in the community. *Journal of Gerontology, 37,* 323–329.

Pfeiffer, E. (1975). A short portable mental status questionnaire for the assessment of organic brain deficit in elderly patients. *Journal of the American Geriatrics Society, 23,* 440–441.

Public Law 89–97 (1965). *Social Security Amendments, Medicare, Title 18, Insurance for the Aged.* Washington, DC: U.S. Government Printing Office.

Public Law 100–203 (1987). *Omnibus Budget Reconciliation Act, Subtitle C, Nursing Home Reform.* Washington, DC: U.S. Government Printing Office.

Rabinovich, B., & Cohen-Mansfield, J. (1992). The impact of participation in structured recreational activities on the agitated behavior of nursing home residents: An observational study. *Activities, Adaptation, and Aging, 16,* 89–98.

Reifler, B. V., Larson, E., Teri, L. (1986). Dementia of the Alzheimer's type and depression. *Journal of the American Geriatric Society, 34,* 855–859.

Reifler, B. V., & Teri, L. (1986). Rehabilitation and Alzheimer's disease. In S. J. Brody and G.E. Ruff (Eds.), *Aging and rehabilitation: Advances in the state of the art.* New York: Springer.

Reisberg, B., Ferris, S. H., & Franssen, E. (1985). An ordinal functional assessment tool for Alzheimer's-type dementia. *Hospital and Community Psychiatry, 36,* 593–595.

Reisberg, B., Ferris, S. H., Leon, M. J., & Cook, T. (1982). The global deterioration scale for the assessment of primary degenerative dementia. *American Journal of Psychiatry, 139,* 1136–1139.

Rentz, D. (1991). The assessment of rehabilitation potential: Cognitive factors. In R. Hartke (Ed.), *Psychological aspects of geriatric rehabilitation.* Gaithersburg, MD: Aspen.

Reynolds, C. F., Perel, J. M., Kupfer, D. J., Zimmer, B., Stack, J. A., & Hoch, C. H. (1987). Open trial response to antidepressant treatment in elderly patients with mixed depression and cognitive impairment. *Psychiatry Research, 21,* 111–122.

Rogers, J. (1993), Clinical trial of indomethacin in Alzheimer's disease. *Neurology, 43,* 1609–1611.

Ross, G., Petrovitch, H., & White, L. (1997). Update on dementia. *Generations,* Winter, 22–26.

Rovner, B. W. (1994). What is therapeutic about special care units? The role of psychosocial rehabilitation. *Alzheimer's disease and Associated Disorders, 8* (1), 355–359.

Rovner, B. W., Kafonek, S., Filipp, L., Lucas, M. J., & Folstein, M. F. (1986). Prevalence of mental illness in a community nursing home. *American Journal of Psychiatry, 143,* 1446–1449.

Rovner, B. W., & Katz, I. R. (1992). Psychiatric disorders in the nursing home: A selective view of studies related to clinical care. *International Journal of Geriatric Psychiatry, 7,* 75–82.

Rubin, E., Drevets, W., & Burke, W. (1988). The nature of psychotic symptoms in senile dementia of the Alzheimer type. *Journal of Geriatric Psychiatry and Neurology, 1,* 16–19.

Rubin, E. H., & Kinscherf, D. A. (1989). Psychopathology of very mild dementia of the Alzheimer's type. *American Journal of Psychiatry, 146,* 1017–1021.

Sarno, J., Sarno, M., & Levita, E. (1973). The functional life scale. *Archives of Physical Medicine and Rehabilitation, 54,* 214–220.

Scalen, S., & Reisberg, B. (1992). Functional assessment staging (FAST) in Alzheimer's disease: Reliability, validity, ordinality. *International Psychogeriatrics, 4,* 66–69.

Schneider, L. (1995). Efficacy of clinical treatment for mental disorders among older persons. In M. Gatz (Ed.), *Emerging issues in mental health and aging.* Washington, DC: American Psychological Association.

Schuman, J., Beattie, D., & Steed, D. (1981). Geriatric patients with and without intellectual dysfunction: Effectiveness of a standard rehabilitation program. *Archives of Physical Medicine and Rehabilitation, 62,* 612–618.

Snowdon, D., Greiner, L., Mortimer, J., Riley, K., & Markesbery, W. (1997). Brain infarction and the clinical expression of Alzheimer disease: The nun study. *Journal of the American Medical Association, 277* (10), 813–817.

Squire, L. (1986). Mechanisms of memory. *Science, 23,* 1612–1619.

Squire, L. (1987). *Memory and brain.* New York: Oxford University Press.

Steffes, R., & Thralow, J. (1987). Visual field limitation in the patient with dementia of the Alzheimer's type. *Journal of the American Geriatrics Society, 35,* 189–193.

Stern, Y., Albert, S., & Sano, M. (1994). The dependence scale. *Journal of Gerontology, 49,* 216–222.

Storandt, M., Botwinick, J., Danziger, W. L., Berg, L., & Hughes, C. P. (1984). Psychometric differentiation of mild senile dementia of the Alzheimer type. *Archives of Neurology, 41,* 497–499.

Sullivan, E., Sagar, H., Gabrieli, J., Corkin, S., & Growdon, J. (1989). Different cognitive profiles on standard behavioral tests in Parkinson's disease and Alzheimer's disease. *Journal of Clinical Experimental Neuropsychology, 11,* 799–820.

Swearer, J. M., Drachman, D. A., O'Donnell, B. F., & Mitchell, A. L. (1988). Troublesome and disruptive behaviors in dementia: Relationships to diagnosis and disease severity. *Journal of the American Geriatrics Society, 34,* 784–790.

Tatemichi, T., Sacktor, N., & Mayeux, R. (1994). Dementia associated with cerebrovascular disease, other degenerative diseases, and metabolic disorders. In R. D. Terry, R. Katzman, & K. L. Blick (Eds), *Alzheimer disease.* New York: Raven Press.

Teri, L., Borson, S., Kiyak, H. S.(1989). Behavioral disturbance, cognitive dysfunction, and functional skill. *Journal of the American Geriatric Society, 37,* 109–116.

Teri. L., & Logsdon, R. (1991). Identifying pleasant activities for Alzheimer's disease patients: The pleasant events schedule—AD. *Gerontologist, 31* (1), 124–131.

Teri, L., Logsdon, R., Wagner, A., & Uomoto, J. (1994). The caregiver role in behavioral treatment of depression in dementia patients. In E. Light, G. Niederehe, & B. Lebowitz

(Eds.), *Stress effects of family caregivers of Alzheimer's patients: Research and interventions*. New York: Springer.

Teri, L., Rabins, P., Whitehouse, P., et al. (1992). Management of behavior disturbance in Alzheimer's disease: Current knowledge and future directions. *The American Journal of Alzheimer's Care and Related Disorders, 6,* 77–88.

Teri, L., & Wagner, A. (1992). Alzheimer's disease and depression. *Journal Consulting Clinical Psychology, 60,* 379–391.

Terry, R. D., Katzman, R., & Beck, K. (Eds.). (1994). *Alzheimer disease*. New York: Raven Press.

Thralow, J., & Rueter, M. (1993). Activities of daily living and cognitive levels of function in dementia. *American Journal of Alzheimer's Care and Related Disorders and Research,* Sept.–Oct., 14–19.

Tulving, E. (1972). Episodic and semantic memory. In E. Tulving & W. Donaldson (Eds.), *Organization of memory*. New York: Academic Press.

Tulving, E. (1983). *Elements of episodic memory*. New York: Oxford University Press.

Tulving, E. (1985). How many memory systems are there? *American Psychologist, 40,* 385–398.

U.S. Senate, Special Committee on Aging (1991). Aging America, trends and projections, 1991 edition. Washington DC: DHHS Pub. 91–28001.

Visser, H. (1983). Gait and balance in senile dementia of Alzheimer's type. *Age and Aging, 12,* 296–299.

Vitaliano, P. P., Breen, A. R., Albert M. S., Russo, J., & Prinz P. N. (1984). Memory, attention, and functional status in community residing Alzheimer type dementia patients and optimally healthy individuals. *Journal of Gerontology, 39,* 58–64.

Vitaliano, P. P., Rosso, J., Breen, A. R., Vitiello, M. V., & Prinz, P. N. (1986). Functional decline in the early stages of Alzheimer's disease. *Journal of Psychology and Aging, 1,* 41–46.

Webster, R., Thompson, D., Bowman, G., & Sutteon, T. (1988). Patient's and nurses' opinions about bathing. *Nursing Times, 84* (37), 54–57.

Weinberger, M., Samsa, G., Schmader, K., Greenberg, S., Carr, D., & Wildman, D. (1992). Comparing proxy and patient's perceptions of patient's functional status: Results from a geriatric outpatient clinic. *Journal of the American Geriatrics Society, 40,* 585–593.

Welsh, K., Butters, N., Hughes, J., Mohs, R., & Heyman, A. (1992). Detection of abnormal memory decline in mild cases of Alzheimer's disease using CERAD neuropsychological measures. *Archives of Neurology, 48,* 278–281.

Welsh, K., Butters, N., Hughes, J., Mohs, R., & Heyman, A. (1992). Detection and staging of dementia in Alzheimer's disease: Use of the neuropsychological measures developed for the CERAD. *Archives of Neurology, 49,* 448–452.

Wolinsky, F., & Johnson, R. (1991). The use of health services by older adults. *Journal of Gerontology, 46,* 345–357.

Wolinsky, F., Johnson, R., & Fitzgerald, J. (1992). Falling, health status, and the use of health services by older adults: A prospective study. *Medical Care, 30,* 587–597.

Yasavage, J. A, Brooks, J. O., Taylor L., & Tinkleberg, J. (1993). Development of aphasia, apraxia, and agnosia and decline in Alzheimer's disease. *American Journal of Psychiatry, 150,* 742–747.

Zanetti, O., Bianchetti, A., Frisoni, G., Rozzini, R., & Trabucchi, M. (1993). Determinants of disability in Alzheimer's disease. *International Journal of Geriatric Psychiatry, 8,* 581–586.

Zarit, S., Orr, N., & Zarit, J. (1985). *The hidden victims of Alzheimer's disease: Families under stress*. New York: New York University Press.

Zarit, S., Reever, K., & Bachman-Peterson, S. (1980). The burden interview. *Gerontologist, 20,* 649–656.

Zimmerman, S., & Magaziner, J. (1994). Methodological issues in measuring the functional status of cognitively impaired nursing home residents: The use of proxies and performance based measures. *Alzheimer's Disease and Associated Disorders, 8,* 281–290.

Generic for All Populations

CHAPTER 8

Cognitive Disabilities Model: How to Make Clinical Judgments

Claudia K. Allen, MA, OTR/L, FAOTA, and Tina Blue, OTR/L

Introduction

Clinical judgments should implement the value of occupational therapy services, and theories should make it easier to apply sound clinical judgment The development of The Cognitive Disabilities Model was done by sorting through and selecting information from occupational therapy, philosophy, the neurosciences, psychology, anthropology, medicine, and observations of clients. Selected information had to enhance the fulfillment of valuable occupational therapy services. Targeted services are those services thought to have genuine merit, with intrinsic and enduring qualities that uphold the abiding worth of the profession.

In practice, occupational therapists should know how to:

1. Deal with function as it is related to doing actions, activities, and roles
2. Consider the whole person
3. Use remaining abilities in the least restrictive environment
4. Compensate for limitations
5. Provide a just right challenge
6. Provide a sense of contentment during most treatment sessions
7. Pursue goals selected by the client and their long-term caregivers that make sense to them
8. Be realistic and practical
9. Recognize individual differences as well as cultural, ethnic, gender, and age differences
10. Provide caregiver education
11. Collaborate with the multidisciplinary team
12. Be reliable and accountable for excellence in the quality of care
13. Be sensitive to the hopes for a quality of life after a disease, illness, or injury.

These general values are noble and should be implemented in everyday practice. As a body of knowledge, the cognitive disability concepts are organized to facilitate the implementation of these services.

More specific recurrent themes are elaborated on throughout the chapter: what to do when the medical condition would improve anyway; how to treat when a stable, long-term disability is identified; and how to help the long-term care giver. The themes were selected because they are areas of current practice that are the most difficult to implement and document. The chapter has two goals: to describe a general theoretical approach and to suggest solutions, within the general approach, to current problems.

Sequence of Abilities

People with cognitive disabilities are those whose ability to think and feel has been impaired by a medical problem. The impairment in thinking and feeling is observed in behavior. Their actions, activities, and role performances are normal in some ways but not in others. Therefore, therapists can infer that their ability to think and feel is nonimpaired in some ways, and impaired in other ways. To understand and empathize with how a disabled person is thinking and feeling, a sequence of cognitive abilities is used to explain the severity of the disability.

The original scale had six cognitive levels, from coma (0) to normal (6) (Allen, 1985). Within a few years of that publication, it became apparent that a six-point scale was too short, so a decimal system was added and named the *Modes of Performance.* Each of the original cognitive levels has five modes of performance (x.0, x.2, x.4, x.6, x.8). Adding the modes of performance and counting only the even numbers provide 26 modes of performance, ranging from 0.8 to 6.0. The longer scale is sensitive to smaller changes in ability to function that have important clinical consequences. The rating criteria describe differences in what the person pays attention to, with the resulting motor behavior and speech performance. The cognitive levels and modes are referred to as the Allen Cognitive Levels (ACL). The ACL serve as a global measure of ability to function as well as a global measure of the severity of a functional disability (Allen, Earhart, & Blue, 1992, 1996).

To make the scale even longer, the odd number can be used. On the scale the preceding odd number can be used to give partial credit when a person pays attention to cues but cannot translate the information into motor or speech performance. For example, x.1 is partial credit for x.2 (Allen, Earhart, & Blue, 1992, 1996). When the odd numbers are added, the scale can be stretched to a 52-point scale. One judges the sensitivity of a scale by evaluating the length of the rating criteria. As of this writing the odd numbers are not used very often, so the rest of the chapter is restricted to the even numbers.

Pattern of Performance

The scale is used to identify qualitative differences in a pattern of performance. No single isolated behavior on a standardized test is deemed sufficient to obtain an ACL score. Several observations are necessary to say that a pattern of best ability to function has been identified. A long scale of qualitatively distinct patterns of performance is necessary to detect small, but important changes in pat-

terns of best ability to function. Best ability to function is the use of optimal mental processes to guide occupations that are as nearly normal as possible. Occupations employ a pattern of performance to do actions, activities, and roles.

Scales are incredibly important because everything that the therapists does is based on the scale. Treatment methods are based on the therapist's assessment of ability to function. Methods that are too high or too low will not work effectively. Too often the ability to function is assessed intuitively by master clinicians. The ACL seeks to articulate the intuitions of master clinicians. These clinicians have the advantage of working with people who have trouble doing ordinary activities. The complexity of ordinary human thought becomes apparent in the difficulties that cognitively disabled clients have in doing ordinary activities. Master clinicians are skilled at circumventing these difficulties and finding ways to use remaining abilities.

Abilities identify the mental processes and resulting behaviors that are still working normally. Limitations are the mental processes and resulting behaviors normally expected, given the person's age, education, and functional history, but not present. Abilities and limitations are determined by the person's place on the scale. If the person is functioning at ACL 4.4, all abilities described between ACL 0 and ACL 4.4 are assumed to be present. The limitations are those abilities described at ACL 4.6 and above to ACL 6.0. Because the same point on the scale identifies assets and limitations, the ACL can be used to measure the ability to function and the severity of a disability. The best ability to function minimizes the severity of the disability as much as possible, and predicts an expected pattern of performance in occupations.

Underlying Mental Structures

The operation of the mental structure is inferred by noting the stimulus that captures attention and the response in the form of motor and speech performance. Limitations are avoided by modifying the task to eliminate the need to use unavailable abilities or by trying a different activity. A match between the person's best ability to function and the demands of the activity provides a just-right challenge. The desired experience for the disabled person is a sense of contentment, to be happy with who they are and what they are doing. The sense of contentment occurs when the demands of the activity match the person's best ability to function. Best ability to function engages optimal mental structures.

Mental structures are universal thought processes that people use to guide their behavior. The flexibility in human actions and activities can be reduced to a minimum number of underlying mental operations, like matching by color and shape. Color and shape can be found in a lot of different objects, but the underlying mental operation of matching is the same. The work of developmental psychologists, like Jean Piaget and Noan Chomsky, is helpful in identifying underlying mental structures. The reduction of human occupations to underlying mental structures is necessary because of the enormous range of human actions, activities, and roles. To analyze the cognitive complexity of everything that people do would be an overwhelming project. The identification of underlying mental structures, like sorting objects by color, provides a parsimonious means of analyzing many occupations.

Psychological development also provides a natural sequence for improvement in ability to function. The disabled person's abilities and limitations are derived from an understanding of how mental structures emerge during psychological development. When the normal development literature failed to explain mental structures that are important to the functional abilities of the disabled person, the ACL has added abilities to the developmental framework.

The sequence of ability to function is used to organize the sequence of treatment goals and associated methods. The sequence can also be used to measure treatment effectiveness when an improvement in overall ability to function is expected. A person's place on the scale can be used to determine the level of care required and in selecting the least restrictive environment. The least restrictive environment should maximize the use of remaining abilities while protecting the disabled person from hazardous encounters with limitations.

Allen Battery

The Allen Battery provides resources for assessing and treating a cognitive disability and for educating caregivers about the level of assistance required. The battery includes (1) instruments for an initial assessment, (2) projects to monitor change while the condition is improving, (3) activities of daily living to set up a home program for people with a residual disability, (4) information for caregivers, to educate them about the need for assistance, and (5) resources to make documentation easier.

Instruments for an Initial Assessment

Initial screening tools are used to get a first impression of the person's general ability. The sensory stimulation kits and two leather lacing tests can be used for screening purposes. The Sensory Motor Stimulation kits are used with low-functioning clients: ACL 0.8 to 3.2. Between ACL 3.0 and 5.8 therapists use the leather lacing tests referred to as the Allen Cognitive Level Screen (ACLS) and the Large Allen Cognitive Level Screen (LACLS). Start with the small one and switch to the large one when visual impairments or hand tremors are affecting performance. Research on the leather lacing screens suggest that interrater reliability can be readily achieved and should be demonstrated by all clinicians (Allen, Earhart, & Blue, 1992). Interrater reliability should be a regular part of fieldwork experiences so that new therapists can report scores with credibility. Test–retest is not a problem in levels 1 through 4 because clients do not remember what they are taught. In level 5 clients report that they remember what they are taught and may get an artificially high score when retested.

If a person has the use of only one hand, the therapist holds the leather piece for the client and asks the client to do the stitches. When people lose the use of their dominant hand, their performance is slower with the nondominant hand. Because the ACLS and LACLS are not timed tests, this is not a problem. The ACLS and the LACLS do however, detect a focal deficit in imagining a line. The client does not know which piece of leather lacing to use or which hole to go through next. When this occurs, further testing is essential to distinguish between a focal versus a global deficit. No other problems with the validity of the test have been detected. Age, gender, and educational background do not seem to distort the data. Correlations with other measures of illness, disability, and intelligence have been, by and large, as expected (Allen, Earhart, & Blue, 1992).

Projects to Monitor Change

The Allen Diagnostic Module (ADM) is a collection of sensory stimulation kits and craft projects used to verify the assessment of ability to function. The ADM Manual describes the setup and scoring of performance of these actions and activities (Allen, Earhart, & Blue, 1992).

With the lower functioning clients, the first impression is verified by sensory stimulation methods. Craft projects are the tools of choice to verify the cognitive levels with higher functioning clients (ACL 3.0 to 5.8). When crafts are refused or not feasible, therapists can verify the cognitive level with activities of daily living. Craft projects are preferred because it easier to observe new learning with them. Activities of daily living (ADL) are overlearned habits, and it is easy to be misled into thinking the person is functioning better than he or she is. The external environment is in a constant state of change, and predictions about how a person will function outside the highly controlled therapy environment are thought to be best made when observing new learning.

For people with a physical disability, ADL can pose a different problem. When new ways of doing ADL must be learned, relearning must replace old habits. Relearning is harder than new learning. As much as possible, craft projects are adapted to compensate for the physical disability so that new learning can be fairly observed. When a person has hemiplegia and trouble with standing balance, problems with dressing can have several explanations. Tabletop craft projects eliminate many of the physical explanations and eliminate the difficulties with relearning.

When the person's ability to function is improving, the ADM is used to measure change. Probes are cues given to see if improvement has occurred.

Each treatment session begins by matching cues to the most recent ability to function. Probes attempt to direct attention to cues usually noticed at the next highest mode of function. If the client does not notice the cue spontaneously, the therapist attempts to direct attention to a cue from the higher mode. When there is no spontaneous or prompted attention to a cue from a higher mode, the condition has not improved. Improvement in the ACL score must occur in a reasonable period of time. For most conditions improvements can be detected within 2 weeks. The scale is so sensitive that many improvements will be detected from 1 day to the next.

Activities of Daily Living for a Home Program

Once the condition has stabilized, the therapist's attention is directed toward the activities of daily living. The goal is to set up a maintenance program that is as nearly normal as possible. A description of a recent typical day is obtained from the client during an interview. If lower functioning clients cannot describe a typical day, a family member or friend may provide the information. Without a family member, the therapist relies on the universal activities of daily living. The recent typical day describes what was normal for the individual. Treatment goals aim at making life with a disability as nearly normal as possible.

A few vital activities that all people do have been analyzed on the Routine Task Inventory (RTI), even though the number of these activities are recognized as minuscule compared to the range of human activity. The RTI includes an analysis of the following ADL: grooming, dressing, bathing, walking and exercising, eating, toileting, taking medication, using adaptive equipment, housekeeping, preparing and obtaining food, spending money, shopping, doing laundry, traveling, and telephoning (Allen, Earhart, & Blue, 1992; Allen, Earhart, Blue, & Therasoft, 1996). This list of realistic activities has been generated according to what most people regard as normal daily and weekly chores, saving therapists the trouble of repeating the same analysis. When the most common activities are not appealing to an individual, therapists should use the descriptions of abilities to analyze activities that are meaningful to the individual (Allen, Earhart, & Blue, 1996).

The Cognitive Performance Test (CPT) was designed as a standardized test to examine a person's mental operations while doing ADL. Procedures for doing six activities have been identified : dressing, shopping, making toast, telephoning, washing, and traveling. Telephoning, for example, asks the person to take a local phone book and call to find the price of a gallon of white paint. The advantage of the CPT is that it is a practical activity with a shared purpose (Burns, 1992). These practical purposes may make more sense than craft projects to some of the cognitively disabled. There still is, however, an element of simulation to the CPT assessments. Some of the concrete clients, for example, will argue that they do not want any paint. A more flexible and dynamic approach to the CPT is being developed. Therapists constantly confront the need to modify assessment activities so that they have meaning to clients, without losing the validity of their assessments.

Caregiver Education Materials

The most common accidents and injuries are listed by the modes of performance in Allen, Earhart, and Blue (1996) and in the computer software (Allen, Earhart, Blue & Therasoft, 1996). Therapists can use these resources in a variety of ways: initial evaluations and discharge recommendations placed in the client's chart, handouts given to caregivers, or in-services given to team members. A tremendous amount of education about the risks associated with a cognitive disability needs to be done. The following discussion offers suggestions about how to approach the different educational needs.

The accidents and injuries that occur in the normal population are the most frequent reasons for requiring emergency services (firefighters, paramedics, hospital emergency rooms). These accidents and injuries can happen to anybody, but the cognitively disabled are at a greater than average risk. Therapists cannot predict what will happen, like a fall that results in a broken a hip. Therapists can only say that there may be an increased proba-

bility that the person might fall and might break a hip.

Lack of attention to environmental cues increases the risks associated with the cognitive modes. Therapists use the lists of safety precautions to warn clients and caregivers about increased risk. The lists are written in fifth grade English and can be given to caregivers. When the natural course of the disease, or history of noncompliance with treatment, indicates that a future change in ACL is expected, therapists may issue two warnings. The first warning matches current ability to function and the second predicts important changes expected in the future.

Very few people understand what a cognitive disability is and how it can affect daily life. Clients, friends and relatives, and other medical professionals all have a tendency to ignore, rationalize, and deny a long-term cognitive disability. Excuses for difficulties in doing any single activity can always be found. Because accidents and injuries can happen to anybody, it is easy to ignore an increase in probability. Therapists can issue warnings, but the decision to take the risk is usually made by someone else. Before a warning is issued, therapists should be careful to substantiate the presence of a disability, as a pattern of performance.

One problem with identifying patterns of performance is that the lists tend to be very long, making them tedious to read and write. Some resources are available to help solve the problem. A software program that can be used for chart documentation and caregiver education is especially helpful in realistically describing patterns that are the potential consequences of long-term cognitive disabilities (Allen, Earhart, Blue, & Therasoft, 1996). If a computer is not available, checklists can be made from the lists of safety precautions for each mode, as has been done for ACL 4.0 in Appendix A (Allen, Earhart, & Blue, 1996).

Caregivers often find it difficult to distinguish between cannot and will not. The natural inclination is to say that a deficiency is motivational and blame the client for the behavioral problem. By telling caregivers what to expect, therapists can reduce some of these conflicts. Therapists can select safety warnings that are a concern for the individual. The warnings are meant to identify an increased probability that the person might do something, like forget to turn off the stove. If and when the problem does occur, the caregiver will recognize it as an expression of the underlying disability.

Members of the multidisciplinary team also have a natural inclination to think that mental problems are motivational. A vast amount of professional jargon can be used to blame the client for behavioral problems and treatment failures. The cognitive levels can be used to change team attitudes. When the team members understand that the problem is a question of cannot, instead of will not, they often are nicer to the client. Environmental compensations can be put in place to reduce the problem behavior, and realistic treatment goals can be established and met. The cognitive levels can be used as an indication of the need for physical and cognitive assistance (see Appendix B). The need for assistance suggests a level of care. Medicare percentages and descriptive terms are used as a way of translating the cognitive levels into a national guideline for functional outcomes. When used correctly, the cognitive levels counter negative value judgments with realistic expectations. Therapists should collaborate with other members of the team in establishing expectations and designing compensations.

By understanding the client's best ability to function, therapists are in a position to advocate for the client's right to use their remaining abilities. The least restrictive environment identifies the place where those abilities can be used safely. Environmental compensations can be made to protect the disabled from hazards and create a less restrictive environment. When caregivers understand what the person can do, and cannot do, they are better prepared to treat the disabled person with the dignity they deserve.

The dictionary definition of rehabilitation confuses family members who are struggling to understand what a cognitive disability means. Rehabilitation is usually defined as the restoration of ability to function in a normal or near normal manner. This definition of rehabilitation can produce some unrealistic expectations about what rehabilitation service providers can do. Clients and families may hope that rehabilitation service providers will restore the ability to function, and as long as services are provided the hope may be sustained. The natural course of the disease tells therapists how much restoration of ability to function to expect, and for how long. Educating family members about the natural course of the disease that leaves a residual disability exposes the tragedy that will have an impact on their lives.

A major legal problem occurs when the client, family, or doctor decides to do an activity anyway, ignoring the therapist's warnings. When attempting to reduce risks, therapists need to be careful about not assuming responsibility for taking the risk. A car, as the extreme example, is a lethal weapon. The legal decision to drive is not made by the therapist. The therapist can warn against driving altogether or suggest situations that would reduce probable hazards. The therapist cannot predict or prevent traffic accidents. To a lesser extent the same legal and ethical problems occur with living situations, finances, and child care. Therapists are in a position to make recommendations and collaborate with long-term caregivers, who are the final decision makers.

Research

A lot of work has been done to improve the credibility of the components of the Allen Battery, with the most studies done on several versions of the screening tools (ACLS). Most of the quantitative studies have used correlations to establish the strength of the association between measures. The strongest correlation is reported as r = + or −1.0. For reliability, the r number should be higher than + or −.80. The r for validity is usually lower, between .30 and .70. A small p represents the statistical significance, with the customary minimum at .05, meaning that the result may be incorrect 5 out of 100 times. Lower p numbers are better, reducing the number of incorrect results. N is the number in the sample; larger Ns increase the confidence in the study.

Interrater reliability has always been high. The original six cognitive levels were used in the first studies that found nearly perfect interrater reliability (r = .99, N = 32, range of levels 2–6). At that time the ACLS was used to place clients in a group that matched their score; the predictive validity was r = .76, N = 23 (Moore, 1978). Newman (1989) examined the next version of the ACLS and found a percentage of agreement between two raters of

95.2% (N = 21). Test–retest reliability for Newman's sample of chronic schizophrenic patients was r = .75 (N = 22, p. 01). Partida (1992) looked at the interrater reliability of the large and small ACL with a small sample (N = 4) and two raters, finding perfect reliability. Howell (1993) found similar interrater reliability with the most recent version of the small ACLS (r = .91, p<.0001, N = 20). Eight raters trained by Penny, Musser, and North (1995) achieved an impressive r = .98. The first step in establishing a credible use of the Allen Battery is to be sure that the rating of the screening tool is accurate. These studies suggest that therapists and their students should be able to establish accurate interrater reliability.

Kehrberg (1992) reported significant correlations between the large leather lacing and the small one, with higher associates with the senile dementia population (r = .95, p<.001) than the control subjects (r = .58, p<.001). The client population was more impaired when gender and test order were controlled. With both sizes, both the dementia population and the controls over the age of 75 did not do as well as those under 75.

Validity is the extent to which a test measures what it says it measures, in this case cognitive processes, global ability to function, and severity of a disability. The ACLS has been correlated with well-known instruments commonly used with a variety of diagnostic categories to check the validity of the scale. The most widely used cognitive measure is the Wechsler Adult Intelligence Scale (WAIS), which is often reported as verbal, performance, and full-scale intelligence (IQ). Katz (1979) found a moderate correlation between the Block Design and the ACLS (r = .45, p<.001). Mayer (1988) used all of the subtests of the WAIS to clarify the type of information processing that is related to adaptation. The strongest correlations were between the ACLS and the Block Design and Object Assembly (r = .729, p<.0001). Performance IQ also showed a high correlation with the ACLS (r = .55, p<.0003). The most enlightening use of the WAIS was to divide the test into crystallized and fluid abilities. Fluid abilities "subsume information processing functions such as attention, perception, flexibility, and problem-solving. Crystallized abilities are dependent on previous training, education, and acculturation (e.g., vocabulary)" (Mayer, 1988,

p. 176). The correlations with fluid abilities gave credence to the notion that a pattern of performance in adapting to a changing environment was being tested. No significant correlations were found with vocabulary, arithmetic, or picture completion, which are part of crystallized intelligence that is influenced by cultural background. This has been further supported by a lack of significant correlations with age, sex, education, occupation, work history, or socioeconomic status in several disabled populations. While these demographic factors do influence intelligence in normal populations, the benefits of cultural experiences do not overcome difficulties in processing the information necessary for planning and problem-solving with new information (Alsberg, 1987; Averbuch & Katz, 1988; Breeding, 1993; Camp & Person, 1987; David & Riley, 1990; Gokey, 1986; Heimann, Allen, & Yerxa, 1989; Herzig, 1978; Heying, 1983; Howell, 1993; Josman & Katz, 1991; Kaeser, 1992; Katz, 1979; Katz, Josman, & Steinmetz, 1988; Mayer, 1988; Moore, 1978; Newman, 1987; Partida, 1992; Penny, Musser, & North, 1995; Richards, 1983; Shapiro, 1992; Skinner, Denton, & Levy, 1989; Williams, 1981; Wilson, Allen, McCormack, & Burton, 1989).

Shapiro's (1992) finding that leather lacing did not correlate with the Perceptual Memory Task (PMT), but did correlate with Visual Motor Integration (VMI), was surprising. A deeper look at underlying mental processes was required. The input of PMT is similar to the Block Design of the WAIS, using colored blocks and increasingly complex designs printed on cards. With the PMT, subjects are given cards for 10 seconds, and then the designs are removed. To match or recognize a pattern, subjects must store an image of the design. The formation and storage of images are not required with leather lacing. With leather lacing people are given examples of stitches to copy or match. With the VMI, subjects are also given geometric patterns to copy. Shapiro's study suggests a need to look beyond the input of visual and auditory cues and consider the underlying mental processes that must be applied to the cues.

The relationship between leather lacing and hand dexterity has been investigated, using the Purdue Pegboard, without a significant correlation as expected. With a sample of depressed patients the time to complete the ACL was used to successfully remove the ceiling effect on the ACLS, which has been a problem with other studies of depression (Carmel, Katz, & Modai, 1996). When the major problem is slowness, or loss of energy, timing the ACLS may provide objective data.

The relationship between leather lacing and verbal abilities has also been studied. David and Riley (1990) found modest correlations between the ACLS and the Shipley Institute of Living Scale, which is a paper-and-pencil test for choosing synonyms and writing responses to a sequence of terms. With N = 57, modest correlations were found with vocabulary, r = .25, p<.02; abstraction, r =.35, p<.001; and IQ, r = .31, p<.005. A stronger correlation was found with the Symbol Digit Modalities Test, which times the translation of novel geometric shapes into written responses (r = .52, p<.001). As suspected, leather lacing is more related to novel learning of perceptual motor tasks than to abstract reasoning and verbal abilities. A similar modest correlation was found between leather lacing and the Social Interaction Test (SIT) (Penny, Musser, & North, 1995). The total SIT correlation was r = ~.32, p<.01; nonverbal r = ~.27, p<.03; conversation r = ~.32, p<.01; voice quality was not significant, r = ~.16. A low ACLS score was associated with reduced social competencies. The scales go the opposite directions, which explains the expected negative correlations. While there is a relationship between what people say and what people do, the relationship is modest.

In an effort to examine the cognitive abilities that emerge during Piaget's period of concrete operations, the Riska Object Classification (ROC) was developed with interrater reliability at r =.83, p<.01. The structured part of this test required too great a leap in cognitive abilities and has not produced significant correlations. The spontaneous portion has been more productive, with a significant association with leather lacing, education, occupation, and social position in a nondisabled population (Williams, 1981). Wilson (1985) also found a significant correlation between the spontaneous portion of the ROC and leather lacing (r = .66, p<.001) and the Mini-Mental Status Exam in her population with senile dementia (r = .90, p<.001). In a study of depressed people, Katz (1979) found significant correlations with leather

lacing (r = .42, p<.001) and the Block Design portion of the WAIS (r = .60, p<.0001). The results of the early studies with the ROC were uneven, suggesting that the developmental continuum needed to be replaced with a different way of organizing our understanding of cognitive abilities. Katz began to work on this by developing a series of class inclusion questions that were found to differentiate significantly between psychiatric patients and normal controls (Katz, Josman, & Steinmetz, 1988; Tolchinsky-Landsmann & Katz, 1988). The ROC is also included as part of the Loewenstein Occupational Therapy Cognitive Assessment (Katz, Itzkovich, Averbuch, & Elazar, 1989; Cermak, Katz, McGuire, Greenbaum, Peralta, & Maser-Flanagan, 1995). The convenient explanation of regression to lower levels of development, in a sequence taken from normal children, was not working. The differences between the way disabled people think, as distinguished from normal children and adults, needed clearer explanations.

Some differences between a psychological view of intelligence and an occupational therapy view of function are emerging from these studies. Psychological tests of intelligence tend to include words, concepts, paper-and-pencil tasks, and even when visual cues are used they must be processed and stored in a sequential manner within a timed period. As a whole, psychological tests have a strong tradition in favoring the left-hemisphere abilities. Leather lacing, crafts, and ADLs probably favor the right hemisphere's contribution to visual spatial abilities. Visual spatial cues are demonstrated and copied while doing an activity. Learning may be instantaneous or acquired through practice in doing the activity. Right-hemisphere processes prepare people for immediate action, containing spontaneity not seen in left-hemisphere processes. Shapiro's (1992) discussion of different responses to the tests she used provides insight into these differences. Because both hemispheres are important, an effort has been made to include both types of ability in the description of the modes to provide a global view of ability to function (Allen, Earhart, & Blue, 1992).

The idea that the scale measured the severity of a disability was first investigated with the Brief Psychiatric Rating Scale; the concurrent validity with the ACLS was r = .53 at admission and r =

.43 at discharge (Moore, 1978). In another sample with a schizophrenic population, Newman (1987) found a correlation with the Global Assessment Scale (r = .46, p<.01, N = 34). Differences between schizophrenic, depressed, and control populations were found in California, and replicated in Israel (Katz, 1979; Katz & Heimann, 1990; Williams, 1981). Heying (1983) expanded the investigation of the ACLS to senile dementia, finding a correlation with the Mini-Mental Status Exam (r = .66, p<.001, N = 33). The results were replicated by Wilson (1985) with N = 20 and r = .59. The Cognitive Performance Test has been used to predict institutionalization in low-functioning patients and trace the functional decline and death in years for people with senile dementia (Burns, 1992). At the other end of the age range, emotionally disturbed boys showed decreased ability to do leather lacing in a school in New York (N = 24). A moderate correlation with Developmental Test for Visuomotor Impairment (r = .44, p<.04) was found on a test designed to screen children for neurological impairments and learning disabilities (Shapiro, 1992). Breeding (1993) found a difference between age groups in a study of normal six- to nine-year-olds from a school with parents in high socioeconomic status (N = 84). The ACLS has been used to differentiate between adolescents, 12- to 18-years-old, with psychiatric disorders (N = 49) and controls (N = 29) matched for age, sex, education, and place of residence (Katz, Josman, & Steinmetz, 1988; Josman & Katz, 1991). In nondisabled adults 18 to 65, Williams (1981) found a positive correlation between ACLS and social, position based on education, social and occupational status as determined by the Hollinghead's Two-Factor Index of Social Position. Cultural factors influence cognitive ability in normal populations but have not had an impact on the disabled scores. The cognitive levels do correlate with well-known measures of the severity of a variety of mental disorders.

The relationship between activities that therapists typically use in practice and leather lacing has also been examined. Newman (1987) found a correlation (r = .63, p<.01) with the Task Oriented Assessment of the Bay Area Assessment of Functional Performance. The study of activities of daily living was started by Heying's (1983) finding of a high correlation (r = 82, p<.001) with the Physical Self-Maintenance Scale and Instrumental Activities of Daily Living Scale presented by Lawton and Brody (1969). Lawton and Brodys activities of daily living were modified and turned into a quantitative measure by Heimann (1985), in the form of the Routine Task Inventory (RTI). Heimann studied psychiatric outpatients, finding an ACLS correlation with the total RTI of r = .64, p<.001 (Heimann, Allen, & Yerxa, 1989). The test–retest reliability of the RTI was established at r = .99, p<.0001 and interrater reliability was established at r = .99, p<.001 (Heimann, 1985). Wilson (1985) found similar test–retest reliability after a 2-week interval (r = .99, p<.0001). Wilson described a community-based sample of people with senile dementia, finding an ACLS correlation with the RTI similar to Heimann's at r = .56, p<.01 (Wilson, Allen, McCormack, & Burton, 1989). Gokey (1987) found a modest correlation between leather lacing and the RTI (r = .44, p<.006). The strength of the correlation between leather lacing and activities of daily living was given an in depth investigation by Gokey (1987), Heimann (1985), and Wilson (1985), leading to the suggestion that eating is one level lower than all other activities. Gokey (1987) found that the RTI had a stronger correlation with working than leather lacing did in a sample of schizophrenic patients. In a comparison of the RTI correlations with leather lacing and classification abilities, a distinction between motor and verbal abilities began to emerge (Gokey, 1987; Heimann, 1985; Wilson, 1985). The safety concerns implicit in the RTI received their first explicit investigation by Alsberg (1987) finding an association between leather lacing and the errors made while making macaroni and cheese in a sample functioning at ACL 4 and 5. Burns (1992) translated six tasks from the RTI into a Cognitive Performance Task, finding a correlation with the Mini-Mental Status Exam (r = .67, N = 77). At four weeks with the CPT, interrater reliability was r = .91 (N = 18) and test–retest was r = .89 (N = 36). The strength of the validity correlations was not great, suggesting that prior experience, motivation, social situations and underlying mental processes can have important influences on ADL.

The investigation of craft activities was initiated by Kaeser (1992), showing improved performance when activities are matched to the cognitive level.

The sample was elderly persons with dementia doing tiling tasks. Subjects at cognitive level 3 performed better on level 3 tiling activities than on a level 4 tiling activities (F(1,14) = 125, p<.001). As expected there was significance difference in the way the level 4 subjects performed on the level 3 and 4 activities.

The first controlled research investigation of treatment effectiveness has been completed in Israel with two groups of schizophrenics in post-acute care. The research group (N = 11)was given activities from the ADM that matched their ability to function and probed for higher abilities. The control group (N = 8) was in a sheltered workshop with tasks given according to the work to be done. Both groups showed a significant improvement on the RTI (z = 2.80, p<.005 for research; z = 2.52, p<.01 for control), but the research group showed a higher gain. The research group showed a significant improvement on the ACLS (z = 2.52. p<.01) but there was no significant improvement in the control group (z = .13). Although the sample size is very small, the study supports the idea that greater gains may be made when the therapist's treatment methods match the capacities of the client (Raweh, 1996).

These quantitative studies have shaped the understanding of the psychological mechanism that explains ability to function. Confidence in using the cognitive levels to describe the severity of the disability in varied populations has been enhanced. Respect for what the person can do, will do, and may do has been heightened because what the person can do explains only a limited percentage of the variance. With the disabled populations, the overwhelming conclusion is that cultural background, as studied with the demographic variables, does not compensate for the severity of a cognitive disability.

Target Population

Three populations are targeted when developing resources for the Allen Battery. The first population is expected to experience a rapid improvement in their ability to function. In neurology the diagnostic categories include cerebral vascular accidents, traumatic head injuries, and craniotomies. The toxicity with delirium that is expected to clear may

also show a marked improvement in the ACL. Affective disorders, especially depression, show rapid change as the new psychotropic drugs work faster and better. The psychotropic drugs are not as effective with schizophrenia, taking several weeks to produce a change of two or three modes. The ACL measures the change and explains the meaning of the person's current ability to function to other caregivers.

The second population has a long-term cognitive disability. The ACL score can be permanent or characterized by progressive decline. A great deal of emphasis has been placed on members of this population because they are not a popular group. Few supports are available to them and their caregivers. The second focus is on providing environmental compensations for clients who do not have the mental capacity to understand their cognitive disability, generalize from the treatment situation to the community, or use remedial skills effectively. Activities are analyzed to identify the underlying mental abilities required to do the task. The client's best abilities are matched to the demands of the activity. Environmental compensations need to be invented and checked to be sure they work safely when people have a limited capacity to learn to adapt. With severe and persistent mental disorders, realistic and relevant actions and activities are still possible. Skilled therapy services are required to set up the environmental conditions needed to elicit the use of best remaining mental abilities.

A wide range of diagnostic categories can describe a long-term cognitive disability. With the elderly the most common diagnoses are Alzheimer's disease and other dementias, cerebrovascular disease (CVD), and Parkinson's disease. Onset of the disease seen with adults include schizophrenia, major affective disorders, aneurysms and brain tumors, and multiple sclerosis. Young adults and adolescents are most likely to have traumatic brain injuries (TBI). Epilepsy begins between 3 and 15 years of age. Cerebral palsy and mental retardation are present at birth. The age of onset affects prior knowledge (Finger & Stein, 1982). With an older onset, people have the benefit of learning with a normal brain, and prior knowledge can be used to compensate for a disability. A younger onset limits the amount of information that is apt to be stored in long-term memory. Simple things like knowing how to tie shoelaces can have a big impact on a home program.

The third population targeted by the model is the long-term caregivers. Environmental compensations for a cognitive disability depend on caregiver education. Compensations for a dysfunctional brain often require the help of another person to supply the cues that the person is able to process. After the therapist figures out what a person's best ability to function is, time must be spent in educating long-term caregivers in how to continue to elicit the client's best ability to function. With low-functioning clients, caregivers are apt to be overwhelmed by what the client cannot do and have trouble coming up with ideas about what they can do. With a moderate degree of disability there is a tendency to think that not doing something is volitional: they could do it if they wanted to. With a mild disability there seems to be an increased risk for substance abuse if remaining abilities are not used constructively. Occupational therapists can be a tremendous help in clarifying expectations and suggesting activities that can be done successfully. Life with a cognitive disability goes on, and therapists contribute by making sure that the quality of that life is as good as it can be. Sustained and constructive improvements in the quality of life frequently depend on the long-term caregiver.

Underlying Assumptions

Theories contain a number of very abstract concepts that influence the way a conceptual model is constructed and then applied in practice. Because these assumptions have a tendency to be wrong, and mess up applications in ways that are hard to identify, an effort is made to make these assumptions as explicit as possible. The concepts that have formed a foundation for the construction of the sequence of abilities and the Allen Battery are discussed below.

Measurement versus Treatment

Clinical experience has led to the conclusion that the traditional separation between evaluation and

treatment does not work. The separation is easy to teach, and the billing office likes it, but in practice the distinction is often artificial. The separation does not work for the same reasons that standardized tests do not work. The quality of life and the quality of performance are influenced by a variety of factors that cannot be adequately specified by standardized evaluation procedures. To get the client's best score on a test, therapists need the freedom to use their treatment techniques to modify test procedures for the individual situation. The goal in using the Allen Battery is to determine the person's best ability to function. Therapists must combine evaluation and treatment techniques. The danger is that best ability will not emerge under the rigidity of highly controlled, standardized conditions (Polkinghorne, 1992). Treatment techniques need to be consistently applied to the evaluation process.

Additional problems influence the artificial split between assessment and treatment. There is a normal variation in best ability to function, according to time of day and how invested people are in the activity that they are doing. We all have lower functioning moments and give less than our best ability to low-priority activities. In addition, in acute conditions all kinds of medical problems can have a temporary influence on ability to function (fatigue, fever, pain, toxicity). The result is that for all practical purposes an assessment is never finished. Therapists evaluate all the time.

Evaluation and treatment occur continuously and simultaneously. This dynamic interaction has been built into the Allen Battery. It is assumed that therapists are always doing both and need guidelines for both processes. When research was first done with the ACLS and the LACLS, standardized testing procedures were followed. After the development of the dynamic process used in the ADM, a more flexible process has been applied to the ACLS and the LACLS with no apparent compromise to the clinical usefulness of the screening tools.

The method of inquiry developed by Piaget and Inhelder has influenced the development of the Allen Battery. These developmental psychologists asked children: What do you think will happen when _____ occurs? Why? Occupational therapists ask questions about ability to function:

Is yours like mine? How is it different? Can you fix it? The method of inquiry is similar: asking the subjects to tell us what they are thinking about the world. The difference in the content of the questions reflects their place in life. Children are trying to figure out how the world works. Disabled adults are trying to be as nearly normal as possible.

At each point in the process, therapists are trying to determine the person's best ability to function. Therapists share the hope that the disabled will be able to function as nearly normal as possible. The cues and prompts that improve performance are noted so that others can help the person engage their best ability to function. To understand the best ability to function of a cognitively disabled person, one must have an understanding of how they are thinking.

The assessment and treatment processes seek to identify simple, basic mental structures that will allow a therapist to understand how a conscious but mentally disabled person is thinking and feeling. We must assume that what they think and feel is both similar to and different from the way we think and feel. The versatility of the mind in perceiving the moment, drawing on memories of prior knowledge, and anticipating future events is described by the ACL. It is assumed that subjective thinking and feelings guide behavior, no matter how simple the action, as long as a person is awake or out of a coma. The central nervous system (CNS) is assumed to guide conscious behavior even though a brain location for consciousness is unknown. Consciousness is thought to be the overall function of the CNS that guides behavior as people think about objects and events, both internal and external. A person's understanding of objects and events can be accurate or inaccurate, and therapists need ways of understanding how a mentally disabled person is thinking (Searle, 1990).

Function

Luria (1966) provides a wonderful history of all the different ways that functioning has been defined throughout the history of Western civilization. The range of definitions can go from the proper action of the synapse between brain cells, to the whole person, or even extended to the functioning of a social system. How function is defined has a big impact on what a field of study does. The Cognitive Disabilities Model targets the whole person. The whole person is a conscious organism that uses thinking to understand objects and events. The conscious organism uses the capacity to think and feel in order to function. The capacity to function is composed of underlying mental processes that can be brought to conscious attention when necessary or may be used automatically. The redness of a tomato, for example, can be an automatic assumption or a deliberate consideration. The perception and interpretation of color is an example of an underlying mental process (Searle, 1990). Underlying mental processes guide all intentional behavior.

To function is to do the occupations that are normal for the individual. These occupations take place in an ever changing environment. The human mind has incredible versatility in adapting to multiple environments that are in a state of flux. Environmental compensations are required when the disabled mind cannot adapt to constant changes in situations and circumstances. A limited capacity to think is pervasive, spreading out through every aspect of the person's life. Therapists generally assume that disabled people want to function as nearly normal as possible, to do the occupations that are normal for them. When normal is not possible, therapists need to understand how the disabled person is thinking. To see the world through the eyes of a disabled person, therapists take note of the stimuli that capture attention. Therapists are trying to infer what information is capturing and sustaining the disabled person's attention. Information that does not even capture attention is not processed. Information that captures and sustains attention may be processed accurately or inaccurately. When information is processed accurately, an ability is identified. Inaccurately processed and ignored information is identified as a limitation.

The ability to function is primarily controlled by the brain. When the brain is operating as a total unit, it is referred to as the global capacity to function. The ability to function is the versatility of the conscious organism to use the brain to guide motor and speech performances. When motor and speech performances are equivalent, the Cognitive

Disabilities Model identifies one overall ability to function. When there is a discrepancy between motor and speech performance, two abilities to function may be identified. The brain has two major operating units, roughly analogous to the left and right hemispheres, that control motor and speech behaviors. Damage to one hemisphere can make performance uneven and necessitates two global assessments of ability to function.

The most thoroughly pervasive influence on ability to function is determined by how the brain is working as a total unit, with the next major determinate being the units for motor and speech performances. To deal with function, occupational therapists should be concerned with the most pervasive influences on the capacity to function. The capacity to function identifies what the person can do: the occupations that are realistic for the individual.

Whole Person

To treat the whole person, the major parts of the human functioning need to be identified. The traditional biological, psychological, and social components are adopted and simplified into what the person can do, will do, and may do. What the person can and cannot do is rooted in the biological pathology of the brain that causes a cognitive disability. Realistic activities are those things that the person is able to do after the effects of the disease, illness, or injury are known. The Cognitive Disabilities Model provides lists of realistic activities.

The Allen Cognitive Levels (ACL) are a sequence of abilities used to analyze activities to identify realistic occupations. Cognitive abilities are thought to be universal, cross-cultural, and handed down through evolution. During normal growth and development the sequence in which cognitive abilities emerge is genetically programmed into the deoxyribonucleic acid (DNA). In children, brain pathology can put a ceiling on normal development. With an adult onset disability, abilities to learn new information may be lost. An adult who has had a normal development may remember how to do activities learned in the past (like writing) and these potential abilities are identified and used as much as possible. Lists of abilities to learn new

information are sequenced according to cognitive development and used to analyze the cognitive complexity of actions, activities, and roles. Lists of occupations and safety precautions are generated by the activity analysis (Allen, Earhart, & Blue, 1996). These lists are realistic examples of what the person can do.

Therapists can share these lists with clients and their caregivers by showing them the lists or explaining them to them. Individuals can make selections from these lists according to their priorities and personal preferences. Occupations that are relevant to the individual usually follow predictable patterns that are influenced by age, gender, culture, and ethnicity. People generally want to be as nearly normal as possible. Therapists avoid making too many assumptions about what is relevant to a given individual and recognize that the final decision about the meaningfulness of an activity rests with the individual. What the person will do is determined by the individual.

The trouble with lists of realistic activities for the cognitively disabled is that they may not contain activities the person would normally want to do, like driving, working, socializing, getting married, and having children. The cognitively disabled rarely understand why common activities may not be realistic for them. They do understand, however, that they are being deprived of activities that they consider normal for them. Over a longer period of time they may interpret their situation in ways that do not acknowledge their limitations. When it is not possible to correct their perceptions or change their realities, therapists focus their attention on realistic activities. The craft projects presented in the ADM are designed to be as nearly normal and attractive as possible. Actions and activities that might be insulting or upsetting are avoided. Simple activities that do not appear to be childish are hard to design, but deemed worth the effort. Because a person's best ability to function is most apt to be applied to an activity that appeals to the individual, the person's interest and motivation must always be taken into consideration.

Economic and social factors influence what a person may do by determining which activities are possible. For the cognitively disabled, another person may be needed to plan, schedule, initiate, sequence through, and clean up after the activity.

The goodwill of people in their social support system may be essential to sustaining the person's ability to function. Caregiver education is an important part of treating the whole person so that other people know how to sustain abilities. The biggest problem with caregiver education is in identifying disabilities that may or may not be permanent. Family members who are trying to plan for their loved ones want to know if the client will get better or worse and how long the disability will last. We do not have very good answers to these questions. The natural course of the disease provides the best information. Too often the literature lacks objective, longitudinal studies about changes in ability to function over a given period of time. Mortality rates can frequently be found in the literature, but mortality provides little information about what changes to expect in daily activities. The cognitive levels can be used to educate caregivers about what to expect now, but it can be very difficult to help them anticipate what to expect in the future. Long-term caregivers may have to adjust to changes in ability to function as they occur.

Human nature is a common topic in philosophy, with different orientations placing more or less emphasis on what a person can, will, and may do. The nature versus nurture controversy in psychiatry is an example of a philosophical debate that placed a dichotomy between biology and the environment. These either/or positions are diminishing. The position taken by the Cognitive Disabilities Model is to recognize all three aspects of human nature and to vary the emphasis according to the severity of the disability and the clinical situation.

Theoretically, a broadly based scale is required that can be easily adapted to a comprehensive view of everyday life. A broadly based scale allows therapists to analyze the cognitive complexity of any activity a client wants to do. To pursue goals selected by the client and their care givers that make sense to them, therapists must be prepared to analyze any occupation. Individual differences in the priorities that people place on activities are to be expected. Priorities that are influenced by differences in cultures, ethnicity, gender, and age are also expected to influence the application of the scale. The ACL scale, describing what a disabled person can do, is not expected to stand alone, and should be used in conjunction with what the person will do and may do.

Biologically-based Scale

The cognitive levels describe the capacity to think that is constrained by a medical condition. In many ways, the cognitive levels work like the age of a child. The age of a normal child tells us what to expect about the child's global ability to function. Age predicts motor and speech performance. The developing human brain learns to process information in a sequence that is genetically programmed into the DNA. We know, for example, that a child must learn to recognize geometric shapes and line orientation before learning to write the alphabet, and we have age norms for these expectations. The same sequence continues to operate with brain pathology. The age norms, however, can be thrown off by brain pathology so that the chronological age of the person does not tell us what to expect. Maturational age can also be misleading because an older person has extra experience and prior knowledge and may have had normal or special intellectual capacities at one time. A different scale is required that describes the development sequences but is not tied to age. In general, the Allen Cognitive Levels follow an innate, universal, and global sequence of ability to do computatively complex, everyday activities. The scale has a strong biological basis that makes it possible to apply to groups of people with different diagnoses. Any medical disorder that affects global capacity to function may be assessed and treated. Therapists are expected to use clinical judgment to further adapt occupations for additional medical impairments.

The construction of the ACL began in 1970 by modifying Piaget's description of the psychological processes that unfold during the first 2 years of life (Ginsberg & Opper, 1969). Piaget's structural approach to information processing continues to influence the model. Chomsky's identification of a universal grammar has also contributed confidence in seeking to describe innate mental structures. The goal in scale development is to identify mental abilities that emerge in an evolutionary, predetermined sequence and may be expressed in any cultural circumstance. The underlying mental structures should be applicable to a wide range of occupations. The sequence in which these mental structures develop is universal. The advantage provided by structuralism is that deep, historical time is responsible for the sequence of abilities. This avoids the problem of placing our own value judgments on which abilities to learn are better than others. Normal growth and development can be studied to see the natural progression of abilities to learn (Cook & Newson, 1996). Anthropology has also contributed to the construction of the scale by identifying human universals found in all cultures. Ethology has contributed knowledge about consciousness. The neurosciences continue to help clarify the distinction between focal and global deficits. The best resources, however, have always been observations of client behavior. Many observations not found in the literature were described and included in the scale in the sequence produced by natural healing, medication effectiveness, or progressive decline. Occupational therapists have the advantage of studying accidents of nature and seeing how medical conditions influence everyday activities. The cognitive complexity of everyday life becomes apparent as we watch people struggle to do what is normally taken for granted.

Historically, developmental psychology emerged from an interest in how intelligence predicts academic performance. The ACL developed out of an interest in how behavioral changes are associated with a changing medical condition. The ACL has been tied to everyday occupations and not tied to a definition of intelligence associated with academic performance. The behavior of interest to occupational therapists occurs in a real world of objects, people, and relations. An effort must be made to identify thinking and learning behaviors that are important in everyday life. Mental structures that are the most deeply rooted in evolutionary time may be more deeply rooted in the biology of the human brain and still available to the most severely disabled. Behaviors that are seen early in human development may be spared by severe brain pathology. Therapists look for mental structures that survive brain pathology. When mental structures are still working, therapists apply

their understanding of activity analysis to help people use remaining abilities in everyday life.

Information Processing System

The construction of the modes of performance follows a conceptual model modified after the work of Anderson (1992). A deliberate effort has been made to keep the construction simple and consistent by selecting major elements that have the biggest impact on ability to adapt to a changing environment. Therapists can observe some of the internal and external cues that initiate the information processing system and the output in the form of actions, activities, and roles. Therapists have to draw inferences about what is going on inside of the information processing system. The essential elements of information processing are attention, information processing speed, verbal/propositional representations, visual spatial representations, short-term memory, and long-term memory. These elements are combined into an information processing system that guides each mode of performance. The same basic framework is used for every mode.

Attention

Attention is the key that opens the door to the information processing system. The content of what the person pays attention to activates the information processing system. Mental activity is evident in movement of the eyes. Watch a person's eyes to see if a person is paying attention and processing the content. The internal and external environment offers sensory cues that may or may not capture attention. The sequence in which sensory cues capture attention is thought to be built into the DNA. Attention activates the information processing system, and the content of the cues defines the modes of representation. Universal motor and speech behaviors result from these mental representations. Attention to placing objects in a row, for example, can be applied to blocks, pegs, cookies, or clams. The mind is keeping track of the notion of row, and the objects are interchangeable. The objects do have to be something that can be placed in a row, but there are hundreds of variations in what the objects are. The content of thought is any object that can be placed in a row. The content of thought is an operation of the mind that organizes cues. Attention identifies the biological origins of complex mental functions that are mediated by anatomical structures and physiological processes of the central nervous system. From attention, therapists begin to draw inferences about how the disabled mind is working.

Processing Speed

The speed in which information is processed is remarkably consistent over years of intelligence testing of healthy subjects (Anderson, 1992). Brain pathology can alter the normal rate. A few disorders speed up the rate and produce symptoms like hyperactivity, pressured speech, and a flight of ideas. Most disorders slow the rate, with the slowest speeds associated with the most severe disabilities. The circuits that are still working seem to be gummed up, and a response to a cue can take 20 seconds or longer. At abnormal speeds only the simplest routine activities can be implemented, irrespective of the latent powers of the rest of the brain. Psychotic depressions, for example, slow the processing speed, and people say they do not have the energy to solve problems. When, however, antidepressants return processing speed to normal, the latent powers of the brain return to normal. With progressive diseases, like Alzheimer's, the person's normal speed gradually diminishes and does not return. Mania is characterized by a flight of ideas and pressured speech that suggests a rapid information processing speed that is slowed by medication. Different rates are characteristic of different diagnoses and vary in the way medications normalize these rates. Because slowing down is far more common, the description of the modes gives a reduced rate.

Verbal/Propositional Representations

Verbal/propositional representations are formed in the left hemisphere and guide speech performance. Speech performance includes all of the communication activities like reading, writing, talking, and listening. Aphasia is the classic symptom associated with damage to the speech centers. The predominant cues for speech are auditory (Anderson, 1992). These representations are processed in a logical sequence that is governed by the passage of time. What people say they do is usually sequential and logical. Therapists frequently note a difference between what disabled people say they will do and what is actually observed during performance. The discrepancy can be explained, in part, by the differences in the way the two hemispheres process information. With a healthy brain people use verbal propositional abilities to anticipate effects and inhibit motor actions.

Visual Spatial Representations

What people do is guided by visual spatial representations. Visual spatial representations are predominate in the right hemisphere, which guides motor performance. Motor performance includes gross and fine motor activities like mobility and doing things with one's hands. Motor performance combines information from the body with environmental cues. Visual cues are the predominant cues. Visual spatial representations are processed simultaneously to form sensations, perceptions, spatial estimates, and images. What people do is governed by a burst of insight into the situation. That is why there is often a difference between what people say they do and what they actually do. The differences in how the information is processed favor a spontaneous response to visual spatial representations that can be inhibited by anticipations of dangers. The ability to inhibit spontaneous responses is impaired by the mildest of cognitive disabilities, producing impulsive behavior and poor judgment. Spontaneous behavior has good survival value for the species, but therapists observe the consequences of not being able to override spontaneous actions.

Memory

Memory was added to Anderson's model because it is a major consideration with an adult onset of a cognitive disability. Long-term memory evaluates the use of prior knowledge. The frequently asked question is "Have you ever done anything like this before?" Activities that have been done the most are most apt to be remembered with brain pathology. When one activity looks better than the general pattern of performance, it is usually due to long-term memory. Memories are stored all over the cerebral cortex, and a lot of individual differences in accessing prior knowledge are expected. Prior knowledge can be tapped to identify special abilities that are not available to the general population of disabled people.

Short-term memory looks at whether the person can remember what he or she is doing now or did just a few minutes ago. When cognitively disabled people cannot remember what they are doing, assistance is required to get them through an activity. Other cognitively disabled people can solve a problem but a few minutes later cannot remember how they did it. If a new skill cannot be stored in short-term memory, it will not be transferred into long-term memory for later use. Difficulties with learning, and frustration on not being able to remember, create a tendency to stop trying. Problems with memory are a common complaint with the cognitively disabled that may be a specific problem with short-term memory or a global deficit. The therapist should observe new learning with an ADM project to identify the specific problem.

Framework for Each Mode

In describing the Allen Cognitive Levels some similarities between the modes can be explained. Each mode is conscious, voluntary, dynamic, and flexible. Each mode is built around the same cognitive framework consisting of attention, processing speed, verbal/propositional abilities, visual spatial abilities, and memory. Each mode is an integrated information processing system, built on the same architectural plan, but with different building materials. The building materials are the contents of the modes, like the colors and shapes that capture attention. The contents specify that cues capture attention and are processed by verbal and motor abilities and at what speed. Twenty-six information processing systems are described, from ACL 0.8 to

ACL 6.0. These information processing systems are arranged in a hierarchical sequence, which is essential for the application of an information processing model. The continuum is necessary in order to determine whether the condition is getting better or worse, to identify the relative severity of different diagnostic categories, and to study the natural courses of disease processes.

Each mode is a general-purpose mechanism that is sensitive to an identified type of input and associated with identified motor and speech behaviors (Anderson, 1992; Fodor, 1983). Where we depart from Anderson, Fodor, and other prominent psychologists is by placing the modes in a hierarchical sequence, like a developmental scale. Fodor's modules are encapsulated and domain specific, resembling Luria's functional domains. Information processing is subdivided into various parts, and there is no way to see how the system is working as a whole or to compare information processing systems. Too many important clinical questions are neglected by encapsulating domains without a hierarchy. Encapsulated domains may be most useful with mild cognitive disabilities, as described below under the heading Awareness of a Disability.

Global and Focal Deficits

As long as the ACL can be accounted for by one number, the ability to function is fairly easy to understand. The normal brain has a global ability to function, and some disease processes usually have an even effect on overall ability to function (schizophrenia, depression, mania, Alzheimer's disease, dementia). The brain is complicated and hemisphere damage can require two ACL scores. Some brain injuries (CVA, craniotomy, head injury) affect one hemisphere more than the other, producing two different general abilities to function. We are still explaining how brain pathology can influence a global ability to function. Global deficits can occur for a variety of additional medical reasons such as toxicity, focal deficits occurring in many locations, or damage to large areas of the brain. When people want to know what effects brain damage has on performance, assessment of overall ability to function is required. The Cognitive Disabilities Model explains how brain pathology influences global ability to function.

Focal deficits have an isolated effect on performance. By themselves, focal deficits, like retrograde amnesia, do not affect overall ability to function. Discrete lesions are studied in the neurosciences and are often reported in the client's chart. Luria's functional areas, for example, are concerned with focal deficits. Luria's classification system includes the following discrete functions: motor, acoustico-motor, cutaneous and kinesthetic, visual, mnestic, speech, writing and reading, arithmetic, and intellectual processes. These are isolated functional abnormalities that are related to separated regions of the brain. The ACL does not address focal deficits, which are left to the expertise of other disciplines. When a number of focal deficits have a cumulative effect on performance, the ACL may be helpful. The distinction between a global and a focal deficit is not always clear. When in doubt, use the ACL assessment to make sure that a hidden global deficit is not missed.

Application of the Allen Cognitive Levels

The setting that a therapist works in can influence the assessment of the ACL. The following discussion describes factors that can influence the therapist's ability to observe patterns of performance. The predominant factors that influence application are:

- evaluating improvements in functional outcomes
- observing long-term patterns of performance with adult onsets
- accounting for childhood onsets
- allowing for individual differences in patterns of performance.

Evaluating Improvements in Functional Outcomes

The sequence of change in ability to function can be learned from observing the performance of people with acute medical conditions. The improvements of psychiatric clients from multiple cultures can be a wonderful resource for identifying change in universal modes of representation. The improvements of clients healing from strokes, head injuries, and craniotomies contribute to the recognition of motor and speech abilities as two types of abilities to function. The decline of people with dementia can contribute to the understanding of the lower levels. As the medical condition of the brain improves or declines, observations are obtained of the sequence of the deep biological hardware of the brain that programs human behavior. Helping the cognitively disabled do activities of daily living places occupational therapists in an ideal position to identify the complex cognitive modules that normal people take for granted. The best population to study is psychiatric clients because the disease process is not confounded by additional physical disabilities or the medical complications associated with aging populations. Observations of psychiatric clients are the easiest way to learn to use the scale. The scale can be used to measure improvements associated with psychotropic drugs that may occur in days or weeks.

Observations of people with CVA and TBI are more difficult because of the confounding physical disabilities and general weakness. With a recent onset, rapid change in the ACL score is common. Therapists can follow these improvements with the ACL and use additional treatment methods for range of motion and endurance.

The greatest difficulty in applying the ACL to populations that are improving is describing the skill of the therapist. Many of these improvements will happen, with or without therapists. The explanation of the importance of the improvements requires a therapist. Therapists can use the ACL as an objective assessment of whether a functional improvement has or has not occurred. There is a lot of wishful thinking surrounding acute conditions that requires objective assessment. The interpretation of improvements, or the lack of improvement, are important to maximize the functional outcomes of acute care and plan for any needed rehabilitation and long-term care. The therapist should use the ADM to assess improvement, and the RTI and computer software to interpret the meaning of a disability.

Observing Long-Term Patterns of Performance with Adult Onset

A consistent pattern of activity performance is easier to learn from people who have a stable medical condition. The therapists may have an opportunity to observe performance in several different activities. The confusion associated with Parkinson's disease, Alzheimer's disease and the other dementias, multiple sclerosis, and epilepsy produces an ACL score that may be consistent for weeks, months, or even years. Whenever the ACL score is consistent, or fluctuating around a baseline, environmental compensations for a home program should be developed. The RTI lists 14 activities that people do. Improvements can be made by checking to see if performance is consistent. An activity that is below the others is a good candidate for improvement.

Many of these diseases are characterized by a progressive decline in ability to function. Therapists can learn about the characteristics of decline: Is it consistent across all activities? If not, what factors seem to prevent decline? A decline in ability to function is an indication for a reevaluation and a different home program.

Accounting for Childhood Onsets

A childhood onset of a cognitive disability makes it much harder to design environmental compensations because the child did not have the benefit of learning with a normal brain. Most of the abilities identified by maturational age are taken from intelligence tests used to predict academic performance. The abilities described in the modes of performance were selected to analyze everyday activities. For children who may not have much academic success, the ACL abilities may help to develop skills that are more practical and realistic than reading and writing. When universal cognitive abilities fail to develop, a ceiling effect on all further development may have been reached. The ACL can be used to objectively measure when these ceilings have and have not been reached. A constant ACL score over a period of months would suggest a ceiling, while an improving ACL score would suggest that a ceiling has not been reached. The ACL may also be used to set treatment goals and select methods that match the child's current ability to function.

Allowing for Individual Differences in Patterns of Performance

The sequence of universal abilities can be confounded by individual differences in intelligence unless some clear distinctions are made. Individual differences are composed of the speed of the basic processing mechanism and specific processors that elaborate on motor and speech behavior (Anderson, 1992). The speed of information processing seems to be controlled by the disease process, which obscures individual differences and is not a clinical problem. A good vocabulary can be misleading and is usually seen in a person with a good educational history. The therapist should use the projects in the ADM to clarify global abilities and distinguish between motor and verbal abilities.

A person who has worked with his or her hands a lot can also have misleading motor skills, but these are usually related to a particular type of activity. Most individual differences encountered with the cognitively disabled are stored in the client's long-term memory. Prior knowledge tends to be encapsulated and applied to specific activities. Specific elaborations can be thought of as the software that the person may have used in the past. An individual difference has a narrow application (Anderson, 1992). Therapists can expect to see a narrow application of an individual difference when the disabled person performs better in one action or activity than in all others. The amount of practice and skill the person has had with similar actions or activities influences retention of abilities; the more a skill is used the better it is retained. Individual differences usually explain behaviors that do not fit into the overall pattern of performance.

Care must be taken not to base assessments and predictions on isolated abilities. The Allen Cognitive Levels attempt to predict performance in computationally complex everyday activities based on general pattern of performance. An isolated, individual ability can misinform the prediction of everyday patterns of performance. Caregivers naturally hope that the cognitively disabled will be able to do "simple routines" better than they can. An isolated ability is frequently seized upon as evidence for an erroneously optimistic prediction. A general and consistent pattern of performance should serve as a basis for predictions, especially when the predictions are used to make discharge recommendations, to protect the safety of the disabled person and the community.

Skilled Services

There are three ways that occupational therapists are reimbursed. The medical condition of the client determines the type of services provided: (1) The medical condition is improving and the ability to function is also improving; (2) the medical condition is stable and no immediate change in the ability to function is expected; and (3) the long-term medical condition has slowly improved or progressed, or actual performance is worse than it should be given the person's ability to function. As long as the client is improving, therapists can be confident that they are providing reimbursable, skilled services. Conditions 2 and 3 are less clearly defined as skilled services, and the provision of these services is inconsistent. The Cognitive Disabilities Model aims at providing services to all three types of medical conditions. The Medicare guidelines contain the clearest definitions of skilled services and indicate the need for services with all three conditions. Services that are consistent with Medicare will be suggested.

Improving

When the medical condition is improving, direct service providers expect improvements in ability to function. Medicare uses medical necessity as admission criteria and states that "significant practical improvement in a reasonable period of time" must be expected (Foto, 1996). The Cognitive Disabilities Model interprets a significant improvement as an increase in a mode of performance, as measured as x.2 on the Allen Cognitive Level scale. The diagnosis and time since onset are used to estimate the natural course of the disease and the

expected amount of improvement on the ACL. Most improvements are expected within 3 to 6 months after brain surgery or injury. The treatment goals are stated as measurable functional outcomes (Allen, Earhart, & Blue, 1992, 1996; Allen, Earhart, Blue, & Therasoft, 1996).

Medicare uses a percentage to measure a decrease in the amount of physical and/or cognitive assistance. The general descriptions of the cognitive levels have been translated into consistency with the Medicare measures of assistance (see Appendix B). The need for physical assistance is for mental disorders with one global score and may be increased with physical disabilities. The length of the ACL scale provides a sensitive measure of small improvements that may be rapidly occurring and fluctuating with acute conditions. The interrater reliability of all therapists using the scale can be readily established by having two therapists independently fill out the rating sheets included in the Allen Battery assessments. Treatment methods include prompts for improvements in ability to function. Third-party payers are naturally skeptical about unreliable measures of improvement because of the temptation to inflate improvements to justify services. Therapists must be fair and objective in reliably assessing ADL improvements.

The natural healing process and medications may be the cause of the improvements. Third-party payers recognize alternative explanations for improvement. The Cognitive Disabilities Model does not hold therapists accountable for being the cause of improvement. The meaning of the improvement in terms of activity performance is explained by the therapist. Clients are discharged from skilled services when the client has returned to his or her premorbid level of function, when no more improvement in ability to function is expected, or when reports of improvement in ability to function are not having an impact on client care.

Stabilizing

"A safe and effective maintenance program" should be established when the medical condition has stabilized (Foto, 1996). Home programs are set up for people who must learn to live with a disability. There may be a slight fluctuation in the ACL score (4.2, 4.4, 4.2, 4.4, 4.4, 4.2), but the fluctuation is hovering around a baseline. To protect the client's safety, the home program is set up to match the person's ability to function, or for the lowest ability when function is fluctuating. The activities included in a home program are selected by the client and the caregiver. Common causes of accidents and injuries while doing activities have been analyzed to generate lists of safety concerns for each mode of performance (Allen, Earhart, & Blue, 1996; Allen, Earhart, Blue & Therasoft, 1996). The goal is to warn caregivers about possible problems that have a greater than ordinary chance of occurring. Caregivers are guided in providing assistance to protect the client and the community. The length of time that it takes to provide caregiver education often depends on the caregiver's capacity to learn and experience in providing assistance to a cognitively disabled person. Clients are discharged when activities can be done safely and are practical. If the therapists learns that the activities are unrealistic, unsafe, or not sustainable, the treatment goals should be changed or the client should be discharged.

Changing

A change in the home program can be expected when a change in the ACL occurs. Recovery and sparing may slowly occur with head injury or brain surgery, producing an improved ACL score. Progressive decline associated with Alzheimer's disease and dementia may slowly reduce the ACL score. When these changes are noted, a periodic reevaluation is indicated to see if a maintenance program needs to be modified (Foto, 1996). The safety lists should match the client's current mode of performance. Activities are still selected by the client and caregiver. When a change in ability to function is expected, caregiver education should include examples of behavior that indicate a need for another periodic evaluation and a new home program.

Paradigm Shift in Cognitive Rehabilitation

Much of current practice is driven by identifying problems and measuring improvement by a de-crease in the evidence of the problem. The problem-oriented record forced this paradigm on therapists. As a result, clients are confronted with what they cannot do. In the problem-oriented paradigm, treatment success is caused by the therapist's pushing the client to do better. If the client does not get better, it must be because the therapist was not skilled enough to get the client to try harder. A good therapist, in this oversimplified view of rehabilitation, will restore all clients to their pre-morbid level of functioning. The problem-oriented paradigm is easy to explain to the lay public and inexperienced students, but in reality the treatment sessions may be frustrating for the client and the therapist. The theoretical mistake is in viewing the therapist as the cause of improvement. If the improvement is going to happen anyway, there is no reason to push the client and make treatment uncomfortable. If the improvement is going to happen anyway, the number, duration, and intensity of the sessions may influence physical endurance but not influence the rate of cognitive recovery. Confrontations with one's problems makes people uncomfortable, and the reason for pushing people into irritating situations needs to be clearly stated.

Is there ever any reason to make the client uncomfortable? Yes, when the improvement would not happen anyway or would not be detected any other way. Improvements that would probably not happen anyway are increases in endurance, range of motion, and strength, and the discomfort should be within the limits of the client's tolerance for discomfort. Sometimes the therapist realizes that improvements are possible but really not necessary. Improvements are necessary when they affect practical aspects of the person's daily life and can be sustainable after discharge. Some improvements in the client's cognitive ability to function will not be detected unless the therapist probes for a higher mode. Probes are suggested in the Allen Battery for the next mode and can usually be evaluated in a few seconds. If the client can process the higher information, expectations are raised. If not, information at the current capacity is accepted. Prolonged probing for the next mode is not recommended because it creates unnecessary frustration and resistance to treatment. The mark of a good therapist is in knowing when it is necessary to push clients and reserving that skill for special circumstances. Most of the time therapists are able to use the client's remaining abilities to provide an opportunity to experience a sense of contentment.

The paradigm shift is from pushing people to overcome problems to helping people use their abilities. When improvements are happening anyway, therapists explain what the improvements mean in relation to the client's occupations. When *no* more improvements are occurring, therapy is *not* finished. Abilities need to be translated into a practical and sustainable home program. Caregivers need to be educated about the type of assistance the client will need now and what to look for in the future. Plans need to be made and verified to protect the client's safety in the discharge environments. Some of the most beneficial outcomes of skilled services are in knowing how to elicit remaining abilities in real life situations. The focus on causing improvements or reducing problems tends to result in confrontations with limitations, followed by premature discharge. Therapists have an opportunity to advocate for the client's right to use their remaining abilities safely, in the least restrictive environment. A paradigm shift that focuses on abilities is required to do that.

Awareness of a Disability

The subjective meaning of cognitive disability can have tremendous impact on whether or not the person benefits from remedial treatment methods. Awareness of a disability and anticipation of secondary effects are present at ACL 5.6 and 5.8. People with a mild disability have the best chance of generalizing and using remedial skills. Remedial skills teach exercises that must have some meaning. Anticipation of secondary effects is based on an abstract concept of what might happen. Generalization is an anticipation of how a problem might be avoided. To generalize, the person must be aware of a problem, anticipate when it might happen, and implement the remedial methods. Generalization is a high level, abstract mental process. Remediation is apt to be most effective when the person has some awareness of a problem and has some capacity to anticipate future problems.

Most clients are unaware of the extent and seriousness of their cognitive disability. Between ACL 5.0 and 5.4 most people are defensive and tend to blame other people, objects, or events for their difficulties. Learning is bound to the material objects they are working with and is not guided by abstract inferences about the properties of objects or events. If they are also blaming other people or objects for their problems, they see no reason for learning generalizable skills. Remedial skills may not be used consistently enough to be safe and effective. The therapist or a work supervisor will have to warn them about all potential dangers. Remedial skill training may be most effective in the client's permanent residence or work location, where dangers can be anticipated and controlled. Assistance with the application of encapsulated skills may be necessary in every activity where application is beneficial. The generalization is done by the therapist because the inferences required to see the benefits of the application are understood by the therapist, not the client. The mildly disabled are not able to anticipate safety hazards or secondary effects.

The defensiveness observed in level 5 is absent between 4.6 and 4.8, and there is no general awareness of a problem, only an isolated awareness of a need for assistance now. Between ACL 4.8 and 4.0, people are so bound to the perceivable moment that the thought of applying a generalizable skill does not make sense, even when explained to them. Remedial skills may be taught through repetitive drilling in exercises that are meaningless to the individual. In the beginning of training, remedial skills may not be spontaneously applied from one session to the next, using the same materials. Weeks and months or drilling may be required for rote performance using the same type of materials. These people are usually compliant and will tolerate tedious drilling. The outcome is a splinter skill that may be valued in a permanent placement or in isolated circumstances. When no practical value can be sustained outside the treatment setting, repetitive drilling is not recommended.

Environmental compensations can be made for those people who do not generalize or use remedial skills effectively. Environmental compensations are made by changing the way directions are given, providing adaptive equipment, and altering the environmental cues. The lists of abilities are used to analyze the mental structures required to do occupations. Directions and cues are modified to match the client's best ability to function. Directions and cues that are beyond the client's ability to understand must be eliminated. Caregivers are taught how to give directions and organize cues. The storage of self-care and household supplies and the removal of hazardous tools and toxins are listed safety concerns for each mode of performance. The most common causes of household accidents and injuries have been analyzed because they have a greater than average chance of occurring with a cognitive disability (Allen, Earhart, & Blue, 1996). Although these safety lists are quite long, the human environment is so varied that therapists should expect to encounter objects and events that have not been analyzed. When that occurs, therapists can use the lists of abilities to analyze additional objects and events. The lists of abilities give a partial understanding of what to expect in a new activity but will probably not predict everything that could possibly happen. Be alert for some surprises that could be dangerous. The safest environmental compensations are made by observing performance in the setting where the activity will be done.

Coordination with Other Scales of Global Ability

To coordinate occupational therapy services with other professionals, the ACL can be used in conjunction with other scales. The strongest correlations are expected with global scales of ability to function. Table 8-1 identifies expected associations. The needs for physical and cognitive assistance are the measures of improvement found in the Medicare Guidelines. The physical assistance codes (independent, standby, minimum, moderate, and total) are reported as percentages. The same terminology and percentages are used for the cognitive assistance codes (Medicare Guidelines: HCFA Pub.13–3). The intensity of assistance usually associated with the ACL is described in Appendix B. The degree of physical assistance is for a global cognitive disability, without a physical disability, like Alzheimer's disease. When a physical

disability is present, like a CVA, the amount of physical assistance expected will increase. This is a change in clinical reasoning for some therapists in cognitive rehabilitation. Assess the ACL first and determine how much of the need for physical assistance is explained by a global inability to function. Then increase the percentage of physical assistance according to additional physical impairments (hemiplegia, broken bone, nerve damage). The most severe and persistent needs for assistance are explained by global mental processes. Effective treatment methods and discharge plans are most apt to be determined by a sensitive global assessment of ability to function. Improvements in physical abilities can be limited by an inability to learn exercises and compensatory techniques.

For cognitive assistance, the percentages given by Medicare are 100, 75, 50, 25, 10, and 0, providing a 6-point scale. It is a 6-point scale because there are 6 rating criteria published in the Medicare Guidelines. While the numbers span from 0 to 100, the interrater reliability of the use of the intermediate numbers is not credible because criteria for their use do not exist. The ACL identifies 26 rating criteria that have been translated into the Medicare percentages to expand the Medicare scale. If you use the additional Medicare numbers (marked with * in Table 8-1), back them up with the ACL numbers.

The Rancho Head Trauma levels are commonly used with traumatic head injury, from signs of coming out of a coma (I) to mild head injuries (VIII). The ACL and the Rancho levels share a common origin: Piaget's description of the six sensorimotor stages of psychological development. The Rancho scale added two lower levels to describe coming out of a coma. The agitation described in Rancho level IV seems to be a symptom of recovery from head injury. The other descriptions seem to be closer to universal abilities that can be seen with other diagnostic categories (Hagan, 1982; Hagan & Malkmus, 1979).

The Global Deterioration Scale (GDS) was developed through observing the decline seen with Alzheimer's disease. The onset of the disease is so subtle that scores 1 through 3 are rarely seen by therapists. Scores 4 through 7 are frequently seen. This disease process is thought to be distinguished by memory problems (Reisberg, Ferris, Leon, &

Table 8-1
Comparison of ACL with Other Global Scales

ACL	Medicare Cognitive Assist.: %	Medicare Physical Assist: %	Rancho Head Trauma	GDS	FIM ADL	FIM Eat	GAS	GAF	Age
0.8	100	100	I			1			0–1 mo
1.0	99*		II						1–5
1.2	98*		III						4–8
1.4	96*	75				2			4–10
1.6	92*								4–10
1.8	88*	50				3			5–12
2.0	84*	25	IV	7					9–17
2.2	82*	15							10–20
2.4	78*	10		1			1–10		
2.6	75					4			12–23
2.8	70*							1–10	
3.0	64*		V				11–20	11–21	18–24
3.2	60*						21–30		
3.4	54*			6	2		31–40	21–30	
3.6	50				3	5	41–50		3 yr.
3.8	46*				4			31–40	
4.0	42*	8*	VI	5	5	6–7	51–60		4
4.2	38*				6–7				5
4.4	34*						61–70		6
4.6	30*		VII	4				41–50	
4.8	25						71–80		
5.0	22*	6*							7–10
5.2	18*	4*					81–90		11–13
5.4	14*	2*		3				51–60	14–16
5.6	10	0	VIII	2			91–100	61–80	17
5.8	6*							81–90	
6.0	0			1				91–100	18–21

*Percentages added to Medicare Guidelines to correspond to the ACL scores.

Cook, 1988). The ACL may be able to identify how information that captures attention is processed. The GDS may identify problems in not being able to remember what has been processed and stored.

The Functional Improvement Measure (FIM) was developed to measure the treatment effectiveness of rehabilitation (Hamilton, Granger, Sherwin et al., 1987). The FIM measures a reduction in the burden of care, as a percentage of effort that the client applies to doing an activity. Recent developments have added cognitive components, as improvements in verbal abilities. Eating and the other ADL are displayed in Table 8-1. Eating has a separate column because on the ACL scale eating is one cognitive level lower that the other ADL. Eating is the first activity that people can do when coming out of a coma and the last activity to fade away with progressive diseases. ADL, as described on the FIM, have a ceiling effect. A person may be independent in doing self-care activities but not be safe at home.

The Global Assessment in Function (GAF) is Axis V of the Diagnostic and *Statistical Manual of Mental Disorders* (DSM IV), 4th edition (1994). DSM IV deals with psychiatric disorders and the scale reflects the higher functional abilities seen with these populations. Independent living and role performance are common concerns that are addressed by the scale. *DSM III* used the Global Assessment Scale (GAS) in Axis V, but the ceiling was too low for mild psychiatric conditions (1980). The GAS is still used with the developmentally delayed.

Maturational Age (MA) is probably the most widely used scale and the easiest for the lay public to understand as a prediction of ability to function. MA does not account for past experience and prior knowledge, which must be factored in with adult onsets and older children.

Case Studies

The first four case studies will use the FIM and GDS because of their wide use in cognitive rehabilitation. The FIM is used to investigate admission and discharge criteria, so the ACL components will emphasize that clinical application. Treatment goals and methods that correspond with the GDS

will be used to illustrate setting up a functional maintenance program. Memory problems detected on the GDS will be used with the ACL to show how the two scales work together to validate discharge recommendations. The last case illustrates the use of the ACL to objectively understand a persistent disability with a psychiatric case.

Use of the ACL and FIM: Two Case Studies

The following two cases depict how the ACL and FIM can be used to describe the client's physical and functional abilities in activities across disciplines in a subacute rehabilitation setting. The scores obtained at admission and discharge will be highlighted to allow comparisons between the two scales. The two cases were selected to demonstrate common rehabilitation problems. Case 1 was admitted for a physical problem with an unknown cognitive problem that had a significant impact on his functional outcome. Case 2 is a left hemiplegia following a CVA, requiring two ACL scores. The cases are followed by a discussion of the two scales.

(1) Walter: Surprisingly Low ACL

This 82-year-old man was admitted to subacute rehabilitation to increase functional abilities following a bowel obstruction. He had a permanent colostomy installed for bowel management, with no other pertinent medical history identified in the chart. Prior to his acute bowel problems, Walter reported that he lived independently with his legally blind sister in an apartment with three front steps. He stated that he prepared his own meals, drove his car, and did the grocery shopping. There was no one available to verify his functional history. He planned to return home to live with his sister.

Initial Evaluation

Physical abilities were within normal limits for the upper extremities. Sitting balance was fair and standing/walking balance was poor related to lower body weakness and poor endurance. Walter had glasses and with these, his vision was within normal limits. No hearing aid was required for hearing within normal limits. Score on the LACLS was 3.8, alerting the therapist to potentially serious cognitive impairments.

Verification of the 3.8 ACL score was done during the next few days by observing performance in his ADL training program, observing performance with the Cognitive Performance Test activities, and having him do a placemat from the ADM. In all situations he was required to use familiar skills, integrate new information with material objects, and move his body in space and time. He knew he was in the hospital, day, and date. He could not remember his therapists' names or schedule of therapies, even when posted and repeatedly pointed out. Personally he was good-natured, co-operative, pleasant, and polite. With ADL re-training he needed step-by-step demonstrations, with no ability to initiate or formulate a sequence of steps. He would politely agree with the need to follow safety precautions, but retention of new information was very poor, requiring constant cueing to protect his safety.

The following ACL scores were completed by the occupational therapist. The FIM scores were completed by nursing (RN), physical therapy (PT), speech therapy (ST), and occupational therapy (OT). Major rating criteria are identified for each activity.

FIM	ACL	Activity: Rated Behavior
5	3.8	Eating: Independent with set-up and someone to initiate opening packages.
5	4.0	Grooming: Needs set-up for time of day to brush teeth, cues to shave sides of face, chin; cues to comb back of head.
4	3.8	Bathing: Needs set-up for time of day, supplies; cues to hidden areas, back, armpits, feet; cues to use supports for balance with supervision for safety.
4	3.8–4.0	Upper Body Dressing: Needs set-up for time of day; sequences self at a slower than normal rate. Needs adjustments of garments in back.
3	3.8	Lower Body Dressing: Needs set-up and help to adjust movements to don/fasten pants and put on shoes.
4	3.8	Toileting: Independent with urinal with occasional cues to fasten/zip pants.
5	3.8	Bladder Management: Set-up urinal.
1	4.0	Bowel Management: Total assistance. Knows he needs a colostomy but unable to understand explanation. Unable to monitor self for potential difficulties or learn new sequence of actions to care for unfamiliar device.
4	3.8	Transfers: Bed/Chair/Wheelchair: Needs contact guard to steady and cue to sequence of actions, lock wheelchair brakes, push up on arms to stand, steady self on rail and not grab onto caregiver.
3	4.0	Walk: Uses a front wheeled walker and needs constant cuing to avoid hazards for 50 feet. Needs flat surface and no pedestrian traffic.
2	4.0	Propel Wheelchair: Follows a straight line for 150 feet; Needs assistance of 1 person with corners, locking brakes, energy conservation.
2	4.0	Stairs: Needs assistance of one person to go up and down 4 to 6 stairs. Unsafe to use walker to transfer from stairs/safety rails.
3	3.8	Comprehension: Needs moderate prompting to verify discomfort and answer questions about basic daily needs. Nods head as if understanding new ADL verbal directions and requires motor cues to follow directions. Follows verbal cues to continue an action.
5	3.8	Expression: Able to articulate clearly but unable to express abstract or complex ideas.

FIM	ACL	Activity: Rated Behavior
5	4.0	Social Interaction: Friendly and pleasant. Social greetings and signs of rank are used. Needs cues to take turns.
2	3.8	Problem-Solving: Needed maximal direction more than half the time to initiate, plan, or complete ADL. 24 hour supervision to set-up supplies, complete steps, check results. He would think an activity was done with inadequate results. Does not remember new information or make new motor adjustments to safely compensate for physical impairments. Poor awareness of disability and potential long-term needs. Can not be depended on to ask for assistance when needed.
2	3.8	Memory: Able to recall familiar ADL sequences with cues but does not recall recent motor adjustments in ADL.

The FIM scores show a wide variation while the ACL scores are fairly consistent. The FIM is designed to reflect the increased burden of care when a part of the body is impaired. The pattern of performance is evident in the ACL scores. At admission, the higher ACL scores in a couple of activities is a good prognostic sign, suggesting that a higher ability to function may emerge.

Treatment

Walter was seen for 3 weeks by OT, PT, and ST to maximize functional abilities for returning home safely. His cognitive disability did have an impact on his ability to compensate for his physical impairment in all of his ADL. His endurance improved to a rating of fair, with good sitting balance and fair standing balance. He continued to require constant cueing to ambulate safely and effectively with a front wheel walker. Carry over of safety and energy conservation techniques was poor. His tolerance for sitting was 1 hour, and a standing tolerance of 10 minutes.

His ACL score did improve to 4.0, with the associated improvements in goal-directed activity performance. He was able to put pieces together to form a design or pattern, take turns, match visual cues, and sort silverware. He could remember the purpose of the activity and sequence himself through the steps. He recognized when he needed

help and asked for assistance. He prepared a simple, familiar stove top meal but required complete setup of supplies in visible locations, cues to turn stove on/off, and assistance to clean up.

OT and ST co-treated in a hands-on problem-solving environment using activities from the CPT and crafts from the ADM. Opportunities to really use reading comprehension, follow new instructions in new learning situations, and retain new information were provided. Because Walter was pleasant, with good social interactions and expression, performance in new activities that required comprehension, problem-solving, and memory were deemed essential to accurate discharge planning.

His ability to initiate and complete fundamental self-care improved as his energy and functional mobility increased, but he required repeated cueing and orientation to set himself up, including getting his clothing from the closet and drawers. He was unable to learn to use the usual long-handled dressing aids or the colostomy equipment. The difficulty he had in learning to do activities lead to the suspicion of a secondary diagnosis of dementia.

Functional Outcome

While some improvement on the FIM was noted, the following FIM and ACL scores raised serious questions about his plan to return home.

FIM	ACL	Activity: Behavior
5	4.0	Eating: Independent with setup. Asks for help to open packages
5	4.0	Grooming: Needs setup and cuing to unseen areas.

FIM	ACL	Activity: Behavior
5	4.0	Bathing: Able to initiate and complete practiced sequence with setup. Stands at sink to wash using counter top for support; sits to wash legs and feet. Refuses to shower, stating he never used one. Does not note wet floor.
5	4.0	Upper Body Dressing: Can get clothing with cues and sequences of self through dressing, at slower than normal rate, with assistance to adjust back.
5	4.0	Lower Body Dressing: While seated, initiates and completes sequence. When standing to pull pants up, needs setup and cuing for safety.
6	4.0	Toileting: Independent in using urinal and fastening pants. Uses grab bars for support.
6	4.0	Bladder Management: Stand at toilet or urinal.
1	4.0	Bowel Management: Total assistance to handle colostomy equipment.
5	4.0	Transfers: Requires supervision to lock brakes, lift foot rests.
4	4.0	Wheelchair: Propels self 150 feet over slightly uneven terrain, around corner, under table/sink. Needs assistance in tight spaces.
5	4.0	Front-Wheeled Walker: Walks minimum of 150 feet on flat surface with cues to unseen hazards. Does not look around while walking.
4	4.0	Stairs: Minimal contact assistance of 1 person and constant cues to sequence the use of safety rails, one action at a time, at slower than normal rate.
3	4.0	Comprehension: Recognizes the need for assistance and requires repeated cues and step-by-step demonstrations of compensatory ADL. Unable to follow written directions or diagrams.
5	4.0	Expression: "My legs feel better. I'll be OK at home." Able to clearly express self subjectively when addressed.
5	4.0	Social Interaction: Same as initial evaluation.
2	3.8–4.0	Problem-Solving: Able to sequence self through actions and sustain awareness of goal for the duration of the activity, but needs help to detect errors in new situations. Asks for assistance when he has a problem that interferes with mobility. Requires on-site supervision to recognize and correct other hazards.
2	3.8–4.0	Memory: Remembers over-learned self-care sequences. Short-term memory continues to be severely impaired with poor carry-over of new techniques to compensate for mobility and endurance. Requires prompting more than half the time.

After a home safety evaluation, it was determined that his mobility would not be safe in the home due to cognitive impairment and decreased endurance. There were many obstacles in rooms and doorways and a generally unclean environment. He also could not climb the front steps. He still requires total assistance with his colostomy and is not a candidate for device training. His sister cannot provide the necessary assistance to do ADL. The team recommended a skilled nursing facility near his neighborhood, with structured activities and a functional maintenance program.

Discussion

On admission this client looks like he needs to learn to manage his colostomy, but his reduced ability to learn is the major problem. No improvement in bowel management was made, as is predicted by his ACL score. The FIM is good at detecting the improvements that occurred in bathing, upper and lower body dressing, toileting, bladder management, transfers, use of the wheelchair/walker, and stairs. The goals and methods used to produce these improvements match the ACL score. Small improvements not detected by the FIM that were detected by the ACL include eating, comprehension, expression, problem solving, and memory. Grooming and social interaction stayed the same on both scales.

The scales in this case seem to reflect the intent of the authors. The FIM is designed to explain the benefits of rehabilitation services to people outside the agency. The ACL is designed to select treatment goals and methods that are most apt to be effective with a limited capacity to learn. This case illustrates a pattern of performance that experienced therapists use to select effective treatment methods. Because the scales were designed to fulfill different objectives about global ability to function, they can be used in a complimentary fashion.

The FIM seems to be sensitive to improvements in functional activities that are explained by a reduction in the need for physical assistance. The FIM detects physical improvements and their implications for reducing the burden of care that are not detected by the ACL. The ACL seems to be sensitive to small changes in cognitive ability that are not detected by the FIM. Physical Medicine and Rehabilitation has a tradition of emphasizing the need for physical improvements and reduction in the need for physical assistance. The cognitive problems that Walter has are not unusual, and should not be treated as a surprise. Cognitive problems should be screened for in all cases.

(2) Melvin: Two ACL Scores

Melvin was selected to illustrate the difference between verbal and motor abilities when there is damage to one hemisphere, but little or no damage to the other. Cerebrovascular Accidents (CVA) are the most common cause of two patterns of performance. A right CVA was selected because strong verbal abilities frequently mislead caregivers into thinking that little disability is present. Focal perceptual impairments and left neglect are frequently detected, but the impact that the damage has on global ability to function is poorly understood.

Melvin was a 72-year-old male with a medical diagnosis of 2 weeks status post Intracerebral Bleed resulting in left hemiplegia, decreased balance and endurance, and perceptual and cognitive impairments that severely interfered with his ability to function. He was bowel and bladder incontinent and required a nasogastric tube for nutrition due to

dysphagia. Medical history included diverticulitis and suspected prostrate carcinoma, for which he was scheduled for surgery. Prior to onset of the CVA, Melvin was independent for ADL, living in a one-story home without steps. He was right-hand dominant. He used to be a radio announcer and still enjoyed word games and other written and computer activities. His goal was to get his hands working so he could get back to his computer.

Initial Assessment

Physical abilities followed a common clinical picture. Passive range of motion was within normal limits for all extremities. The right side was within normal limits for strength, endurance, coordination, and sensation. The left arm was flaccid with severely impaired sensation cutaneously and kinesthetically, and the arm went into a flexion synergy when he yawned. The left leg had poor selective movement and increased extensor tone. Sitting and standing balance were poor. Endurance was fair minus. Vision was functional with his glasses and hearing was within normal limits.

Orientation was intact for person and place but not date. He knew he was in the rehabilitation unit and tried to cooperate with the therapists. He could be cued to check the clock and calendar to orient himself. Severe left neglect required cueing 75% of the time during activities. When doing activities he was extremely disorganized and distractible, easily frustrated, and agitated with labile affect.

A sticker card from the ADM was used to observe spatial and sequencing problems. As expected, he neglected the left side of the card. He also had trouble placing the stickers in a row, discriminating between the stickers according to size, shape, or color, placing stickers in the boxes printed around the perimeter of the card, and repositioning stickers when errors were identified. ACL score for the sticker card was 3.4. He knew he was supposed to be making a card and was aware of the trouble he was having doing a simple task. The experience seemed to be traumatizing; he became frustrated, agitated, and demanded to be taken to his room. He refused to attend Diagnostic Crafts for the next 2 weeks.

Potential motor apraxia and agnosia problems

were ruled out by observing self-care activities. He could discriminate between objects and use the associated action suggested by self-care supplies (washcloth and tooth brush). Self-care was consistent with ACL 3.4. Speech therapy reported more success with written and verbal tasks. His level of orientation, goal-directed questions, ability to remember some names and his awareness of his physical disability suggested a verbal ACL of at least 4.0, possibly even a 4.2. The initial ACL and FIM are listed below, with the ACL divided into verbal (ACL.V) and motor (ACL.M) performance.

FIM	ACL.V	ACL.M	Activity: Behavior
1		3.2	Eating: NG tube. Identifies knife, fork, spoon
2		3.4	Grooming: Needs stabilization to sit. Spontaneously grasps and uses correct repetitive action to comb, use electric razor, without noting effects. Needs cues to left side.
2 & 1		3.4	Bathing: Able to pick up washcloth and wash one spot of upper body or right side. Needs total assistance to wash right hand. Poor sitting balance and motor control required total assistance for lower body.
1		3.2	Upper Body Dressing: Able to grasp garment and attempt familiar action. Total assistance required to compensate for physical impairments.
1		3.0	Lower Body Dressing: Able to grasp garments while lying in bed. Total assistance required to compensate for physical impairments.
1	4.0		Toileting: Foley catheter and diaper. Unable to recognize need to void, but understood need for assistance.
1	4.0		Bladder Management: Relies on catheter.
1	4.0		Bowel Management: Relies on diapers and total assistance.
1		3.4	Transfers: Total assistance with 2 helpers. Aware of goal but unable to change actions needed for physical impairments. Becomes impulsive, anxious, and frustrated.
1		3.4	Walk/Wheelchair: Unable to walk. Propels wheelchair short distance with right arm, not foot. Needs cues to operate brakes with right hand and to look to the left 75% of the time.
2	4.2	3.4	Comprehension: Talks about inability to use left hand but unable to understand how limited actions affect activities. Distractibility requires re-direction to simple activities 50% of the time.
4	4.2		Expression: Melvin has a large vocabulary and uses it to articulate ideas related to basic daily needs. When distracted, he requires minimal prompts to re-focus conversation.
3	4.2		Social Interaction: When under stress or in unfamiliar situations he becomes frustrated and loses his temper without apology to staff or his wife. He interrupts others, relates conversation to self and demands assistance without regard for others.
1	4.0	3.4	Problem-Solving: Able to generate verbal directions for next step in familiar self-care tasks but unable to translate into effective motor sequence. He can say what to do, but cannot do it. Solved routine motor problems less than 25% of the time. Tended to do an associated repetitive action without looking at effects.
1	4.0	3.4	Memory: Recognizes and names a few staff members. Remembers goal of activity and verbally states next step. Cannot do next step in familiar ADL sequence or new motor action in simple activity/ADL without total assistance.

The distinction between verbal and motor abilities explains Melvin's problems with social interactions. When therapists asked him to do motor actions above his capabilities, he used his verbal abilities to defend himself. He could excuse his difficulties to do self-care and mobility activities with his recognition of his physical disability. The sticker cards removed the excuse, and the perceptual/cognitive problem was clear to the client and the therapist. Activities like bathing, dressing, and mobility were confounded by his loss of balance. Grooming was confounded by over learning or not caring. Crafts exposed the problem that was causing the frustration and lability.

Treatment

Twelve weeks of healing and rehabilitation were characterized by improvements in his lower extremities, decreased perceptual difficulties, and a decrease in the discrepancy between his verbal and motor abilities. At the time of discharge from sub-acute care his verbal ACL was 4.8 and motor ACL was 4.4 with glimmers of 4.6. He learned to use lists to compensate for decreased memory and anxiety. Lists were used to help him practice adaptive techniques for ADL. He learned to monitor the return of his visual spatial abilities with crafts. Despite verbal confirmations that he understood safety precautions, Melvin fell twice during the last week in trying to get out of bed to reach the telephone.

Functional Outcome

At the time of discharge his left arm had increased flexor tone but was edematous, painful, and non-functional. His wife was given a home program to minimize pain and prevent contractures. The result of improved activity performance are reported in the FIM and ACL scales.

FIM	ACL.V	ACL.M	Activity: Behavior
5		4.6	Eating: Needs setup and close supervision to decrease impulsivety while eating mechanical soft diet. Uses a rocker knife to cut.
5		4.4	Grooming: Needs setup and occasional cues to shave left side.
2 & 3		4.4	Bathing: Wife will bathe. Needs moderate assistance to bath impaired left arm. Requires bed bath and can roll from side to side for trunk and legs.
5		4.6	Upper Body Dressing: Requires setup and standby assistance for dynamic balance. Cuing for safety on edge of bed while following written step-by-step directions for one handed don/duff of pull-over shirt. Requires daily repetitive drilling to learn directions.
4		4.6	Lower Body Dressing: Needs setup and standby assistance to dress while lying in bed, with written directions to sequence steps. Uses Velcro to fasten shoes. Minimal assistance with fastening pants.
3		4.6	Toileting: Bowel incontinent and initiates requests to change diapers. Pulls up pants by bridging and rolling from side to side. After using urinal, requires assistance with fasteners.
4		4.4	Bladder Management: Uses urinal; needs assistance to empty.
4		4.4	Bowel Management: Incontinent.
4		4.4	Transfers: Requires intermitten cuing to set wheelchair brakes, minimal contact assistance to steady and identify hazards, 25% cuing to left side.
2 & 3		4.4	Walk/Wheelchair: Walks with a quad cane and 1 person 50 feet; propels wheelchair on right side a minimum of 150 feet with assistance in small spaces. Needs constant cuing to look around.

FIM	ACL.V	ACL.M	Activity: Behavior
1		4.4	Stairs: Needs 2 people to assist going up/down 4 stairs with cuing to left.
4	4.8	4.4	Comprehension: Understands and executes a written or verbal instruction specifying a single action. Requires prompting 25% of time to refer to written directions for dressing and recording thoughts to ease anxiety. Memorizes new directions by rote.
5	4.8		Expression: Ability to express basic daily needs clearly. Impaired ability to express complex or abstract ideas.
5	5.0		Social Interaction: Good when able to tell a narrative story without time constraints. Tends to argue, blame others for errors or refuses to do an activity if stressed, unfamiliar, or problematic.
3	4.8	4.4	Problem-Solving: Inflexible in following written directions about new information and seeks verification. Matches a sample for size, shape, color, 4 objects, linear measure, and direction. Able to self-detect errors from a sample and seek assistance. Poor problem-solving with three dimensional objects, new problems that require inferences or anticipation of primary or secondary effects. Cannot inhibit impulsive or dangerous actions.
4	4.8	4.4	Memory: Reads and follows a schedule without cues and follows inflexibly. Stores lists of new information related to an activity and verbally repeats 75% but does only 50%. Required 2 weeks of daily drilling with written prompts to learn adjustments in dressing self. Remembers supply locations day to day.

Melvin went home with his wife, who was educated in transfer techniques and proper body mechanics. Home health was to follow up with a trial of bowel control training and adapted use of his computer. A 3-in-1 commode and hospital bed were ordered. Social services recommended family therapy and respite care. Melvin still has a tendency to lose his temper when frustrated or to become labile. His wife was instructed on how to watch for signs of depression that he is at a greater than average risk for with his awareness of his loss of premorbid abilities and the need to adjust his daily activities.

Discussion

Melvin demonstrates the emotional turmoil that can accompany an awareness of a cognitive disability. When verbal abilities are better than motor abilities this pattern of awareness may be seen. Verbal propositional abilities provide the concepts necessary to compare current activities with past performance. The opposite is not apt to occur. When motor abilities exceed verbal abilities, the person is not apt to have the concepts necessary to form a catastrophic reaction.

Comparing ACL and FIM Scores According to the Two Case Studies

The ACL and FIM scores are displayed in columns so that the readers can see what a pattern of performance looks like. Patterns of ACL performance are usually pretty consistent. When one or two scores are higher than the rest, those higher scores may be a good prognostic indicator that ability to function will improve. The other likely explanation for a score that is higher than the rest is individual differences. If a high priority is placed on an activity or the person has done a similar activity a lot in the past, an isolated activity can be higher than the rest. This is not so apt to happen with the ADL reported on the FIM, because ADL are over learned. The consistency in the scores on the ACL are explained by the underlying mental processes. The underlying mental processes allow therapists to know what to expect from one activity to the next. Walter's scores are consistent across all activities. Melvin's pattern of performance is clarified by dividing motor and verbal mental processes. The FIM scores are not expected to be consistent because the scores respond to impairments of parts of the body.

As a measure of the severity of a disability, these two cases reveal a problem with the FIM. The two cases were not selected for this reason, but the problem was suspected. The problem is that not enough weight is given to the impact of a cognitive disability. The total scores for the ACL and FIM at admission and discharge are compared on Table 8-2. The FIM scores for Walter were 59 (admission) and 73 (discharge). Melvin's scores were lower: 24 at admission and 63 at discharge. At discharge, Melvin's FIM scores was worse than Walter's. However, Walter never could sequence himself through a modified activity, which is why he never learned to manage his colostomy. Melvin can use lists to learn a modified activity through repetitive drilling, which is why he is a candidate for bowel training. From this perspective, Melvin is not as disabled as Walter. A problem also exists in claims about the amount of improvement Walter made on the FIM. The behavioral descriptions suggest that very modest gains were made, and these gains might have been made in an even shorter length of stay. As a measure of the severity of a disability, the total scores for the ACL are nearly identical at admission: 66 and 65.8. A noticeable improvement is detected as discharge for Melvin (86.6) but not for Walter (68). The ACL numbers are saying that the severity of Walter's disability did not change much, but Melvin's did. The ACL numbers match the behavioral descriptions better than the FIM numbers. The FIM may be a better measure of the burden of care than the severity of a disability.

The low scores on the FIM (1-4) are rated by a percentage of effort and are presumed to be the percentage of physical effort. Attempts to correct the loading for physical effort have been made by adding the verbal activities to the FIM. These efforts have not gone far enough. The functional outcomes that rehabilitation professionals produce are obtained by teaching adaptations. These outcomes are primarily constrained by the client's incapacity to learn what is taught. A cognitive disability is a terribly onerous and persistent contributor to the severity of a disability and a constraint on functional outcomes.

Use of the ACL and GDS in Designing Maintenance Programs: Two Case Studies

The Global Deterioration Scale (GDS) is frequently used to guide functional maintenance programs in skilled nursing facilities. Rehabilitation professionals have been doing quarterly screenings on these residents and noting any decline in status or any potential for improvement in functional areas. Therapists establish baselines, design successful activities, and teach activity directors and designated nursing personnel how to carry out a maintenance program. Case 3 was selected to demonstrate how the ACL and the Allen Battery can be used with the GDS to design a functional maintenance program for a client with end-stage Alzheimer's disease. Case 4 looks at how memory problems influence the use of the ACL to make discharge recommendations.

(3) Louis: Functional Maintenance Program

Louis is 83 years old with a primary diagnosis of Alzheimer's disease and secondary diagnoses of Chronic Obstructive Pulmonary Disease and hypertension. Past medical history include pneumonia and tachycardia. Progressive decline during the last 2 months noted by nursing and the client's wife include: increased agitation (hitting, kicking, punching staff while trying to do care), decreased memory for recognizing loved ones, decreased and less intelligible verbalizations, bowel and bladder incontinence, and impaired functional mobility. The physician ruled out any new diagnosis and concluded the decline was probably an exacerbation of the Alzheimer's disease. Haldol was prescribed and an associated decrease in agitation and increase in cooperation has been observed without

Table 8-2

Total and Average Scores on the FIM and ACL for the Two Cases at Admission and Discharge

	Admission	Discharge
FIM		
Walter	59 (average = 3.47)	73 (average = 4.29)
Melvin	24 (average = 1.41)	63 (average = 3.5)
ACL		
Walter	66 (average = 3.88)	68 (average = 4.0)
Melvin	65.8 (average = 3.66)	86.6 (average = 4.56)

side effects. Tension is building between his wife and the nursing staff. His wife visits every day at lunch time and insists on feeding him, which he could do himself with setup and supervision. Then his wife tries to get him to brush his teeth, which he cannot do. When she yells at him to "try harder," Louis gets agitated and upset, leaving nursing with a disturbed client when his wife goes home. Conflicts like this often stimulate a referral to OT.

Initial Functional Assessment

The client has hearing aids in both ears, in good working order. Vision is within normal limits to do the following: locate food and cup, see a person across the room and return a wave, briefly manipulate objects, grab onto rails, bars, and furniture to stabilize self. Caregiver has to pry hands off of rails and bars despite repeated verbal prompts. Client is able to gesture and speak short phrases which are usually unintelligible and out of context. He inconsistently recognizes his wife. He is not ambulatory and spends time in a Gerichair that is too big and causes him to slide down and to the right at an awkward angle. Ability to function seems to decline while in the Gerichair: flattened affect, decreased recognition of his wife, no spontaneous movement, ACL = 1.6. With correct positioning in the Gerichair, he is able to hit, catch, and throw a ball and balloon, use bean bags to hit a basket. Spontaneous grasp and release of objects was tried but not observed. Appropriate positioning raised ACL to 2.8. A high-backed wheelchair and pummel cushion were ordered to maintain head/trunk alignment, hips in at 90 degrees of flexion, and improve level of functioning while sitting.

Louis stands with maximal assistance, grabs onto bars for stability while being bathed and dressed. His grasp of material objects is inconsistent: comb or washcloth held at eye level. Directives are required to push limbs through garments and sequence actions.

Louis picks up a spoon or cup and eats and drinks without being cued. Spills are not noticed and size of bits is not regulated. Eating is messy when he attempts to put food in open containers or other objects that distract him from eating. With a usually good appetite, he eats nearly 100% of his plate every day.

Best ability to function is ACL 2.8, which is apt to decline if poorly positioned. Glimmers of ACL 3.0 were seen with efforts to grasp grooming objects, suggesting that further improvements with consistent positioning might be possible. GDS score is 7: needs assistance to sit up correctly in a chair.

Treatment

After a few days, Louis was positioned in his new wheelchair, with noticeable improvements in his verbal and motor responses: gestures, smiles, and more consistent recognition of his wife. His cooperation with caregivers was accompanied by vocalizations that were largely unintelligible or out of context, but he seemed to enjoy the "conversation." The improvement that positioning made was explained to those who help him with bathing, dressing, and grooming. They were told to probe for ACL 3.0 by holding garments and supplies at eye level and encouraging familiar actions with hand-over-hand assistance. If he showed any signs of distress, they were to rescue him immediately by doing the action for him.

A role for his wife at lunch time was designed by teaching her how to reduce the distractions that created the messy eating. She agreed to sit at her husband's side out of his view, and wipe his mouth as needed. She would present the food items, one dish or course at a time, with packages opened and fluids poured in cups half full. She would precut any resistive food that escaped the kitchen uncut but give him an opportunity to cut with the edge of his spoon. She would also bring a favorite food item each day (e.g., nectarine) and give it to him at the end of the meal. The food item always brought a favorable response and gave them a chance to connect. The difficulties in using a toothbrush and other previously familiar objects were explained to her, and she agreed to ask the nurses before she tried anything new. The nursing staff was taught the same food and environmental compensations. Both she and the nursing staff were pleased with the arrangement as it met everyone's needs and did not distress the client.

When proper positioning in the wheelchair was consistent, best ability to function was tested. Cues ranged from ACL 3.0 to 3.4. His ACL score increased from 2.8 to 3.2 in the first session with the new wheelchair. He used a washcloth to wash his hands, put clothespins on a stick, randomly placed pegs in holes, and did not put as many things in his mouth as he had in the past. As treatment progressed the therapist also discovered that he could draw by following a contrasting line on paper. When his wheelchair brakes were unlocked, he could push and pull against the edge of the table in a gentle and soothing rocking motion. He seemed to enjoy catching, batting/throwing objects and using bean bags best of all. He could sustain an active interest in these types of activities for 15 to 20 minutes until he became distracted or uncomfortable.

Functional Maintenance Program

The activities director was provided with the following list of activities that Louis could successfully in his wheelchair. These activities provide maximal cognitive assistance to initiate and sustain actions and sequence the steps of the activity. The goals were selected to match his best ability to function and individualized from those suggested for his mode.

Goals:

A) Client will give expected functional response to interact with objects and people 75% of the time with signs of increased comfort and enjoyment as evidenced by cooperation to complete activities, relaxed and engaged mood, increased affective range(smiling), and increased verbal responses.

B) Client will preserve muscle strength, endurance, and maintain bone integrity by participating in two activities daily for at least 15 minutes.

Methods:

With verbal directives and demonstrations:
Rhythmic activities for both hands (scarf. Towel, plastic tube).
Bean bags to toss at a target.
Songs with associated actions (clapping, swaying, foot tapping/stomping)

Ball positioned to kick.
Safe objects to grasp, release, throw, hit.
Objects to use in a back and forth motion (pen, pencil, sandpaper, brush)
Familiar objects to name (Reminiscing boxes, magazine, scrap book).
Household objects to name and handle.
Demonstration to imitate active range of motion.

Interdisciplinary Care Plan

The problems were selected from the those identified in the client's chart. The goals and approaches match his best ability to function. Goals and methods are suggested in Allen, Earhart, & Blue (1996) and individualized for the client as follows.

Problem #1: Bathing, grooming and dressing deficit due to cognitive and physical impairments related to medical condition.

Goals:

A) Client will maintain stability, grasp self-care objects, and do familiar back and forth actions with hand-over-hand assistance and directives to perform bathing, oral hygiene, and grooming.

B) Client will maintain stability, grasp, and begin correct actions to put on familiar garments with cueing.

C) Client will cooperate with care giver assistance to complete bathing and dressing safely 100% of the time.

Methods:

A) Position in wheelchair or shower chair; offer washcloth, comb, toothbrush and tooth paste at eye level, initiate familiar back and forth motions. Provide physical guidance and assistance as needed to complete actions.

B) Position in wheelchair. Hand garment to client and direct to move when appropriate, providing physical guidance and assistance as needed to complete actions.

C) Prevent falls be removing unstable furniture that might be grabbed onto for support.

Prevent confusion and resistance by allowing plenty of extra time to change from sit to stand and feel secure in new position.

Prevent reduced circulation by dressing in loose fitting clothes and checking for skin redness.

Disciplines: Nursing and occupational therapy.

Problem #2: Self-feeding deficit due to severe cognitive impairments related to medical condition.

Goal:

Client will initiate and sustain actions to use spoon, cup to feed/drink safely to provide adequate nutrition/hydration 100% of the time with setup and supervision.

Methods:

A) Open packages, pour liquids, precut resistive food into bite-size pieces, put bib on.

B) Present one course at a time, in front of client.

C) Provide opportunities to cut soft food with edge of spoon.

D) Prevent choking by removing non-edibles from mouth, monitoring size of bites scooped on spoon, avoiding stringy or hard to chew foods.

E) Prevent spills by filling cup half full.

F) Prevent burns by restricting access to hot foods and fluid until cool.

G) Allow wife to assist with the above process with supervision.

Disciplines: Nursing, dietary, and occupational therapy.

Discussion

The GDS gives the therapist a rough idea of how well the client is functioning, but it is not sensitive to smaller changes in ability. The difference that proper positioning made in his ability to eat and cooperate with self-care is detected by the ACL. The ACL provides the goals and methods that are apt to be effective for the even numbered modes of performance. Sufficient detail is given to spell out the approaches to client care that can be understood by caregivers who may not have much training or experience. The functional maintenance program contains goals and methods that are environmental compensations for residual cognitive disabilities.

(4) Maud: Memory Problems

Memory problems can be focal or global deficits. Amnesia is a focal deficit that does not usually affect global ability to function, and is rarely seen by therapists. The memory problems associated with Alzheimer's disease are global, making assessment and discharge recommendations difficult. The following case was selected to demonstrate how a global memory problem can be added to the ACL score as an additional impairment.

Maud is 74 years old with a primary diagnosis of Alzheimer's dementia with delusions. Diagnosed with Alzheimer's disease 5 years ago, she has been living alone, with the family checking in on her. She has been driving, cooking, and attending church activities. Prior to admission to subacute rehabilitation, she was in a psychiatric unit for 10 days, her first psychiatric admission. Her first psychotic episode included severe agitation, paranoid delusions, suicidal ideation, depressed mood, and confusion. She was started on a trial of Respiradol and Buspar. Having never received psychiatric care before, the family was interviewed for a history of mental illness. Maud has a life-long behavior pattern consistent with hypomanic features and an aunt with Bipolar Disorder. The transfer to subacute rehabilitation was for further titration of her medication and discharge planning. The family hopes that she will be able to return home.

The initial ACL is to assist with medication titration, expecting further improvements in her ability to function as the medications take effect. Once the ACL stabilizes, it will be time to think about the discharge plan.

Initial Evaluation

No physical impairments were noted: vision and hearing were within normal limits; very strong and mobile. Too mobile, in fact. During the first 2 nights she climbed over the bed rails and wandered through the halls looking for her daughter and making attempts to leave the facility. Her mood was very labile, changing quickly from elevated and smiling to irritable and anxious without identifiable provocation. Retention of new information was no more than 5 seconds, when attention could be focused. No paranoid or suicidal ideations were reported.

Her initial ACL score was made by observing ADL performance on the unit as she refused to talk to the therapist. She was not goal-directed, could not initiate, sequence, or complete familiar self-care actions, refused to shower or change her clothes, and ignored safety warnings. She frequently rifled through her roommates drawers, taking things and misplacing things in odd places. ACL = 3.4; GDS = 6, and these scores are consistent with each other.

Progress at 1 Week

Nursing reports that Maud has less anxiety, no lability and is generally cheerful, with good social and verbal skills. She recognized and enjoyed visiting with her daughter but still does not know where she is in time and space. She has agreed to change her clothes before retiring at night and has stopped trying to leave the facility. She continues to be severely disoriented, thinking that she is at home, work, on her way to a social event and frequently looking for her purse and car keys. GDS = 5, slightly improved.

Occupational therapy observations in ACLS, self-care and ADM projects obtained a score of ACL = 4.4. While showering, she was cooperative with redirection and assistance to cue for safety hazards. She could do the rest of her self-care independently with setup and cueing to initiate. She does not initiate a self-care routine, which is lower than would be expected at ACL 4.4. A slight improvement in short-term memory was seen in her ability to sustain a goal for about 10 to 15 minutes to get dressed, do a craft project, and collate papers. Attention span at ACL 4.4 in usually one hour. Memory aids were not used: the calendar placed in her room and a schedule of her activities

were not referenced or remembered. Topographical orientation is improving: she can find her bedroom door with her name on it and her bed, when within 100 feet. While she shows ACL 4.4 abilities, her memory problems are having a detrimental affect on her performance.

Progress at 2 Weeks

Maud's mood stabilized into a cheerful, slightly elevated and playful affect, without anxiety. Her GDS score also stabilized at 5, with severe disorientation in time and space. The ACL score showed a few glimmers of 4.6, but these abilities are not functional given her memory problems. She still cannot remember what she is doing longer than 15 minutes, and use of memory aids has not improved. Self-care still must be initiated for her and she needs standby assistance to solve new problems in self-care and craft projects from the ADM. Her cheerful mood reflects her comfort in a facility that protects her safety and gives her the cues she needs to use her best ability to function. Because of her memory problems, it was determined that she should continue living in a facility with 24 hour supervision and a functional maintenance program.

(5) Charles: Small Changes in a Chronic Disability

Schizophrenia produces a global disability that gets better and worse form time to time. The most frequent cause for getting worse is thought to be a common problem with poor compliance in taking medications. Even when the medications are taken, some people get worse for known and unknown reasons. During an acute hospitalization a small change in ACL score may be seen, but there seems to be a ceiling on how much better many of these people will get. The modes seem to be sensitive enough to detect a slow, progressive decline over a period of a few years. The following case was selected to illustrate the persistence of the affects of this disease.

Charles was 42 years old and had his first break at the age of 23, after 2 years in college and a tour in the Army. His delusions center around a belief that the Vietnamese put a bullet in his head, and the bullet is used by the Vietnamese to control his thoughts. Between the ages of 23 to 32 he lead a nomadic existence, hitchhiking around the western states and going in and out of private and public psychiatric hospitals. At age 32, he was hospitalized in this facility and started on prolixin, which is given as a shot and released over a period of 2 weeks. At the time of admission he was agitated, bordering on violent (punching walls) with paranoid delusions. The retrospective chart review suggested that he was a ACL 4.0 when first seen in OT and stabilized at ACL 4.4 at discharge. A prolixin shot has been given every 2 weeks by his doctor, who has maintained him as an out-patient, with minimal delusions and no agitation unless he drinks beer. Beer makes him uncontrollable, and he has hit a few people, but not so severely as to require hospitalization or an arrest. He has been maintained in the community, living first in a board and care, then with his mother, alone in an apartment, and currently with his girl friend and her mother. He has not been able to work or attend school for any extended period to time since his first onset. He is supported by Social Security Insurance and a caring mother, who is active in the Alliance for the Mentally Ill.

A new psychotropic drug that has fewer side effects and reports of improving ability to function is being tried (Olazibine). The affects are being monitored in outpatient OT 3 times a week for 3 weeks. On admission he preferred the seat selected by many paranoid clients, which is at a small table in a distant corner where the rest of the group can be observed with little social interaction. Admission ACLS score was 4.5. While fringing the ADM placemat he was able to adjust the pressure (ACL = 4.6) but was unable to cross the midline (ACL = 4.4). During the second week he started sitting at the larger table with other clients and would stop working to talk to them, and he offered to get a cup of coffee for a lady in a wheelchair. Social conventions were followed in a courteous, pleasant manner with a few hints on spontaneity. Performance on the ADM projects was a steady ACL = 4.8 during the third week. When asked, he said that the new drug was better because "it is easier for me to think." He thanked the therapist for seeing him and said he had really enjoyed

making the projects. The meaning of the change was documented and explained to the treating physician.

Discussion

The ACL scale had to be lengthened to pick up these small changes in ability to function. As with this case, many small changes do not influence the social/welfare supports that clients require. The changes are, however, experienced as important to the quality of life of the client and their loved ones. The ACL can be used to validate a small change and guard against the temptation to hope that a whole new life style is now possible. The hopes, wishes, denial, and rationalizations that surround the implications of a cognitive disability can be very emotional. The case illustrates how the ACL can be used to objectively clarifying the meaning of small changes in the severity of a disability.

Note about the Case Studies

These cases were selected to reflect common clinical observations. Admission and discharge measures were highlighted in the first two cases. The use of a sensitive scale to select and explain treatment methods was the focus of the last three cases. Confounding variables were left out, but in reality they are always present. Therapists use their conceptual models to help explain confounding variables.

Theory Development

The recognition of similarities between Piaget's description of the stages of sensorimotor development and the mental processes that guided the performance of psychiatric patients formed the first step in knowledge development (Allen, 1982; Ginsberg & Opper, 1969). The need to develop a conceptual model was identified by two factors: difficulties in explaining the value of psychiatric occupational therapy and the deinstitutionalization of the chronically mentally ill. In 1975 and 1976 the Executive Board of the American Occupational Therapy Association sponsored a mental health task force to study the problems in that area of practice. As the chair of the task force, Allen thought that the difficulties could all be traced to weaknesses in the literature. The unique knowledge and skill of the psychiatric occupational therapist was ambiguous, at best. At the same time, the homeless effects of deinstitutionalization were becoming apparent in California. The mentally ill would leave their board and care homes and opt to live on the street. By 1980, 15 to 20 thousand mentally ill were thought to be living on the streets of Los Angeles. Many of them rotated through Los Angeles County/University of Southern California Medical Center's Psychiatric Hospital, where the model was developed. The model emerged in a social context that often denied, or had trouble explaining, the presence of a cognitive disability. The need to educate people about the disability and put the necessary protections in place was the primary motivation. Occupational therapists were thought to be a prime profession for assuming this responsibility because they were practically the only group watching what the clients were doing.

The titration of psychotropic drugs provided a natural laboratory for observing people who were getting better and worse, which was the primary topic in team meetings led by biologically oriented psychiatrists. Impressive studies demonstrating biological correlates with psychiatric diseases led to a rejection of psychoanalytic explanations and an acceptance of a disease model. The disease model provided an opportunity to dispense with the mind/body split that had separated occupational therapy into those treating the physically disabled and those treating the mentally ill (Allen, 1985). The potential for unification was there, but it took a decade to figure out how to organize the knowledge. Several efforts were made to get physical and cognitive disabilities on one scale, and finally succeeded (see Table1). The trick was to measure the cognitive disability first, which gives a certain amount of physical disability, and then add any other physical problems. To broaden application from psychiatric and dementia cases, a view of function was required that incorporated cognitive and physical disabilities.

The research studies helped to sort through the huge number of psychological performance components suggested by developmental and cognitive psychology. The limitations of following a developmental frame of reference became apparent by comparing control groups to disabled populations. There are some similarities and many differences between normal populations and disabled populations. The limitations of disabled people suggest psychological mechanisms that are assumed in healthy subjects. The psychological mechanisms that disabled adults are able to use needed to be identified, prioritized, and classified according to their influence on everyday activities. Cognitive psychology suggested many mechanisms that were related to academic performance or beyond the capacity of many disabled people. Borrowing concepts from developmental and cognitive psychology has its limitations, because accidents of nature involve a unique set of psychological mechanisms.

While a lot was learned from leather lacing, the screening test was never meant to be an outcome measure. The clinical use of the measure suggested the need to expand the scale and to develop additional assessments.

The first efforts to organize the assessments after leather lacing were the Expanded Activity Analysis (Allen & Earhart, 1987), the first version of the RTI, and the CPT (Burns, 1992), using the six cognitive levels. The modes made it necessary to change the activity analysis, design, instructions, and rating of craft projects and the RTI (Allen, Earhart, & Blue, 1993). The RTI and the CPT made it necessary to better explain "best ability to function" and "patterns of performance." The emphasis on functional outcomes heightened an awareness of a need to deal with safety in long-term care situations. All of this needed to occur within a conceptual framework that accounted for individual differences without sacrificing group data. The framework outlined above is an effort to respond to the research findings and clinical needs. The deficiencies in standardized testing procedures required a new philosophy of science that was built into the ADM. A lot of effort has gone into the measurement of ability to function. The reasoning was that reliable, valid, and sensitive measurements needed to be established before any questions about treatment effectiveness could be addressed. Finally we have enough tools to begin to look at these questions. More comprehensive assessments will probably be required. The discussion turns to how future measurements and associated treatments might be developed.

Unresolved Theoretical Concerns

Developing a theoretical base that would look at the subjective experiences of the whole person to improve the quality of life of a cognitively disabled person has met many obstacles and few resources. Whole fields of study that seem like they ought to be beneficial to cognitive rehabilitation are often deficient when it comes to assessing and improving everyday life of the cognitively disabled. The quality of life is a subjective experience, but subjective experiences have been outlawed in many disciplines during the 20th century. Modern science has emphasized standardized tests that inhibit flexibility. Gradually these problems are being recognized and efforts are being made to resolve them. The following is a review of some of the obstacles and projections of future theoretical developments, with some personal opinions about bodies of knowledge that have not been worth the time and effort, and those that have been a marvelous help.

Learning

Behavioral psychologists placed a taboo on conscious thoughts, feelings, and beliefs. The meaning of an activity to the individual and their loved ones gets lost in the stimulus-response approach to conditioning. Some treatment techniques, like chaining, have been taken from this body of knowledge but hardly seem to be worth the trouble it takes to find them. The work of behavioral psychologists has not been very helpful in the quality of life because their field of study has been so narrowly defined.

Piaget's work on the process of adaptation, using the equilibrium principle to define assimilation and accommodation and explain how learning occurs, has been disappointing too (Haroutunian, 1983). Struggling to understand Piaget's interpretation of the equilibrium principle was not worth the effort because it did not help improve a person's ability to function. Learning may be pro-

grammed into the child's genetic material, and the ability to learn may be followed by teachers and developmental psychologists, but they do not know how to cause a change in the capacity to learn. They can measure associated changes in development, but their methods are not causal. Maturational age can provide a sequence for the development of abilities that are cross-cultural and universal. Many of the abilities that humans take for granted—bipedal walking, communicating, flexible tool use, and anticipating secondary effects—are very complex. Development of complex, universal abilities is probably genetically transmitted and not taught. When normal development does not occur or severe brain pathology removes these abilities to learn, we do not know how to teach the development of complex, universal abilities. Developmental psychology has been used to help identify a sequence of abilities, but occupational therapy must develop its own change in ability to learn.

The developmental sequence can be used to monitor changes while they are occurring. The natural course of the disease can be used to determine whether the ability to function is apt to get better or worse and the rate in which change may occur. For more than a decade Allen has looked for, but not found, a credible theory of learning that could guide therapists in raising a person's ability to function. Without a theory of learning, therapists can follow changes in the biological condition but are uncertain about how to cause change in the complex capacity to learn. The sad fact is that the capacity to learn can reach a limit, which is not normal, and no more improvement will occur. At that point, it is time to set up a home program and do caregiver education so that remaining abilities can be used in the least restrictive environment. When the ceiling has been reached, and under what conditions therapists should say that has occurred are uncertain and need to be clarified.

Remediation and Environmental Compensations

Psychoanalysts assumed that the brain could heal itself by changing what a person thinks or does.

Sigmund Freud's assumption is firmly entrenched in cognitive rehabilitation with the remedial approaches, which assume that the brain can repair or reorganize itself (Neistadt, 1990). The assumption turned out to be incorrect with major psychiatric diseases. What happens if it is also incorrect in cognitive rehabilitation? The alternative is an adaptive approach, which is implemented through environmental compensations. Some natural healing does occur after brain injury, and some associated improvement in ability to function will probably occur. This theoretical base assumes that some improvements will happen anyway, especially with a recent onset. Other biological explanations for change in ability to function are acknowledged. What the person thinks or does may, or may not, enhance these biological explanations for changes in ability to function. A scale is required that can be used as a sensitive measure in controlled studies to find out which improvements in ability to function really do happen anyway. For changes that would happen anyway, do occupational therapy services influence the rate or amount of change? If the answer is no, (and I suspect the answer is yes and no) environmental compensations are important things for therapists to do. What is required is a measure that is sensitive enough to detect both types of change, the ones that will happen anyway and the ones that therapists produce. It is hoped that the length of the ACL scoring criteria will be sensitive enough to detect small but important changes that would not happen anyway.

The psychoanalytic assumption leads to addressing a question that may turn out to be of no practical importance to occupational therapists. The choice between remediation and environmental compensation should not be based on ambiguous beliefs about how the brain may or may not repair itself. The choice between treatment methods should be based on the functional outcome for the client. The ACL can be used to measure the outcome with the functional activities described in the RTI. Therapists do not need to wait for a better understanding of what is happening with the biology of the brain. Therapists can observe behavior and see if performance is improving or not. The concern about the biology of the brain may be misleading, diverting attention away from functional outcomes.

Our guess is that the client's lack of understanding of a cognitive disability is a major obstacle for both remediation and environmental compensation. That is why the Cognitive Disabilities Model focuses on caregiver education. A sustained functional outcome may depend on the long-term care giver. To select treatment methods therapists should look at the environmental circumstances required to sustain improvements.

The study of a decline in ability to function is not a popular topic. Gerontology indicates that most of the decline associated with aging occurs after the age of 85. Progressive diseases are the other known cause of decline. This decline is acknowledged, and as it occurs assistance should be provided in setting up a new home program and providing caregiver education. A periodic evaluation for establishing a different maintenance program is needed whenever there has been a decline in the overall pattern of performance. As the risks for accidents and injuries increase with a decline in ability to function, more needs to be learned about effective preventions.

Human Thoughts and Feelings

In a strange way, the theory of natural selection has been detrimental to the understanding of everyday activities. The evolutionary adaptiveness of behavior has the behavioral and biological scientists stuck on reproduction and child rearing activities. Other activities that are important to humans and animals are given scant attention When the criteria for the correctness of a point of view are limited to such a narrow range of activities, as reproduction and childrearing, the theory has little to offer about the quality of life. A new theory of evolution is needed that deals with a broader range of activities, social relations, and the creative use of the mind. Stories of evolution could offer more information about the historical use of the mind, but the intentional and creative elements of thinking are ignored by natural selection (Ingold, 1993). As this problem gains recognition, there is hope that biologists will have more to offer about our understanding of human nature.

Neuropsychological concepts tend to dominate much of cognitive rehabilitation. The problem is that neuropsychology is driven by its own agenda. Luria (1966) for example, was interested in identifying the relationships between functional brain systems and local brain lesions. Occupational therapists are interested in the actions, activities and roles that people want to do. Occupations are a complex combination of both discrete and indistinguishable functions of the brain. The neuropsychological approach was rejected because its purpose is to understand the biology of the brain as related to the parts of behavior that can be isolated. Occupational therapy must develop its own unique approach to understanding how the disabled brain integrates information to guide everyday occupations.

Cognitive psychology expanded the stimulus-response used in behavioral psychology to include an input, throughput, and output for information processing. The trouble is that all the throughputs tend to be in pieces, as attributes of thinking. These parts of thinking are not put together but are scattered like pieces of a jigsaw puzzle. To understand others we need to know how they think and feel, to know what life is like subjectively. Behavioral scientists have avoided subjective mental experiences, and one seldom sees much about what is intended, believed, thought, felt, wished, or desired (Griffin, 1992). The subjective experiences of a conscious individual must be addressed to help people obtain a meaningful quality of life. Much of cognitive psychology was not helpful because the relationships between an attribute of thought, a subjective experience, and a functional activity are unknown. The notable exception is the work of Anderson (1992), who did a wonderfully informative synthesis of developmental and cognitive psychology, getting both fields of study down to their essential elements. His work is used to articulate an underlying information processing system.

Anthropologists and ethologists have created a vast literature about cultural and animal differences and have recently begun to look at similarities. Human universals are especially useful in suggesting potential behavioral norms. Culturally biased value judgments can be avoided through the identification of universal human behaviors. Comparing the cognition of humans to other species has not been as productive because consciousness has been avoided in comparative cognition (Roitblat, 1987). Disciplines that avoid consciousness do not have much to say about the quality of life. Ethology is struggling to deal with consciousness, and many of the issues raised concerning how animals feel and think are instructive (Griffin, 1992). The studies of primate thinking have identified so many differences between humans and monkeys that primate skills had to be excluded from the theoretical base (Cheney & Seyforth, 1990; Gibson & Ingold, 1993).

The study of disabled cognition presents therapists with a unique database. The mental structures that disabled humans use to do ordinary occupations provide an excellent means for understanding the complexity of human thoughts and feelings. Our favorite "body and knowledge" comes from what has been learned from observing clients and asking them questions about what they are thinking.

Conclusion

The clinical judgment required to apply the Cognitive Disabilities Model requires an understanding of how changes in ability to function are influenced by changes in the medical condition of the client. While the medical condition is changing, the therapist's expertise is required to explain how various medical conditions do, and do not, influence overall ability to function. Once the medical condition has gotten as good as it is going to get for now, the therapist sets up a functional maintenance plan. A good maintenance program needs to be realistic, relevant, and sustainable. The person's ability to function determines what is realistic. From a list of realistic activities, the client decides what is relevant. Activities that are sustainable are often determined by the caregiver assistance that is available. Caregiver education is an important part of setting up a sustainable functional maintenance program.

Therapists use their knowledge to provide a way of understanding how a mentally disabled person is feeling and thinking. Therapists understand the versatility of the mind that remains intact: a mind that can perceive the moment, draw on memories of prior knowledge, and anticipate future events. As long as the person is awake and out of a coma, therapists assume that subjective thinking and feelings guide behavior, no matter how simple the action. As long as the CNS is working there is some understanding of objects and events. No matter how confused and distorted the person's logic is at times, therapists can reach for and find positive efforts that make sense. A good intention for doing an action, activity, or role can always be found and taught to other caregivers.

References

Allen, C. K. (1982). Independence through activity: The practice of occupational therapy (psychiatry). *American Journal of Occupational Therapy, 36*, 731–739.

Allen, C. K. (1985). *Occupational therapy for psychiatric diseases: Measurement and management of cognitive disabilities.* Boston: Little, Brown.

Allen, C. K. (1987a). Occupational therapy: Measuring the severity of mental disorders. *Hospital and Community Psychiatry, 38*, 140–142.

Allen, C. K. (1987b). Eleanor Clarke Slagle Lectureship–1987: Activity, occupational therapy's treatment method. *American Journal of Occupational Therapy, 41*, 563–575.

Allen, C. K. (1988). Cognitive Disabilities. In S. C. Robertson (Ed.), *Focus: Skills for assessment and treatment.* Bethesda, MD: American Occupational Therapy Association.

Allen, C. K. (1989a). Treatment plans in cognitive rehabilitation. *Occupational Therapy Practice, 1*, 1–8.

Allen, C. K. (1989b). Psychiatry. In T. Malone (Ed.), *Physical and occupational therapy: Drug implications for practice.* Philadelphia: Lippincott.

Allen, C. K. (1990). Development of a research tradition. *Mental Health Special Interest Section Newsletter.* Bethesda, MD: American Occupational Therapy Association.

Allen, C. K.(1991). Cognitive disability and reimbursement for rehabilitation and psychiatry. *Journal of Insurance Medicine, 23*, 245–247.

Allen, C. K. (1994). Creating a need-satisfying, safe environment: Management and maintenance approaches. In C. B. Royeen (Ed.), *AOTA self-study Series: Cognitive rehabilitation.* Bethesda, MD: American Occupational Therapy Association.

Allen, C. K. (1996). *Allen cognitive level test manual (with kit included).* Colchester, CT: S & S/Worldwide.

Allen, C. K., & Allen, R. E. (1987). Cognitive disabilities: Measuring the social consequences of mental disorders. *Journal of Clinical Psychiatry, 48*, 181–191.

Allen, C. K., Earhart, C. A., & Blue, T. (1992). *Occupational therapy treatment goals for the physically and cognitively disabled.* Bethesda, MD: American Occupational Therapy Association.

Allen, C. K., Earhart, C. A., & Blue, T. (1993). *Allen Diagnostic Model manual.* Colchester, CT: S & S/Worldwide.

Allen, C. K., Earhart, C. A., & Blue, T. (1996). *Understanding the modes of performance.* Ormond Beach, FL: Allen Conferences, Inc.

Allen, C. K., Earhart, C. A., Blue, T., & Therasoft. (1996). *Allen cognitive level documentation (software).* Colchester, CT: S & S/Worldwide.

Allen, C. K., Foto, M., Moon-Sperling, T., & Wilson, D. (1989). A medical review approach to Medicare outpatient documentation. *American Journal of Occupational Therapy, 43*, 793–800.

Allen, C. K., & Robertson, S. C. (1993). *A study guide of occupational therapy treatment goals for the physically and cognitively disabled.* Bethesda, MD: American Occupational Therapy Association.

Alsberg, D. (1987). *Safety implications of cognitive disabilities: Using cognitive theory as an adjunct to discharge planning.* Unpublished master's thesis: Rush University, Chicago.

American Psychiatric Association. (1980) *Diagnostic and Statistical Manual of Mental Disorders: DSM III* (3rd ed.). Washington, DC: Author.

American Psychiatric Association. (1994). *Diagnostic and Statistical Manual of Mental Disorders: DSM IV* (4th ed.). Washington, DC: Author.

Anderson, M. (1992). *Intelligence and development: A Cognitive theory.* Cambridge, MA: Blackwell.

Averbuch, S., & Katz, N. (1988). Assessment of perceptual cognitive performance comparison of psychiatric and brain injured adult patients. *Occupational Therapy in Mental Health, 8*, 57–71.

Breeding, C. J. (1993). Performance of six to nine year old children without disability for the Allen cognitive level test, expanded version. Unpublished master's thesis, University of Southern California, Los Angeles.

Brown, D. E. (1991). *Human universals.* Philadelphia: Temple University Press.

Burns, T. (1990). The cognitive performance test: A new tool for assessing Alzheimer's disease. *OT Week.* December 27. Bethesda, MD: American occupational Therapy Association.

Burns, T. (1992). Cognitive performance test. In C. K. Allen, C. A. Earhart, & T. Blue. *Occupational therapy treatment goals for the physically and cognitively disabled.* Bethesda, MD: American Occupational Therapy Association.

Camp, C., & Peterson, C. (1987). *A comparison of cognitive level and adaptive behavior in an adult sample with mental retardation.* Unpublished master's thesis, San Jose State University, San Jose, California.

Carmel, R., Katz, N., & Modai, I. (1996). Construct validity of the Allen cognitive level (ACL) test: Relationship of cognitive level to hand dexterity in a group of adult inpatients suffering from major depression. *Israel Journal of Occupational Therapy, 5*, 230–231.

Cermak, S. A., Katz, N., McGuire, E., Greenbaum, S., Peralta, C., & Maser-Flanagan, V. (1995). Performance of Americans and Israelis with cerebral vascular accident of the Loewenstein occupational therapy cognitive assessment battery. *American Journal of Occupational Therapy, 49*, 500–506.

Cheney, D. L., & Seyfarth, R. M. (1990). *How monkeys see the world: Inside the mind of another species.* Chicago: University of Chicago Press.

Cook, V., & Newson, M. (1996). *Chomsky's universal grammar: an Introduction* (2nd ed). Cambridge: Blackwell.

Data Management Service (1987). Guide for the Use of the Uniform Data Set for Medical Rehabilitation. Buffalo, New York: Data Management Service of the Uniform Data System for Medical Rehabilitation.

David, S. K., & Riley, W. T. (1990). The relationship of the Allen cognitive level test to cognitive abilities and psychopathology. *American Journal of Occupational Therapy, 44,* 493–497.

Earhart, C. A., & Allen, C. K. (1988). *Cognitive disabilities: Expanded activity analysis.* Authors.

Eibl-Eibeesfeldt, I. (1989). *Human ethology.* New York: Aldine de Gruyter.

Finger, S., & Stein, D. B. (1982). *Brain damage and recovery: Research and clinical perspectives.* New York: Academic Press.

Fodor, J. A. (1983). *The modularity of mind.* Cambridge, MA: MIT Press.

Foto, M. (1996). Nationally speaking—Delineating skilled versus nonskilled services: A defining point in our professional evolution. *American Journal of Occupational Therapy, 50,* 168–170.

Gibson, K. R. (1993). Tool use, language and social behavior in relation to information processing capacities. In K. R. Gibson & T. Ingold, (Eds.), *Tools, language, and cognition in human evolution.* Cambridge: Cambridge University Press.

Gibson, K. R., & Ingold, T. (Eds.). (1993). *Tools, language, and cognition in human evolution.* Cambridge: Cambridge University Press.

Ginsberg, H., & Opper, S. (1969). *Piaget's theory of intellectual development: An Introduction.* Englwood Cliffs, NJ: Prentice Hall.

Gokey, M. A. (1986). *The relationship between cognitive level and daily functioning in persons with chronic schizophrenia.* Unpublished master's thesis; San Jose State University, San Jose, California.

Griffin, R. D. (1992). *Animal minds.* Chicago: University of Chicago Press.

Hagen, C. (1982). Language-cognition disorganization following closed head injury: A Conceptualization. In L. E. Yexler. *Cognitive rehabilitation: Conceptualization and intervention.* New York: Plenum Press.

Hagan, C., & Malkmus, D. (1979). Intervention strategies for language disorders secondary to head trauma. American Speech-Language-Hearing Association Convention Short Course, Atlanta.

Hamilton, B. B., Granger, C. V., Sherwin, F. S., et. al. (1987). A uniform national data system for medical rehabilitation. In M. J. Fuhrer (Ed.), *Rehabilitation outcomes: Analysis and measurement.* Baltimore: Paul H. Brooks.

Haroutunian, S. (1983). *Equilibrium in the balance: A study of psychological explanation.* New York: Springer-Verlag.

Health Care Financing Administration (n.d.) *Medical hospital manual 10* (HCFA Pub. 13-3, Section 3906). Bethesda, MD: Department of Health and Human Services.

Heimann, N.E. (1985). *Investigation of the reliability and validity of the routine task inventory with a sample of adults with chronic mental disorders.* Unpublished master's thesis, University of Southern California, Los Angeles.

Heimann, N. E., Allen, C. K., & Yerxa, E. J. (1989). The routine task inventory: A tool for describing the functional behavior of the cognitively disabled. *Occupational Therapy Practice, 1,* 67–74.

Herzig, S. I. (1978). *Occupational therapy assessment of cognitive levels as predictors of the community adjustment of chronic schizophrenic patients.* Unpublished master's thesis, University of Southern California, Los Angeles.

Heying, L. M. (1983). *Cognitive disability and activities of daily living in persons with senile dementia.* Unpublished master's thesis, University of Southern California, Los Angeles.

Howell, T. F. (1993). *The Allen cognitive level test–1990: Reliability studies with the depressed population.* Unpublished master's thesis, University of Florida.

Ingold, T. (1993). Tool use, society, and intelligence. In K. R. Gibson, & T. Ingold (Eds.). *Tools, language, and cognition in human evolution.* Cambridge: Cambridge University Press.

Josman, N., & Katz, N. (1991). Problem-solving version of the Allen Cognitive Level (ACL) test. *American Journal of Occupational Therapy, 45,* 331–338.

Kaeser, D. S. (1992). *Cognitive disability theory as a basis for activity analysis for elderly persons with dementia.* Unpublished master's thesis, Western Michigan University; Kalamazoo.

Katz, N. (1979). *An occupational therapy study of cognition in adult inpatients with depression.* Unpublished master's thesis, University of Southern California, Los Angeles.

Katz, N., & Heimann, N. (1990). Review of research conducted in Israel in cognitive disability instrumentation. *Occupational Therapy in Mental Health, 10,* 1–15.

Katz, N., Itzkovich, M., Averbuch, S., & Elazar, B. (1989). Loewenstein occupational therapy cognitive assessment battery for brain injured patients: Reliability and validity. *American Journal of Occupational Therapy, 43,* 184–192.

Katz, N., Josman, N., & Steinmetz (1988). Relationship between cognitive disability theory and the model of human occupation in the assessment of psychiatric and nonpsychiatric adolescents. *Occupational Therapy in Mental Health, 8,* 31–43.

Kehrberg, K. (1992). Part II: The Large ACL. In C. K. Allen, C. A. Earhart, & T. Blue. *Occupational therapy treatment goals for the physically and cognitively disabled.* Bethesda, MD: American Occupational Therapy Association.

Kehrberg, K. (1993). *Large Allen cognitive level test manual (with kit included).* Colchester, CT.: S & S/Worldwide.

Lawton, M. P., & Brody, E. M. (1969). Assessment of older people: Self-maintaining and instrumental activities of daily living. *Gerontologist, 9*, 1179–186.

Levy, L. L. (1986) A practical guide to the care of the Alzheimer's disease victim. *Topics in Geriatric Rehabilitation, 4* (4), 53–66.

Levy, L. L. (1992). The use of the cognitive disability frame of reference in rehabilitation of cognitively disabled older adults. In N. Katz (Ed.), *Cognitive rehabilitation: Models for intervention in occupational therapy.* Stoneham, MA: Butterworth-Heinemann.

Luria, A. R. (1966). *Higher cortical functions in man* (2nd ed.). New York: Basic Books.

Mayer, M. A. (1988). Analysis of information processing and cognitive disability theory. *American Journal of Occupational Therapy, 42*, 176–183.

Miller, R. (1987). *Meaning and purpose in the intact brain: A philosophical, psychological and biological account of conscious processes.* New York: Clarendon Press.

Moore, D. S. (1978). *An occupational therapy evaluation of sensorimotor cognition: Initial reliability, validity, and descriptive data for hospitalized schizophrenic patients.* Unpublished master's thesis, University of Southern California, Los Angeles.

Mosey, A. C. (1994). Working taxonomies. In C. B. Royeen (Ed.) *AOTA self-study series: Cognitive rehabilitation.* Bethesda, MD: American Occupational Therapy Association.

Neistadt, M. E. (1990). A Critical analysis of occupational therapy approaches for perceptual deficits in adults with brain injury. *American Journal of Occupational Therapy, 44*, 299–305.

Newman, M. (1987). *Cognitive disability and functional performance in individuals with chronic schizophrenic disorders.* Unpublished master's thesis, University of Southern California; Los Angeles.

Partida, A. (1992). *Reliability and validity of two alternate versions of the Allen cognitive level test among adults with mental illness.* Unpublished master's thesis, University of Southern California, Los Angeles.

Penny, N. H., Musser, K. T., & North, C. T. (1995). The Allen cognitive level test and social competence in adult psychiatric patients. *American Journal of Occupational Therapy, 49*, 420–427.

Polkinghorne, D. E. (1992). Postmodern epistemology of practice. In S. Kabale (Ed.), *Psychology and postmodernism.* London: Sage.

Raweh, D. (1996). *Treatment effectiveness of the cognitive disabilities theory of Allen with adult schizophrenic outpatients:*

A primary study. Unpublished master's thesis, Hebrew University of Jerusalem, Israel.

Reisberg, B, Ferris, S. H., Leon. M. J., & Cook, T. (1982). The global deterioration scale for assessment of primary degenerative dementia. *American Journal of Psychiatry, 139*, 1136–1139.

Reisberg, B. (1986). Functional assessment staging with annotations. *Geriatrics, 41*, 30–46.

Richards, G. E. (1983). *Evaluation of the Allen cognitive level test as an occupational therapy assessment tool.* Unpublished master's thesis, West Chester State College.

Roitblat, H. L. (1987) *Introduction to comparative cognition.* New York: W. H. Freeman.

Searle, J. R. (1990a). Consciousness, exploratory inversion, and cognitive science. *Behavioral and Brain Sciences,* 585–642.

Searle, J. R. (1990b). Who is computing the brain. *Behavioral and Basic Sciences, 13*, December: 632–642.

Shapiro, M. E. (1992). Application of the Allen cognitive level in assessing cognitive level functioning in emotionally disturbed boys. *American Journal of Occupational Therapy, 46*, 514–520.

Skinner, S., Denton, P., & Levy, B. (1989). *A descriptive study of inpatient schizophrenic functioning in occupational therapy open clinic and task group.* Bethesda, MD: American Occupational Therapy Foundation.

Tolchinsky-Landsmann, L., & Katz, N. (1988). Concrete to formal thinking: Comparison of psychiatric outpatients and a normal control group. *Occupational Therapy in Mental Health, 8*, 73–94.

Wilkerson, D. L., Batavia, A. I., & DeJong, J. D. (1992). Use of functional status measures for payment of medical rehabilitation. *Archives of Physical Medicine and Rehabilitation, 73*, 111–120.

Williams, L. R. (1981). *Development and initial test of an occupational therapy object-classification test.* Unpublished master's thesis, University of Southern California, Los Angeles.

Wilson, D. S. (1985). *Cognitive disability and routine task behaviors in a community based population with senile dementia.* Unpublished master's thesis, San Jose Sate University; San Jose, California.

Wilson, D. S., Allen, C. K., McCormack, G., & Burton, G.(1989). Cognitive disability and routine task behaviors in a community-based population with senile dementia. *Occupational Therapy Practice, 1*, 58–66.

World Health Organization. (WHO) (1980). *International classification of impairments, disabilities, and handicaps.* Geneva, Switzerland: Author.

Habor UCLA Med Center 1000 W Carson St. Torrance, Ca. 90509

Occupational Therapy
Discharge Summary

12/20/96

Prepared by: Claudia Allen
Updated by: Claudia Allen

Patient Name Cva, Recenta   **Number**   **ACL Level: 4.0**

ABILITIES

Patient's Abilities ACL: 4.0

DESCRIPTION OF PATIENT'S ABILITIES: The person's best ability to function at this time has been observed in the following behaviors:

Pays Attention to Activity to be Done
** Aware of activities with a sequence of steps: beginning, middle, and end for a sequence of steps to complete an activity.
** Looks at samples of designs, patterns from nature (flowers, animals, geometric shapes, household item).
** Notices objects in plain sight, within arms reach.
** Recognizes familiar possessions, new possessions, supplies used in self-care routines.
** Remembers information about 1 or 2 activities that have a high priority for the individual.
** Aware of friendly social greetings and signs of social rank.

Motor Control of Doing Routine Activities
** Sequences own actions and sustains awareness of goal for the duration of the activity.
** Does not spontaneously look at the sample; notes when shown.
** Does not set up to do an activity or clean up when finished.
** Does self-care routines without cues. Sets own priorities for preferred activities and learns location of supplies.
** Recognizes errors in size, shape, or color when asked; may not choose to correct the error, may repeat the error, or abandon the task if not helped. Asks for assistance.
** Recognizes day/night rhythms for doing activities. Measures passage of time by activity completion and may be disoriented to date and time of day.
** Recognizes a physical disability and the need to compensate.
** Uses understanding of pattern to but pieces together to form a design, matches the sample.

Verbal Communication by Remembering Current and Past Activities/Possession
** Self-generates verbal directions for next step in familiar task.
** Compares objects using words such as same, equal, or uses word opposites (high/low, good/bad).
** Asks another person for assistance.
** Shows obedience to authority or a verbal defense of self, "I like it like that."
** Gives or shares possessions; owner has the right to use the object first and shares only when possession is acknowledged.
** Identifies with group membership, with negative attitudes toward outsiders.
** Engages in verbal conflict as ritualized fighting: dehumanizing, belittling, accusing. or laughing at others.
** Differentiates between man made and natural objects.
** Uses names for classifying members of family, kin, generations.
** Recognizes cultural taboos for rape, murder, violence, copulation, and relieving self in public.
** States awareness of typical times for eating, feasting, showing hospitality to others, greeting people and customary day/night rhythms to daily life.

Submitted by: _____ Date: 12/20/96
                        Claudia Allen

Habor UCLA Med Center 1000 W Carson St. Torrance, Ca. 90509	**Occupational Therapy** **Discharge Summary** 12/20/96

Prepared by: Claudia Allen
Updated by: Claudia Allen

Patient Name Cva, Recenta   **Number**   **ACL Level: 4.0**

SAFETY PRECAUTIONS

ACL USED FOR PATIENTS
SAFETY PRECAUTIONS: 4.0

SAFETY PRECAUTIONS FOR THIS PATIENT: The following suggestions are ways of preventing common problems that have a greater than average chance of occurring.

MOVING/WALKING
** In a hospital bed, put the rails down to prevent falls by attempting to climb over rail.
** Prevent getting lost by escorting on one or two new routes until learned, pointing out hazards.
** Prevent accidents by escorting while walking in traffic and preventing from stepping in front of cars.
** Prevent falls by pointing out stairs, curbs, uneven surfaces; avoid walking on gravel, wet, or slippery surfaces.
** Prevent falls by restricting access to steep, narrow, or circular stairs.
** Prevent falls by installing grab bars in bathroom and where dressed.
** Prevent falls by carrying items up and down stairs, using a hand rail.
** Prevent injury, overexertion, or lack of effectiveness by supervising exercise program and anticipating potential complications.

BATHROOM ACTIVITIES
** Prevent embarrassment by checking clothing adjustments and assisting with fasteners.
** Prevent getting lost by escorting to new bathroom when otherwise independent.
** Prevent toileting emergencies by reminding to go ahead of time.
** Remind to bathe at a routine time each day and place necessary supplies in plain sight within arms reach. May need help getting shampoo out of back of hair.
** Prevent flooding by checking to see that the water is turned off.
** Prevent falls by not walking on wet, slippery floor and making sure that all needed items are in tub/shower. Install a nonskid rug on floor tiles and wipe up water spills/drips.
** Prevent falls in bath tub by making sure that the bath mat is pushed down tight.
** Prevent falls after seated in tub by assisting with balance and sequence of movements to get out of the tub.
** Prevent electrical shock or burns by removing electrical appliances from the bathroom sink area (radio, hair dryer, curling iron, razor, stereo.)
** Prevent allergies, chemical reactions, and fires by checking precautions on grooming supplies before independent use. Watch while using straight razor, nail clippers or scissors, mascara if unsteady hands, fingernail polish or any other product that requires timing.
** Prevent confusion and resistance by allowing 2 to 3 times the usual rate to bathe and groom, as well as get dressed.
** Avoid missed hair and nail appointments by making and reminding to keep appointments.

DRESSING
** Avoid conflict and confusion by grouping clothes into outfits and limiting selections. Remove clothing that does not fit or causes embarrassment.
** Prevent falls by removing loose-fitting shoes or slippers.
** Avoid embarrassment by assisting with clothing selections.

Habor UCLA Med Center 1000 W Carson St. Torrance, Ca. 90509	**Occupational Therapy** **Discharge Summary** *12/20/96*

Prepared by: Claudia Allen
Updated by: Claudia Allen

Patient Name Cva, Recenta   **Number**   **ACL Level: 4.0**

EATING

** Prevent frustration by precutting food. Allow 2 to 3 times usual time to eat. Open packages. Follow food preferences by limiting choices to 3 specific possibilities.
** Prevent waste or neglect by opening food containers and pouring liquids.
** Prevent spills by filling cup half full. Remind to check for hot food and fluid and to wait until cool.
** Prevent burns by allowing preparation of cold snack or sandwich.
** Restrict access to food if on a restricted diet, by keeping out of sight.
** Prevent adverse reaction to medications by knowing side effects and possible complications and reporting to doctor.
** Prevent poor compliance with taking medication by handing measured liquids and pills to the person and checking swallowing.
** Prevent overdose by storing medications out of sight in child-proof containers.
** Prevent running out of medications by checking on supply and renewing prescriptions.

HOUSEKEEPING

Injury

** Consider the value of monitoring the individual with a night light, home intercom system.
** Organize self-care supplies in a cupboard or drawer with items used daily in plain sight. Remove unnecessary, poisonous, or burnable items. Avoid changes in packaging that can be confused with another product, such as liquid soap for hand lotion.
** Remove access to power tools, flammables, toxins, cutting tools (knives, saw, shovel), and hot tools (iron, glue gun, stove, coffee pot).
** Do not leave alone to supervise the care of a child or a pet.
** Do not leave alone to prepare hot food that could burn or catch on fire.
** If a stove is used, check to be sure the stove is turned off, move pot holders, paper, and anything else that could burn away from heat, turn pot handles toward stove, and carry boiling water.
** Restrict access to driving a motor vehicle.

Falls
** Anchor down electrical cords, tape down curled or frayed rugs, and restrict access to wet or highly polished floors.
** Remove unstable chairs, tables, towel racks that might be grabbed onto for support.
** Remove clutter from stairs, clothing from banisters and hand rails, and repair deteriorating steps.
** Prevent climbing to reach something by replacing light bulbs, taking things in and out of cupboards, washing windows and curtains, hanging pictures, painting walls/woodwork.

Fires
** Take out the trash, remove stacks of papers and paper boxes. Make sure papers and burnable materials are not stored under stairs.
** Put a screen in front of the fireplace. Clean fireplace, chimneys and flues regularly.
** Prevent starting a fire with fluid, gas, or paraffin.
** Prevent burns by restricting possible contact with high heat sources.
** Remove electrical cords draped over or near a heat source and frayed cords.

Habor UCLA Med Center
1000 W Carson St.
Torrance, Ca. 90509

**Occupational Therapy
Discharge Summary**

12/20/96

Prepared by: Claudia Allen
Updated by: Claudia Allen

Patient Name Cva, Recenta   **Number**   ACL Level: 4.0

** Turn appliances off during a power outage, ground plugs, remove excessive appliances from a circuit/outlet, and replace fuses with correct limit on amperage.
** With an electric blanket, prevent use of a hot water bottle or an extra blanket to avoid electric shock or burns.
** Check cigarettes for smoldering ashes, not smoking in bed, and not leaving ash tray on chair arm.
** Check butane by not storing near a heat source, in sunlight, or near hot water pipes.
** Install and maintain smoke detectors, fire extinguisher.
** Plan and rehearse an escape route and an alternative route.
** If a fire occurs, close windows and doors and get out. If in doubt, get out.

Robbery
** Supply with daily spending money and manage all other finances.
** Remove valuables from plain sight in front of door, window, car seat. Secure doors and windows at front, back, and sides.
** Etch identification numbers on valuables, hide cash in a consistent but unusual place.
** Protect security by using a peep hole with chain lock and checking to see who has been buzzed through a security system.
** When leaving home, leave a light on in the living room and locate a spare house key.
** Prepare "no" statements for strangers and verify the identity of public officials.
** Rehearse not giving name and address to strangers.
** Call the head office to verify the identity of salesman.
** Limit telephone access to a few important numbers and monitor expense, interrupting others.

WORK AND SOCIAL RELATIONS
Prevent unrealistic expectations and social conflict that have a greater than average chance of occurring by
** Supervising by showing how to do a new activity, one step at a time. Do not depend on signs or posted notes as reminders.
** Avoiding reading to get new information or remind of what to do
** Limiting working hours to 2-3 hours per day.
** Allowing 2 to 3 times normal rate to get job done.
** Having someone in the area to watch while working.

PHYSICAL DISABILITY
** Use a sliding board to transfer from bed to chair to toilet.
** Use an overhead trapeze with cueing to hold body off bed.
** Prevent decreased mobility by clearing space for wheelchair access, using offset door hinges and furniture leg extenders.
** Prevent frustration by allowing to propel wheelchair forward and back using the rims. Assist with turning corners.
** Assist with active range of motion by reminding to do exercises to prevent deformities.
** Provide constant cueing to use overhead pulley and parallel bars.
** With high blood pressure, remind to stand up slowly and assist with getting out of a hot tub slowly.
** Use raised toilet seat, toilet support, bedside commode.
** Use safety belt to stand and walk if balance is unsteady.

<table>
<tr><td rowspan="3">

Habor UCLA Med Center
1000 W Carson St.
Torrance, Ca. 90509

</td><td>

**Occupational Therapy
Discharge Summary**

12/20/96

</td></tr>
</table>

Prepared by: Claudia Allen
Updated by: Claudia Allen

Patient Name Cva, Recenta   **Number**   **ACL Level:** 4.0

** Use bath chair with arms, or tub/shower bench, hand-held shower head.
** May benefit from a telephone amplifier.
** Provide built-up eating and writing utensils, weighted writing utensils.
** With the use of one hand, provide wash mitt, suction hand brush.
** Install door knob extenders.
** Assist with putting on ankle/knee brace.
** Provide pick-up walker, wide-base quad cane.
** Provide a male urinal.
** Provide an adapted shaving cream dispenser.
** With poor vision, provide a magnifier.

Submitted by: _____ Date:12/20/96
Claudia Allen

Appendix B

MODES	COGNITIVE ASSISTANCE REQUIRED	PHYSICAL ASSISTANCE REQUIRED
1.0 1.2	100% - The person requires 24-hour nursing care to turn the body to prevent bed sores and hook up artificial feeding. Total cognitive assistance (100%) is required to position, bathe, and clothe the person who is bedridden. A response to sensory stimulation may be obtained through any of the senses. You may individualize sensory stimulation by using cues that are strong, distinctive, and relevant to the person's functional history.	100%: - One or more people are required to perform all physical activities.
1.4	96% - The person requires 24-hour nursing care to feed a soft diet, place on bed pan, check for skin redness, bathe, and groom. Sensory stimulations are located and tracked as location changes. Individual ideas from person's past may focus attention.	100% - Requires total physical assistance of 1 or more persons with most activities. 75% physical assistance with eating and oral hygiene.
1.6	96% - The person requires 24-hour nursing care to feed a soft diet, place on bed pan, check for skin redness, bathe, and groom. Sensory stimulations to parts of the body capture attention. Individual cues from person's past history may also focus attention on body parts.	100%: - Requires total physical assistance of 1 or more persons with most activities. 75% physical assistance with eating and oral hygiene and moving in bed.
1.8	88% - The person requires 24-hour nursing care to sustain feeding self, engage in exercises, bathe and groom. 88% total cognitive assistance is required to place cup and spoon in hand and establish a routine for voiding and bathing. Sensory stimulation engages the arms in movements but trunk balance is not dependable and may require support.	50%: - Sit up/down, stand, pivot transfer. 100% physical assistance of a wheel chair for moving around with support to sustain sitting position.
2.0	84% - The person requires 24-hour nursing care to assist in moving from bed to chair to toilet. 84% maximum cognitive assistance is required to act as a contact guard during transfers and to initiate and sustain all self-care activities. Sensory stimulation is required to bear weight and balance while sitting and standing. Individual preferences in bed position, favorite chair, and toileting location can be honored	25% - Is required to sit up/down, stand, and pivot transfer. 50% Physical Assistance from wheel chair or arm chair to sustain sitting position. Put bed rails up to keep from rolling out of bed. For exercises, use a safety belt for sitting and standing exercises

MODES	COGNITIVE ASSISTANCE REQUIRED	PHYSICAL ASSISTANCE REQUIRED
2.2	82% - The person requires 24-hour nursing care to sit and stand safely or prevent standing if unable to bear weight. 82% maximum cognitive assistance to initiate and sustain self-care activities is required. Touching and naming parts of the body reduces the burden of care. Individual preferences for the way things feel to the person can be honored.	15% - To sustain balance when changing position from sit to stand and maintain sitting position while being dressed, bathed, groomed. A lap tray or table may be used for support when seated in a chair with solid arms. Put bed rails up to prevent rolling out of bed
2.4	78% - Requires 24-hour nursing care to prevent wandering off and getting lost and insure safe toileting, bathing and grooming. 78% maximum cognitive assistance is required to initiate and sustain self-care activities and prevent falls. Walks in indicated direction for activities of daily living. Indicates individual preferences for large, rhythmic body movements	10% - Fine motor actions on all objects used in activities of daily living. Physical barriers or alarms to prevent getting lost and attempting to walk on anything other than flat surfaces. Put bed rails down to prevent attempts to climb over the top
2.6	74% - The person needs 24-hour nursing care to escort to activities of daily living, point out stairs and curbs, assist with toileting, bathing, grooming, and dressing (74% maximum cognitive assistance). Individual differences in where the person wants to go may be honored.	10% Fine motor actions on all objects used in activities of daily living. Physical barriers or alarms to prevent getting lost and attempting to walk on anything other than flat surfaces. Put bed rails down to prevent attempts to climb over the top
2.8	70% - The person needs 24-hour nursing care to assist with bathing, grooming, and dressing and make sure objects used for support are stabile. 70% maximum cognitive assistance is required to point out stairs, edge of bathtub, to provide food, and to bathe. Individual preferences in what is used for support may be honored (grab bars, rails, counters).	10% Fine motor actions on all objects used in activities of daily living. Physical barriers or alarms to prevent getting lost and attempting to walk on anything other than flat surfaces without an escort. Put bed rails down to prevent attempts to climb over the top.
3.0	64% - The person needs 24-hour nursing care to place safe objects in front of the person and assist with toileting, bathing, grooming, and dressing. 64% moderate cognitive assistance is required to elicit and sustain habitual motions for self-care. Individual preferences for handling different objects may be honored.	10% Fine motor actions on all objects used in activities of daily living. Physical barriers or alarms to prevent getting lost and attempting to walk on anything other than flat surfaces without an escort. Put bed rails down to prevent attempts to climb over the top
3.2	60% - The person needs 24-hour nursing care to place objects in from of the person and assist with toileting, bathing, grooming, and dressing. One to one supervision requires 60% moderate cognitive assistance to sustain actions. Individual preferences in what the person likes to move may be honored.	10% - Fine motor actions on all objects used in activities of daily living. Physical barriers or alarms to prevent getting lost and attempting to walk on anything other than flat surfaces without an escort. Put bed rails down to prevent attempts to climb over the top

MODES	COGNITIVE ASSISTANCE REQUIRED	PHYSICAL ASSISTANCE REQUIRED
3.4	54% - The person needs 24-hour nursing care to sequence through the routine steps of toileting, bathing, grooming and dressing. 54% moderate cognitive assistance is required to go to the next step in self-care activities. Individual preferences for repetitive actions that the person likes to do may be honored	10% Fine motor actions on all objects used in activities of daily living. Physical barriers or alarms to prevent getting lost and attempting to walk on anything other than flat surfaces without an escort. Put bed rails down to prevent attempts to climb over the top
3.6	50% - The person needs 24-hour supervision to provide the supplies needed for activities of daily living, sequence through the steps of toileting, bathing, grooming, and dressing, and remove access to dangerous objects. 50% moderate cognitive assistance is required to finish all steps and check results. Individual preferences for the effects that repetitive actions have on objects may be honored.	10% - Fine motor actions on all objects used in activities of daily living. Physical barriers or alarms to prevent getting lost and attempting to walk on anything other than flat surfaces without an escort. Put bed rails down to prevent attempts to climb over the top
3.8	46% - The person needs 24-hour supervision to get supplies out for all activities of daily living, to check results, and to remove dangerous objects. The person may think that an activity is finished when the results are inadequate. 46% moderate cognitive assistance is required to complete self-care and protect from harm. Individual preferences for using up supplies can be honored.	10% Fine motor actions on all objects used in activities of daily living. Physical barriers or alarms to prevent getting lost and attempting to walk on anything other than flat surfaces without an escort. Put bed rails down to prevent attempts to climb over the top
4.0	42% - The person needs 24-hour supervision to remove dangerous objects and solve problems due to minor changes in routine activities. May fix self a cold snack or sandwich. 42% minimum cognitive assistance requires on-site supervision to recognize and correct hazards. Individual preferences in doing 1 or 2 important activities may be honored.	8% - Fine motor actions on all objects used in activities of daily living.
4.2	38% - The person needs 24-hour supervision to remove dangerous objects outside of the visual field and to solve problems arising from minor changes in the environment. The person may spend a daily allowance, walk to familiar locations in the neighborhood, or follow a simple, familiar bus route. 38% minimum cognitive assistance is required to recognize and correct hazards in routine activities.	8% - Fine motor actions on all objects used in activities of daily living.

MODES	COGNITIVE ASSISTANCE REQUIRED	PHYSICAL ASSISTANCE REQUIRED
4.4	34% - The person may live with someone who does a daily check on the environment, removing any safety hazards and solving problems when minor changes in the home occur. May be alone for part of the day with a procedure for obtaining help by phone or from a neighbor. May have a daily allowance and go to familiar places in the neighborhood. 34% minimum cognitive assistance is required to set-up new activities and clean-up after routine activities.	8% - Is needed to assist with fine motor activities
4.6	30% - The person may live alone with daily assistance to monitor personal safety and provide a daily allowance. Bills and other money management concerns require assistance. Reminders may be required to do household chores, attend familiar community events, or any other additions to household routines (30% minimum cognitive assistance	8% - Is needed for fine motor activities.
4.8	26% - The person can live alone with daily assistance to monitor safety and check problem solving effectiveness. The person may get to a regularity scheduled community activity without assistance. With a job coach the person may succeed in supportive employment. 26% minimum cognitive assistance is required to set-up new activities and verify results.	8% - Is needed for fine motor activities.
5.0	22% - The person may live alone with weekly checks to monitor safety and check problem solving effectiveness. With a job coach the person may be able to work in support employment. Independence in attending regularly scheduled community activities may be expected. 22% standby cognitive assistance is required to anticipate environmental hazards and prevent social conflict	6%- Is needed for fine motor activities.
5.2	18% - The person may live alone with weekly checks to monitor home safety and assist with finances. 18% standby cognitive assistance is required to anticipate hazards and prevent social conflict. Individual preferences may be honored in improving the appearance of material objects.	4% - Is needed for fine motor activities.

MODES	COGNITIVE ASSISTANCE REQUIRED	PHYSICAL ASSISTANCE REQUIRED
5.4	14% - The person may live alone and work in a job with a wide margin of error. 14% standby cognitive assistance is needed to anticipate hazards and prevent industrial accidents. Individual preferences for improving the appearance of activities can be honored.	2% - Is needed for fine motor activities.
5.6	10% - The person may live alone or with family and work in situations where hazards are consistent and predictable. 10% cognitive assistance is required to point out hazards that are a secondary effect of actions. May be relied on to follow safety precautions consistently with training.	0% - No Physical Assistance
5.8	6% - The person may live and work independently. 6% standby cognitive assistance is needed to plan for the future, anticipate the need for joint protection, functional positioning, and the consequences of fatigue.	0% - No Physical Assistance
6.0	0% - The person can live and work independently. No cognitive assistance is needed.	0% - No Physical Assistance

CHAPTER 9

A Dynamic Model for Cognitive Modifiability:
Application in Occupational Therapy

Naomi Hadas-Lidor, MA, OTR, and Noomi Katz, PhD, OTR

In the first part of this chapter, the theoretical base—the principles of Feuerstein's Dynamic Approach for Cognitive Modifiability in the evaluation and treatment of cognitive deficits—is presented, including its relationship and relevancy to occupational therapy. In the second part, we describe clinical applications in occupational therapy using Mediated Learning Experience and Instrumental Enrichment. The examples we discuss refer to intervention with clients following brain injuries, clients suffering from psychiatric disorders, adolescents with adaptation difficulties following physical disability and social deprivation, as well as immigrant mothers native to Russia's Caucasus Mountains.

Theoretical Base

The Dynamic Approach for Cognitive Modifiability, as well as its assessment and treatment, was developed by Reuven Feuerstein and colleagues between 1950 and 1960 in Israel. Feuerstein's (1979, 1980) work is based on extensive experience with Israeli adolescents who demonstrated mental retardation in intellectual performance due to their diverse cultural origins, disrupted lives, and limited opportunities to learn. His work provided the foundation for a general theory of cognitive competence, coupled with a technology for assessing learning potential (i.e., Learning Potential Assessment Device, LPAD). Feuerstein's emphasis in this approach is on improving functional deficits in the cognitive process through Mediated Learning

Experience (MLE) and Instrumental Enrichment (IE).

In general this approach is concerned first with the ability to learn and solve problems; second, with examining why this ability fails to develop during early childhood in the absence of environmental enrichment; third, with focusing on systematic learning mediated by a caring adult; and fourth, with how much later than generally thought possible, identified cognitive deficits can be remediated by a formal instructional program.

This method of intervention started in the 1950s with the evaluation and treatment of adolescents suffering from cultural deprivation. Later, it was adapted to populations with learning disabilities, Down's syndrome, and autism. On the other hand, it was also adapted to normal populations in industrial settings, especially in France (Avanjini, 1990).

During the past 15 years the approach has been used and adapted by Israeli occupational therapists with various client populations, such as clients following brain injuries, psychiatric and geriatric clients, adolescents with behavioral problems, and more recently with mothers native to the Caucasus who immigrated to Israel.

The Philosophy:
Concept of Cognitive Modifiability

Instrumental Enrichment and the LPAD represent an active modification approach as opposed to passive-acceptance of the performance problems seen in clients with retarded cognition (Feuerstein,

1980). One characteristic of the former approach is the goal of changing the individual by providing him or her with the means to successfully adapt to his or her environment. In contrast, the passive-acceptance approach focuses on changing the environmental conditions to adapt to the low performance level of the mentally retarded individual.

The central issue is whether the individual is regarded as an open or closed system, since the implications of this view are far ranging. Advocates of the active modification approach think of the individual as an open system that is receptive to change and modification. In this framework, modifiability is considered to be the basic condition of human beings. The individual's manifest level of performance at any given point in his or her development cannot be regarded as fixed or immutable, much less a reliable indication of future performance. This viewpoint has been expressed through the rejection of IQ scores as a reflection of a stable or permanent level of functioning. Instead, and in accordance with the open system approach, intelligence is considered a dynamic self-regulating process that is responsive to external environmental intervention. The view of the human being as an open system is utilized in various occupational therapy theoretical approaches most obvious in the Model of Human Occupation (Kielhofner, 1985, 1995).

The assumption that the human organism is open and amenable to change demands a very different method of assessment and evaluation, whose purpose is to evaluate the individual's capacity to learn, and hence, to be modified. The purpose of assessment is to reveal the potential of the individual and identify the deficient processes that may be impeding development. Treatment may then be directed at correcting deficiencies, by which the individual will be able to change the course of his or her development.

The aim of the program is to modify the individual's cognition by changing his or her internal structures rather than by changing only the environment. To appreciate this process-oriented approach, the therapist should specify the kinds of changes the program will aim to produce. The term "cognitive modifiability" was chosen to convey the idea of a process of continuous and self-regulated change set into motion by the program. In the

individual with mental retardation, the final process in reversing his or her low manifest level of performance is to cause a diversion from his or her current pattern of development, which requires an active interaction between the individual and sources of external and internal stimulation. Once activated, the dynamics of modifiability propel the individual along a course of development that could not otherwise be anticipated on the basis of his or her previous performance. Among other factors, cognitive modifiability is a product of highly specific experiences and learning and is a means of adapting to the environment. The survival of any organism depends on its ability to adapt. For the human organism, successful adaptation involves the ability to respond not only to a constant and stable environment, but also to situations and circumstances that are constantly changing.

The belief that intervention causes structural change is similar to the sensory integration theory in occupational therapy, where changes are assumed to occur within the central nervous system causing adaptive responses to the environment (Ayers, 1979; Fisher, Murray, & Bundy, 1992). Toglia (1989, 1991, in this book) presents a Dynamic Interactional Approach to Cognitive Rehabilitation that is based on the same assumptions. In contrast, Cognitive Disabilities Theory (Allen, 1985; Allen, Earhart, & Blue, 1992; Allen & Blue, in this book) is based on the assumption that occupational therapy intervention centers on adapting the task and the environment to the client's current capabilities. This direction also agrees with current approaches in rehabilitation (Anthony, Cohen, & Farkas, 1990; Giles, in this book; Neff, 1985).

The Theory of Mediated Learning Experience

The theory of Mediated Learning Experience (MLE) is the underlying theoretical basis for the concept of cognitive modifiability. The basic assumption in this theory is that the major factor causing cognitive differences among people is the MLE. Deficit or lack of MLE is a stronger explanation than any etiologic differences.

Feuerstein conceives the development of cognitive structures in the organism as a product of two interactions between the organism and its environment: direct exposure to sources of stimuli and mediated learning. The first, and the most universal modality is the organism's direct exposure to all sources of stimulation that it receives from the very earliest stage of development. This exposure changes the organism by affecting its behavioral repertoire and its cognitive orientation. These changes in turn affect its interaction with the environment, even when the environment itself remains constant and stable. Direct exposure to stimuli continues to affect the learning of the organism throughout its life span, to the extent that the stimuli present are varied and novel.

The second modality, which is far less universal and is characteristic of human beings, is Mediated Learning Experience (see Figure 9-1). When discussing this, we refer to the way in which stimuli emitted by the environment are transformed by a "mediating" agent (e.g., a parent, teacher, or therapist). This mediating agent, guided by his or her intentions, culture, and emotional investment, selects and organizes the world of the stimuli for the client (i.e., student). The mediator selects stimuli that are most appropriate and then frames, filters, and schedules them. He or she determines when certain stimuli appear or disappear and ignores others. Through this process of mediation, the cognitive structures of the clients are affected. The client acquires behavior patterns and learning

sets, which in turn become important ingredients of his or her capacity to become modified through direct exposure to stimuli. Since direct exposure to stimuli over time constitutes the greatest source of the individual's experience, the individual's cognitive development is influenced significantly by whether or not the individual has sets of strategies and repertoire that permit him or her to efficiently use this exposure.

Conceptually the role of the mediator is in some ways similar to the role of the occupational therapist as a facilitator in the original occupational therapy philosophy and habit formation (Meyer, 1922, reprinted 1977; Slagle, 1922), as well as in the Model of Human Occupation (Kielhofner, 1985; 1995), and in the Sensory Integrative Approach (Ayers, 1979; Fisher et al., 1992).

The relationship between MLE and direct exposure to stimuli, the two modalities for the development of cognitive structures, can be set forth as follows: The more often and the earlier an individual is subjected to MLE, the greater will be his or her capacity to efficiently use and be affected by direct exposure to sources of stimuli. On the other hand, the less MLE the developing individual is offered, in terms of both quantity and quality, the lower his or her capacity will be to be affected and modified by direct exposure to stimuli. Feuerstein and Feuerstein (1991) outline 12 parameters that describe the quality of the MLE. The three main

---

Figure 9-1

Mediated Learning Experience Model
(From Feuerstein and Feuerstein, 1991, with permission).

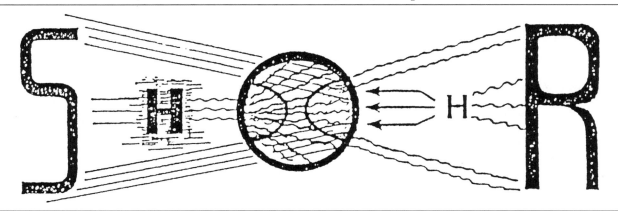

necessary parameters of the MLE are intentionality and reciprocity, transcendence, and mediation of meaning.

■ *Intentionality and reciprocity:* MLE requires a degree of intentionality on the part of the mediator. The voluntary nature of the mediated interaction is evident in certain well-defined instances. The purpose is to increase the intentionality of the recipient and raise his or her awareness of the ways he or she acts.

■ *Transcendence:* An interaction that provides mediated learning must be also directed toward transcending the immediate needs or concerns of the client by venturing beyond the here and now, in space and time. The premise of the approach is that working on transcendence is an integral part of the process of intervention. Transcendence, in terms of the ability to make generalization, is done according to MLE during the process of intervention.

■ *Mediation of meaning:* In contrast to the first two parameters, mediation of learning deals mainly with the energetic dimensions of the interaction (i.e., with why things happen or are done). It raises the individual's awareness and understanding and makes explicit the implicit reasons and motivations for doing things. Mediation of meaning focuses on the interaction of the individual with the environment and aims to increase his or her ability to make choices.

The remaining nine parameters, unlike the first three, are not necessary conditions of MLE but rather are considered reinforcing parameters (Feuerstein & Feuerstein, 1991). The intentionality of the mediator and the transcendent (i.e., generalization) nature of mediated interaction is directed toward building new cognitive structures and broadening the individual's system of needs for functioning.

An individual may lack MLE because of the following two main reasons: first, the nature of the individual's environment (i.e., poverty, cultural deprivation, and disturbed families); second, the individual's condition at a given point in his or her development (i.e. learning disabilities, brain injuries, emotional disturbances, and mental retardation). The lack in MLE has the same manifestations regardless of the cause or diagnosis.

The goal of any intervention based on MLE is always to restore a normal pattern of development. The purpose of MLE, as reflected in the Instrumental Enrichment (IE) program, is never to train the individual merely to master a set of specific skills that will enable him to function only in a limited way. Instead the goal is to change the cognitive structures of the low performer and to transform him or her into an autonomous, independent thinker capable of initiating and elaborating actions. Thus the focus is not on a functional approach but more on a cognitive remediation approach (Neistadt, 1990). Within the intervention process, the therapist works directly on helping the individual mediate structural generalizations.

In short, the goal set for the cognitively low performers according to the theory of MLE is adaptation to a normal environment, as opposed to adapting the environment to meet the specific needs of these performers.

For example, Klein (1991) developed an intervention program (i.e., More Intelligent & Sensitive Child—MISC), which aims to help parents enhance the cognitive development of their young children using the MLE principles, in order to prepare them to benefit from future learning (Klein & Hundeide, 1989).

In a different way, Kushnir (1996) discusses the preventive intervention program, which she carried out with healthy mothers, native to the Caucasus, who immigrated to Israel. She describes the unique characteristics of this ethnic group and the crisis and changes they experienced in Israel. The aim of the intervention program, according to Feuerstein's theory, was to improve both the adjustment of the mothers to the new cultural environment and the quality of the mother–infant interaction. In turn, this would enable a Mediated Learning Experience, which would improve the children's cognitive modifiability.

In another example, Moreno (1996) describes the treatment process of a 20-year-old man who suffered from brain injury for 3 years. The treatment followed all 12 components of Mediated Learning Experience and adapted the principles to the special needs of the client and his physical difficulties.

Tzuriel and Eiboshitz (1992) investigated the efficacy of the Structural Program of Visual-Motor Intervention (SP-VMI) with preschool disadvantaged and special education children. The SP-VMI is based on the theoretical perspectives that emphasize developmental principles and needs for mastery of perceptual-motor skills in relation to writing and reading skills (i.e., Gesell and Montessori), and on the MLE theory that stresses mediation of metacognitive strategies and an active-modificational approach. The major findings of their study show that children in the experimental group significantly improved their performance from pre- to postintervention on perceptual-motor tests, measure of cognitive modifiability, and adjustment categories. The improvement on the dynamic test of the Rey Complex Figure was significantly higher for the disadvantaged children in the experimental group as compared to the parallel subgroups among the control group. The findings, in general, confirm the efficacy of the SP-VMI and support the integration of MLE processes with perceptual-motor training.

These examples suggest that the MLE concepts are practical and adaptable regarding the prevention–rehabilitation continuum with a variety of client populations.

The Learning Potential Assessment Device

The dynamic assessment approach was developed to alter the cycle of failure the low performer experiences in the classical intelligent tests (i.e., a static assessment approach). The measurement and re-measurement of an individual's existing capacities should be abandoned in favor of first inducing and then assessing the individual's modified performance within the test situation. By assessing modifiability, we must focus on the cognitive functions found to be directly responsible for the demonstrated deficiencies. We must also continually remember that these deficiencies experienced by the client at the input and output phases of the mental act may be attributable to motivational and/or emotional components, and do not necessarily reflect that the individual has a deficient elaboration capacity.

Four major components are changed in the learning potential assessment device (LPAD) when it is compared to classic assessment, including:

1. The structure of test instruments (i.e., intelligence tests were analyzed for their components and divided into various graded exercises
2. The test logistics and testing procedures (i.e., first, the relationship of tester–testee were transformed into teacher–student or therapist–client, as described in the MLE, and second, the assessment was not timed—only the length of the whole process was considered
3. The interpretation of the results (i.e., the focus is on the change process and the individual's investment in it, and no score is given)
4. The general orientation of the test (from product to process).

The goals of a dynamic cognitive evaluation are

1. To assess an individual's modifiability when he or she is confronted with conditions that aim at producing a change in him or her
2. To assess the extent of the observed modifiability in terms of both the functional levels made accessible to the individual through the process of modification and the significance of the levels he or she attained in the hierarchy of cognitive operations
3. To determine how much intervention was necessary to bring about a given amount or type of modification
4. To determine how much significance the modification achieved in one area can have for other general areas of functioning
5. To search for the individual's preferred modalities that represent areas of relative strength and weakness in terms of both his or her existing inventory of responses and preferred strategies for achieving the desired modification in the most efficient and economical way.

In using the LPAD, the therapist is not interested in passively collecting data about skills the client may or may not possess. Rather the therapist assesses general learning modifiability by measuring the individual's capacity to acquire a given principle, learning set, skill, or attitude, depending on the specific task at hand. The extent of modifiability and the amount of treatment investment necessary to bring about the change are assessed, respectively by:

1. Measuring the client's capacity, first to grasp and then to apply these new skills to a variety of tasks progressively more distant from the one in which the principle was taught
2. Measuring the amount of explanation and training investment required in order to produce the desired result.

The significance of the attained modification is measured by the client's developing patterns of behavior that prove his or her efficiency in areas other than those that were actively modified by the training process.

The use of this dynamic approach in assessment assumes that the individual represents an open system that may undergo important modifications through exposure to external and/or internal stimuli (Lidz, 1987). However, the degree of the individual's modifiability through direct exposure to various sources of stimulation is considered to be a function of the quantity and quality of mediated learning experience.

In the context of this theoretical model of cognitive modifiability, intelligence is defined as the capacity of the individual to use previous experiences when adapting to new situations. The emphasis is on the use of previously acquired experiences. One can measure an individual's modifiability only by using dynamic assessment, which attempts to substitute for the missing experiential background using a concrete and focused intervention, and by providing the client with the opportunity to demonstrate his or her growing capacities in a progressive way following the focused intervention.

For example, one of the tests used in the LPAD is the *Complex Figure Drawing Test* (Rey-Osterrieth in Lezak, 1995), which consists of a complex geometric figure with both internal and external details. The figure is a composite of 18 elements. The subject must first reproduce the complex figure from the stimulus model and then, after a latency period, reproduce it from memory. In the LPAD, if the subject did not perform the test maximally,

the examiner provided appropriate mediation for the correct drawing of the complex figure, and the subject then needed to repeat the first two stages of drawing. The examiner then calculated the presence and accuracy of the details within the figure drawings, in order to form a final quantitative evaluation. Each of the 18 characteristics of each element received one point for correct shape and proportionality and one point for correct location or placement. Each of the phases, except for the learning-mediation phase, received a total score. The score, which allowed for a maximum of 36 points for each phase, followed the same pattern of scoring outlined by Lezak (1995).

An examination of the structuring and organization of the figure drawings resulted in a final qualitative evaluation. A scoring system of one (most rational) to seven (least rational) indicated a general, overall level of performance. Types of performance were classified according to intellectual habits, rapidity of reproduction, and the precision of the result.

Goals of the assessment are

■ to assess the subject's capacity to organize and structure a complex figure
■ to assess the subject's quality and precision within the complex figure drawing
■ to assess the subject's level of organization and visual memory, according to the quality of the reproduction of the complex figure, following a latency period of three minutes
■ to assess the subject's modifiability, through evaluating the quality, organization, accuracy, and completeness of the complex figure drawing, following mediation
■ to assess the subject's process of structuring and organizing a complex figure.

The following two test performances provide examples of changes that occurred after mediation.

Example 1:
23-Year-Old Occupational Therapy Student

The test proceeded in the following four stages: Copy-design, memory, mediation, and copy-design and memory. Figures 9-2 and 9-3 show the

Figure 9-2

Example 1:
RCF memory production before mediation.

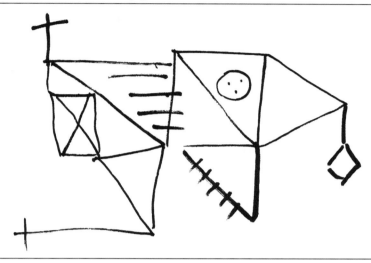

Note: Originals are in colors.

Figure 9-3

Example 1:
RCF memory production after mediation.

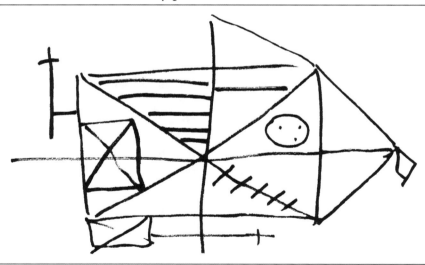

memory production before and after mediation. Comparison of the two memory trials showed:

1. Slower execution occurred on the first trial (1½ minutes), as opposed to the second trial (1 minute).

2. The general perception of the structure was that it included a large rectangle with internal divisions only during the second trial.

3. Sequential work was not present in the first trial. The work occurred in episodes and jumped from place to place, without any clear

pattern or method. In the second trial, we saw work in a logical sequence, through the organizing of shapes according to size (i.e., a larger rectangle preceded a smaller triangle). The second stage of this trial involved dividing the figure, and the third stage consisted of building up the components internally and externally.

4. In the first trial, the student remembered eight out of 18 items, while in the second, she remembered 17.

5. The number of inaccurate answers in constructing the figure was very high in the first trial, as opposed to only three at the second trial.

Example 2:
30-Year-Old Woman, Who Suffered from Schizophrenia

The test proceeded in the following four stages: Copy-design, memory, mediation, and copy-design and memory. Figures 9-4 and 9-5 show the memory production before and after mediation. Comparison of the two memory trials showed the following:

1. The client's first attempt at executing the task was very poor, in terms of the number of items that she remembered and their organization. The second attempt, after mediation, showed improvement in the areas of organizational ability, general perception of the rectangular and triangular shapes, and perception of the internal divisions within the rectangle.

2. While the client remembered approximately two out of 18 items in the first trial, she remembered 13 items in the second.

3. Accuracy was difficult to evaluate in the first trial, but was very good (almost error free) in the second.

These two examples showed that, after mediation, clear learning and improvement occurred, which thus provided the learning potential needed for further intervention.

Theoretical discussions and studies related to dynamic assessment have increased during the past years. Some of them present theoretical dilemmas of the assessment (Beasley & Shayer, 1990; Buchel & Scharnhorst, 1993; Brown, Campione, Webber, & McGilly, 1992), while others report research results. Day and Cordon (1993) compared school children achievement between standard tests and the LPAD assessment and found higher achievement among children assessed on the LPAD. Kaniel (1992) examined the mediation effect on performance and distribution of errors in the Raven Progressive Matrices Test and found improved performance. Similar results were found also by Burns, Delclos, Vye, and Sloan (1992) and by Guthke (1992). Additionally in several works related to reading ability, clinical experience suggests that the LPAD is useful for diagnosing and understanding of dyslexia (Brozo, 1990; Carney & Cioffi, 1990; Carney & Cioffi, 1992; Grisseman, 1993).

There is an increase of data to support the use of dynamic assessment in general and the LPAD specifically, and more applications are seen also in occupational therapy as exemplified in the assessments developed by Toglia (in this book).

Instrumental Enrichment—An Intervention Program for Cognitive Modifiability

We present Instrumental Enrichment (IE) in this chapter as an intervention strategy for the redevelopment of cognitive structures in the cognitively low performer. It is designed as a direct and focused approach to those processes that, because of their absence, fragility, or inefficiency, are responsible for poor intellectual performance, irrespective of underlying etiology. The IE program consists of more than 500 working pages of paper-and-pencil exercises, divided into 15 sections (see table 9–1). Each part focuses on a specific cognitive deficiency but can also address the acquisition of many other learning prerequisites. This structured approach assists the therapist/teacher in his or her choice of the materials to be taught/used and in their sequence of presentation. By knowing the focus of each section, the therapist/teacher is able to select and match specific material to the needs and deficits of particular clients/student. Intervention is either individual or in groups and takes place in approximately three to five sessions per week (Feuerstein, 1979).

Figure 9-4

Example 2:
RCF memory production before mediation.

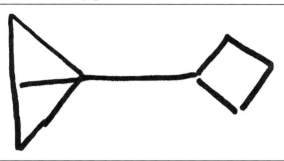

Figure 9-5

Example 2:
RCF memory production after mediation.

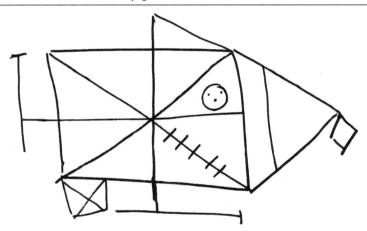

The major goal of IE is to increase the individual's capacity to be modified through direct exposure to stimuli and experiences that occur throughout life and with formal and informal learning opportunities. In order to attain this major goal, the following six subgoals should serve as guidelines for the construction of the IE program and its application:

1. Correcting the deficient functions in order to change the structure of the cognitive behavior

2. Acquiring basic concepts, labels, vocabulary, operations, and relationships necessary for IE as represented by the content of the materials, which themselves are purposely content-free

3. Developing (producing) intrinsic motivation through habit formation. To verify that whatever is taught will become part of an active repertoire, spontaneously used by the individual, one has to verify that the need for its use will be an intrinsic one rather than a response to an extrinsic system

Table 9-1
Instrumental Enrichment Materials

Nonverbal tools	*Tools requiring independent reading and comprehension skills*
1. Organization of dots	11. Categorization
2. Analytic perception	12. Instructions
3. Illustrations (cartoons)	13. Temporal relations
	14. Transitive relations
Tools requiring limited vocabulary	15. Syllogism
4. Orientation in Space I	
5. Orientation in Space II	*Additional tools*
6. Orientation in Space III	1. Absurdities
7. Comparisons	2. Analogies
8. Family relations	3. Convergent and divergent thinking
9. Numerical progressions	4. Illusions
10. Stencil design	5. Language and symbolic comparisons
	6. Maps
	7. Auditory and haptic discrimination

4. Producing reflective, insightful processes in the student/client as a result of his or her confrontation with both failing and successful behaviors in the IE tasks

5. Creating task-intrinsic motivation, which has two aspects, including the enjoyment of a task for its own sake and the social implication of succeeding in a task that is difficult even for independent adults

6. Providing the cognitively low-performing individual with a self-identity that sees himself or herself as capable of generating information and ready to function as such, as a result of this self-perception.

In the Dynamic Approach for Cognitive Modifiability outlined above, evaluation and treatment are interwoven and undertaken together during intervention.

Instrumental Enrichment in Occupational Therapy and Target Populations

Instrumental Enrichment in Israel has been used with adult populations for the past decade (Katz & Hadas, 1995). It is used mainly by occupational therapists who specialize in rehabilitation of adolescent and adult populations with various dysfunc-

tions (physical, cognitive, emotional, behavioral). IE is used in conjunction with evaluation and treatment of daily living skills (ADL), vocational/professional skills, and social skills, as well as during transition from the hospital to the community.

The goals of the occupational therapist in this approach are twofold: improvement of underlying structures, and adaptation of the person to his or her environmental circumstances. IE is utilized in all three of the following phases of rehabilitation: medical rehabilitation, transitional setting of rehabilitation, and vocational and social rehabilitation in the community. Regardless of etiology, IE is used with populations who suffer from cognitive, emotional, and/or adaptational dysfunctions. Table 9-2 presents the goals and methods of treatment with these populations.

In the next section, we will provide examples of the treatment process according to IE within an occupational therapy framework among the following four populations (see Figure 9-6):

1. Clients following brain injury, who suffered from cognitive deficits during rehabilitation

2. Clients who suffered from psychiatric or emotional disorders and were in a transitional rehabilitation setting

3. Children suffering from ADHD and emotional problems

	Table 9-2	
	The Use of Instrumental Enrichment in Different Populations	
Type of Dysfunction	**Treatment Goals**	**Treatment Methods**
Cognitive	The improvement of dysfunctional skills: perception, thinking and memory processes	Individual
Emotional	The improvement of personal and interpersonal behavior, and of cognitive flexibility	Group and individual
Adaptational	The improvement of social and cognitive skills; the development of coping mechanisms for adaptation to reality	Mainly individual

4. Adolescents with adaptational difficulties in a community rehabilitation center.

Cognitive Treatment for Brain-Injured Clients Using Instrumental Enrichment in a Rehabilitation Center

The Loewenstein Hospital is a major rehabilitation center in Israel that treats traumatic head injuries that typically result from accidents or various tumors. The average age of the clients is young, about 30 years old. Clients are transferred to the Loewenstein Hospital from acute-care hospitals immediately after intensive medical treatment is terminated. They arrive with different levels of independence and confusion—from clients bedridden or sitting in a wheelchair but unable to stand, dress, eat, or wash unassisted, to those seemingly independent, that is, able to get around the hospital and get to treatment sessions on their own.

The treatment of clients at this point revolves around the area of deficit and is adapted to the needs of the injured client at any given moment (Katz, Hefner, & Rueben, 1990; Najenson, Rahmani, Elazar, & Averbuch, 1984). The emphasis here is on treatment, not on education, so the use of the enrichment tools is not exactly as in the IE program. An instrument is not followed through all of its exercises. An impaired skill will be exercised with suitable parts (i.e., working pages) from different sections. Exercises not from the enrichment program but at the same level and style may be added. The multitude of materials at graded

levels enable systematic and broad treatment of a specific deficit.

Instrumental Enrichment and Spatial-Orientation Problems

The treatment relates to the following four aspects: the individual's physical ability to perform daily living activities; the place (table) where he or she works on the pages of the Instrumental Enrichment program, the immediate surroundings (i.e., hospital, ward), and the nonimmediate surroundings (i.e., city, country). The tools of the enrichment program used in treatment are organized in ascending order of difficulty as follows (see Table 9-1):

Orientation in Space I, II, and III: Spatial orientation has three sections that intervene directly in one of the most commonly observed deficiencies of the cognitively disabled performer: his or her limited use of articulated, differential, and representational spatial dimensions. The first of the three sections deals with spatial orientation relative to one's own body, using one's own movements for the frame of reference. The second part adds dimensions of topological space (i.e., on, above, below, up, down, between). The third part deals with an external and stable reference system, the cardinal points of the compass, which is then combined with the first two reference systems. These three parts are directed primarily toward the creation of specific strategies for differentiating the

Figure 9-6

IE intervention in occupational therapy
(Hadas-Lidor 1996, used with permission from *IJOT*).

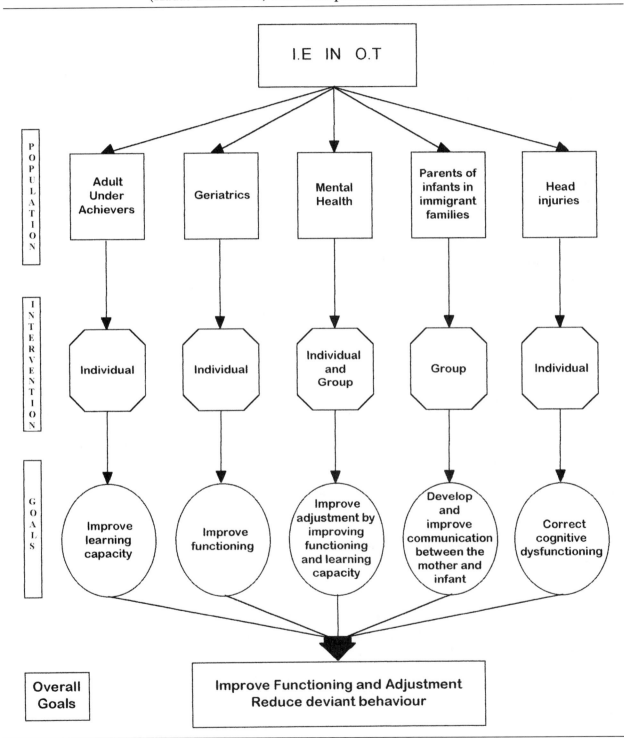

spatial frame of reference from other criteria. They also introduce and demonstrate the relativity of certain systems versus the stability of others.

Organization of Dots: Each of the 26 working pages of organization of dots contains 14 to 18 exercises. The teacher/therapist provides the learner/client with ample opportunities to engage in various functions, to understand the role they play in the specific exercises, and to become aware of the roles these activities play in their own motor behavior. The motor aspect of the task is to identify and outline, within an amorphous cloud of dots, a series of overlapping geometric figures such as squares, triangles, diamonds, and stars. The molecular components of the task are numerous and reflect a wealth of elements that can directly challenge the difficulties experienced by the cognitively low-performer. The exercises therefore are addressed to the correction of a variety of deficient cognitive functions including projection of virtual relationships, conservation of constancy, visual transport, precision and accuracy, summative behavior, planning and restraint of impassivity, discrimination, and segregation of proximate elements.

Analytic Perception: The analytic perception part consists of 38 working pages. The first unit includes such tasks as subdividing a simple or complex whole into its parts, summing the number of the components, and finding parts that are identical to the given standard within a complex whole. To find a part, the individual must allow sufficient time to completely and accurately perceive the part, transport it visually (or through interiorization) into the field, and engage in a systematic search. In the exercises of the second unit, the parts of a whole are identified, categorized, and summed. Tasks involve seeking strategies for the recognition, registration, and inclusion of the relevant components of a whole. In the third unit, tasks deal with constructing wholes based on identifiable parts and the closure of figures on a gestalt test by deducing the parts that are missing and identifying them in another setting. The last unit provides subjects with practice in constructing new wholes from the union of some of the parts. Tasks range from pure perceptual exploration to transposition and transformations of the elements.

Instrumental Enrichment in the Development of Thought Processes

The treatment begins with the simple and moves to the more complex; from single to multiple, from the individual to the whole community. The IE tools include stimuli in three areas: visual, verbal, and numerical. The IE sections used in the treatment of thought processes from simple to complex are as follows.

Comparisons: Comparisons deal with the development of spontaneous comparative behavior. Comparative behavior is the most elementary building block of relational thinking and, therefore, a primary condition for any cognitive process that will transcend mere recognition and identification. The comparisons part consists of 22 working pages. The first unit introduces the subject to the concept of commonality and differences in pictorial and verbal modalities. In the exercises, the subject must compare two items on discrete dimensions, which start with size, form, number, and spatial and temporal concepts, and conclude with abstract attributes not immediately perceived (such as function, composition, and power). In the second unit, the subject compares objects to a standard along several dimensions simultaneously. In the exercises of the third unit, the learner is required to establish classes.

Categorization: Categorization is designed to deal with the lack of, or impairment of, the learner's ability to elaborate on gathered data by use of hierarchically higher mental processes, for the organization of the data into superordinate categories. Classification is based on successful comparison, differentiation, and discrimination. The categorization part consists of 31 working pages, divided into units and graded according to levels of complexity. The instrument is presented through the use of verbal, pictorial, schematic, and figural modes. It is based on skills and procedures learned in comparisons and leads into the instrumental syllogism section.

Numerical Progressions: The major focus of this part is to train the learner to search for the rules that form the basis of certain experienced events and into the relationships existing between them.

Transitive Relationships: The transitive relations part has 23 working pages. It focuses on drawing inferences of new relationships from those existing between object and/or events that can be described in terms of "greater than," "equal to," and "less than." In the first five pages of this part, the subject is introduced to the concept of ordered sets and the signs used to designate relationships. In the first exercise, he or she is offered strategies for ordering the data and encoding it in such a way as to have the coded information present in the visual field.

Representational Stencil Design: The representational stencil design is an advanced level in the instrumental enrichment program. It capitalizes on functions acquired in the other parts (e.g., organization of data, analytic perception, comparisons, categorization, spatial orientation, and temporal relationships) and permits their application to situations that require rather complex levels of representational internalized behavior. The representational stencil design part consists of working pages that require the learner to construct mentally, and not through motor manipulation, a design identical to that in a colored standard. Colored stencils, some of which are solid and some of which are cut out, are printed on a poster. The learner mentally recreates the given design by referring to the stencils that must be used, and by specifying the order in which they must be superimposed on each other.

In summary, the adaptation of IE to the treatment of people suffering from head injuries requires that:

1. *The treatment is individualized.* It must be adapted to each person according to his or her specific deficits and conditions.
2. *The treatment focuses on cognitive skill* through using the whole range of materials. Working through all parts of the instrument is not significant; it is more important to use stimuli that are appropriate to the specific deficit.
3. *The treatment is progressive and very slow* through sometimes, out of necessity, adding similar exercises to the treatment, even if they are not part of the enrichment program.
4. *The treatment uses illustration when necessary.* For example, in the spatial orientation working

pages, sometimes the therapist must build a three-dimensional model (e.g., with a Lego® set), or cut out a figure of a person from cartoon and stand it up to provide a concrete illustration. To help in the analysis and synthesis exercises, the therapist must cut out the parts and help to assemble them again into a design.

Instrumental Enrichment for Psychiatric Clients: Group Treatment

Shalvata Psychiatric hospital in Israel includes a halfway rehabilitation unit for client evaluation and preparation for rehabilitation in the community. Most often the clients treated in the unit have had a history of psychiatric hospitalization and have been diagnosed with various types of schizophrenia. Ages of the population range from 18 to 40 years. The main goal of the unit is to prepare clients for social and vocational rehabilitation in the community. The enrichment program within this unit usually takes place in groups of four to five clients.

There are three objectives of treatment. The first involves improving the client's cognitive ability and flexibility through using existing skills, focusing on the process of adaptation to changing situations, and learning problem-solving techniques, such as those related to decision making, organization, and planning. Second, treatment focuses on improving the client's social skills and helping him or her integrate into a work group, specifically by moderating impulses, developing the ability to listen as well as to accept orders and criticism, and finally, establishing the ability to express one's self. Third, treatment tries to raise the client's awareness of his or her strengths and weaknesses, and to learn how to use one's assets for adaptation.

To demonstrate a group process, we will describe an example of a group session that centered on awareness to work needs. Page 9 from the comparison section of the IE program was utilized (see Figure 9-7). The purpose of this exercise is to help the client automatize comparisons, perceive the basis for classification, and correct his or her episodic grasp of reality. The client learns to find similarities and differences between objects, events, and ideas. He or she learns to use concepts and

Figure 9-7

Working page 9, Comparison section of Feuerstein IE program.

Name _____

9

Circle the word or words that describe what is common between the sample picture on the left and each of the pictures in the same row.

Sample Picture

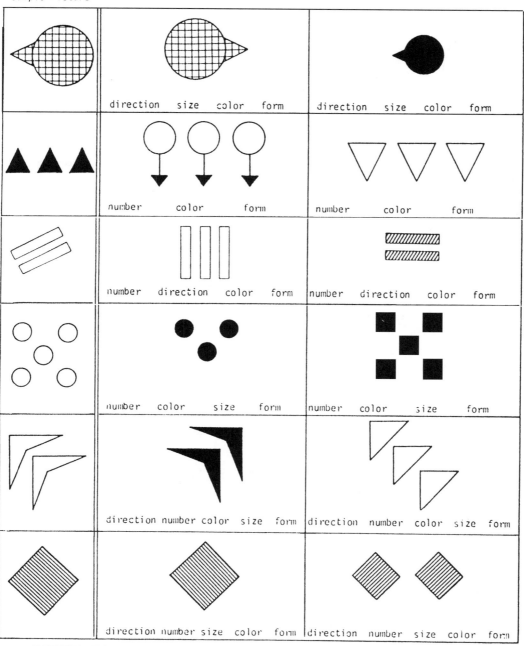

Comp 9

to identify the most essential or characteristic dimensions, while ignoring the irrelevant.

The activity of the group included three parts. First, the task was performed as given on the page. Each person received a working page and had to complete it individually. Second, criteria were suggested and opened to discussion during the session. For example, the therapist discussed with the group the concept of objective and subjective criteria, and the explanations and interpretations of these terms by the people in the group were used. *Objective* was defined as "something that I am not involved in," or "something that is not dependent on me." Following the individual work, a group discussion was conducted on the need for criteria when making a choice or decision. For example, participants used objective criteria (i.e., color, shape, size, material, and weight) and subjective criteria (i.e., taste, goal, and need) to understand when and why one among them would compare two ashtrays on the table. This led to the third activity in which at the group's suggestion, participants made a list of things that "we can choose in life" such as car, mate, house, school, furniture, where to live, profession, and workplace. Out of the initial list, they further decided to make a list of criteria in order to choose a workplace; they included subjective criteria and compared each other's criteria to the group's (Table 9-3).

Intervention of this kind allows therapists to raise the individual's awareness of himself or herself to his or her needs at any given moment and in comparison to the rest of the group. As Tzuriel (1991) states, the affective motivational factors play an important role in the reciprocal interaction of MLE and cognitive modifiability.

The treatment was based on two goals: forming an awareness of the practical necessity for activating the cognitive functions treated by this tool, and the spontaneous use of cognitive skills for the purpose of adaptation or preparation for the work role. It is interesting to note in Table 9-3 that the needs of belonging, love, and security (i.e., second and third in Maslow's hierarchy of needs) are the most important needs for all members of the group. Only one participant pointed out the highest need in the hierarchy—self-actualization—as important to him. The causal relationship between needs and cognitive functions was recently stated by Rand (1991). He incorporates the concept of need as one component in an integrative model based on MLE. Need is defined as "an internalized energizing psychological system which is function bound" (p. 80).

Instrumental Enrichment with a Child Suffering from ADHD

Goldwasser and Hadas-Lidor (1996) presented the case of Jimmy, a 10-year-old boy who experienced lengthy periods of mild obsessive behavior at moments of pressure and anxiety, which necessitated admission to a children's mental health clinic. He also had a history of difficulties with learning, reading, and writing. Although a neurological examination concluded that Jimmy suffered from ADHD,

Table 9-3

The Needs That Work Fulfills and Their Importance in the Eyes of Participants in the Rehabilitation Group

		Participants				
Needs	Maslow's Hierarchy	1	2	3	4	5
Able working hours; pay, good conditions	Basic needs	+	0	0	+	−
Tenure, security, safety	Security needs	+	+	+	+	+
Good personal relations, pleasant atmosphere	Love needs	+	+	+	+	+
Evaluation and acceptance	Evaluation needs	−	0	−	0	+
Interest, advancement development	Self-actualization needs	0	0	−	−	+

Note: The first list of needs was compiled by the group participants. The second list is according to Maslow's hierarchy of needs for comparison. The scales is as follows: + very important; − not important; 0 of little importance.

he did not receive any medicinal intervention. During the intake discussion, he suffered from lapses in his chain of thought and had a tendency toward perseverance (e.g., repeating words and sentences a number of times). Sometimes he stopped in the middle of a sentence and could not remember what he wanted to say. He suffered from compulsive behavior (e.g., compulsive organization and tidiness at home and in class) and from an overemphasized need for perfection in terms of writing individual letters. He often occupied his time with attempts in finding connections between different objects. Throughout all his behavior, he typically displayed a significant amount of fear and lack of self-confidence.

Following his initial evaluation and diagnosis, we decided to treat Jimmy with IE and withhold medication. At first, the treatment plan focused on his low self-image and lack of confidence, and later on his specific functional difficulties. According to Jimmy, his low self-image was a result of difficulties in reading and writing at school. He thought that his parents were disappointed in him, even though it appeared that they had accepted and supported him.

We began treatment with the aid of analytic perception, an important component of the IE program. Its main aim is to teach strategies, to organize and analyze the conceptual field, to differentiate between its various parts, and to divide the whole according to specific goals. Additional goals for Jimmy were to exercise the skills of reconstructing a given field, as well as to build a field through practice from the start. In reference to character makeup, the aim of this tool was to encourage changes in Jimmy's opinion, attitude, and motivation for performance for his own sake and within the environment, through developing various cognitive strategies.

The specific goals that we chose in treating Jimmy's low self-image through the use of analytic perception tools were:

1. To increase his awareness of the fact that every part is a whole within itself
2. To increase his awareness that it is possible to create new wholes by combining different parts
3. To increase his awareness that each part is essen-

tially arbitrary, and is dependent on the needs and goals at a given time and place.

Jimmy received the exercise on page 1 of the analytical perception section (see Figure 9-8). In the first stage, he performed the task according to the following instructions: "On the left-hand side of the page, list the number of different parts that form the shape, and on the right-hand side, draw each part in a different color." He then needed to respond to the following question: "If you were given one of the small parts that made up the whole, would you be able to know or guess what the overall shape was?" In his first attempt, Jimmy initially answered affirmatively. He then covered the whole shape, exposed a small part, and began to participate in a second chance at the question. Next, he looked repeatedly at the piece, and eventually concluded that he could not predict the appearance of the final shape by simply looking at the original, single piece. In other words, when the individual views and overemphasizes the part as being a whole in itself, it becomes impossible to learn from the part what the total and final shape will be.

Next, Jimmy needed to choose one of the shapes from the analytic perception exercises and to relate to it as though it represented the pieces that are found in each one of us. He had to define each part, as well as identify which aspect of his personality or daily life roles each represented. Some examples of his responses were: He found reading and writing difficult ; he enjoyed drawing and participating or observing sports; he was a pupil at school as well as his mother's son, and so forth. Jimmy chose the shape that was composed of nine parts, among which he was content with seven, but defined two as being problematic (i.e., his functioning at school and his reading and writing). In a follow-up question, he was unable to label any piece as being the biggest, and he answered that he felt good about many parts. Jimmy realized that, normally, he thought in generalities (i.e., that the moment he viewed one part as bad, he saw everything as bad), and that he was unable to isolate his feelings or events.

At this stage, however, he arrived at a cognitive understanding that more good parts existed than parts with which he could not live. This allowed him

Figure 9-8

Working page, Analytical Perception section of Feuerstein IE program
(Goldwasser and Hadas-Lidor, 1996, with permission from *IJOT*).

Color each section a different color.	Place a number in each section.

Into how many sections has the whole been divided? 4

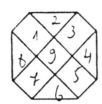

Into how many sections has the whole been divided? 9

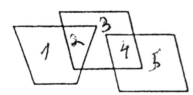

Into how many sections has the whole been divided? 5

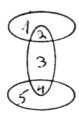

Into how many sections has the whole been divided? 5

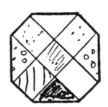

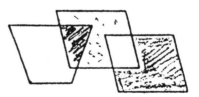

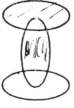

Analytic Perception – 1

to become more sensitive to his weaker side, without feeling threatened about his overall performance.

We discussed the possibility that, in time, the weaker points that were problematic today would lessen. In other words, each part would become arbitrary and dependent on the needs and goals of a specific time and place. Even if Jimmy found it difficult today to cope with and overcome learning difficulties within the school framework, his new understanding of reality would lead him to a positive self-image and eventually to changes in his functioning in the classroom and at home.

The Importance of Instrumental Enrichment for Clients Suffering from Emotional Disorders

In the case of clients with emotional disorders, the IE performs the following functions: (1) focuses on behavioral elements, both personal and interpersonal; (2) helps the individual relate to others through group treatment; (3) emphasizes integration processes and awareness and utilization of one's capabilities; and (4) intervenes through following an order of the working pages according to clients' needs (although pages are often chosen out of order to best suit the needs of the group).

Instrumental Enrichment with Clients Who Exhibit Adaptational Difficulties

The rehabilitation center in Herzeliya is one of 20 community vocational rehabilitation centers in Israel that serve a heterogeneous population of age, type of injury, and gender. The common denominator for this population is the limitation of employment. The client's dysfunction can be cognitive, emotional, physical, developmental/learning, related to cultural deprivation, or any combination of the above.

The rehabilitation center has a number of activity centers, including diagnosis and reality-oriented workshops that aim to develop vocational skills, production workshops on different levels, as well as secretarial, sewing, and cooking workshops. The interdisciplinary team that works at the center includes social workers, psychologists, counselors, occupational therapists, and placement specialists.

At the center, two major goals of rehabilitation were identified. The client should be able to work in the community either in the open market or in a partially sheltered or completely sheltered workshop. The client will be able to live independently in the community.

Some of the clients in the workshops also receive a few extra hours of treatment per week based on the enrichment program. They learn basic general educational subjects and, as with everyone else, have sessions with a social worker. The success of enrichment therapy depends on optimal coordination between the various team members.

The goals of enrichment in this framework are as follows:

1. To improve cognitive flexibility and adaptability (this capacity to change will enable the rehabilitation client to adapt to the work reality in his or her community)
2. To improve and enhance the client's work habits, including his or her ability to follow a time schedule, to produce an end result, to accept orders and criticism, and to work independently.

With these goals in mind, the therapist chooses from the following areas of the IE working pages, in addition to organization of dots, orientation in space, analytic perception, and transitive relations which have already been described. Additional areas such as family relations and cartoons are very rarely used.

Temporal relations: This area is geared toward retraining the person's perception of time and his or her capacity to register processes and order temporal relationships.

Instructions: Instructions is one of the few sections in the whole program in which verbal factors play an important and central position. Language is emphasized as a system for both encoding and decoding processes on a variety of levels. These range from simple labeling after recognition to the use of inferred instructions deduced from combining given instructional codes and presented stimuli. The individual must read and carry out instructions and use the three phases of the mental act in the following systematic and orderly way: *input*—gathering of the data; *elaboration*—ordering the object in the required relationship; and *output*—carrying out the instruction by drawing the required figures.

Syllogism: The mastery of this concept indicates an ability to engage in both inductive and deductive reasoning under highly abstract conditions.

Case Example of an Adolescent Client

One example of treatment involves an adolescent with a mild physical disability since birth and social deprivation that were expressed as adaptational difficulties. Eli was 15 years old when he started coming to treatment. He was born in Yemen, the third of five children. His father is a plumber, and his mother is a kindergarten teacher's helper. Eli has had a deformation in his right hand from birth. He is considered the least successful or the "black sheep" of the family. He attended a regular school until the seventh grade and was then referred to neuropsychological and vocational evaluation. The main assessment results indicated that he has psychomotor restlessness. For example, he uses his right hand only to assist the left; he works quickly but not efficiently; he tires easily; he works impulsively; and he follows only short assignments or tasks. His shape perception is normal, as are his perception of models and memory of simple material. He has more difficulty when planning is required. His thought processes are concrete, yet his logical thought is deficient, and he works on a trial and error basis and has no self-criticism.

The team's recommendations following the evaluation were that Eli should be given simple and short tasks that could be changed easily, and that he should also be provided with cognitive training. The first phases of rehabilitation included production workshops for habit training, a study program in basic education, and a two-part enrichment plan to treat Eli's behavior problems (impulsivity, low self-esteem) and his cognitive problems (use of strategies, complexity and oral material, attention, and concentration).

At the beginning of treatment, Eli would hide his right hand and talk very little (and then with a limited vocabulary). His self-expectations were very low—to be a production line worker. While talking, he would not make direct eye contact. His gaze was "scattered," not focused, and he worked inefficiently.

The second phase of rehabilitation included transferring Eli to the secretarial workshop due to both his request and our evaluation results that indicated his potential to learn. In his studies, he was busy gaining basic knowledge and learning new terms, learning to read and write, and improving his ability to formulate sentences and summarize material.

In the enrichment program with Eli we used working pages from the organization of dots; analytical perception; categorization—the knowledge of general terms; instructions—the treatment of impulsivity, concentration, and receiving orders; cartoons—language improvement; and numerical progression. After a year of treatment in the center and at Eli's request, he was enrolled in secretarial school. Two years later, Eli is currently working as a teller in a bank. He is independent and does not receive any treatment.

Instrumental Enrichment is important in a community rehabilitation center for the following reasons:

1. The work must be coordinated with the other aspects of treatment that the client is receiving.
2. The focus is on adaptation to a general setting, especially to a work environment.
3. The order of the IE sections is not binding; the choice of working pages is according to the treatment subject.
4. The treatment is individualized.

The population in the center is very heterogenic, and sometimes small groups can be formed to emphasize interpersonal relationships and working together.

Research on Instrumental Enrichment

Research studies have traditionally centered on children and adolescents with learning disabilities, mental retardation, and cultural/social deprivation. Burden (1987) and Savell et al. (1986) reviewed the research studies conducted in reference to Instrumental Enrichment treatment effectiveness in the 1970s and early 1980s. The first studies that were performed in the 1970s are reported by Feuerstein (1970). They focused on adolescents who immigrated to Israel from North Africa. The studies attempted to show the effectiveness of the IE program with a pre–post design and a matched control group, which received enrichment in general content areas (the GE group). Their findings showed significant differences in the experimental group over the control group in nonverbal IQ tests. No significant improvement was evident in self-concept in either of the groups. However, the original studies were criticized for problems in their methodology and data analysis.

The largest body of data was collected in the United States during the late 1970s within five large centers among various populations (Burden, 1987). The findings reinforce the original study's results, showing significant increase of IQ scores (especially on the Raven Matrices) following the IE program. In addition, the effects on noncognitive measures (self-esteem, motivation, locus of control, and the approach to problems) were reported to increase the following of the IE program (Savell et al., 1986).

In the 1990s, there is an increase in studies concerning IE intervention with various populations. Juliobo, Malicky, and Norman (1995) show that metacognition of young readers improved during the IE intervention. Sanz de Acedo Lizarraga (1991) discusses the impact of IE intervention on literacy as well as metacognition in written composition. Several studies reported about IE intervention with healthy populations, such as engineers (Alwis & Seng Seok Hoon, 1993), high school students (Strang & Shayer, 1991) and gifted children (Braude, 1994; Kaniel & Reichenberg, 1990; Kaniel & Reichenberg, 1992).

The mutual relations between IE and intelligence is the subject of two studies. Blagg (1991) examined whether intelligence can be improved with IE intervention, and Church (1994) conducted a longitudinal study of the effect of Feuerstein's IE program on intersensory integration, academic achievement, and referral for special education program.

In all of these works, the IE program seemed to have an impact. This was also found by Hadas-Lidor in a recent study investigating the effectiveness of cognitive dynamic treatment through the use of Instrumental Enrichment in mentally ill adults. The subjects included 60 clients who suffered from schizophrenia and required treatment at a rehabilitation day center. The clients were randomly assigned into two groups, one utilized IE as treatment, and the other treated clients according to traditional groups. Length of treatment and time in the day during a week was equal for both groups. The study was a pre–post quasi-experimental design and lasted for half a year. The following variables were measured before and after treatment: cognitive performance, self-concept, and daily functioning. The results following treatment showed significant differences between the study group and the control group in the areas of cognitive performance and daily functioning, within both the home and work environments. No significant differences were found regarding self-concept. This study, which is the first treatment effectiveness study within adults suffering from schizophrenia, has important implications, as it suggests both that the IE program is effective and that clients suffering from schizophrenia can improve in their cognitive skills as well as everyday functioning.

In summary, the theory behind and the practice of the IE program and the LPAD dynamic assessment are still under development, and research studies are being conducted in many countries worldwide and by different professionals. The dynamic approach has also been recommended for inclusion in the framework of cognitive rehabilitation in the adult brain-injured population (Groverman et al., 1985; Hadas-Lidor, 1996; Toglia, 1989; Toglia, 1991).

Summary

The theory of Cognitive Modifiability is composed of the following three main elements: the concept of cognitive modifiability, the approach to treatment (MLE), and the instruments of assessment and treatment (LPAD, IE environments). The theory of cognitive modifiability is, first and foremost, an approach to understanding the relationships between the individual and other persons, and (only afterwards) is it a treatment method. The Learning Potential Assessment Device (LPAD) is a tool that enables us not only to assess the cognitive potential of the clients, but to assess their ability to modify and to adjust. The IE program is special in that it is *optimistic* (it supports the belief that everyone has the potential to learn and change in every situation, if the right way is found), *holistic* (it considers all aspects of the person, such as cognitive, emotional, and behavioral), and *flexible* (it can be applied to all ages, to different needs, and within various treatment settings). Instrumental Enrichment agrees with occupational therapy philosophy and rehabilitation. It relates to the person as a whole despite his or her disabilities and tries to improve the individual's quality of life and self-esteem. Environment refers to the framework of the person's life, and it is important that this environment be suited to his or her needs and abilities in his or her present situation (Hadas-Lidor, 1996).

Implications for Further Development in Occupational Therapy

As mentioned earlier, much research has been performed on children and adolescents. Only a few studies exist on the effectiveness of the LPAD and Instrumental Enrichment with adult disabled populations and further research is needed. Qualitative methods might be utilized in such studies, as they are appropriate for understanding treatment outcomes of this dynamic intervention process (Burden, 1990). Theoretically, it is important to continue the conceptual work of integrating the philosophy and theory of cognitive modifiability and Mediated Learning Experience with occupational therapy principles. Clinically, it is important to analyze tasks and try to combine the IE materials with evaluation and treatment tools and methods utilized in occupational therapy.

References

Allen, C. K. (1985). *Occupational therapy for psychiatric diseases: Measurement and management of cognitive disabilities.* Boston: Little, Brown.

Allen, C. K., Earhart, C., & Blue, T. (1992). *Occupational therapy treatment goals for the physically and cognitively disabled.* Bethesda, MD: American Occupational Therapy Association.

Alwis, W., & Seng Seok Hoon, A. (1993). Thinking skills for engineers: Mediated learning with knowledge-rich tasks. *Aeeseap J. of Engineering Education, 23,* 61–66.

Anthony, W., Cohen, M., & Farber, M. (1990). *Psychiatric rehabilitation.* Boston: Center for Psychiatric Rehabilitation.

Avanjini, G. (1990). Pedagogies de la Mediation. Autour du P.E.I. programme d'Enrichissement Instrumental du Professeur Reuven Feuerstein. Lyon, Depot Legal: Chronique Sociale.

Ayers, J. (1979). *Sensory integration and the child.* Los Angeles: Western Psychological Services.

Beasley, F., & Shayer, M. (1990). Learning potential assessment through Feuerstein's LPAD: Can quantitative results be achieved? *The International Journal of Dynamic Assesment and Instruction, 1,* 2.

Blagg, N. (1991). *Evaluation of I.E. in England—can we teach intelligence? A contribution evaluation of Feuerstein's I.E. program.* Hillsdale, NJ: Erlbaum.

Braude, G. (1994). *I.E. in technical highschool for disadvantaged adolescents.* South Africa: University of Witwatersrand.

Brown, A. L., Campione, J. C., Webber, L. S., & Mcgilly, K. (1992). Interactive learning environments: A new look at assesment and instruction. In R. Bernard Gifford and M. C. O'Connor (Eds.). *Changing assesments: Alternative views of aptitude, achievement and instruction. Evaluation in education and human services.* Boston: Kluwer.

Brozo, W. G. (1990). Learning how at-risk readers learn best—A case for interactive assessment. *Journal of Reading, 33,* 522–527.

Buchel, F. P., & Scharnhorst, U. (1993). The learning potential assessment device (LPAD): Discussion of theoretical and methodological problems. In J. H. M. Hamers, K. Sijtsma, & A. J. J. M. Ruijssenaars (Eds.) *Learning potential assessment: Theoretical, methodological and practical issues.* Amsterdam/Lisse: Swets and Zeitling.

Burden, R. (1987). Feuerstein's Instrumental Enrichment Programme: Important issues in research and evaluation. *European Journal of Psychology of Education, 11,* 3–16.

Burden, R. (1990). Whither research on I.E.? Some suggestions for future action. *International Journal of Cognitive Education and Mediated Learning, 1,* 1.

Burns, M. S., Delclos, V., Vye, N. J., & Sloan, K. (1992). Changes in cognitive strategies in dynamic assessment. *International Journal of Dynamic Assessment and Instruction. 2,* 45–54.

Carney, J., & Cioffi, G. (1990). Extending traditional diagnosis in the dynamic assessment of reading abilities. *Reading Psychology, 11,* 177–192.

Carney, J., & Cioffi, G. (1992). The dynamic assessment of reading abilities. *International Journal of Disability, Development and Education, 39,* 107–114.

Church, S. L. (1994). *A longitudinal study of the effect of Feuerstein's I.E. on intersensory integration, academic achievement and referal for special education program.* Norman: University of Oklahoma.

Day, J. D., & Cordon, L. A. (1993). Static and dynamic measures of ability: An experimental comparison. *Journal of Educational Psychology, 85,* 75–82.

Feuerstein, R. (1970). A dynamic approach to the causation, prevention, and alleviation of retarded performance. In H. C. Haywood (Ed.), *Socio-cultural aspect of mental retardation.* New York: Appleton-Century-Crofts.

Feuerstein, R. (1979), in collaboration with Y. Rand and M. B. Hoffman. *The dynamic assessment of retarded performers: The learning potential assessment device, theory, instruments, and techniques.* Baltimore: University Park Press.

Feuerstein, R. (1980), in collaboration with Y. Rand, M. B. Hoffman, & R. Miller. *Instrumental enrichment: An intervention program for cognitive modifiability.* Baltimore: University Park Press.

Feuerstein, R., & Feuerstein, S. (1991). In R. Feuerstein, P. S. Klein, & A. J. Tannenbaum, *Mediated Learning Experience.* London: Freund.

Fisher, A. G., Murray, E. A., & Bundy, A. C. (1992). *Sensory integration: Theory and practice.* Philadelphia: Davis.

Goldwasser, S., & Hadas-Lidor, N. (1996). Instrumental Enrichment with children suffering from emotional and cognitive problems, and social difficulties. *Israeli Journal of Occupational Therapy, 5,* E37–50.

Grisseman, H. (1993). Diagnostical implication in new understanding of dyslexia. *Schweizerische Zeitscohrift fur Psychologie Revue Suisse de Psychologia, 52,* 205–229.

Groverman, A. M., Brown, E. W., & Miller, M. H. (1985). Moving toward common ground: Utilizing Feuerstein's model in cognitive rehabilitation. *Cognitive Rehabilitation,* May/June, 28–30.

Guthke, J. (1992). Learning tests: The concept, main research findings, problems and trends. *Learning and Individual Differences, 4,* 137–151.

Hadas-Lidor, N. (1996). Feuerstein's theory of cognitive modifiability and its applications to occupational therapy. *Israeli Journal of Occupational Therapy, 5,* E1–15.

Juliobo, M., Malicky, G., & Norman, C. (1995). *Metacognition of young readers in an early intervention program.* Alberta, Canada: University of Alberta.

Kaniel, S. (1992). The effect of mediation on performance and distribution of errors in the Raven Progressive Matrices test. *International Journal of Cognitive Education & Mediated Learning, 6,* 17–24.

Kaniel, S., & Reichenberg, R. (1990). Dynamic assessment and cognitive program for disadvantaged gifted children. *Gifted Education International, 7,* 9–15.

Kaniel, S., & Reichenberg, R. (1992). Instrumental Enrichment—effects of generalization and durability with talented adolescents. *Gifted Education International, 8,* 128–135.

Katz, N., & Hadas, N. (1995). Cognitive rehabilitation: Occupational therapy models for intervention in psychiatry. *Psychiatric Rehabilitation Journal, 19,* 29–37.

Katz, N., Hefner, D., & Rueben, R. (1990). Measuring clinical change in cognitive rehabilitation of clients with brain damage: Two cases, Traumatic Brain Injury and Cerebral Vascular Accident. *Occupational Therapy in Health Care, 7,* 23–43.

Kielhofner, G. (Ed.). (1985). *A model of human occupation, theory and application.* Baltimore: Williams & Wilkins.

Kielhofner, G. (Ed.). (1995). *A model of human occupation, theory and application* (2nd ed.). Baltimore: Williams & Wilkins.

Klein, P. S. (1991). Moral assessment and parental intervention in infancy and early childhood: New evidence. In R. Feuerstein, P. S. Klein, & A. J. Tannenbaum (Eds.), *Mediated Learning Experience (MLE) Theoretical, Psychosocial and Learning Application.* London: Freund.

Klein, P. S., & Hundeide, K. (1989). *More intelligent and sensitive child (MISC): A training manual.* Norway: University of Oslo.

Kushnir A. (1996). Mediated intervention with mothers natives of the Caucasus who immigrated to Israel. *Israeli Journal of Occupational Therapy, 5,* E105–126.

Lezak, M. (1995). *Neuropsychological assessment* (2nd ed.). Baltimore: Williams & Wilkins.

Lidz, C. S. (1987). *Dynamic assessment: An interactional approach to evaluating learning potential.* New York: Guilford Press.

Meyer, A. (1922, reprint 1977). The philosophy of occupation therapy. *American Journal of Occupational Therapy, 31,* 10, 639–642.

Moreno C. (1996). Feuerstein's mediated learning and instrumental enrichment: Applications in occupational therapy intervention: A case study. *Israeli Journal of Occupational Therapy, 5,* E152–158.

Najenson, T., Rahmani, L., Elazar, B., & Averbuch, S. (1984). An elementary cognitive assessment and treatment of the craniocerebrally injured client. In B. A. Edelstein & E. T. Couture (Eds.), *Behavioral assessment and rehabilitation of the traumatically brain damaged.* New York: Plenum Press.

Neff, S.W. (1985). *Work and human behavior* (3rd ed.). New York: Aldine.

Neistadt, M. (1990). A critical analysis of occupational therapy approaches for perceptual deficits in adults with brain injury. *American Journal of Occupational Therapy, 44,* 299–304.

Rand, Y. (1991). Deficient cognitive functions in non-cognitive determinants—An integrating model: Assessment and intervention. In R. Feuerstein, P. S. Klein, & A. J. Tannenbaum, *Mediated Learning Experience.* London: Freund.

Sanz de Acedo Lizarraga, R. (1991). Learning to think: Metacognition in written composition. *International Journal of Cognitive Education & Mediated Learning, 5,* 15–32.

Savell, J. M., Twohig, P. T. & Rachford, D. L. (1986). Empirical status of Feuerstein's "Instrumental Enrichment" (FIE) technique as a method of teaching thinking skills. *Review of Educational Research, 56,* 4, 381–409.

Slagle, E. C. (1922). Training aids for mental clients. *Archives of Occupational Therapy, 1,* 11–17.

Strang, J., & Shayer, M. (1991). Enhancing high school students' achievement in chemistry through a thinking approach. *International Journal of Science Education, 15,* 319–337.

Toglia, J. P. (1989). Approaches to cognitive assessment of the brain injured adult: Traditional methods and dynamic investigation. *Occupational Therapy Practice, 1,* 36–57.

Toglia, J. P. (1991). Generalization of treatment: A multicontext approach to cognitive perceptual impairment in adults with brain injury. *American Journal of Occupational Therapy, 45,* 501–516.

Tzuriel, D. (1991). Cognitive modifiability, mediated learning experience and affective motivational processes: A transactional approach. In R. Feuerstein, P. S. Klein, & A. J. Tannenbaum. *Mediated Learning Experience.* London: Freund.

Tzuriel, D., & Eiboshitz, Y. (1992). Structured program of visual–motor integration (SP–VMI) for preschool children. *Learning and Individual Differences, 4,* 103–124.

PART 2

General Topics

CHAPTER 10

Cognitive Changes in Later Life: Rehabilitative Implications

Linda L. Levy, MA, OTR/L, FAOTA

Most older adults experience detectable changes in some areas of cognitive function as they age (Kausler, 1991, 1994; Salthouse, 1991). Fortunately, the effect of these changes on cognitive, functional, and behavioral competence is small; the majority of older persons remain active and productive until a very old age (Howieson, Holm, Kaye, et al., 1993). Yet, for the rehabilitation population, such changes in cognitive function are likely to necessitate knowledgeable adjustments in traditional rehabilitation protocols and strategies. This chapter will provide an overview of the most consistently documented cognitive changes that accompany normal aging and will highlight implications for rehabilitation professionals. At the outset, it should be recognized that cognitive changes do not occur uniformly in all persons or at given ages (Schaie, 1990). Consequently, there is no reason to assume that all older adults undergo cognitive decline with age, even if many of them do.

Memory

The most intensely studied cognitive process in aging is memory. Before we can identify the specific nature of changes that occur with age, it is important to review some basic concepts.

Memory is a basic cognitive function that is exceedingly complex. It builds upon attention (information needs to be attended to before it can be remembered) and includes the ability to learn information through any of the senses, to retain it for variable periods of time, and then to retrieve

the information when needed. Memory and learning are difficult to differentiate. Learning involves the acquisition of new information; memory involves the retention of that information. Clearly, there can be no memory if learning has not occurred first, and learning has no meaning without memory.

A number of theoretical models have been proposed about how memory operates. Some focus on the process of learning and memory; others focus on the structure of memory stores. Information processing theorists (Cerella, 1990; Best, 1989) describe memory in terms of three basic processes in which we engage when we try to learn and remember information: attending and taking in new information through the senses (learning/encoding), interpreting and retaining it for variable periods of time (encoding/storage), and then accessing the information when needed (retrieval). Structural information processing theories (Atkinson & Shiffrin, 1968) focus on the ways in which information is stored and organized in the brain.

The most influential structural theory of memory was developed by Atkinson and Shiffrin (1968). It proposes that memory involves the processing of information in three distinct types of memory storage systems: sensory memory, primary (short-term) memory, and secondary (long-term) memory. According to this theory, information must first pass through sensory memory in order to reach primary (short-term) memory, and then pass through primary (short-term) memory in order to enter secondary (long-term) memory. (Note that the theorists suggested that the terms *short-*

term memory and *long-term memory* be relabeled *primary memory and/or working memory* and *secondary*, respectively, to avoid confusion with the more conventional use of these terms.)

Sensory memory stores exact replicas of stimuli impinging on each of the senses in sensory registers. Sensory memories last for a brief period—from less than a second (in the case of a visual sensory memory) to as long as 4 seconds (in the case of auditory sensory memory). Information can be retrieved from sensory memory by attending to it, whereupon it is transferred into the primary (short-term) store.

Primary memory has a very small capacity and is quite brief: It can hold up to seven (plus or minus two) items of information (Miller, 1956) for conscious processing, and it can store this material for up to 30 seconds, unless maintained by repeating the information to ourselves, a process known as *mental rehearsal*. (The average memory span for words is five. For digits it is about seven or eight). Units of information beyond seven (plus or minus two) are lost by displacement by new information or decay, the fading of information over time. A classic example of primary memory is remembering a telephone number long enough to dial it. If one needs to remember the number for later use, then the number needs to be converted, or "encoded," in the form of concepts that can be stored and eventually recalled. Otherwise, the information will only get as far as short-term memory and will be forgotten in 5 to 10 seconds. Primary memory is also known as *working* or *immediate* memory and is often equated with consciousness. It is typically assessed by the digit span, the ability of an individual to repeat accurately a series of numbers presented by the examiner.

Secondary (long-term) memory is considered the "memory bank," the largest component of the memory system. It is the repository of information that was learned as recently as minutes ago (converted from primary memory), as well as very remote long-term memories. Secondary (long-term) memory stores information in terms of abstract symbols—primarily words but also images. Advances in positron-emission tomography (PET) scan technology reveal that anatomically the brain is constantly changing as it learns and remembers; specifically, conversion of primary memory into secondary memory is accompanied by demonstrable growth of new connections between neurons. Secondary memory has unlimited capacity, retains information permanently, and requires that information be analyzed and organized for storage and for later retrieval.

In order for stored information to be useful, it must be retrievable, i.e., accessible on demand. This process requires new information to be stored by associating it with other relevant information already been stored in secondary memory. These associations then serve as cues for retrieval of that information. Information can be retrieved in two ways: recall or recognition. *Recall* requires search and retrieval of information from storage without the use of any externally provided, orienting (or association) cues. In contrast, *recognition* requires information in storage to be matched with external orienting (or associational) cues. Clearly, recall is a more demanding test of retrieval than recognition: recalling the name of the current Speaker of the House is more difficult than recognizing his name when it is presented along with several others.

Tests for "recent" recall include the ability to remember the therapist's name for periods of 5 to 10 minutes in the face of distraction and/or orientation to time and place—items that must be learned daily. Tests for "recent" recall are particularly significant because they are often used in determining learning potential. Tests for "remote" recall include personal wedding dates, current events from the past, and/or lists of past presidents.

Experimental data on memory demonstrate only slight changes in learning/encoding processes prior to the age of 65, after which there is noticeable decline. The evidence is consistent that aging increases the amount of time it takes to perceive and retrieve information; in addition, central nervous system activity slows with age, and there are significant differences in the speed with which information is processed. Hence, older adults require more time and effort than younger people to learn/encode and retrieve an equivalent amount of new information (Perlmutter, et al., 1987; Poon, et al, 1980; Poon, et al. 1986). Concurrently, concentration is more easily disrupted; recalling a word, name, or thought may take longer (this is a memory lapse, not, as is often feared, a memory loss); older adults have greater difficulty with divided attention; and learning new information takes longer. Nonetheless, learning/encoding can be enhanced by practice or repetition and by efforts to enhance the association of new information with that already in storage (Smith, 1980; Zachs, 1982). Additionally, there is evidence that many of the factors that disadvantage elders at this stage of information processing can be reversed such that ultimately there is minimal decline in the ability to learn (Gounard & Hulicka, 1977). Reversible factors include *pace* (allowing sufficient time for the older adult to respond)(Witte, 1975), *diminished motivation* (secondary to increased caution, response reluctance, increased anxiety, and/or disinterest in content)(Botwinick, 1967; Eisdorfer, 1968), *reduced "depth" of information processing* (merely skimming the material rather than subjecting it to more meaningful analysis)(Craik, 1977), *decreased use of memory enhancing strategies* (mnemonic devices such as visual images)(Rowe & Schnore, 1971), and *sensory impairment* (mitigated by compensatory strategies for visual and auditory deficits). Thus, although information processing theorists propose a model of age-related changes in learning/memory performance based on decrements, they also suggest that these decrements can be compensated for.

Structural processing theorists have found age-related decrements in the sensory memory store (Craik, 1977; Craik & Jennings, 1992), although they are considered to be of limited practical significance. (Note that the sensory memory store represents pure visual or auditory input and is likely to be adversely affected by sensory changes.) Similarly, age differences in primary (short-term/working/immediate) memory are minimal (Craik, 1977; Woods & Britton, 1985; Craik & Jennings, 1992). As a result, one can expect that older adults will be able to attend to, perceive, and briefly retain small amounts of information within the normal span of seven (plus or minus two) items with little difficulty, if not distracted.

It is at the level of secondary (long-term) memory that significant age-related deficits have been documented, findings that are consistent with those of the processing theorists. Beginning around age 50, older adults appear to have more difficulty with retrieval of information from secondary storage (Crook & West, 1990). Although they perform

almost as well as their younger counterparts on recognition tests (at least until their late 80s), older adults do not fare as well when using recall mechanisms (i.e., no associative cue in the environment) to retrieve information. This deficit worsens over time (Craik & Jennings, 1992; Albert, 1988). The oft bemoaned "Why did I come into this room?" phenomenon illustrates this difficulty. Curiously, very long-term memory ("tertiary" or "remote" memory) appears not to be affected until well after the age of 70 (Weingartner & Parker, 1984).

The difficulty with recall is considered to be a problem of retrieval rather than one of encoding or storage. This is because recall requires the individual to independently "call up" information that was previously learned, organized (i.e., encoded), and stored for future retrieval; recognition provides the individual with the item itself as an orienting cue to search memory and retrieve the information. Hence, the cues provided in recognition tests compensate for deficient retrieval strategies and provide means to retrieve information that was previously stored (encoded). The implication here is that older adults who experience difficulties in retrieving previously acquired information benefit from cues (Craik & Jennings, 1992). Compensatory cues can include the use of notes, lists (Burack & Lachman, 1996), and calendars; redundant cuing (i.e., simultaneous oral and written instructions); and whenever possible, questions posed in recognition rather than in recall form (i.e., "Was your last appointment Monday or Wednesday?" rather than "When was your last appointment?").

When accompanied by concerns of diminished performance of desired life activities in otherwise healthy older adults, this secondary memory deficit is described as "age-related cognitive decline" (Caine, 1993). The term *age-related cognitive decline* has replaced the older terms *age-associated memory impairment* (AAMI)(Albert, 1988; Crook et al, 1986; Larrabee et al., 1992) and *benign senescent forgetfulness.* Such concerns may include problems remembering newly learned facts or names of new acquaintances, difficulties remembering tasks on a list, misplacing objects, forgetting telephone numbers, or forgetting what one intended to do minutes after deciding to do it. Although not always definitive, these concerns are distinguished from dementia by their minor severity, by their nonprogressive nature, and by the fact that they do not significantly interfere with social or occupational functioning. Research is leading to the development of cognitive intervention strategies to help the older adult compensate for any adverse effects of age-related cognitive decline on daily life functioning (Crook, 1986; Kausler, 1989; Scogin, Storandt, & Lott, 1985; Larrabee et al., 1992; Willis & Schaie, 1994; Fogler & Stern, 1994; Riley, 1995; Gordon, 1995).

As is apparent from this discussion, mild forgetfulness (*age-related cognitive decline*) can be considered a part of a normal pattern of aging, and, given the current state of our knowledge, is not cause for undue concern. Most investigators consider such changes in cognitive function benign and neither progressive nor significantly disabling. A caveat, however: Hasher and Zacks (1988) have proposed a theory of breakdown in inhibitory mechanisms in short term-memory that has been implicated in both normal healthy aging and Alzheimer's disease. In addition, a recent study provides disconcerting, albeit preliminary, evidence that dementia may constitute one extreme on a continuum of cognitive decline (Brayne et al., 1995). This raises questions about whether individuals with cognitive impairment go on to develop dementia if they live long enough or whether there actually is a subgroup whose cognitive impairment does not progress. Clearly, these are findings that bear watching.) In contrast, moderate to severe memory difficulties (i.e., repeated or permanent forgetting of recent, personally relevant facts; the gist of conversations with significant others; or past knowledge and skills) are not normal and should be brought to the attention of a medical provider. Significant memory difficulties most often signal a reversible medical problem, such as untreated hypertension, diabetes, anemia, thyroid dysfunction, malnutrition, infection, dehydration, or, the most common cause of reversible memory impairment, adverse drug reactions/interactions (Perlmutter et al., 1987) Medications commonly associated with memory disturbances include anti-diabetics, anti-anxiety agents, anti-hypertensives, anti-psychotics, stomach acid suppressants, tricyclic anti-depressants, and anti-Parkinson's agents (Morrison & Katz, 1989; AHCPR, 1996). Significant memory difficulty may also be indicative of

a major disease process, such as major depression (depression affects the memory of an older adult more than that of a younger person), alcohol abuse, or, less commonly, dementia. (For those 65 to 75, the risk of Alzheimer's disease is 3% to 6%; after age 80, the risk is considerably higher—at least 16% (Breteler et al., 1992). Also of importance is the finding that those older adults who express concerns about memory lapses are more likely to be either depressed or suffering from a treatable medical condition than demented (Feher et al., 1991; Thompson et al., 1987; Kahn et al. 1975). Generally, older adults with dementia are unaware of their lapses, are unconcerned about them, or attribute them to other causes. They tend not to remember what it is that they forgot.

Cognitive Screening Instruments

The most widely used screening instrument when cognitive impairment is suspected in older adults is the Mini-Mental State Exam (MMSE) (Folstein, Folstein, & McHugh, 1975) (See Appendix 1). Other frequently used instruments include the Blessed Orientation-Memory-Concentration Test (BOMC)(Katzman et al., 1983), the Blessed Information-Memory-Concentration (BIMC) test (Katzman et al., 1983), and the Short Portable Mental Status Questionnaire (SPMSQ)(Pfeiffer, 1975). The MMSE provides specific norms for older adults (Crum, Anthony, Bassett, & Folstein, 1993), has excellent test-retest reliability (Folstein, Folstein, & McHugh, 1975; Tombaugh & McIntyre, 1992), validity (Folstein, Folstein, & McHugh, 1975; Tombaugh & McIntyre, 1992), sensitivity (Tombaugh & McIntyre, 1992; Bachman, Wolf, Linn, et al., 1993) and is the most comprehensive of cognitive screening tests. A broad range of cognitive abilities are assessed, including memory (i.e., immediate and recent recall of three items and response to questions related to temporal orientation), language (i.e., naming common objects, repeating a linguistically difficult sentence, following a three-step command, and writing a sentence), spatial ability (i.e., copying a two-dimensional figure), and set shifting (i.e., performing serial sevens or spelling the word "world" backwards). Table 10-1 presents an overview of cognitive components mea-

Table 10-1

Components of Cognition Measured by Selected Tests				
Components of cognition measured	MMSE	BIMC	BOMC	SPMSQ
Immediate memory	X			
Short-term memory recall	X	X	X	X
Abstract thinking judgment				
Aphasia	X			
Apraxia	X			
Agnosia	X			
Constructional Ability	X			
Concentration	X	X	X	X
Orientation	X	X	X	X
Spatial ability	X			
Requirements for testing				
Verbal responses	X	X	X	X
Reading ability	X			
Writing ability	X			
Mathematical ability	X			X
Motor ability	X			
Vision	X			

Note: MMMSE = Mini-Mental State Examination. BIMC = Blessed Information-Memory-Concentration Test. BOMC = Blessed Orientation-Memory-Concentration Test. SPMSQ = Short Portable Mental Status Questionnaire.

sured by the most commonly used brief cognitive tests (adapted from White & Davis, 1990).

The MMSE (Appendix 1) requires no test specific training, can be administered by a variety of clinicians with general skill and knowledge of test administration, and takes approximately 10 minutes. To reiterate, however, it is a screening tool, not a diagnostic tool. It is especially useful in providing a baseline to monitor the course of cognitive impairment over time. Longitudinal follow-up after assessment of cognitive decline is probably the most important diagnostic procedure for differentiating Alzheimer's disease from normal aging (AHCPR, 1996). If a trigger raises concern about cognitive performance, it is important to establish a baseline to facilitate determination of cognitive decline over time.] A score of less than 24 out of a possible 30 points is generally recommended as indicative of cognitive impairment (Anthony et al., 1982), albeit "of unknown origin," warranting referral for a more comprehensive evaluation by a medical provider. For example, before a diagnosis of dementia is entertained, an older adult's low MMSE score is interpreted within the context of other clinical data, such as informant-based history of cognitive decline, evidence of impairment in IADL, educational background, assessment for depression, sensory impairment, or factors other than dementia that may account for impaired performance (AHCPR, 1996).

Occupational therapists should note that the functional status assessment is particularly important in detecting early stages of the disease (Morris et al., 1991; Wilder et al., 1994). Specifically, the Functional Activities Questionnaire (FAQ)(Pfeffer, Korosaki, Harrah, Chance, & Filos, 1982) has been identified as the most useful measure to discriminate between older adults with and without cognitive impairment (AHCPR, 1996). The FAQ is an informant-based measure of functional abilities that provides performance ratings on 10 higher order ADL. Levels of performance are rated as follows: dependent=3, requires assistance=2, has difficulty but does by self=1, and independent=0. A total score is computed by summing scores across the 10 items. Scores range from 0 to 30, and a cut-point of 9 (dependent in three or more activities) is recommended (AHCPR, 1996). Table 10-2 pro-

Table 10-2

Functional Activities Questionnaire

Individual Items on the Functional Activities Questionnaire

1. Writing checks, paying bills, balancing checkbook.
2. Assembling tax records, business affairs, or papers.
3. Shopping alone for clothes, household necessities, or groceries.
4. Playing a game of skill, working on a hobby.
5. Heating water, making a cup of coffee, turning off stove.
6. Preparing a balanced meal.
7. Keeping track of current events.
8. Paying attention to, understanding, discussing TV, book, magazine.
9. Remembering appointments, family occasions, holidays, medications.
10. Traveling out of the neighborhood, driving, arranging to take buses.

Source: From Pfeffer et al., 1982.

vides a listing of the 10 activities considered by this instrument.

Finally, it should be recognized that cognitive screening and tracking instruments are limited in providing information useful for determining rehabilitation potential for patients with cognitive impairment.

Speed of Information Processing/Reaction Time

One of the most consistent findings in the study of aging is that speed of information processing and reaction time declines with advancing age (Salthouse, 1985, 1991; Shock, 1985). This is found on a variety of experimental tasks ranging from the simple (how long does it take to press a button after a light goes on) to the complex (how fast can one write). The decrement increases with the complexity of the task and response and is more pronounced in tasks requiring psychomotor rather than verbal responses. Overall, the speed with which older adults perform such tasks decreases approximately 20% for simple tasks and can reach 50% or more for complex tasks (Schaie and Willis, 1996; Cerella, 1990). Most of the psychomotor slowness observed in very old age is likely a product of this decline. In addition, this slowing been linked to higher order cognitive processes like reasoning and abstraction (Salthouse, 1991).

The generalized slowing of information processing/reaction time does not appear to be primarily a function of peripheral nervous system factors (e.g., sensory acuity, speed of peripheral nerve conduction, or speed of movement once the response is initiated)(Botwinick, 1984). Rather, as indicated above, it appears to reflect a basic change in the speed with which the central nervous system processes information. The cause for this slowing has been attributed to disruptions of connections within the neural network, increasing the time required to process information as individuals age (Cerella, 1990; Salthouse et al., 1996. See Levy, 1996 for an overview of age-related neurological changes.)

Yet, there is evidence that average reaction times are faster among active older adults than among nonathletic younger adults (Spirduso & MacRae, 1990; Spirduso & Clifford, 1978; Woollacott, 1988), that reaction time is better in older adults who engage in physical activity than in those who are sedentary (Stelmach & Worringham, 1985), and that reaction times can be significantly improved by physical exercise (Botwinick, 1978; Stelmach & Worringham, 1985; Emery, Burker, & Blumenthal, 1992). Since exercise increases blood flow to the brain, increases the amount of oxygen in the blood, and may even affect the structure of neural tissue, these factors are also implicated in age-related changes in reaction time (Schaie & Willis, 1996; Birren & Fisher, 1992; Birren, Woods, & Williams, 1980).

Intelligence

One of the more controversial issues in gerontology is whether intelligence declines with age. Intelligence is not a unidimensional concept; it includes a variety of intellectual abilities (i.e., verbal, numerical, reasoning, spatial relations, memory), and is extremely difficult to measure or even to define. The most influential measure of global or general intelligence in use today is the Weschler Adult Intelligence Scale (WAIS). The WAIS includes a verbal scale and a performance scale that are combined to assess intelligence quotient (IQ). As measured by the WAIS, intelligence quotient (IQ) remains stable into the mid fifties or early sixties and thereafter decreases with advancing age, a finding that is consistent among studies (Hertzog & Schaie, 1988). So, while debate continues about whether intelligence actually declines with age, there is general agreement that people perform worse on intelligence tests as they grow older.

It is important to take note, however, of the differential rates in decline and stability with advancing age seen in the various categories of intellectual ability on the WAIS. Specifically, the performance scale, which measures for example, the speed of copying a picture, shows earlier and significant decline. The verbal scale, which measures information retention, vocabulary, and comprehension, remains fairly steady. The differences between these two scales has been found so often that the phenomenon is known as the "classic aging pattern" (Botwinick, 1978; Kausler, 1991).

There is a growing consensus that traditional intelligence tests are not an appropriate measure of intellectual functioning in older adults. The fact that speed of response is given great weight in these tests clearly puts older people at a disadvantage. There are also compelling arguments that declines demonstrated by the WAIS may reflect well-documented slowing of information processing/reaction time (reflecting biological changes of the central nervous system) rather than decline in intellectual ability (Schaie, 1989; Salthouse, 1985).

Horn and Cattell (1967) and Cattell (1963) offered one of the first theoretical explanations for this differential decline by proposing two general kinds of "intelligence": crystallized and fluid. Fluid intelligence involves the "mechanics" of intelligence, such as memory capacity, speed of processing, efficiency of receptors, and elementary cognitive operations. It operates by the mechanics of information processing and is believed to decline with increasing age. Crystallized intelligence involves the "pragmatics" of intelligence (Staudinger, Cornelius, & Baltes, 1989). It is measured by using tests of vocabulary, information, and mechanical knowledge, and reflects content-rich, pragmatic knowledge systems that have been acquired through years of education and acculturation. It is believed to remain stable or increase at least up to about age 70 (Balota & Duchek, 1988; Pryse-Phillips, 1989; Kausler, 1991) and may show additional increase through self-directed learning and education (Hayslip & Sterns, 1979). These age trends are similar to the WAIS "classic aging pattern," since the verbal scale deals primarily with crystallized intelligence and the performance scale emphasizes fluid intelligence.

The continuing debate about intelligence in aging has resulted in greater appreciation for the fact that conventional methods of measuring intellectual abilities have not always been sensitive to the skills actually used by older adults in everyday life. Increasingly, theorists argue that the intellectual functioning of older adults is more accurately assessed in the context of the social/cultural and life-stage demands of older adulthood than by youth based standards of intellectual functioning (WAIS). Labouvie-Vief (1985, 1989) argues that formal operational thinking is well suited to adolescence and young adulthood, when considering all options equally is desirable; however by midlife and beyond, decisions must be made on the basis of prior commitments and appreciation of consequences for all real persons involved. From this perspective, cognitive maturity and adaptation are more relevant conceptualizations of intellectual capacity in older adulthood (Cornelius & Caspi, 1987; Schaie, 1990; Willis & Baltes, 1980).

This recognition is providing impetus to the development of new testing methods, such as age-relevant intelligence tests, which include measures of the more pragmatic aspects of intelligence. In large part, these efforts focus on assessing "everyday cognitive competence," i.e., the practical intelligence required to carry out those complex tasks of daily living (IADL) considered essential for living on one's own in society (Willis, 1996a; Diehl, Willis, & Schaie, 1995). Willis and colleagues (Willis, 1996b; Willis & Marsiske, 1993) have recently constructed a psychometrically-based Everyday Problems Test (EPT) to assess the older adult's ability to solve complex tasks of daily living. This test assesses pragmatic intelligence using printed material associated with each of the seven IADL domains (taking medications, managing finances, shopping for necessities, using the telephone, managing transportation, preparing meals, and housekeeping) (Fillenbaum, 1985). For example, the older adult is shown the label for an over-the-counter cough medicine and asked the maximum number of teaspoons to be taken in a 24-hour period. Although steps toward defining or measuring age relevant intelligence are still in early stages (Willis, 1996a, 1996b), the effort holds promise.

Cognition and Health

An emerging body of literature is investigating the relationship between cognition and health and illness in older adults. The major hypothesis is that cognition in healthy older adults remains relatively intact, whereas cognition in those with chronic disease processes shows precipitous declines (Schaie, 1990; Launer et al. 1995). Empirical evidence lends support to this premise, particularly with reference to chronic disease processes such as hypertension, cardiovascular disease, and diabetes (Siegler & Costa, 1985; Elias, Elias, & Elias, 1990; Elias et al., 1993; Schaie, 1990; Sands & Meredith, 1992), as well as with self-reported pain (e.g., osteoarthritis) (Parmelee, Smith, & Katz, 1993). In these studies, health consistently emerged as a more important variable in predicting cognitive decline than chronological age. The implication here is that changes in cognitive function (typically, memory) might more usefully be viewed as potentially modifiable manifestations of disease and/or manifestations of changes in physiological functioning.

Cardiovascular diseases, specifically hypertension and heart disease, are of particular interest to cognitive psychologists because these conditions so frequently tend to be associated with lower levels of cognitive performance (Elias, Elias, & Elias, 1990; Elias et al., 1990; Elias & Marshall, 1987).

There is ample evidence that the more serious cardiovascular conditions (atherosclerosis and cerebrovascular disease) increase the risk and extent of cognitive decline. Not only has it been shown that untreated hypertension is inversely related to cognitive functioning, that is, those with high untreated blood pressure scored lower on cognitive tests (Elias et al., 1993); there also is evidence that medications that prevent subtle brain changes due to hypertension, low blood pressure, and elevated blood sugar have an important impact on the occurrence of cognitive impairment (Launer et al., 1995).

At the same time, longitudinal studies demonstrate that older adults experience a marked decline in IQ only a few years or months from death (Riegel & Reigel, 1987; Kleemeier, 1962; Berkowitz, 1965; Steuer et al., 1981). These observations have led to the terminal drop hypothesis, which proposes that time prior to death, rather than time since birth, predicts intellectual decline. In this view, there may be little or no cognitive decline until physiological deterioration occurs in the final years of life. This premise is supported by observations that marked declines in verbal abilities predict imminent death (Jarvik, 1962; Jarvik & Falek, 1963).

These emerging findings about the relationship between health and cognition open the possibility that age is an indirect marker of physiological disease and/or health problems that may influence cognitive performance (Ferrucci et al., 1993). Consequently, age-related cognitive change may not be inevitable and may represent an underlying pathological process of some kind (Sliwinski et al., 1996; Salthouse, 1989). Indeed, there is evidence that some older adults show no decline in test scores even into their nineties (Jarvik, 1988; Verhaeghen, 1993; Hill et al., 1995). It may well be that healthy older adults who maintain an active physical and intellectual life will show little or no loss of cognitive abilities unless (or until) confronted with serious disease.

The corollary to the hypothesis of disease and cognitive decline with age is that the preservation of health may preserve cognitive abilities. In addition to aforementioned evidence about the benefits of normalizing blood pressure, there is evidence that physical exercise is related to both the maintenance and improvement of cognition in older adults. Active older adults perform better on a variety of cognitive measures than their sedentary peers (Clarkson-Smith & Hartley, 1989; Stones & Kozma, 1989). Exercise has also been shown to improve memory performance (Dustman, Ruhling, & Russert, 1984; Hassmen, Ceci, & Backman, 1992), even with the cognitively impaired (Powell, 1974; Diesfeldt & Diesfeldt-Groenendijk, 1977). In addition, researchers have identified institutionalized older adults with some degree of cognitive impairment as a particularly appropriate target group for demonstrating the psychological benefits of physical activity (Morgan, 1989). Notwithstanding, an important implication to consider here is that the level of physical activity inherent in conventional occupational therapy protocols may itself provide ancillary cognitive benefit.

These findings have additional implications for rehabilitation. Given the preponderance of chronic disease (and especially cardiovascular disease) within rehabilitation settings, it is probable that this cohort of older adults will experience more than the usual amount of age-related cognitive change. Because traditional rehabilitation protocols typically require patients to learn new procedures, carry over learning from one day to the next, and retain these gains upon returning home, it is likely that older adults involved in traditional rehabilitation protocols will derive benefit from approaches that help compensate for "age-related" (and/or "health-related") cognitive change. (Here, "traditional" rehabilitative protocols are contrasted with protocols targeted for those with cognitive impairment. Note that these compensatory strategies, listed in the section below, need also to be considered to enhance the teaching and learning of older adult caregivers, who themselves may also be frail.

Implications for the Rehabilitation Professional

To accommodate age-related changes in learning and memory and to thereby optimize rehabilitation potential of older adults in traditional rehabilitation settings, occupational therapists need to consider the following:

1. New information is processed more slowly; present new information more slowly.

2. Information is retrieved more slowly from long-term memory; provide more response time.

3. Recognize that older adults are especially susceptible to stress and anxiety in learning situations, which itself can impede new learning. Learning is significantly enhanced in a supportive environment where anxiety is reduced.

4. Limit background noise, interruptions, and other distractions that may compete for the individual's attention. This includes distractions such as talking to the older adult who is attempting a new task. Minimize nonessential information.

5. Older adults do best when tasks are self-paced and not timed. Allow individuals to pace their own learning. This often means reducing content in a given time period to offer greater clarity, specificity, and depth, and to allow the older adult means to compensate for sensory impairment and increased cautiousness. Provide self-paced instructional materials to serve as additional memory cues whenever possible.

6. Cue redundantly. For maximal effect, use auditory and visual information together. Learning is facilitated when older adults hear and see new information at the same time. Use large print on a blackboard, whenever possible. Prepared written materials (handouts) best assist in learning when they are very similar to what is being taught orally.

7. Increase the rehearsal of information to be committed to memory. Repeat information in order to increase information storage.

8. Recognize that information and skills that are directly relevant and meaningful to the individual are more likely to be learned and remembered. Precede teaching with an assessment of the individual's interest in what will be taught, what the individual already knows, and what the individual thinks he or she needs (or does not need) to know.

9. Personalize teaching sessions; associate new information with known information. New learning or techniques are best retained and retrieved when they build on previous ways of

doing things. Begin with statements such as "what I want you to do is similar to. . ."

10. Instruct individuals in the use of various associational strategies or "mnemonic techniques," (visual images, verbal associations, etc.) which may be used to better organize material for storage.

11. Recognize that a broad range of medications adversely effect the individual's response time and/or ability to recall information. Patience and understanding are essential to reduce anxiety that can further interfere with learning.

12. Encourage "thinking aloud" (Giambra & Arenberg, 1980) when the individual practices a new skill, to determine if principles taught are being applied correctly and to provide for rehearsal and repetition of new information.

13. Vision or hearing difficulties experienced by most older adults and can impede learning by limiting the amount of information the individual receives (in sensory memory) to eventually store in secondary memory. Present information using methods that compensate for the probable sensory problems of older adults (e.g., increased intensity, yet glare-free lighting; large print instructional materials; lowered voice pitch).

14. Recognize that tasks requiring speed and fine motor coordination place older adults at particular disadvantage. Whenever possible, emphasize tasks that capitalize on their strengths, i.e., judgment and understanding based on experience.

15. Encourage the use of pocket note pads, watch alarms, voice recorders, post-it reminders, or other such aids to help in cuing and keeping track of new information.

16. Above all, encourage the individual to keep exercising—intellectually AND physically. There is ample evidence that building cardiovascular endurance can itself improve cognitive abilities. The usual recommendation is a brisk walk for 20 minutes several times a week.

Conclusion

Although controversy and debate continue in the area of cognition and aging, some general conclusions appear to be warranted by the available evidence. On average, there appears to be an age-related decline in cognitive performance. Many cognitive functions appear not to begin to decline until the mid-fifties or sixties, especially those involving verbal ability, and these declines tend to be small. There are important exceptions, however, with regard to information processing speed, psychomotor skills, and certain aspects of memory (especially recall), wherein declines are mild but more significant. Declines in these areas tend to be accentuated in less healthy, albeit cognitively intact, older adults, and are likely to necessitate modifications in the teaching and learning elements of traditional rehabilitative protocols. So, while losses in some cognitive abilities are probable with increasing age and more likely with pathology, these losses are benign and neither progressive nor disabling; they are not of sufficient magnitude to interfere with daily relationships, function, or quality of life. Cognitive impairment sufficient to compromise relationships, function, or quality of life is most likely to be caused by an adverse drug interaction or a reversible medical condition. This degree of impairment may also signal a disease process such as depression (the most likely alternative), or, when progressive, dementia.

At the same time, there is evidence that some cognitive competencies may actually increase with aging (e.g., crystallized intelligence). In addition, there is promising evidence that in healthy older adults cognition may remain relatively stable throughout the later years.

References

Agency for Health Care Policy and Research (November, 1996). *Recognition and initial assessment of Alzheimer's disease and related dementias.* Clinical practice guideline No. 19. Rockville, MD: U.S. Department of Health and Human Services, Public Health Service, Agency for Health Care Policy and Research. AHCPR Pub. No. 97-0702.

Albert, M. S. (1988). Cognitive function. In M. S. Albert & M. B. Moss (Eds.), *Geriatric Neuropsychology.* NY: Guilford Press.

Anthony, J. C., LeResche, L., Niaz, U., Von Korff, M., & Folstein, M. (1982). Limits of the "Mini-Mental State" as a screening test for dementia and delirium aging hospital patients. *Psychological Medicine, 12,* 397–408.

Atkinson, R. C., & Shiffrin, R. M. (1968). Human memory: A proposed system and its control processes. In K. Spence & J. Spence (Eds.), *The psychology of learning and motivation*, Vol. 2. NY: Academic Press.

Bachman, D. L., Wolf, P. A., Linn, R. T., Knoefel, J. E., Cobb, J. L., Belanger, A. J., White, L. R., & D'Agostino, R. B. (1993). Incidence of dementia and probable Alzheimer's disease in a general population: the Framingham study. *Neurology, 43,* 515–519.

Balota, D. A., & Duchek, J. (1988). Age-related differences in lexical access, spreading activation, and simple pronunciation. *Psychology and Aging, 3,* 84–93.

Berkowitz, B. (1965). Changes in intellect with age: IV. Changes in achievement and survival in older people. *Journal of Genetic Psychology, 107,* 3–14.

Best, J. B. (1989). *Cognitive psychology.* St Paul: West Publishing.

Birren, J. & Fisher, L. (1992). *Aging and slowing of behavior: Consequences for cognition and survival.* In T. Sonderegger (Eds.), *Psychology and aging.* Nebraska Symposium on Motivation, 1991. Lincoln, NE: University of Nebraska Press.

Birren, J. E., Woods, A. M., & Williams, M. V. (1980). *Behavioral slowing with age: Causes, organization, and consequences.* In L. W. Poon (Ed.), *Aging in the 1980's.* Washington DC: American Psychological Association.

Botwinick, J. (1967). *Cognitive processes in maturity and old age.* NY: Springer.

Botwinick, J. (1978). *Aging and behavior* (2nd Ed.). New York: Springer.

Botwinick, J.(1984). *Aging and behavior: A comprehensive integration of research findings.* NY: Springer.

Brayne, C., Gill, C., Paykel, E., Huppert, F., & O'Connor, D. (1995). Cognitive decline in an elderly population—A two wave study of change. *Psychological Medicine, 25,* 673–683.

Breteler M. M. B., Claus J. J., Van Duijn C. M., Launer L. J., & Hofman A. (1992). Epidemiology of Alzheimer's disease. *Epidemiology Review, 14,* 59–82.

Burack, O., & Lachman, M. (1996). The effects of list-making on recall in young and elderly adults. *Journal of Gerontology, 51B,* 226–233.

Caine, E. D. (1993). Should aging-associated cognitive decline be included in DSM-IV? *Journal Of Neuropsychiatry and Clinical Neuroscience, 5,* 1–5.

Cattell, R. B. (1963). The theory of fluid and crystalline intelligence. *Journal of Educational Psychology, 54,* 1–22.

Cerella, J. (1990). Aging and information-processing rate. In J. E. Birren & K. W. Schaie (Eds.), *Handbook of the psychology of aging* (3rd ed.). NY: Academic Press.

Clarkson-Smith, L. & Hartley, A. A. (1989). Relationships between physical exercise and cognitive abilities in older adults. *Psychology and Aging, 4,* 183–189.

Cornelius, S. W., & Caspi, A. (1987). Everyday problem solving in adulthood and old age. *Psychology and Aging, 2,* 14–153.

Craik, F. I. (1977). Age differences in human memory. In J. E. Birren & K. W. Schaie (Eds.), *Handbook of the psychology of aging.* Cincinnati: Van Nostrand Reinhold.

Craik, F. I., & Jennings, J. (1992). Human Memory. In F. Craik & T. Salthouse (Eds.), *Handbook of memory disorders.* Chichester: Wiley.

Crook, T. H., & West, R. L. (1990). Name recall performance across the adult lifespan. *British Journal of Psychology, 81,* 335–349.

Crook, T., Bartus, R. T., Ferris, S. H., Whitehouse, P. J., Cohen, G. D., & Gershon, S. (1986). Age-associated memory impairment: Proposed diagnostic criteria and measures of clinical change-Report of a National Institute of Mental Health Work Group. *Developmental Neuropsychology, 2,* 261–265.

Crum, R., Anthony, J., Bassett, S., & Folstein, M. (1993). Population based norms for the mini-mental status examination by age and educational level. *Journal of the American Medical Association, 269,* 2386–2391.

Diehl, M., Willis, S., & Schaie, K. W. (1995). Older adults competence: Observational assessment and cognitive correlates. *Psychology and Aging, 10,* 478–491.

Diesfeldt, H. & Diesfeldt-Groenendijk, H. (1977). Improving cognitive performance in psychogeriatric patients: The influence of physical exercise. *Age and Aging, 6,* 58–64.

Dustman, R., Ruhling, R., & Russell E. (1984). Aerobic exercise training and improved neuropsychological function of older individuals. *Neurobiology and Aging, 5,* 35–42.

Eisdorfer, C. (1968). Arousal and performance: Experiments in verbal learning and tentative memory. In G. A. Tallend (Ed.), *Human aging and behavior.* NY: Academic Press.

Elias, M. F., Elias, J. W., & Elias, P. K. (1990). Biological and health influences on behavior. In J. E. Birren & K. W. Schaie (Eds.), *Handbook of the psychology of aging* (3rd ed.). NY: Academic Press.

Elias, M. F., & Marshall P. H. (Eds.) (1987). *Cardiovascular disease and behavior.* Washington, DC: Hemisphere.

Elias, M., Robbins, M., Schultz, N., & Peirce. T. (1990). Is blood pressure an important variable in research on aging and neuropsychological test performance? *Journal of Gerontology, 45,* 128–135.

Elias. M. F., Wolf. P. A., D'Agostino, R. B., Cobb, J. & White, L. (1993). Untreated blood pressure is inversely related to cognitive functioning: The Framingham Study. *American Journal of Epidemiology, 138,* 353–364.

Emery, C., Burker, E., & Blumenthal, J. (1992). Psychological and physiological effects of exercise among older adults. In K. W. Schaie (Ed.), *Annual Review of Gerontology and Geriatrics.* NY: Springer.

Feher, E. P., Mahurin, R. K., Inbody, S. B., Crook, T. H., & Pirozzolo, F. J. (1991). Ansognosia in Alzheimer's disease. *Neuropsychiatry, Neurophysiology, and Behavioral Neurology, 4,* 136–146.

Ferrucci, L., Guralnik, J., Marchionni, N., Costanzo, S., Lamponi, M., & Baroni, A. (1993). Relationship between health status, fluid intelligence, and disability in a non-demented elderly population. *Aging, Clinical and Experimental Research, 5,* 435–443.

Fogler, J., & Stern, L. (1994). *Improving your memory: How to remember what you're starting to forget.* Baltimore: Johns Hopkins Press.

Folstein, M. F., Folstein, S. E., & McHugh, P. R. (1975). "Minimental state: a practical method for grading the cognitive state of patients for the clinician. *Journal of Psychiatric Research, 12,* 189–198.

Giambra, L., & Arenberg, D. (1980). Problem solving, concept learning, and aging. In L. W. Poon (Ed.), *Aging in the 80's.* Washington D.C.: American Psychological Association.

Gordon, B. (1995). *Memory: Remembering and forgetting in everyday life.* New York: Mastermedia.

Gounard, B. R., & Hulicka, I. M. (1977). Maximizing learning efficiency in later adulthood: A cognitive problem-solving approach. *Educational Gerontology: An International Quarterly, 2,* 417–427.

Hasher, L., & Zacks, R. (1988). Working memory, comprehension, and aging: A review and a new view. In G. Bower (Ed.), *The psychology of learning and motivation,* Vol 22. NY: Academic Press.

Hassmen, P., Ceci, R., & Backman, L. (1992). Exercise for older women: Training method and its influences on physical and cognitive performance. *European Journal of Applied Physiology, 64,* 460–466.

Hayslip, B., & Sterns, H. L. (1979). Age differences in relationships between crystallized and fluid intelligence in problem solving. *Journal of Gerontology, 34,* 404–414.

Herzog, C., & Schaie, K. W. (1988). Stability and change in adult intelligence: Simultaneous analysis of longitudinal means and covariance structures. *Psychological Aging, 3,* 122–130.

Hill, R., Grut, M., Wahlin, A., Herlitz, A., Winblad, B., & Backman, L. (1995). Predicting memory performance in optimally healthy very old adults. *Journal of Mental Health and Aging, 1,* 57–67.

Horn J. L. & Cattell, R. B. (1967). Age differences in fluid and crystallized intelligence. *Acta Psychobiologica, 26,* 107–129.

Howieson, D., Holm, L., Kaye, et al. (1993). Neurological function in the optimally healthy oldest old: Neuropsychological evaluation. *Neurology, 43,* 1882–1886.

Jarvik, L. F. (1962). Biological differences in intellectual functioning. *Vita Humana, 5,* 195–203.

Jarvik, L. F. (1988). Aging of the brain: How can we prevent it? *Gerontologist, 28,* 739–747.

Jarvik, L. F., & Falek, A. (1963). Intellectual stability and survival in the aged. *Journal of Gerontology, 18,* 173–176.

Kahn, R., Zarit, S., Hilbert, N., et al. (1975). Memory complaint and impairment in the aged. *Archives of General Psychiatry, 32,* 1569–1573.

Katzman, R., Brown, T., Fuld, P., Peck, A., Schecter, R., & Schimmel, H. (1983). Validation of a short orientation-memory-concentration test of cognitive impairment. *American Journal of Psychiatry, 140,* 734–739.

Kausler, D. H. (1989). Impairment in normal memory aging: Implications of laboratory evidence. In G. C. Gilmore, P. J. Whitehouse, & M. R. Wycle (Eds.), *Memory, aging and dementia.* NY: Springer.

Kausler, D. H. (1991). *Experimental psychology, cognition, and human aging* (2nd ed.). NY: Springer-Verlag.

Kausler, D. H. (1994). *Learning and memory in normal aging.* San Diego: Academic Press.

Kleemeier, R. W. (1962). Intellectual change in the senium. *Proceedings of the Social Statistics Section of the American Statistical Association, 1,* 290–295.

Labouvie-Vief, G. (1985). Intelligence and cognition. In J. E. Birren & K. W. Schaie (Eds.), *Handbook of the psychology of aging* (2nd ed.). NY: Von Nostrand Reinhold.

Labouvie-Vief, G. (1989). *Cognitive functioning in the middle years.* In S. Hunter & M. Sundel (Eds.), *Midlife myths: Issues, findings, and implications.* Newbury Park, CA.: Sage.

Larrabee, G., McEntee, W., Youngjohn, J & Crook, T. (1992). Age associated memory impairment: Diagnosis, research, and treatment. In M. Bergener, K. Hasegawa, S. Finkel, & T. Nishimura (Eds.), *Aging and Mental disorders: International Perspectives* (p. 134–149). NY: Springer.

Launer, L., Masaki, K., Petrovitch, H., Foley, D., & Havlik, R. (1995). The association between midlife blood pressure levels and late-life cognitive function. *JAMA, 274 (23),* 1846–1851.

Levy, L. (1996). Biological Changes in Older Adults. In *The Role of Occupational Therapy With The Elderly (ROTE)* (2d ed.). Bethesda, MD: American Occupational Therapy Association.

Morgan, K. (1989). Trial and error: Evaluating the psychological benefits of physical activity. *International Journal of Geriatric Psychiatry, 4,* 125–127.

Morris, J. C., McKeel, D. W., Storandt, M., Rubin, E., Price, J., Grant, E., Ball, M., & Berg, L. (1991). Very mild Alzheimer's disease: Informant-based clinical, psychometric, and pathologic distinction from normal aging. *Neurology, 41,* 469–478.

Morrison, R. L., & Katz, I. R. (1989). Drug-related cognitive impairment: Current progress and recurrent problems. *Annual Review of Gerontology and Geriatrics, 9,* 232–279.

Parmelee, P. A., Smith, B., & Katz, I. R. (1993). Pain complaints and cognitive status among elderly institution residents. *Journal of the American Geriatrics Society, 41,* 517–522.

Perlmutter, M., Adams, C., Berry, J., Kaplan, M., Person, D., & Verdonik, F. (1987). In K. W. Schaie & K. W. Eisdorfer (Eds.), *Annual Review of Gerontology and Geriatrics,* Vol. 7. NY: Springer.

Pfeffer, R., Kurosaki, T., Harrah, C., Chance, J., & Filos, S., (1982). Measurement of functional activities in older adults in the community. *Journal of Gerontology, 37,* 323–329.

Pfeiffer, E. (1975). A short portable mental status questionnaire for the assessment of organic brain deficit in elderly patients. *Journal of the American Geriatrics Society, 23,* 440–1.

Poon, L. W., Fozard, J. R., Cermak, L. S., Arenberg, D., & Thompson, L. (Eds.). (1980). *New directions in memory and aging.* Hillsdale, NJ: Erlbaum.

Poon, L. W., Gurland, B., Eisdorfer, C., Crook, C., Thompson, T., Kasniak, A., & Davis, K. (Eds.) (1986). *Handbook for the clinical assessment of older adults.* Washington DC: American Psychological Association.

Powell, R. (1974). Psychological effects of exercise on the psychiatric state of institutionalized geriatric mental patients. *Journal of Gerontology, 29,* 157–161.

Pryse-Phillips, W. (1989). Examination of the highest cerebral functions in the elderly. *Seminars in Neurology, 9* (8), 561–568.

Riegel, K., & Riegel, R. (1972). Development, drop, death. *Developmental Psychology, 6,* 306–319.

Riley, K. P. (1995). Bridging the gap between researchers and clinicians: Methodological perspectives and choices. In R. L. West & J. Sinott (Eds.), *Everyday memory and aging: Current research and methodology.* New York: Springer-Verlag.

Rowe, E. J., & Schnore, M. M. (1971). Item concreteness and reported strategies in paired associate learning as a function of age. *Journal of Gerontology, 26,* 470–475.

Salthouse, T. A. (1985). Speed of behavior and the implications for cognition. In J. E. Birren & K. W. Schaie (Eds.) *Handbook of the psychology of aging* (2nd ed.). New York: Von Nostrand Reinhold.

Salthouse, T. A. (1989). Age-related changes in basic cognitive processes. In M. Storandt & G. R. VandenBos (Eds.), *The adult years: Continuity and change.* Washington, DC: American Psychological Association.

Salthouse, T. A. (1991). *Theoretical perspectives on cognitive aging.* Hillsdale, NJ: Erlbaum.

Salthouse, T., Hancock, H., Meinz, E., & Hambrick, D. (1996). Interrelations of age, visual acuity, and cognitive functioning. *Journal of Gerontology, 51B,* 317–330.

Salthouse, T., Hancock, H., Meintz, E., & Hambrick, D. (1996). Interrelations of age, visual acuity, and cognitive functioning. *Journal of Gerontology, 52,* 317-330.

Sands, L. P., & Meredith, W. (1992). Intellectual functioning in late midlife. *Journal of Gerontological and Psychological Science, 47,* 81–84.

Schaie, K. W. (1989). Perceptual speed in adulthood; Cross sectional and longitudinal studies. *Psychology and Aging, 4,* 443–453.

Schaie, K. W., & Willis, S. (1996). *Adult development and aging* (4th ed.). Harper Collins: New York.

Schaie, K. W. (1990). Intellectual development in adulthood. In J. E. Birren & K. W. Schaie (Eds.), *Handbook of the psychology of aging* (3rd ed.). NY: Academic Press.

Scogin, F., Storandt, M., & Lott, R. (1985). Memory skills training, memory complaints, and depression in older adults. *Journal of Gerontology, 40,* 562–568.

Shock, N. W. (1985). Longitudinal studies of aging in humans. In C. E. Finch & E. L. Schneider (Eds.), *Handbook of the biology of aging* (2nd ed.). NY: Von Nostrand Reinhold.

Siegler, I. C., & Costa, P. T. (1985). Health behavior relationships. In J. E. Birren & K. W. Schaie (Eds.), *Handbook of the psychology of aging* (2nd ed.). NY: Von Nostrand Reinhold.

Sliwinski, M., Lipton, R., Buschke, H., & Stewart, W. (1996). The effects of preclinical dementia on estimates of normal cognitive functioning in the aged. *Journal of Gerontology, 51,* 217–225.

Smith, A. (1980). Age differences in encoding, storage, and retrieval. In L. W. Poon, J. R. Fozard, L. S. Cermak, D. Arenberg, & L. Thompson (Eds.), *New directions in memory and aging.* Hillsdale NJ: Erlbaum.

Spirduso, W. W., & Clifford, P. (1978). Replication of age and physical activity effects on reaction and movement time. *Journal of Gerontology, 33,* 26–30.

Spirduso, W. W., & MacRae, P. G. (1990). Motor performance and aging. In J. E. Birren & K. W. Schaie (Eds.), *Handbook of the psychology of aging* (3rd ed.). NY: Academic Press.

Staudinger, U., Cornelius, S., & Baltes, P. (1989). The aging of intelligence: Potentials and limits. *Annals of the American Academy of Political and Social Science, 503,* 43–59.

Stelmach, C. E., & Worringham, C. J. (1985). Sensorimotor deficits related to postural stability: Implications for falling in the elderly. In T. S. Radebaugh et al., (Eds.), *Clinics of geriatric medicine.* Philadelphia: Saunders.

Steuer, J., LaRue, A., & Blum, J. (1981). "Critical loss" in the eighth and ninth decades. *Journal of Gerontology, 36,* 211–213.

Stones, M. J., & Kozma, A. (1989). Age, exercise, and coding performance. *Psychology and Aging, 4,* 190–194.

Thompson, L., Gong, V., Haskins, E., & Gallagher, D. (1987). Assessment of depression and dementia during the later years. In K. W. Schaie (Ed.), *Annual Review of Gerontology and Geriatrics,* Vol. 7. NY: Springer.

Tombaugh T. N., & McIntyre, N.J. (1992). The mini-mental state examination: A comprehensive review. *Journal of the American Geriatrics Society, 40,* 922–935.

Verhaeghen, P. (1993). Facts and fiction about memory aging: A quantitative integration of research findings. *Journal of Gerontology, 48,* 157–171.

Weingartner, H., & Parker, E. (1984). *Memory Consolidation.* Hillsdale, NJ: Erlbaum.

White, H., & Davis, P. (1990). Cognitive screening tests: an aid in the care of elderly outpatients. *Journal of General Internal Medicine, 5,* 438–445.

Wilder, D., Gurland, B., Chen, J., Lantigua, R., Encarnacion, P., & Katz, S. (1994). Interpreting subject and informant reports of function in screening for dementia. *International Journal of Geriatric Psychiatry, 9,* 887–896.

Willis, S. (1996a). Everyday cognitive competence in elderly persons: Conceptual issues and empirical findings. *Gerontologist, 36,* 595–601.

Willis, S. (1996b). Everyday problem solving. In J. E. Birren & K. W. Schaie (Eds.), *Handbook of the psychology of aging* (4th ed., pp. 287–307). NY: Academic Press.

Willis, S., & Baltes, P. (1980). Intelligence in adulthood and aging: Contemporary issues. In L. W. Poon (Ed.), *Aging in the 1980's.* Washington DC: American Psychological Association.

Willis, S., & Marsiske, M. (1993). *Manual for the Everyday Problems Test.* University Park, PA.: Pennsylvania State University.

Willis, S., & Schaie, K. W. (1994). Cognitive training in the normal elderly. In F. Forette, Y. Christen, & F. Boller (Eds.), *Cerebral plasticity and cognitive stimulation.* Paris: Fondation Nationale de Gerontologie.

Witte, K. L. (1975). Paired-associate learning in young and elderly individuals as related to presentation rate. *Psychological Bulletin, 82,* 975–985.

Woods, R. T., & Britton P. G. (1985). *Clinical psychology with the elderly.* Rockville MD: Aspen.

Woollacott, M. J. (1988). Response preparation and posture control: Neuromuscular changes in the older adult. *Annals of the New York Academy of Science, 51*(5), 42–53.

Zachs, R. T. (1982). Encoding strategies used by young and elderly adults in a keeping track task. *Journal of Gerontology, 37,* 203–207.

Appendix 1

Mini-Mental State Examination

Maximum Score	Score	
		Orientation
5	( )	What is the (year) (season) (date) (day) (month)?
5	( )	Where are we: (state) (county) (town) (hospital) (floor)?
		Registration
3	( )	Name 3 objects: 1 second to say each. Then ask the patient all 3 after you have said them. Give 1 point for each correct answer. Then repeat them until he learns all 3. Count trials and record. Trials:
		Attention and Calculation
5	( )	Serial 7's. 1 point for each correct. Stop after 5 answers. Alternatively spell "world" backwards.
		Recall
3	( )	Ask for the 3 objects repeated above. Give 1 point for each correct.
		Language
9	( )	Name a pencil and watch (2 points). Repeat the following "No ifs, ands or buts" (1 point). Follow a 3-stage command: "Take a paper in your right hand, fold it in half, and put it on the floor" (3 points). Read and obey the following: Close your eyes (1 point) Write a sentence (1 point). Copy design (1 point).

_____ Total Score
Assess level of consciousness along a continuum

Alert   Drowsy   Stupor   Coma

Instructions for Administration of Mini-Mental State Examination

Orientation

(1) Ask for the date. Then ask specifically for parts omitted, e.g., "Can you also tell me what season it is?" One point for each correct.
(2) Ask in turn "Can you tell me the name of this hospital?" (town, county, etc.). One point for each correct.

Registration

Ask the patient if you may test his memory. Then say the names of 3 unrelated objects, clearly and slowly, about one second for each. After you have said all three, ask him to repeat them. This first repetition determines his score (0-3) but keep saying them until he can repeat all 3, up to 6 trials. If he does not eventually learn all 3, recall cannot be meaningfully tested.

Attention and Calculation

Ask the patient to begin with 100 and count backwards by 7. Stop after 5 subtractions (93, 86, 79, 72, 65). Score the total number of correct answers.

If the patient cannot or will not perform this task, ask him to spell the word "world" backwards. The score is the number of letters in correct order, e.g., dlrow = 5, dlorw = 3.

Recall

Ask the patient if he can recall the 3 words you previously asked him to remember. Score 0-3.

Language

Naming: Show the patient a wrist watch and ask him what it is. Repeat for pencil. Score 0-3.

Repetition: Ask the patient to repeat the sentence after you. Allow only one trial. Score 0 or 1.

3-Stage command: Give the patient a piece of plain blank paper and repeat the command. Score 1 point for each part correctly executed.

Reading: On a blank piece of paper print the sentence "Close your eyes", in letters large enough for the patient to see clearly. Ask him to read it and do what it says. Score 1 point only if he actually closes his eyes.

Writing: Give the patient a blank piece of paper and ask him to write a sentence. Do not dictate a sentence, it is to be written spontaneously. It must contain a subject and verb and be sensible. Correct grammar and punctuation are not necessary.

Copying: On a clean piece of paper, draw intersecting pentagons, each side about 1 in., and ask him to copy it exactly as it is.

Estimate the patient's level of sensorium along a continuum, from alert on the left to coma on the right.

Median Mini-Mental State Examination Score by Age and Education Level

	Education				
	0–4y	5–8y	9–12y	≥12y	Total
18–24	23	28	29	30	29
25–29	25	27	29	30	29
30–34	26	26	29	30	29
35–39	23	27	29	30	29
40–44	23	27	29	30	29
45–49	23	27	29	30	29
50–54	22	27	29	30	29
55–59	22	27	29	29	29
60–64	22	27	28	29	28
65–69	22	27	28	29	28
70–74	21	26	28	29	27
75–79	21	26	27	28	26
80–84	19	25	26	28	25
≥85	20	24	26	28	25
Total	22	26	29	29	29

Agency for Health Care Policy and Research (November 1996). Recognition and initial assessment of Alzheimer's disease and related dementias: Clinical practive quideline No. 19. Rockville, MD: U.S. Department of Health and Human Services, Public Health Service, Agency for Health Care Policy and Research. AHCPR Pub. No. 97-0702.

CHAPTER 11

Metacognition: The Relationships of Awareness and Executive Functions to Occupational Performance

Noomi Katz, PhD, OTR, and Adina Hartman-Maeir, MSc, OTR

With the purpose of introducing the concepts of metacognition and emphasizing their importance in occupational therapy practice and theory, this chapter contains the following parts:

1. A presentation of metacognitive components: awareness and executive functions
2. A review of existing assessments
3. An outline of treatment guidelines
4. Case studies
5. Research findings in adults with neurological dysfunctions
6. An analysis of metacognitive components in the occupational therapy cognitive models, as well as suggestions about integrating metacognitive components in all occupational therapy models for practice.

Occupational performance and cognition are two major factors determining health in general and quality of life. Occupational performance encompasses human functioning in the areas of self-care, work/productivity, and play/leisure (Mosey, 1986; McColl & Pranger, 1994). Cognition is a basic, universal human trait that underlies every human function (Katz, 1992) and is defined as the individual's capacity to acquire and use information in order to adapt to environmental demands (Lidz-Schneider, 1987). Since cognition and occupational performance are closely related, therapists working with individuals with disabilities aim to improve both, in order to improve clients' func-

tional performance with the ultimate goal of living in the least restrictive environment.

Cognition comprises cognitive and metacognitive skills (Katz, 1994a). Metacognition, defined as awareness and executive functions, controls the use of cognitive skills and provides the basis for transfer and generalization of learned skills to daily functioning. Thus metacognition is conceptualized as the link between cognitive skills and occupational performance, as well as between all performance components and occupational performance.

Metacognition is defined as "knowing about knowing." Metacognitive knowledge includes knowledge about ourselves, the tasks we face, and the strategies we employ (Flavell, 1985). Brown (1987) differentiated between "knowing about knowing" (i.e., declarative knowledge wherein an example includes knowing the name of a flower) and "knowing how to" (i.e., procedural knowledge wherein an example is knowing how to ride a bike). Nelson and Narens (1994) proposed a model of metacognition to distinguish between the components of monitoring and control processes. Jarman, Vavrick, and Walton (1995) elaborated on this model and denoted that these components correspond to those of knowledge/awareness of abilities and deficits, and executive functions. Executive functions are the processes of initiating, planning, and regulating task performance. The two components of awareness and executive functions monitor and control activities in all domains of life

(Flavell, 1985) and have been identified as critical determinants to rehabilitation success in adults with neurological dysfunction (Diller & Riley, 1993; Lezak, 1995; Prigatano, 1986).

Metacognition involves higher-order integrative processes, associated mainly with the frontal lobes (Stuss, 1991, 1992). Cognitive and behavioral deficits associated with frontal lobe damage often do not appear on standardized psychological tests conducted in laboratory settings (Damasio & Anderson, 1993), as these executive deficits are evident mainly in functional tasks that by nature require the integration and organization of many skills. Awareness of deficits is analyzed within the context of daily tasks; only through such activities can we truly observe the implications of an awareness deficit. For example, if a person verbally acknowledges a memory deficit but does not make adjustments for this deficit in his or her daily activities, the therapist should conclude that his or her awareness level is not adequate to live independently and safely in the community. Likewise, executive functions can particularly be observed in novel, nonroutine daily tasks, which require a person to actively initiate, plan steps ahead, evaluate performance, and change actions as necessary. Since occupational therapists specialize in occupational performance, they have a unique opportunity to contribute to metacognitive assessment, treatment, and theoretical development.

Metacognitive deficits have been identified in clients following traumatic brain injury, stroke, dementia, and schizophrenia. However, since problems in metacognition can also result from nonneurological origins, such as a lack of information regarding dysfunctions and their consequences or psychological denial, the subject matter can and should be applied to many other client populations.

Metacognitive Components

The literature on metacognition shows a lack of uniformity in the use of metacognitive terminology. Metacognition is sometimes defined exclusively as either awareness or as executive functions, and other times it includes both components without their explicit use or differentiation. The follow-ing discussion is based on neuropsychological literature about metacognitive skills and deficits.

Awareness

"Self-awareness is generally defined as the perception of changes in higher cognitive functions" (Berquist & Jacket, 1993, p. 275). Prigatano and Schacter define self-awareness as "the capacity to perceive the 'self' in relatively 'objective' terms while maintaining a sense of subjectivity" (1991, p. 13). They further state, "Self-awareness or awareness of higher cerebral functions thus involves an interaction of thoughts and feelings" (p. 13). Lezak recently defined self-awareness as a component of volition referring to "awareness of oneself psychologically, physically and in relation to one's surroundings" (1995, p. 651). The term awareness deficit used here implies the inability to recognize deficits or problems caused by neurological origins, excluding psychological denial (Barco, Crosson, Bolesta, Werts, & Stout, 1991; McGlynn & Schacter, 1989).

Unawareness may result from damage to frontal, parietal, or temporal regions of the brain (McGlynn & Schacter, 1989). A distinction has been made between general and specific unawareness that is associated with different neuroanatomical structures. Frontal damage can lead to unawareness of either the global deficit or condition in general or the complex processing deficits, such as problem solving or understanding the social implications of brain injury (Prigatano, 1991). Parietal damage may result in specific unawareness of perceptual or motor deficits, such as seen in hemiplegia and hemianopia (Bisiach & Geminiani, 1991). This type of unawareness has also been termed anosognosia; thus the terms unawareness of deficits and anosognosia are often used interchangeably in the literature. Finally, temporal lesions may cause unawareness of language disorders (Rubens & Garrett, 1991). No matter what factors caused the unawareness, all forms of it have a profound impact on occupational performance.

A hierarchy of awareness levels has been described by Barco et al. (1991) and Crosson et al. (1989) in which intellectual awareness is situated at the base. This level describes the knowledge of deficits and was subdivided into the following areas: basic knowledge pertaining to the existence of a deficit, and knowledge of the functional implications of this deficit. At times problems can be related to either component. For example, a client with intact intellectual awareness after brain injury involving a memory deficit acknowledges that he or she has a memory problem that interferes with shopping tasks. Another client may be totally unaware of memory loss, or he or she may be aware of memory problems but not of their functional implications and the need to overcome them.

The authors further describe the following two additional higher levels titled emergent awareness and anticipatory awareness, which function in the capacity of detecting errors in performance, anticipating problems, and planning strategies for compensation. However, these two levels are in essence part of the executive functions. Intellectual awareness is the knowledge about deficits and how to compensate for them, and emergent and anticipatory awareness relate to the actual doing (i.e., planning and regulating performance). Thus the use of the term awareness by Barco et al. (1991) combines the metacognitive aspects of knowledge/monitoring (awareness) and control (executive process/functions) (Jarman et al., 1995) and appears not to be exclusively limited to awareness.

Executive Functions

Executive functions are considered frontal lobe functions and constitute the dynamic "doing" aspect of metacognition, as opposed to the more static knowledge component of awareness (Ylvisaker & Szekeres, 1989). Stuss (1992) defines the major role of executive functions as the conscious direction of behavior toward a selected goal. Lezak (1982, 1983, 1987) defines executive functions as those capacities inherent in directed, effective activity, including initiating actions, setting goals, planning and organizing behavior, carrying out goal-directed behaviors, using strategies effectively, and monitoring and self-correcting behavior. Recently, Lezak divided the executive functions into four major components: volition, planning, purposive action, and effective performance (1995, p. 650). According to the model proposed by Jarman

et al., executive functions are termed "metacognitive control" and are defined as "the creation or production of cognitive strategies and their use or implementation in various tasks and life situations" (1995, p. 167). According to Winegardner (1992), executive functions allow us to apply specific skills appropriately to novel and nonroutine daily problems and situations. Winegardner emphasized the role of executive functions in novel situations, such as driving a car on wet pavement, as opposed to habitualized automatic activities that do not require the guidance of the executive system, for example, a morning routine of getting dressed. A client with problems in the area of executive functions faced with a new problem will have difficulty initiating, planning, carrying out actions, detecting errors, and changing his or her actions accordingly. It is this level of executive functions that limits a person's ability to be left alone and causes a real safety risk.

The two components of metacognition defined above are interrelated as conceptualized within a hierarchical feedback–feedforward model that includes self-awareness, executive functions, and sensory-perceptual components (Stuss, 1992). For example, awareness of one's strengths and weaknesses is a prerequisite for realistic goal setting and self-regulation of performance. A person with deficits in self-awareness will show incapability of planning appropriately, detecting deficits, and correcting difficulties that stem from them. It is easy to see why metacognitive deficits limit occupational performance.

Existing Assessments

Awareness

Awareness assessments (Table 11-1) include rating scales, questionnaires for clients and caregivers, comparisons of clients' and relatives' ratings of ADL and IADL, predictions and estimations of test performance, and nonverbal awareness in task performance.

Awareness Rating Scales are based on therapists' observations and interactions with clients: The Anosognosia Rating Scale (Bisiach et al., 1986) is a four-point scale describing the type or extent of

Table 11-1
Assessment of Awareness

Instrument	Content, Method, Scale
Awareness Rating Scales:	
Anosognosia Rating Scale (Bisiach et al., 1986)	Questions and observation of awareness during performance 4-point scale; 0-spontaneous, 1-specific questions, 2-demonstration, 3-acknowledgment.
Insight Rating Scale (Toglia, 1993a)	Rating of awareness levels: general to specific awareness of impairments, and functional implications of deficits; rated following performance of activities; 8-point scale: 1-unawareness to 8-full awareness.
Awareness Questionnaires:	
Anosognosia Questionnaires (Cutting, 1978; Starkstein et al., 1992)	Awareness of physical deficits; questions and probing; scoring: use of Bisiach et al. (1986) 4-point scale.
Awareness Interview (Anderson & Tranel, 1989)	Awareness questions: general to specific; 8 questions for motor, thinking, memory, orientation, language, and visual perception; asked before performance; comparison to test performance; 3-point scale.
Awareness Questionnaire (Hibbard et al., 1992)	Same as the above interview with addition of affective domain.
Competency Rating Scale (Prigatano, 1986)	30 questions related to cognitive, physical, emotional, and social difficulties in daily activities; 5-point scale; patient and family 2 parallel forms; awareness rate-comparison between the two reports.
Comparison of clients' and relatives' reports on functional measures:	
DeBettignies et al. (1990) used the Physical Self-Maintenance Scale (PSMS) and IADL. Can be used with other functional measures.	
Comparison of prediction before and estimation after test performance:	
Contextual Memory Test (Toglia, 1993b) & Toglia Categorization Test (1994)	Questions before and after the administration of the tests; scores: size of discrepancy.
Self-Awareness Scale (Pendley, 1993)	Awareness of performance completeness and accuracy; Questions following test performance; 6-point scale: 0-no response to 5-accurate perception of performance.
Nonverbal awareness in task performance:	
(Ramachandran, 1995)	Awareness of physical disabilities; clients have to choose between unimanual and bimanual tasks; score: number of correct choices.

Note: Reprinted with permission from the Canadian Journal of Occupational Therapy, *1997, 64, p. 57.*

inquiry required to elicit awareness responses. The highest score is given for spontaneous report of deficits, and the lowest one for no acknowledgment of deficits. This scale has been used for evaluating awareness of hemiplegia and hemianopia (AHP) in clients post CVA, but is applicable to all other populations. The Insight Rating Scale (Toglia, 1993a) is an eight-point scale describing awareness levels, ranging from unawareness of injury to full awareness of general and specific deficits and their functional implications. The scale was used clinically but no research findings are available yet.

Awareness questionnaires were designed to assess the clients' ratings of their general disability and specific deficits in various domains: The Anosognosia Questionnaire by Cutting (1978) relates to awareness of physical deficits after CVA. Scoring is by the Bisiach four-point rating scale. Research findings revealed significant differences in the incidence of anosognosia in hemiplegia (AHP) in right versus left CVA (Cutting, 1978; Starkstein et al., 1992).

The Awareness Interview (Anderson & Tranel, 1989) comprises eight standardized questions pertaining to awareness of illness in general and to physical and cognitive deficits. Responses for each item are scored on a three-point scale. An awareness index is obtained by calculating the discrepancy between the interview scores and the neuropsychological and physical test scores. Reliability and validity results showed that interrater reliability was .92, and awareness scores significantly differentiated between right and left CVA groups (Anderson & Tranel, 1989; Wagner & Cushman, 1994).

The Awareness Questionnaire (Hibbard et al., 1992) is similar to the awareness interview, yet provides additional questions regarding awareness of affective changes after brain injury. Clients' responses are compared with psychological, neuropsychological, and physical test results. Reliability and validity results showed that interrater reliability was .95, and different awareness patterns were found in right and left CVA groups. A larger percentage of the RCVA group minimized their motor deficits (40%) compared to the LCVA group (18%), and a larger percentage of the LCVA group exaggerated their motor and cognitive deficits (20%, 36%), compared to the RCVA group (8%, 14%). Responses to the awareness interview and questionnaire could also be compared with other objective tests used by occupational therapists, such as the LOTCA (Itzkovich, Elazar, Averbuch, & Katz, 1990) for cognitive deficits or a motor scale for physical deficits.

The Prigatano Competency Rating Scale (PCRS) (Prigatano, 1986) is a structured questionnaire consisting of 30 items related to cognitive, physical, emotional, and social difficulties encountered in daily activities. Two parallel forms are provided

separately, for clients and relatives. They are instructed to estimate the amount of difficulty in task performance on a five-point scale. Awareness is defined as the degree of compatibility between the two reports. The PCRS subclassified individuals following traumatic brain injury into three groups with different levels of awareness. Group membership was correlated with number of lesions based on neuroradiological findings (Prigatano, 1991).

Comparison of Clients and Caregivers Ratings on ADL and IADL Scales. For example, DeBettignies et al. (1990) operationally defined awareness as the discrepancy between clients' and relatives' scores on Lawton and Brody's (1969) Physical Self-Maintenance Scale (PSMS) and Instrumental Activities of Daily Living Scale (IADL). Since assessing the client's awareness of functional status is central to achieving maximal independence, this simple method of assessing awareness should be applied to other functional measures. For example, a comparison of client and caregiver reports on the Functional Independence Measure (FIM) (Granger, 1993) could provide a measure of the client's awareness of his or her functional status.

Comparison of Prediction and Estimation to Test Performance. The Contextual Memory Test (CMT) and Toglia Category Assessment (TCA) are standardized tests for visual memory and categorization (Toglia, 1993b; 1994). They include questions for predicting performance that are administered prior to performing the tests and then proceed with estimation questions. Two awareness scores are calculated by comparing prediction and estimation to actual performance. Research on the CMT was conducted with people following brain injury and healthy populations (Toglia, 1993b). Test–retest reliability for the discrepancy between prediction and recall scores in the brain-injured group was .90. A comparison between healthy and brain-injured discrepancy scores revealed significant differences ($t = -10.79$, $p < .001$). The direction of prediction was also different; the brain-injured group tended to overrate its performance while the healthy group tended to underestimate it.

The Self-Awareness Rating Scale, designed by Pendley (1993), is based on two questions that probe self-perception of accuracy and completeness after test performance. For example, after finishing the Block Design Test, the client is asked, "Did you use all blocks?" to investigate completeness, and "Are the blocks in the right places?" to evaluate accuracy. A six-point scale is scored based on answers to questions, the presence or absence of cues from the examiner, and any action taken by the client to modify his or her responses both for completeness and accuracy. This scale was used in a study of awareness in RCVA and healthy control groups. The two awareness questions were asked after a battery of neuropsychological tests. Interrater reliability showed 90.2% agreement on the awareness scale. The study group demonstrated poorer self-awareness than the control group on each test individually as well as on all of the tests combined.

Non-verbal Awareness in Task Performance. Ramachandran (1995) introduced an innovative method designed to assess implicit awareness of physical disabilities in people with hemiplegia. The client is presented with a series of five choices between unimanual and bimanual tasks coupled with corresponding prizes. The more valuable prizes are always associated with the bimanual tasks. A client with hemiplegia is expected to choose a unimanual task that he or she thinks is within his or her abilities. The score reflects the number of correct choices made in several trials. This method has been investigated in only a few clients with anosognosia and has been found to correlate with a lack of awareness to hemiplegia.

In summary, the majority of instruments used to assess awareness are verbally based. They probe awareness of various performance components, and some additionally address areas of occupational performance, such as ADL and IADL. In general the clients' responses are compared with external criteria, such as family caregiver ratings or test scores. Further research is recommended to understand the awareness of community living tasks in order to determine the safety of people living alone.

Executive Functions

Most cognitive assessments are by nature structured tasks that do not provide the opportunity to assess executive functions. Among the newly developed assessments of executive functions, some relate to all components while others to more specific aspects of executive functions. Table 11-2 lists only assessments developed specifically for measuring executive functions and are divided into tabletop test, functional tasks, and rating scales. In addition, the use of traditional psychological measures, such as the Verbal Fluency Test, the Wisconsin Card Sorting Test, the Tower Tests, or the Rey Complex Figure, are used for assessing components of executive functions (Lezak, 1983; 1995).

The Open Ended Tabletop Test. The Tinker Toy Test (TTT) (Lezak, 1983; 1993; 1995) is a free constructional performance test (i.e., without the constraints of a model). Lezak strongly advocates the necessity of evaluating executive functions in unstructured tasks and situations. Otherwise, Lezak states, it is not possible to observe real initiation, planning, regulation, etc. Scoring of the TTT is based on the number of pieces used, the verbal description of a proper idea, the manner in which the construction was executed, the richness of using the pieces, the complexity, etc. Thus qualitative content measures as well as quantitative aspects are taken into account. Although TTT correlates significantly at r = .50 with measures of constructional abilities, it seems to be sensitive to additional components of executive functions. The TTT was found to be valid in differentiating between groups (i.e., functionally dependent patients, nondependent patients, and healthy controls). The number of pieces used and the complexity of the constructions significantly differentiated between these three groups. The test was also found to predict rehabilitation and employability following head injury (Lezak, 1993, 1995).

Functional Tasks. The Route-Finding Task (Boyd & Sautter, 1993) is an open-ended performance task, designed to assess executive functions in a relevant, real world problem-solving activity of finding a certain place (i.e., an office in a hospital; a class in a school, etc.). The task includes explicit instructions and hierarchical cueing procedures. Performance is scored according to a four-point scale addressing areas of task comprehension, in-

	Table 11-2
	Assessment of Executive Functions
Instrument	**Content, Method, Scale**
Tabletop Test:	
Tinker Toy Test (TTT) (Lezak, 1982; 1995)	Tabletop; free constructional test; scoring: number of pieces; complexity; proper idea, etc.
Functional tasks:	
Kitchen Task Assessment (Baum & Edwards, 1993)	Functional task of making cooked pudding; performance scored on six components.
Woodrow Wilson Route Finding Task (Boyd & Sautter, 1993)	Real world open-ended problem-solving task; scored on six components and overall independence, and checklist of potential problems.
Rating Scales:	
Executive Function Behavioral Rating Scale (Sohlberg & Geyer, 1986)	Observation of performance in everyday activities; scoring three major areas: exception of plans, time management, self-regulation.
The Initiation Log (DePoy et al., 1990)	Observation of performance in activities; six-point initiation scale, from independent initiation to refusal.
Executive Functions Assessment (Pollens et al., 1988).	Observation of performance in everyday activities; eight categories of executive functions are rated on a 3-point scale.

Note: Reprinted with permission from the Canadian Journal of Occupational Therapy, *1997, 64, p. 59.*

formation seeking, direction retention, error detection, and on-task behavior. In addition, an overall total independent score is given and a checklist of potentially contributing problems (in the emotional, interpersonal, communication, perceptual and motoric domains) is suggested.

A reliability and validity study of 31 young adults with head injuries (Boyd & Sautter, 1993) showed high interrater reliability of .94. Concurrent validity was measured by correlating the task with neuropsychological tests of concept formation, hypothesis testing and mental flexibility, perceptual organization, verbal comprehension, and rapid information processing. All measures, except for speed of information processing, correlated significantly with performance on the route-finding task. These findings demonstrate the sensitivity of the task to higher integrative cortical functions and provide evidence of the relationship between laboratory and everyday functional measures of these aspects of cognition.

The Kitchen Task Assessment (Baum & Edwards, 1993; Baum, 1995) is a functional cooking task designed to measure executive function components. Initiation, organization, performance of all steps, sequencing, judgment and safety, and completion are scored on the following four-point scale: independent, required verbal cues, required physical assistance, not capable at all. Reliability and validity were studied with the dementia population. Interrater reliability for the total score was .85 (ranging from .63 for safety to 1.0 for initiation). Validity was supported by KTA scores differentiating between levels of dementia, and significant correlations were found with neuropsychological and functional tests ($r > .60$). The structure of the test was explored through factor analysis, showing the KTA as a unidimensional instrument (i.e., one factor explained 84% of the variance).

Rating Scales. The Initiation Log (DePoy, Maley, & Stranraugh, 1990) is a six-point scale relating to patients' level of initiation in therapeutic activities. The scale ranges from independent initiation of activity, to initiation with various cues to refusal to do an activity. Therapists score the log on a daily or weekly basis and in this way, changes over time are assessed. Results of two single case studies of clients with closed-head injury showed that one subject's score did not change from the time of the pretest to three weeks later, while the second subject's score following treatment changed from 4 to 1 (i.e., independent initiation).

The Executive Function Behavioral Rating Scale (Sohlberg & Geyer, 1986) was developed in order to provide a comprehensive assessment of executive functions. The scale is comprised of three major areas: (1) the selection and execution of cognitive plans in a task, i.e., knowledge of appropriate steps, sequencing, initiation, organization skills, repair, and speed of response; (2) time management, i.e., time estimation, creating time schedules, performance of scheduled activities; (3) self-regulation, i.e., impulse control, perseveration, and environmental dependency. The client is rated after being observed in a wide range of activities.

The Executive Functions Assessment (Pollens, McBratnie, & Burton, 1988) is a form designed to record observations relevant to the executive functions. The assessment includes eight categories: awareness, goal setting, planning, self-initiating, self-inhibiting, self-monitoring, ability to change set, and strategic behavior. Criteria are provided for rating each category on a three-point scale: within normal limits, moderate, and severe. The authors found that the form encouraged their vigilance in observing these behaviors and noting changes over time. The main focus of the observation is on executive functions, yet this assessment incorporates the awareness component as well.

In summary, executive functions are assessed in performance measures and rating scales based on observations. Some, such as the TTT, are based on tabletop performance tasks, while others are based on real life activities. The combination of formal measures and qualitative observational data is recommended for assessment of executive functions (Depoy et al., 1990), and more new, creative, and sensitive assessment techniques are needed that will tap the "in context" aspects of executive functions and determine the environmental conditions that influence occupational performance.

Metacognitive Treatment Guidelines

Cognitive rehabilitation is traditionally divided into two major approaches. The first, remedial, consists of direct retraining or restoration of impaired core areas of cognitive skills. The second, functional or compensatory substitution, teaches clients to use their assets to achieve successful performance despite the presence of underlying cognitive deficits (Ben-Yishay & Diller, 1993; Diller, 1992; Katz, 1994b; Neistadt, 1988; Neistadt, 1990). However, what was not emphasized until recently is that in both the remedial and functional approaches the role of metacognition is essential. Without awareness of a deficit it is difficult to engage a client in remediation. Moreover, if clients are unaware of their deficits, they do not feel the need for or may not be willing to learn compensatory techniques (Ben-Yishay & Diller, 1993; Berquist & Jacket, 1993; Diller & Riley, 1993; Crosson et al., 1989; Prigatano, 1986; Prigatano & Schacter, 1991). Without initiation, planning, or self-regulation, there will be no effective generalization of the retrained or learned skills to support everyday life.

Awareness

The main principle in the remediation of awareness is to provide the client with information about the nature of the dysfunction and its manifestations in task performance. The goal of treatment is to enhance the client's awareness of both his or her deficits and their impact on functional performance. Awareness deficits are perceived as a barrier to engaging clients in any training; achieving understanding of strengths and limitations is seen as prerequisite for other treatments (Ylvisaker, Szekeres, Henry, Sullivan, & Wheeler, 1987).

Treatment guidelines (Klonoff, O'Brien, Chiapello, & Cunningham, 1989) include the provision of initial tasks that target deficits, such that clients can recognize problems without feeling overwhelmed (i.e., tasks that are not too easy and not too difficult); tasks that allow clients to experience improvement with practice; and tasks that allow the therapist and clients to explore strategies for improving performance once the client's level of performance has reached a plateau. Clients should be taught how to score their own performance and to analyze the required underlying skills before they start a task. It is the responsibility of the therapist to provide feedback on the client's performance. Feedback should relate to:

1. Discrepancies between expected and actual performance
2. The benefits and limitations of compensatory strategies they used
3. The variability in their performance
4. The degree of cueing they needed to complete the tasks
5. The potential impact of residual difficulties on their everyday functioning.

Some of the techniques that have been used to facilitate the recognition of problems include videotaping and self-rating scales.

The working alliance between the client and therapist must be emphasized in the remediation of awareness deficits, since the provision of feedback is a central component in treatment. The client's ability to accept and integrate the feedback is dependent on the development of a trusting relationship with the therapist and must be planned to include tasks that are of interest to him or her.

Barco et al. (1991) introduced a two-part treatment method for awareness deficits that includes facilitation and compensation. Facilitation is similar to the remedial guidelines described above. If remediation of awareness fails, then external compensation for unawareness must be implemented. Often clients lack a basic knowledge of their deficits and therefore will not invest themselves in treatment. Even if a therapist succeeds in teaching the clients compensatory strategies, they will not implement changes if they remain unaware. External compensations involve the use of an agent other than the client and/or environmental modifications. For example, a client with dementia of the Alzheimer's type, unaware of the functional implications of his memory deficit, attempted to perform activities beyond his abilities. Attempts at improving his awareness by providing information and feedback concerning his performance failed, as he believed he could manage his life independently and did not see the need for learning compensatory memory strategies. His safety was at risk when he turned on the gas and forgot to light it, or when he went shopping and did not know what to buy or where his money was located. This client was in need of an external agent who would help him manage his affairs and protect him from danger. The external agent is most often a caregiver, a spouse or child, or in some cases a neighbor.

The assessment and treatment of awareness should be the first step in rehabilitation of any deficit. Initially, treatment should be focused on the remediation of awareness deficits, since only with intact awareness can therapy proceed effectively. If unawareness is persistent, then appropriate external compensations need to be applied.

Executive Functions

The importance of the executive functions in rehabilitation has been clearly stated by Lezak: "In the last analysis, . . . the patient's capacity to benefit from rehabilitation training and to apply what is learned depends on the integrity of the executive functions. Skills have minimal value if it does not occur to the patient to apply them, or to regulate their application appropriately, or to correct errors as they come up" (1987, p. 56). The main principle in the remediation of executive functions is to provide the person with opportunities for choice and selection, planning, and self-correction. The treatment goal is to attain independent problem solving.

Remediation typically involves presenting the client with unfamiliar, unstructured open problems. In these situations the client is required to think of a plan of action, implement it, and examine and regulate his or her own performance. Task demands should be graded according to the degree of structure and amount of feedback provided in order to enable gradual improvement (Sohlberg, Mateer, & Stuss, 1993).

Sohlberg and Mateer (1989) developed an intervention model for executive functions comprised of three components: selection and execution of cognitive plans, time management, and self-regulation. Treatment activities are then adapted to address the problematic areas. For example, errand completion through the use of a list may be incorporated into the task as it requires initiation, planning, and organization, or scheduling activities may be utilized as they require time management. Task analyses, with specific and explicit emphasis on executive functions components, are suggested for the first two components of the model.

Behavior modification principles are suggested for treating deficits in self-regulation (i.e., the third component). Behavior modification treatment initially provides explicit cues and performance feedback, and gradually fades and decreases as clients become increasingly aware of their behavior and more able to monitor and regulate their responses. Cicerone and Wood (1987) provide an example of self-regulating strategy training. A self-instructional procedure was taught that required the client to verbalize a plan of behavior using fading cues. Initially the plan was verbalized aloud, then whispered, and finally verbalized internally by the client. The treatment included generalization training (i.e., practicing the strategy in real life situations). This strategy helped the client to overcome impulsive behavior and to improve his planning abilities. This strategy was also used by Fetherlin and Kurland (1989) to increase the functional independence of brain-injured adults.

Finally, a compensatory or functional approach to treating executive functions is advocated if clients do not benefit from task modifications, cues, or performance feedback. Compensation does not assume that independent problem solving or transfer of learning occurs; therefore it involves the training of individual functional activities. The treatment goal is to broaden the client's repertoire of activities that he or she can perform independently in the context of everyday life (Giles, in this book).

Some of the literature on treatment of executive functions combines elements of both awareness and executive functions training, for example in the "Executive Functions Module of the BRAIN-WAVE-R" rehabilitation program (Bewick, Raymond, Malia, & Bennett, 1995). Although designated for the improvement of executive functions, it combines awareness training principles. The module includes exercises in the areas of self-organization, planning, strategy development, cognitive flexibility, time management, etc., advocating the use of comparative rating scales (i.e., therapist-client, prediction, and estimation of task performance) to facilitate self-awareness in these areas.

Case Examples

Case Study 1

Joseph, 76 and single, used to work as a clerk for a government agency and is currently retired. He lives entirely alone in the community and spends most of his time wandering around his neighborhood. He was never married and is not in contact with other family members. He was referred for a cognitive and functional evaluation by his family physician, because of suspected memory loss and dementia of Alzheimer's type (DAT).

Cognitive Assessment

When asked in the awareness interview why he was referred to the clinic he could not answer. He did not spontaneously report any problems in physical, cognitive, or functional areas: "Everything is OK, I can't think of any reason why they asked me to come here." In response to specific questions about physical and cognitive deficits he admitted to having a slight problem with his memory: "Yes, lately I've been having some difficulty remembering things." Yet he denied any functional implication of this problem: "No, this does not affect my life in any way. I just have to get a job and it will get better."

Results of the Cognistat cognitive screening test revealed severe deficits in orientation and memory. His prediction of performance prior to testing and his estimation of performance after testing were much higher than his actual performance.

Functional Assessment

Since it was evident that his awareness level was insufficient, IADL checklists requiring reliable self-report were not applicable; therefore a performance test was required. The Assessment of Motor and Process Skills (AMPS) was used to evaluate his IADL ability. Results revealed adequate motor skills (scores 3 and 4), yet markedly deficient problems in the majority of the process skills (scores 1 and 2). The results of the AMPS predicted that Joseph had severe deficits that would interfere with performance of IADL. A home visit ascertained this prediction. Joseph's apartment was piled with debris, spoiled food, and dirty clothing. He was clearly not able to care for his daily needs. During the visit, he still maintained that he managed just fine. He was not interested in attending a day center or moving to a more sheltered environment.

Summary of Evaluation

It was evident that Joseph had severe cognitive deficits that impacted on his daily life. Since there was no family member to verify his report, his awareness level was measured by comparing his self-report to test performance and functional observation. The discrepancy between his self-report, prediction of his abilities, and actual performance indicated a serious problem in awareness.

Recommendations

1. Involvement of community social services
2. Occupational therapy to address his cognitive deficits.

Treatment:

Community social services were involved immediately. They made contact with him and provided meals to his apartment, yet he was not interested in additional help. He refused to contact his sister or to consider alternative living arrangements, and he continued to insist that all he needed was to find a job. The primary goal of occupational therapy was to enhance his awareness of deficits in order to facilitate the compensation for them.

Treatment comprised mainly both therapist feedback and self-feedback on Joseph's performance in a variety of tasks. Initially tasks were simple tabletop memory games, as they were less threatening than functional activities and results on them are easily measurable. Joseph was asked to predict his performance and then to compare the results with the predictions. The tasks were gradually changed to ones more relevant to his daily life. This was conducted in a very supportive and gradual manner to prevent extreme and overwhelming reactions.

After Joseph's awareness level improved, it was possible to begin compensatory treatment. This included learning the use of a diary and, mainly, accepting the need for a change in his environment.

Results

1. After six sessions, Joseph was willing to attend a day center for cognitively impaired individuals that provides a supportive and stimulating environment, with activities adapted to the cognitive level of each client. He is currently attending the program 3 days a week.
2. He consented to making contact with his sibling who is helping to care for his daily needs.
3. He learned how to use a diary and is able to use it for temporal orientation and making appointments.
4. He has consented to the help offered by social services and his sister and is currently in the process of moving to a more protected living environment.

Commentary

Joseph's condition provides an example of a person with a serious metacognitive deficit. He was not aware of his disease (DAT), was mildly aware of his cognitive deficit (i.e., he acknowledged having a memory deficit after confrontation), and was totally unaware of the functional implications of his condition. As a result of his unawareness and inability to perceive any problems, he was not even able to seek help. The metacognitive assessment targeted this problem very clearly. This case also demonstrates that the metacognitive component in cognitive rehabilitation is the first building block in treatment, which enables the client to further engage himself in rehabilitation.

Case Study 2

Esther is 53 years old, married with three children, and had previously worked as a homemaker. She had undergone a craniotomy after she had hemorrhaged in her left occipital lobe. Initially after surgery she was confused, had a mild right hemiparesis, and a right visual-field deficit, but was released from the hospital two weeks later, appearing independent in ADL. Two months post surgery she complained to her physician that she was unable to "manage things" at home and therefore was referred to occupational therapy.

Cognitive Assessment

In the awareness interview Esther spontaneously spoke about her medical condition and the difficulties she was encountering in her daily life. She could not cook, clean, shop, read, or write as she used to before her stroke. She said that in the beginning her right side was weak, but since that problem was resolved she did not understand why she was unable to manage her life efficiently. When asked if she was experiencing cognitive and visual deficits, she looked bewildered and said, " Maybe, I'm not sure . . . yes I think so."

Results of the Behavioral Inattention Test (BIT) (Wilson, Cockburn, & Halligan, 1987) revealed problems in visual attention. Her score on the conventional tests was 119 (score below 129 is considered an indication of unilateral visual neglect). Analysis of her performance on cancellation tasks revealed two observations. (1) Bilateral omissions occurred, yet more on the right than on the left, particularly on the more demanding attentional tasks (i.e., Star Cancellation). (2) Esther's performance on the behavioral subtests, revealed difficulties scanning pictures, dialing telephone numbers, reading, and copying. Most of her omissions and errors were on the right side. In the copying task she used only the left side of the page.

Functional Assessment

Esther reported moderate difficulty in all areas of IADL in responding to the IADL checklist. The AMPS was administered to analyze which skills were affecting her performance. Results revealed problems in several of the processing skills. Esther did not attend adequately to all aspects of the task or environment, nor did she adequately notice and respond to problems she encountered.

Summary of Evaluation

Esther was aware of the functional difficulties she was encountering and knew that they were a result of her brain surgery, but she was not adequately aware of her visual and attentional deficits that were affecting her functional status.

Treatment

The goals of treatment were:

1. To improve her awareness of visual attention deficits
2. To learn compensatory strategies to address her visual field deficit
3. To improve her attention and compensate for the residual deficits
4. To improve her IADL status.

Treatment initially comprised feedback regarding the test results. Esther was very receptive to the information, claiming that nobody had ever pointed it out to her before. It was easier for her to comprehend her visual, as opposed to attentional, deficits; therefore she was taught about the nature of an attentional deficit and when it would most likely affect her activities. She began to keep a diary in which she recorded the problems she encountered in her daily life. She learned that she had the most difficulty when attempting to do more than one thing at a time, when her children were talking to her while she was cooking, or when the area was cluttered. The process of teaching her about her deficits also included providing her with feedback and teaching her to give self-feedback in tasks that either required varied degrees of attention or combined both visual fields. At the end of the first few weeks of treatment she became adequately aware of her deficits. The next stage involved graded exercises that required attention and visual scanning. The final stage involved the implementation of compensatory strategies for residual deficits, such as turning her head to the right when crossing streets, using her finger to follow the text while reading, and structuring her schedule and environment to prevent overload on limited attentional resources.

Results

After 6 months of treatment, Esther was fully aware of her deficits and was able to perform most IADL independently. She could also predict when she would need assistance from others.

Commentary

This case provides an example of a deficit in intellectual awareness and of specific physical and cognitive deficits following a stroke. Esther lacked knowledge of the less obvious implications of her illness (i.e., visual and attentional deficits) as well as the meaning of them in her everyday life. She became aware of her functional difficulties and was able to seek the necessary assistance. By using metacognitive treatment, the occupational therapist provided the missing link between the illness and the daily problems she was facing. This knowledge was the first step required for subsequent rehabilitation to be effective.

Research Findings

Awareness

Research in clients with brain injuries shows that clients usually underestimate problems in comparison to their relatives and overestimate their abilities in comparison to relatives and staff. Unawareness may persist until 2 to 3 years post injury and is most severe following frontal and parietal lesions. This deficit is seen in clients with traumatic brain injuries (Crisp, 1992; Prigatano, 1991) as well as

in clients after cerebral vascular accidents (CVA), especially with right hemisphere lesions (Bisiach et al., 1986; Hibbard et al., 1992; Wagner & Cushman, 1994).

Research in RCVA has shown that awareness of deficits is strongly associated with unilateral neglect (Pendley, 1993; Azouvi et al., 1996). In addition, unawareness of motoric impairment (anosognosia) at 1 month post stroke predicts poor rehabilitation outcome, 5 months later (Giallanella & Matiolli, 1992).

Some of the same phenomenon are seen in clients with dementia (McGlynn & Kaszniak, 1991; Nebes, 1992) and schizophrenia (Amador, Strauss, Yale, & Gorman, 1991; Cuesta & Peralta, 1994). Clients with dementia usually underestimate their difficulties and overestimate their performance, while interestingly, their appraisal of relatives' performance may remain accurate. An interaction of awareness with cognitive skills was found in dementia, suggesting that both deficits coexist (McGlynn & Kaszniak, 1991; Lopez, Becker, Somsak, Dew, & DeKosky, 1994). Clients with schizophrenia show similar patterns to those with brain injuries with frontal lobe involvement, thus suggesting that unawareness is neurologically based in some of these clients as well (Amador et al., 1991).

Executive Functions

Research findings have indicated an association of executive skills with frontal lobe functions (Burgess & Shallice, 1996; Stuss, 1992). Deficits in the executive functions have been demonstrated in clients with traumatic brain injury, dementia of the Alzheimer's type, schizophrenia, subarachnoid hemorrhage (Tidswell, Dias, Sagar, Sagar, Mayes, & Battersby, 1995), and Huntington's and Parkinson's diseases (Hanes, Andrews, Smith, & Pantelis, 1996).

Case studies in traumatic brain injury show some successful training effects for initiation, self-regulation, and planning deficits (Cicerone & Giacino, 1992; Depoy et al., 1990; Lawson & Rice, 1989). For example, Cicerone and Giacino (1992) use a modified version of the Tower of London task as a training modality to remediate executive functions. Analysis of the performance of six single subjects showed improvement following the self-instructional training, but with much variability among the clients.

Deficits in executive functions have been identified in the population with Alzheimer's disease (Brugger, Monsch, Salmon, & Butters, 1996; Binetti, Magni, Padovani, Cappa, Bianchetti, & Trabucci, 1996). Furthermore, the relationship between executive function deficits and daily activity and self-care has been demonstrated by Baum (1995). Her research acknowledges the major role that executive skills play in activity and self-care of the elderly afflicted with this disease, and highlights the need to train caregivers in the accommodation of executive deficits in order to sustain higher levels of activity.

The population with schizophrenia also has been characterized by executive function deficits (Goldberg, Weinberger, Berman, Pliskin, & Podd, 1987; Green, Satz, Ganzell, & Vaclav, 1992; Sullivan, Shear, Zipursky, Sagar, & Pfefferbaum, 1994). These studies have examined some aspects of the executive functions, mainly using the Wisconsin Card Sorting Test (WCST) (Heaton, 1981). The WCST measures mental flexibility, which is an underlying component of self-regulation. Goldberg et al. (1987) studied 44 clients with schizophrenia who were randomly assigned to three treatment conditions: no instructions, instructions for category shifts, and card-by-card instructions. Subjects were retested 2 weeks later. Only those who received card by card instructions improved their performance markedly in training, but at retesting performance returned almost to baseline in all groups. The authors suggest similarities among clients with frontal lobe damage, reporting, "They seem to perceive the mistakes they make but are unable to use the information to modify their behavior" (p. 1014).

In another study, Green et al. (1992) studied 46 clients with schizophrenia and 20 control subjects with other psychiatric disorders. Significant differences were found between the groups for perseveration errors, number of correct answers, and number of categories in the WCST. After training, improvement in performance on the test was found following a combination of reinforcement and detailed instruction. The authors conclude that this treatment procedure may be necessary to increase mental flexibility.

Studies regarding the area of metacognition of adults with brain dysfunctions appear to be at a beginning stage. Research within the field of occupational therapy should provide data on both the relationship of metacognition to occupational performance and the impact of metacognitive deficits on daily activities. Further validation of assessments and the efficacy of treatment approaches need to be investigated.

Analysis of Metacognitive Components in Occupational Therapy Cognitive Models for Practice

Seven occupational therapy models for cognitive rehabilitation are described in this book. In the past, explicit metacognitive components were rarely incorporated into them, excluding Toglia's (1991, 1992) Dynamic Interactional Model. However, in the updates presented in this book metacognitive components are more prevalent.

Dynamic Interactional Model

Toglia (1991, 1992) presented the first cognitive model in occupational therapy to include variables of awareness and executive functions based on contemporary definitions and conceptualizations. Metacognition, in her writings, refers to two interrelated aspects of knowledge about one's own cognitive processes and the ability to monitor one's own performance. "The skills involved in metacognition include: the ability to evaluate task difficulty in relation to current skills, to plan ahead, to choose appropriate strategies, and to predict the consequences of action and monitor performance" (Toglia, 1992, p. 109). Under the category of control functions, Toglia (1992) lists monitoring, error detection, planning, decision making, and evaluating results.

First, Toglia incorporates awareness evaluation into her Dynamic Interactional Assessment (DIA). Awareness is scored according to three measures: prediction, estimation, and general response. She also suggests interview questions with an insight rating scale (Toglia, 1993a). She then incorporates metacognitive training techniques, such as self-estimation, role-reversal, self-questioning, and self-evaluation, into the Multicontext Treatment Approach, suggesting that these should be integrated into daily treatment activities.

The Multicontext Treatment Approach (Toglia, 1991; in this book) targets the individual's capacity to process, monitor, and use new information flexibly across task situations. Tasks are analyzed according to the levels of transfer that are needed, for example from near transfer (i.e., similar task characteristics) to very far transfer (i.e., daily activities). Deficient processing strategies, such as executive functions (i.e., decreased ability to initiate a plan of action), are identified. Then the targeted strategy is consistently held while task parameters are varied and changed, placing progressively more demands on the impaired processing strategies and the ability to transfer learning. Recently, in the update described in this book, Toglia specifically outlines metacognitive strategies and training techniques, such as anticipation, self-prediction, self-checking and evaluation, self-questioning, time-monitoring, and role-reversal. In general during metacognitive training, the client becomes gradually more responsible for his or her performance. Toglia equates metacognitive and awareness training by focusing on the client's evaluation and monitoring of his or her own performance.

Although Toglia developed her approach for clients following brain injuries, it already has been applied to clients with schizophrenia (Fine, 1993; Josman, in this book), and in essence can be generic to many other populations with CNS dysfunctions, including dementia, Parkinson's disease, and multiple sclerosis.

The Quadraphonic Approach: Holistic Rehabilitation

Within this model, one of the four theoretical frameworks underlying the Quadraphonic Model is the teaching/learning theory. According to Abreu (1992), metacognitive theory is part of teaching/learning, and is especially relevant for clients who function at higher levels, since metacognitive training relies heavily on language communication. The client/learner stage of awareness is considered a major factor influencing the individual's performance. Abreu suggests an awareness and motor learning continuum that illustrates an interface between the stages of both factors (Abreu, 1992).

Abreu (in this book) includes metacognitive evaluation and training in all phases of treatment using questions, cues, and prompts to enhance the client's awareness. Awareness is evaluated by questioning the client before, during, and after testing.

Abreu and Toglia (1987) were the first to introduce a cognitive rehabilitation model for people with brain dysfunctions into occupational therapy. Neuropsychological and information processing literature provides the basis for both models in relation to metacognitive components.

Neurofunctional Model

In his neurofunctional model, Giles (1992) focuses on three major impairment areas as central to developing functional retraining programs: memory, attention, and frontal lobe functions. He states that these deficits are not to be treated directly but are important for therapists' understanding and designing of functional skills programs. Theoretically in this current update, instead of addressing problem-solving deficits, Giles relates directly to frontal lobe deficits. Among the frontal lobe functions, he elaborates on planning and initiation, self-awareness, and metacognitive functioning. Planning and initiation are clearly executive functions, while self-awareness is seen as a failure to accept a "new self" and understand current limitations. For metacognitive functioning he uses the model developed by Nelson and Narens (1994) of the two processes of monitoring and control that were elaborated on earlier. On this basis, Giles incorporates the need to gather information on these areas during the evaluation process and relates to metacognitive control strategies in skills training, suggesting gradual training in independent performance of tasks and knowledge of the parameters involved in the task. In addition, debriefing is used as feedback to raise knowledge of the results.

Cognitive Disability Model

Allen's (1985) Cognitive Disability Model was conceptualized as an information processing system where the throughput—conscious awareness—was used to analyze six cognitive levels according to purpose, experience, process and time. This analysis refers to some aspects of executive function without using the term. It shows a hierarchy from deficits at levels 1 to 3, limited functioning at level 4, partial functioning at level 5, to intact functioning at level 6.

Awareness of deficit as used in this chapter was not previously discussed in the model. It is important to point out that Allen, Earhart and Blue (1992) use the terms *self-awareness disability* (defined as a disturbance in self-care activities) and *situational awareness disability* (defined as a disturbance in understanding relations in daily situations) in very different ways from the metacognitive concept of self-awareness discussed in this chapter and from the recent writing of Allen and Blue in this book.

Allen and Blue acknowledge the impact of awareness of disability to the person's ability to benefit from remedial treatment methods. They present an ascending hierarchy from cognitive levels 5.8 and 5.6 where awareness of disability and anticipation of secondary effects are present; through levels 5.4 to 5.0 where partial awareness exists but people are defensive and tend to blame external causes for their difficulties; at levels 4.8 to 4.0 there is no general awareness to problems only isolated awareness of a need for assistance. The authors discuss the relationships of learning, generalization, and environmental compensations to the extent of awareness and cognitive level.

Integrating Metacognitive Components in Occupational Therapy

Theoretically, metacognition resides in the Cognitive Performance Components as conceptualized in the Occupational Therapy's Domain of Concern (Mosey, 1986) or the Mental Performance Components in the Model of Occupational Performance (McColl & Pranger, 1994). In the Model of Human Sub-Systems developed by USC's Occupational Science (Clark et al., 1991), and identified as influencing occupation, cognition is equated with the information processing subsystem. In this chapter, it is suggested that the cognitive component can be categorized into and then analyzed as two major elements: cognitive skills and metacognitive skills. Each element includes further subcomponents. For example, cognitive skills comprise attention, memory, visual–spatial perception, and categorization skills, whereas metacognitive skills comprise self-awareness and executive functions. However, the importance of metacognition as defined above is in its widespread involvement in other performance components and in all areas of occupational performance and should be considered basic to the performance of daily occupations.

Thus metacognitive components are key elements in occupational performance, without awareness of deficits no treatment will be effective, and without executive functions no learned strategy will be initiated, executed, or regulated. To evaluate these essential components, we have to make observations during occupational performance. Therefore, it is imperative that occupational therapy practice models incorporate contemporary concepts of metacognition into their theoretical base and methods of intervention. Occupational therapists have expertise in observations of tasks performed in daily naturalistic situations. This expertise should be used to integrate metacognitive components into our task or activity analyses. The assessments mentioned earlier can be used in various combinations, depending on the specific circumstances of the client. Metacognitive training should be introduced into our treatment methods. Some beginning work is introduced but more must follow to include the provision of research evidence.

One major difficulty in metacognitive evaluation is the assessment of people who cannot express themselves verbally. In these cases, observations of occupational performance are even more important as indicators of both cognitive and metacognitive skills. Occupational therapists' expertise and focus on nonverbal activities and performance measures can have a major impact on intervention and research.

It is strongly proposed that the constructs of awareness and executive functions as higher-order integrative and control functions should be included in all occupational therapy practice models, and not only in cognitive models, whether biomechanical, sensory integration, or motor learning, to demonstrate occupational therapists' concern with the totality of human functioning. Obviously, specific practice models or frames of reference that focus on cognitive disabilities as major variables for intervention should include metacognitive as well as cognitive assessment and treatment methods.

Occupational performance is the core concept and focus of our profession, but being aware of strengths, deficits, and executive functions is prerequisite for successful functioning in any occupation, task, or activity. In summary, the unique contribution of occupational therapy in cognitive rehabilitation is the use of occupations of self-care, productivity, and leisure to observe and evaluate metacognitive components of awareness, executive functions, and cognitive skills during the performance of tasks. Occupational therapy intervention does not aim to improve cognitive skills for their own sake, but to improve occupational performance through improvement of cognitive components.

Acknowledgment

This chapter was partly published in the *Canadian Journal of Occupational Therapy*, 1997, 64, 53–62, by the same authors.

References

Abreu, B. C. (1992). The quadraphonic approach: Management of cognitive-perceptual and postural control dysfunction. *Occupational Therapy Practice, 3,* 12–29.

Abreu, B. C., & Toglia, J. P. (1987). Cognitive rehabilitation: An occupational therapy model. *American Journal of Occupational Therapy, 41,* 439–448.

Allen, C. K. (1985). *Occupational therapy for psychiatric diseases: Measurement and management of cognitive disabilities.* Boston: Little, Brown.

Allen, D. K., Earhart, C., & Blue, T. (1992). *Occupational therapy treatment goals for the physically and cognitively disabled.* Bethesda, MD: American Occupational Therapy Association.

Amador, X. F., Strauss, S. A., Yale, S. A., & Gorman, J. M. (1991). Awareness of illness in schizophrenia. *Schizophrenia Bulletin, 17,* 113–132.

Anderson, S. W., & Tranel, D. (1989). Awareness of disease states following cerebral infarction, dementia and head trauma: Standardized assessment. *Clinical Neuropsychologist, 3,* 327–339.

Azouvi, P., Marchal, F., Samuel, C., Morin, L., Renard, C., Louis-Dreyfus, A., Jokic, C., Wiart, L., Pradat-Diehl, P., Deloche, G., & Bergego, C. (1996). Functional consequences and awareness of unilateral neglect: Study of an evaluation scale. *Neuropsychological Rehabilitation, 6,* 133–150.

Barco, P. P., Crosson, B., Bolesta, M. M., Werts, D., & Stout, R. (1991). Training awareness and compensation on postacute head injury rehabilitation. In S. J. Kreutzer & P. H. Wehman (Eds.), *Cognitive rehabilitation for persons with TBI.* Baltimore: Brookes.

Baum, C. (1995). The contribution of occupation to function in persons with Alzheimer's disease. *Journal of Occupational Science: Australia, 2,* 59–67.

Baum, C., & Edwards, D. F. (1993). Cognitive performance in senile dementia of the Alzheimer's type: The kitchen task assessment. *American Journal of Occupational Therapy, 47,* 431–438.

Ben-Yishay, Y., & Diller, L. (1993). Cognitive remediation in traumatic brain injury: Update and issues. *Archives of Physical Medicine and Rehabilitation, 74,* 204–213.

Berquist, T. F., & Jacket, M. P. (1993). Programme methodology: Awareness and goal setting with the traumatically brain injured. *Brain Injury, 7,* 275–282.

Bewick, K. C., Raymond, M. J., Malia, K. B., & Bennett, T. L. (1995). Metacognition as the ultimate executive: Techniques and tasks to facilitate executive functions. *NeuroRehabilitation, 5,* 367–375.

Binetti, G., Magni, E., Padovani, A., Cappa, S. F., Bianchetti, A., & Trabucchi, M. (1996). Executive dysfunction in early Alzheimer's disease. *Journal of Neurology, Neurosurgery and Psychiatry, 60,* 91–93.

Bisiach, E., & Geminiani, G. (1991). Anosognosia related to hemiplegia and hemianopsia. In J. P. Prigatano & D. L. Schacter (Eds.), *Awareness of deficit after brain injury.* NY: Oxford University Press.

Bisiach, E., Vallar, G., Perani, D., Papagno, C., & Berti, A. (1986). Unawareness of disease following lesions of right hemisphere: Anosognosia for hemiplegia and anosognosia for hemianopia. *Neuropsychologia, 24,* 471–482.

Boyd, T. M., & Sautter, S. W. (1993). Route-finding: A measure of everyday executive functioning in the head-injured adult. *Applied Cognitive Psychology, 7,* 171–181.

Brown, A. L. (1987). Metacognition, executive control, self-regulation, and other more mysterious mechanisms. In F. E. Weinert & R. H. Kluwe (Eds.), *Metacognition, motivation and understanding.* Hillsdale, NJ: Erlbaum.

Brugger, P., Monsch, A. U., Salmon, D. P., & Butters, N. (1996). Random number generation in dementia of the Alzheimer's type: A test of frontal executive functions. *Neuropsychologia, 34,* 97–103.

Burgess, P. W., & Shallice, T. (1996). Response suppression, initiation and strategy use following frontal lobe lesions. *Neuropsychologia, 34,* 263–273.

Cicerone, K. D., & Giacino, J. T. (1992). Remediation of executive function deficits after traumatic brain injury. *Neurorehabilitation, 2,* 12–22.

Cicerone, K. D., & Wood, J. W. (1987). Planning disorder after closed head injury: A case study. *Archives of Physical Medicine and Rehabilitation, 68,* 111–115.

Clark, F. A., Parham, D., Carlson, M. E., Frank, G., Jackson, J., Pierce, D., Wolfe, R. J., & Zemke, R. (1991). Occupational science: Academic innovation in the service of occupational therapy's future. *American Journal of Occupational Therapy, 45,* 300–310.

Crisp, R. (1992). Awareness of deficit after traumatic brain injury: A literature review. *Australian Occupational Therapy Journal, 39,* 15–21.

Crosson, B., Barco, P. P., Velozo, C. A., Bolesta, M. M., Cooper, P. V., Werts, D., & Brobeck, T. C. (1989). Awareness and compensation in postacute head injury rehabilitation. *Journal of Head Trauma Rehabilitation, 4,* 46–54.

Cuesta, M. J., & Peralta, V. (1994). Lack of insight in schizophrenia. *Schizophrenia Bulletin, 20,* 359–366.

Cutting, J. (1978). Study of anosognosia. *Journal of Neurology, Neurosurgery and Psychiatry, 41,* 548–555.

Damasio, A. R. & Anderson, S. W. (1993). The frontal lobes. In K. H. Heilman & E. Valenstein (Eds.), *Clinical Neuropsychology.* NY: Oxford University Press.

DeBettignies, B. H., Mahurin, R. K., & Pirozzolo, F. J. (1990). Insight for impairment in independent living skills in Alzheimer's disease and multi-infarct dementia. *Journal of Clinical and Experimental Neuropsychology, 12,* 355–363.

DePoy, E., Maley, K., & Stranraugh, J. (1990). Executive function and cognitive remediation: A study of activity performance. *Occupational Therapy in Health Care, 7,* 101–114.

Diller, L. (1992). Neuropsychological rehabilitation. *Advanced Experimental Medical Biology, 325,* 105–114.

Diller, L., & Riley, E. (1993). The behavioral management of neglect. In I. H. Robertson & J. C. Marshall (Eds.), *Unilateral neglect: Clinical and experimental studies.* Hillsdale, NJ: Erlbaum.

Fetherlin, J. M., & Kurland, L. (1989). Self-instruction: A compensatory strategy to increase functional independence with brain-injured adults. *Occupational Therapy Practice, 1,* 75–78.

Fine, S. (1993). Neurobehavioral perspectives on schizophrenia. In J. Van Deusen (Ed.), *Body image and perceptual dysfunction in adults.* Philadelphia: Saunders.

Flavell, J. H. (1985). *Cognitive development.* Englewood Cliffs, NJ: Prentice-Hall.

Giallanella, B., & Matiolli, F. (1992). Anosognosia and extrapersonal neglect as predictors of functional recovery following right hemisphere stroke. *Neuropsychological Rehabilitation, 2,* 169–178.

Giles, G. M. (1992). A neurofunctional approach to rehabilitation following brain injury. In N. Katz (Ed.), *Cognitive rehabilitation: Models for intervention in occupational therapy.* Stoneham, MA: Butterworth-Heinemann.

Goldberg, T. E., Weinberger, D. R., Berman, K. F., Pliskin, N. H., & Podd, M. H. (1987). Further evidence for dementia of the prefrontal type in schizophrenia. *Archives of General Psychiatry, 44,* 1008–1014.

Granger, C. V. (1993). *Guide for the Uniform Data Set for Medical Rehabilitation.* Adult FIM version 4.0. Buffalo, NY: State University of New York at Buffalo.

Green, M. F., Satz, P., Ganzell, S., & Vaclav, J. F. (1992). Wisconsin Card Sorting Test performance in schizophrenia: Remediation of a stubborn deficit. *American Journal of Psychiatry, 149,* 62–67.

Hanes, K. R., Andrews, D. G., Smith, D. J., & Pantelis, C. (1996). A brief assessment of executive control dysfunction: Discriminant validity and homogeneity of planning, set shift, and fluency measures. *Archives of Clinical Neuropsychology, 11,* 185–191.

Heaton, R. K. (1981). *Wisconsin Card Sorting Test Manual.* Odessa, FL: Psychological Assessment Resources.

Hibbard, M. R., Gordon, W. A., Stein, P., Grober, S., & Sliwanski, M. (1992). Awareness of disability in patients following stroke. *Rehabilitation Psychology, 37,* 103–119.

Itzkovich, M., Elazar, B., Averbuch, S., & Katz, N. (1990). *LOTCA Manual.* Pequannock, NJ: Maddak.

Jarman, R. F., Vavrik, J., & Walton, P. D. (1995). Metacognition and frontal lobe processes: At the interface of cognitive psychology and neuropsychology. *Genetic, Social and General Psychology Monographs, 155–210.*

Katz, N. (1992). *Cognitive rehabilitation: Models for intervention in occupational therapy.* Stoneham, MA: Butterworth-Heinemann.

Katz, N. (1994a). Occupation and metacognition. Paper presented at the Research Colloquium, CAN/AM Occupational Therapy Conference, Boston.

Katz, N. (1994b). Cognitive rehabilitation: Models for intervention. *Occupational Therapy International, 1,* 34–48.

Katz, N., & Hartman-Maeir, A. (1997). Occupational performance and metacognition. *Canadian Journal of Occupational Therapy, 64,* 53–62.

Klonoff, P. S., O'Brien, K. P., Chiapello, D. A., & Cunningham, M. (1989). Cognitive retraining after traumatic brain injury and its role in facilitating awareness. *Journal of Head Trauma Rehabilitation, 4,* 37–45.

Lawson, M. J., & Rice, D. N. (1989). Effects of training in use of executive strategies on a verbal memory problem resulting from closed head injury. *Journal of Clinical and Experimental Psychology, 1,* 842–854.

Lawton, M. P., & Brody, E.M. (1969). Assessment of older people: Self-maintaining and instrumental activities of daily living. *Gerontologist, 9,* 179–186.

Lezak, M. D. (1982). The problem of assessing executive functions. *International Journal of Psychology, 17,* 281–297.

Lezak, M. D. (1983). *Neuropsychological assessment* (2nd ed.). NY: Oxford University Press.

Lezak, M. D. (1987). Assessment for rehabilitation planning. In M. Meir, A. Benton, & L. Diller (Eds.), *Neuropsychological rehabilitation.* NY: Guilford Press.

Lezak, M. D. (1993). Newer contributions to the neuropsychological assessment of executive functions. *Journal of Head Trauma Rehabilitation, 8,* 24–31.

Lezak, M. D. (1995). *Neuropsychological assessment* (3rd ed.). NY: Oxford University Press.

Lidz-Schneider, C. (1987). *Dynamic assessment: An interactional approach to evaluating learning potential.* NY: Guilford Press.

Lopez, O. L., Becker, J. T., Somsak, D., Dew, M. A., & De-Kosky, S. T. (1994). Awareness of cognitive deficits and anosognosia in probable Alzheimer's disease. *European Neurology, 34,* 277–282.

McColl, M. A., & Pranger, T. (1994). Theory and practice in the occupational therapy guidelines for client-centered practice. *Canadian Journal of Occupational Therapy, 61,* 250–259.

McGlynn, S. M., & Kaszniak, A. W. (1991). When metacognition fails: Impaired awareness of deficit in Alzheimer's disease. *Journal of Cognitive Neuroscience, 3,* 183–189.

McGlynn, S. M., & Schacter, D. L. (1989). Unawareness of deficits in neuropsychological syndromes. *Journal of Clinical and Experimental Neuropsychology, 11,* 143–205.

Mosey, A. C. (1986). *Psychosocial components of occupational therapy.* NY: Raven Press.

Nebes, R. D. (1992). Cognitive dysfunction in Alzheimer's disease. In F. I. M. Craik & T. A. Salthouse (Eds.), *The handbook of aging and cognition.* Hillsdale, NJ: Erlbaum.

Neistadt, M. E. (1988). Occupational therapy for adults with perceptual deficits. *American Journal of Occupational Therapy, 42,* 141–148.

Neistadt, M. E. (1990). A critical analysis of occupational therapy approaches for perceptual deficits in adults with brain injury. *American Journal of Occupational Therapy, 44,* 299–305.

Nelson, O., & Narens, L. (1994). Why investigate metacognition? In J. Metcalfe & A. P. Shimamura (Eds.), *Metacognition.* Cambridge: MIT Press.

Pendley, A. L. (1993). The effect of right-hemisphere brain damage on self-awareness skills: Diagnostic and therapeutic implications. Unpublished doctoral dissertation, University of Colorado at Boulder.

Pollens, R. D., McBratnie, B. P., & Burton, P. L. (1988). Beyond cognition: Executive functions in closed head injury. *Cognitive Rehabilitation, September–October ,* 26–32.

Prigatano, G. P. (1986). *Neuropsychological rehabilitation after brain injury.* Baltimore: John Hopkins University Press.

Prigatano, G. P. (1991). Disturbances of self-awareness of deficit after traumatic brain injury. In J. P. Prigatano & D. L. Schacter (Eds.), *Awareness of deficit after brain injury.* NY: Oxford University Press.

Prigatano, G. P., & Schacter, D. L. (1991). *Awareness of deficit after brain injury.* NY: Oxford University Press.

Ramachandran, V. S. (1995). Anosognosia in parietal lobe syndrome. *Consciousness and Cognition, 4,* 22–51.

Rubens, A. B., & Garrett, M. F. (1991). Anosognosia of linguistic deficits in patients with neurological deficits. In J. P. Prigatano, & D. L. Schacter (Eds.), *Awareness of deficit after brain injury.* NY: Oxford University Press.

Sohlberg, M. M., & Geyer, S. (1986). *Executive function behavior rating scale.* Paper presented at Whittier College Conference Series, Whittier, California.

Sohlberg, M. M., & Mateer, C. A. (1989). *Introduction to cognitive rehabilitation: Theory and practice.* NY: Guilford Press.

Sohlberg, M. M., Mateer, C. A., & Stuss, D. T. (1993). Contemporary approaches to the management of executive control dysfunction. *Journal of Head Trauma Rehabilitation, 8,* 45–58.

Starkstein, S. E., Fedoroff, P., Price, T. R., Leiguardia, R., & Robinson, R. G. (1992). Anosognosia in patients with cerebrovascular lesions. *Stroke, 23,* 1446–1453.

Stuss, D. T. (1991). Disturbances of self-awareness after frontal system damage. In J. P. Prigatano & D. L. Schacter (Eds.), *Awareness of deficit after brain injury.* NY: Oxford University Press.

Stuss, D. T. (1992). Biological and psychological development of executive functions. *Brain and Cognition, 20,* 8–23.

Sullivan, E. V., Shear, P. K., Zipursky, R. B., Sagar, H. J., & Pfefferbaum, A. (1994). A deficit profile of executive, memory, and motor functions in schizophrenia. *Society of Biological Psychiatry, 36,* 641–653.

Tidswell, P., Dias, P. S., Sagar, H. J., Mayes, A. R., & Battersby, R. D. E. (1995). Cognitive outcome after aneurysm rupture: Relationship to aneurysm site and preoperative complications. *Neurology, 45,* 875–882.

Toglia, J. P. (1991). Generalization of treatment: A multicontext approach to cognitive perceptual impairment in adults with brain injury. *American Journal of Occupational Therapy, 45,* 505–516.

Toglia, J. P. (1992). A dynamic interactional approach to cognitive rehabilitation. In N. Katz, *Cognitive rehabilitation:*

Models for intervention in occupational therapy. Stoneham, MA: Butterworth-Heinemann.

Toglia, J. P. (1993a). Cognitive-perceptual rehabilitation: A dynamic interactional approach. Workshop presented at Cornell University Center, New York.

Toglia, J. P. (1993b). *Contextual Memory Test Manual.* San Antonio: Therapy Skill Builders.

Toglia, J. P. (1994). *Toglia Categorization Assessment Manual.* Pequannock, NJ: Maddak.

Wagner, M. T., & Cushman, L. A. (1994). Neuroanatomic and neuropsychological predictors of unawareness of cognitive deficit in vascular population. *Archives of Clinical Neuropsychology, 9,* 57–69.

Wilson, B.A., Cockburn, J., & Halligan, P.W. (1987). *Behavioral Inattention Test Manual.* London: Thames Valley Test.

Winegardner, J. (1992). Executive functions. In H. Cohen (Ed.), *Neuroscience for rehabilitation.* Philadelphia: Lippincott.

Ylvisaker, M., & Szekeres, S. F. (1989). Metacognitive and executive impairments in head-injured children and adults. *Topics in Language Disorders, 9,* 34–49.

Ylvisaker, M., Szekeres, S. F., Henry, K., Sullivan, D. M., & Wheeler, P. (1987). Topics in cognitive rehabilitation therapy. In M. Ylvisaker & E. M. R. Gobble (Eds.), *Community re-entry for head-injured adults.* Boston: Little, Brown.

CHAPTER 12

Cognitive Rehabilitation Research in Occupational Therapy: A Critical Review

Elizabeth DePoy, PhD, MSW, OTR/L, and Lynn Gitlow, MEd, OTR/L

As illustrated by the breadth of approaches to cognition and cognitive rehabilitation presented in this book, cognition is a critical concern of occupational therapists. Multiple theoretical lenses have been used to explain cognition, to link it to function, and to examine methods by which to facilitate maximum function through cognitive remediation. Moreover, the diversity of people with cognitive impairments treated by occupational therapists render cognitive rehabilitation a complex set of strategies with no specific formula on how to achieve the best outcomes. In 1992, Katz noted that minimal research existed to support cognitive rehabilitation approaches. However, in large part as result of the combination of multiple theoretical lenses and the difficulty in predicting outcome, a significant body of research from occupational therapy and other fields has evolved. In this chapter, we critically examine the research that has supported cognitive intervention in occupational therapy. This overview provides a basis for recommending future methodology to enhance our understanding of cognitive phenomena and the ways in which occupational therapists can implement cognitive rehabilitation intervention to improve occupational performance.

Cognitive deficits are seen across the life span and result from multiple causes. Because of the enormity of the field, the research literature on cognition, cognitive rehabilitation, and functional correlates of cognition is extensive and diverse. We therefore limit our discussion to the global constructs of cognition and cognitive rehabilitation rather than to the subcomponents thereof.

Consistent with the American Occupational Therapy Association (AOTA) *Self-Study Series on Cognitive Rehabilitation,* we define cognition as the "acquisition, processing and application of information to daily life" (Royeen, 1993, p. 9). To organize our discussion of research, we begin with a review of the research literature on the relationship of cognition to function as it is applied to clinical occupational therapy practice. Because much of the clinical research on cognition addresses assessment of cognition and cognitive skills, we present an overview of that body of knowledge and then proceed to classify the research literature on cognitive rehabilitation into four major categories:

1. Research on general stimulation techniques (Green, 1993)
2. Research on substitution and transfer techniques (Green, 1993)
3. Research on behavioral intervention (Green, 1993)
4. Research on systemic intervention.

Finally, based on our review, we offer substantive and methodological suggestions for future research in cognitive rehabilitation.

Although numerous taxonomies have been suggested for classifying approaches to cognitive rehabilitation (Royeen, 1993; Toglia, 1993), we have chosen this taxonomy to organize the research literature into categories that, although not mutually exclusive, are sufficiently diverse from one another to yield clarity while avoiding redundancy. The following definitions clarify each approach to cognitive rehabilitation and to related research.

General stimulation refers to an approach to cognitive rehabilitation that relies on drills and exercises of selected cognitive skills. For example, using computer programs to enhance problem solving would be contained in this category of interventions. Repetition and practice provide the foundation for the general stimulation approach to cognitive rehabilitation. While Prigatano (1987) found minimal improvement in cognition using general stimulation techniques, occupational therapists and other rehabilitation professionals have used stimulation techniques, and in investigating their outcome, have found diverse results as we will discuss below.

Substitution and transfer techniques include interventions that are primarily compensatory. Two types of compensation are promoted through the use of substitution and transfer. The first is functional adaptation and the second is relocation of brain function. Popularized by Luria in the early 1970s (Green, 1993), relocation of brain function involves training alternative areas of the brain to take over functions that were previously controlled by injured brain tissue. Functional adaptation involves personal and environmental adaptations to facilitate function. These interventions are considered in the same category of intervention because adequate and appropriate environmental aids must be used to maximize the success of relocation of brain function. Occupational therapy interventions with persons with traumatic brain injury frequently rely on this category of intervention. For example, individuals with poor short-term memory will be given aids, such as a date book and an alarm watch, so that they rely on visual and auditory brain centers rather than memory to regain the capacity to organize time and complete daily tasks.

The behavioral approach to cognitive remediation relies on substituting external reinforcers for lost internal motivation and behavioral regulation. Positive and negative reinforcement is attached to specified observable actions in order to increase the likelihood of stimulating and maintaining a desired set of behaviors. While there is some mention of behavioral elements in the cognitive rehabilitation literature in the occupational therapy field, few studies on interventions that rely exclu-sively on behavioral techniques were found. An example of a behavioral technique would be the establishment of a token economy to ensure that an individual meets his or her stated objectives for the day.

The systemic approach to cognitive rehabilitation is characterized by a broader focus than the previous three classifications. Rather than focusing on an individual's acquisition of a specific skill or function, a systems approach to rehabilitation is used. Systems may include family, the workplace, school, etc. These systems are modified to improve the cognitive functioning and thus the occupational functioning of individuals with cognitive deficits. Examples of this approach would include instructing family members in techniques of environmental adaptation that enhance the safety of individuals with dementia.

Because occupation is the unique domain of occupational therapy, we posit three heuristics for our review of research:

1. Occupational therapy research in the field of cognitive rehabilitation must address occupational function.
2. Assessment not only must address cognitive skill or process evaluation but must advance beyond skill to examine how the skill deficits and strengths impact occupational function.
3. Occupational therapy intervention research, despite its focus on cognitive skill or process acquisition, must ultimately examine function and an individual's capacity to negotiate his or her living environments.

Consistent with Radomski (1994) and Royeen (1993), the role for occupational therapy in the field of cognitive rehabilitation must be focused on occupational performance linked to functional outcomes.

Moreover, as urged by Nelson (1988), and as we address later in the chapter in more detail, we use the term occupation, rather than activity, to describe the medium through which occupational therapists conduct their work. We use these heuristics to create a lens through which to critically examine current research in cognitive rehabilitation relevant to occupational therapy. (N.B.: This chapter addresses cognitive rehabilitation. Therefore, much of the literature on children is omitted in that it is habilitative rather than rehabilitative.)

Cognition and Function

A full spectrum of views of the relationship between cognition and function has been posited, from the extreme view that cognition and function are one and the same, to the perspective that cognition is a separate phenomenon from function. Because occupational therapy research is primarily clinical, occupational therapy researchers do not typically address the link between function and cognition specifically. Rather, the relationship between cognition and function is embedded within our research and theory. Work on assessment is especially revealing about one's view of the relationship between cognition and function in that implicit within any sound cognitive assessment is a theoretical foundation clarifying the nature of cognition and how it can be accessed and evaluated. We address this point later in this chapter. Consistent with contemporary theory (Kielhofner, 1995), we take the position that cognition is a performance component contained in the mind–body subsystem. Because we suggest that habit maps and routines are a primary domain of occupational therapy, our clinical intervention and thus our research should focus on cognitive performance as a basis for improving occupational function. Congruent with our view, Abreu (in this book) suggests that occupational therapists address both micro- and macro-level perspectives. Micro-level perspectives address subskills or performance skills (attention, memory, categorization, and problem solving), while the macro perspective places cognition, its assessment, and its treatment within a personal–social context. It is therefore not surprising to find, as discussed below in each of the approaches to intervention, that the occupational therapy research literature frequently attempts to examine both cognitive and functional outcomes of cognitive rehabilitation and to integrate these outcomes into the context of the daily lives of those who are receiving occupational therapy intervention.

An excellent example lies in the work of Neistadt (1993) who studied the association between con-

structional skill impairment and meal preparation in a population of individuals with traumatic brain injury (TBI). Her work was important as a bivariate descriptive study and moreover for illuminating the constraints that occupational therapy researchers face in attributing functional outcomes to cognitive intervention.

One might note that all cognitive assessments must observe behavior as a basis for drawing conclusions about cognitive function. However, some assessments, such as those developed by Allen (1985) and Fisher (1993), begin with a global functional task and extract cognitive information, while others, such as the Lowenstein Occupational Therapy Cognitive Assessment (LOTCA) (Katz, Itzkovich, Averbuch, & Elazar, 1989), use specific tasks to assess cognition and then link findings to functional capacity. The ever more popular postmodern inquiry strategies such as narrative are being increasingly integrated into occupational therapy assessment as well (Spencer, Krefting, & Mattingly, 1993; Abreu, in this book).

Allen's (1985, 1992, in this book) work clearly illustrates research that, although aimed at assessment, addresses the link between cognition and function. Her assessments have been extensively scrutinized for reliability and validity with varied findings (David, 1990; Cusick & Harai, 1991). However, Allen's approach to assessment supports the occupational therapy commitment to focus on function. Similarly, Arnadottir (1990) uses functional skills to assess cognition. Activities of daily living (ADL) tasks are the basis for evaluating cognitive strengths and deficits.

The link between cognition and function is inherent in Hartman-Maeir and Katz's important work published in 1995. They conducted an examination of the validity of the Behavioral Inattention Test (BIT) and then advanced their research to ascertain the association between BIT score and function in daily tasks. The authors used associational statistical procedures to examine relationships, and caution should therefore be taken in suggesting predictive validity of the BIT for the functional activities that were found to be significantly related to BIT performance.

As we will discuss below, one criterion that we use to assess the value of research on cognitive rehabilitation for occupational therapy practice is the effort to link cognitive skill assessment and rehabilitation to occupational function. Therefore, efforts to investigate this relationship should be continued within the context of research on assessment and intervention.

We now turn to a discussion of the research in cognitive rehabilitation that has been conducted by occupational therapists or that is important to inform occupational therapy practice. We begin our examination with a discussion of assessment and then move to research in intervention.

Assessment

Much of the research done in the field of assessment focuses on validating and standardizing tools to evaluate cognitive function. The process of developing or creating assessment begins with a clear understanding and definition of the constructs to be assessed. Once lexically defined, the approach to assessment can be specified. It is of critical importance in selecting an assessment to establish the domain of cognition to be assessed, and to clarify the conceptual view of cognition that will be used to guide assessment and subsequent intervention. As we indicated above, this thinking process identifies how the developer of an assessment protocol views cognition and its link to function. Thus, any occupational therapist who is selecting a cognitive assessment should examine the conceptual and empirical foundation of the assessment to ascertain the congruence between what he or she wishes to know and what an assessment actually can reveal about a client. For example, using Toglia's dynamic interactional approach to cognition (Toglia, in this book) would call for global assessment of the capacity to learn and generalize information, while approaching cognition as a cognitive behavioral phenomenon, as suggested by Giles (1994, in this book), would call for assessing the completion of cognitive task performance, incorporating both behavioral and cognitive elements. Each measures cognition, but each views cognition in very different ways. An occupational therapist who would approach intervention by enhancing a client's learning capacity would not obtain sufficient information upon which to plan intervention goals

and strategies by using a cognitive–behavioral assessment.

In the area of assessment, we take the position that both quantitative and qualitative assessments of cognition and related behaviors are necessary to ascertain a holistic understanding of a client's status as well as to evaluate process. Moreover, as we stated above, selection of assessment must be consistent with the view of cognition that is used in intervention and in the establishment of outcome goals and objectives. In the case where quantitative assessments are used, every effort should be made to ensure instrument validity and reliability. Moreover, methodological rigor in the use of qualitative assessment must be upheld as well.

Many assessments of cognitive function have been developed and/or used by occupational therapists. Here, we review selected assessments. Although we do not examine the literature on the Rancho Los Amigos Scale (Rancho Los Amigos Medical Center, 1986) in this chapter, mostly because it was not developed by or specifically for occupational therapists, we mention it because of its frequent use in the assessment of cognitive recovery from traumatic head injury and other brain injuries. It is a scale that views cognitive recovery as a set of behaviors over which one gains increasing control. This scale is of critical importance to occupational therapists because of its use with multiple disciplines and its standardization based on behavioral indicators. Occupational therapists who use it should become familiar with the theoretical foundation on which it is based and on the protocol for assessing cognitive level.

In response to the need for assessments that inform occupational therapists about cognition and function, numerous assessments have been developed and/or are in diverse stages of development. As stated above, much of the research in cognitive rehabilitation has been devoted to assessment and its use in occupational therapy practice. Because an exhaustive overview of cognitive assessments is beyond the scope of this chapter, we present several examples here for illustrative purposes.

Neistadt (1992) demonstrates an efficacious method of examining instrument efficacy. In her work, she examined the reliability and validity of the Rabideau Kitchen Evaluation-R (RKE-R). To assess criterion validity, she tested the association between the WAIS-R block design (Wechsler, 1981) and the RKE-R (Neistadt, 1992). She also conducted reliability studies to ascertain the stability of the instrument. Her careful scrutiny led her to conclude that the test may not be adequate for assessing cognition due to measurement difficulties and problems with interrater reliability. In attempting to norm the test, Neistadt (1992) did find that this test might be better in assessing those with obvious deficits than those with subtle ones. This work is an example of an excellent effort to test the adequacy of occupational therapy assessment of cognition as a basis for improving the accuracy of our clinical assessments. As a result of her study, Neistadt (1992) was able to target the assessment to a limited population and suggested that qualitative observation be added to the RKE-R protocol. Thus, Neistadt's work not only criticized an assessment, but suggested its useful domain and methods by which it could be improved and used.

As introduced briefly above, the work done by Allen (1985; 1992; in this book) on assessment of cognitive function has been central to cognitive assessment in occupational therapy. According to Allen, occupational therapists should evaluate the learning capacity of all clients regardless of diagnosis. "[To] the extent to which a therapist's services depend on the therapist's ability to teach a person how to do something, the therapist should evaluate that person's ability to learn" (Allen, 1992, p. 9). While used widely, Allen's approach to assessment has come under tight scrutiny. As a result, Allen, Earhart, and Blue (1992) have modified the initial Allen Cognitive Level (ACL) and developed new task analysis scales to assess cognition. To date, Allen has developed numerous cognitive assessments. As described by Zemke (1993), when therapists use the term ACL, they are actually referring to four versions of the assessment: the ACL-original, the ACL-expanded, the ACL-problem solving, and the current ACL-90. Allen cautions therapists to be comprehensive in assessing cognitive functional abilities and emphasizes the use of a battery of assessment tools to evaluate cognitive function. Validation and reliability studies have been conducted on these assessments with varying findings regarding psychometric properties.

The Cognitive Performance Test (Allen, Earhart, & Blue, 1992) was developed specifically to assess the functional levels of persons with Alzheimer's disease (Zemke, 1993). This test uses familiar occupational performance tasks such as dressing to assess cognitive function. Burns, Mortimer, and Merchak (1994) studied the test for reliability and validity and found it adequate for the population that was studied.

Allen's work has not only been examined for its efficacy in ascertaining cognitive skills globally, but new efforts have been initiated to assess the cultural relevance of her approaches. For example, Cusick and Harai (1991) examined capacity of the ACL, the Large Cognitive Level (LCL), and the Routine Task Inventory (RTI) to distinguish between subjects with and without disabilities across cultures. Unfortunately, because of design limitations, this small pilot study was unable to yield much more than exploratory questions about the cultural relevance of Allen's tests. However, the study creates a basis for future examination of Allen's work in diverse cultural groups. Scrutiny of the cultural relevance of assessment is an area of occupational therapy research that has been initiated by Katz and Heimann (1990) and should be expanded.

Recognizing the need for the development of assessments for occupational therapy practice, Fisher (1993) developed the Assessment of Motor and Process Skills (AMPS). This tool is an excellent example of an assessment that was designed to link assessment of daily life tasks to their underlying performance skills. The use of Rasch analysis to examine psychometric properties of the assessment tool made it possible for Fisher to develop hierarchically arranged tasks into an assessment linking performance with function. "The AMPS does not evaluate impairments of the mind-brain-body performance subsystem. Instead he or she [the occupational therapist] evaluates how underlying motor and process skill capacities are manifested in the context of performance of simple meal preparation and other household tasks ... Process skills are actions the person uses to logically organize and adapt behavior over time in order to complete a task" (Kielhofner, 1995, p. 235). The AMPS has an impressive array of validation studies, but is limited to intervention in selected instrumental activities of daily living (Kielhofner, 1995). Other functional areas are not tested by the AMPS. The AMPS also relies on client capacity to make a choice of activity and/or to be familiar with an activity. Therefore, it may not be appropriate for persons with memory and/or metacognitive impairments.

The Lowenstein Occupational Therapy Cognitive Assessment (LOTCA), initially developed in the early 1980s, was specifically designed to isolate and observe cognitive components of function. This assessment is supported by excellent standardization efforts, investigating reliability, criterion validity, discriminant validity, and construct validity (Katz et al., 1989). Research to standardize the test as norm referenced was also conducted (Averbuch & Katz, 1991) as well as examination of the degree to which the instrument was influenced by culture (Cermak et al., 1995). The rigor in the development and standardization of this tool allows occupational therapists to use it with confidence and present its findings to other professionals as sound information on clients' cognitive status and improvement.

Expanding assessment and intervention to a dynamic, interactional perspective, Toglia (1992) developed assessments that reflect this strengths-based approach to treating cognition. As reviewed in her chapter in this text, one example of dynamic assessment is the Contextual Memory Test (CMT). Research on this assessment includes efforts to establish normative data as well as efforts to support concurrent validity and reliability. Research on the CMT and other assessments based on the dynamic interactional approach have illuminated the use of these approaches by empirically highlighting their strengths and identifying their limitations.

In addition to global assessments of cognition, some tools have been developed for specific populations. For example, Hopkins, Dixon-Medora, & Krefting (1993) developed the Kingston Geriatric Cognitive Battery (KGCB) to assess cognitive skills in persons with dementia and ascertain their tolerance for other activity. The assessment is divided into three areas: orientation tasks, spatial motor tasks, and language skills. Criterion validity, factor analysis, interrater reliability, and content validity were discussed in the article presenting the psychometric properties of the instrument (Hopkins et al., 1993). The KGCB appears to be an adequate test of cognitive skill, but its link to function, while

mentioned, was not addressed. Nevertheless, the work by Hopkins et al. (1993) provides an excellent example of how occupational therapy assessment should be scrutinized.

In this section, we have discussed selected research on assessment of cognitive function in occupational therapy. Examples of assessments and related research synthesized with an examination of their psychometric properties reveal that assessment is a complex function that requires systemic scrutiny and investigation. It is incumbent on occupational therapists to assure rigor in their assessment processes. Adherence to a standard of rigor ensures that the information upon which treatment decisions and assessment of treatment process and outcome are based is accurate and adequate to inform our focus on occupational function. Several authors (DePoy, Maley, & Stanraugh, 1990; Toglia, 1993; Shimelman & Hinojosa, 1995; Abreu, in this book) have suggested that qualitative assessment be integrated with quantitative measurement of cognition as a foundation for ascertaining elements of occupational function that cannot be ascertained by the use of positivist methods.

Intervention

General Stimulation and Behavioral Techniques

Because the use of general stimulation techniques by occupational therapists is so common, many evaluative questions have arisen about the efficacy of this genre of approaches, and about which techniques yield the most significant functional outcomes. As a result, the body of literature generated to answer these questions is vast. Moreover, because behavioral techniques are frequently used with general stimulation and investigated in the same or similar types of research, and because behavioral techniques in themselves are not used frequently by occupational therapists, we have chosen to address both in one section. To illustrate the nature of research related to general stimulation and behavioral techniques, we have chosen a set of selected studies, and also include the work of Pepin, Loranger, and Benoit (1995) who reviewed the research literature on various approaches to cognitive rehabilitation. Consistent with our literature review, Pepin et al. (1995) note that the research, most of which relies on quasi-experimental design or case study methodology, yields equivocal results and is limited in its capacity to determine if increases in cognitive skill measured in these studies can generalize to daily function. However, even if more stringent designs cannot be enacted because of field constraints, as suggested by DePoy and Gitlin (1994), we support the conduct of systematic inquiry provided that a researcher's claims and conclusions do not exceed the capacity of the design.

First, we discuss the use of quasi-experimental designs to examine outcomes of intervention. Quasi-experimentation frequently is the only choice that occupational therapy researchers have to conduct quantitative studies of their interventions. While these designs are capable of revealing change over time, they are not able to attribute the change to the intervention because of limited control, and in many cases, inability to randomly assign clients to control or experimental groups (DePoy & Gitlin, 1994). However, since this type of design fits within the structure of clinical intervention, it is valuable in documenting change following an intervention and therefore should be considered by occupational therapy researchers when constraints of clinical research prevent the implementation of more controlled designs. Several studies illustrating the use of quasi-experimental design are presented here to demonstrate what they can and cannot tell us.

The study conducted by Brown, Harwood, Hays, Heckman, and Short (1993) is characteristic of many studies in the field. Brown et al. (1993), used a quasi-experimental design to compare the outcomes of a traditional occupational therapy task approach to a cognitive attentional intervention in a sample of individuals with schizophrenia. The study was designed well as a comparison of two interventions with clients being assigned to one of two treatment groups. Interestingly, both groups improved on measured outcomes. However, because no control was used in the design, the extent to which either intervention produced the outcomes cannot be ascertained. While the authors did not obtain empirical support for one approach over the other, this type of comparative design is

valuable to use, once it has been established that the traditional approach in itself yields significantly improved outcomes on the dependent variable. Another strength illustrated by this study was the use of multiple assessments and the attempt to link skill acquisition with volitional areas of function, including self-confidence, motivation, and efficiency.

Similar to Brown et al. (1993), Thomas, Hicks, and Johnson (1994) used a pre–post test, quasi-experimental design to assess the degree to which cognitive retraining techniques learned in a group format were successful in teaching elders with cognitive impairments to improve in upper extremity dressing. The researchers tested four subjects with the ACL-expanded version, the Mini Mental State Examination (MMSE), and the Functional Independence Measure (FIM). Based on descriptive statistical analysis, the authors claimed that improvement occurred on measured outcomes. This work demonstrates an attempt to link cognition to function and highlights efficacious use of standardized assessments for instrumentation. However, the limitations of the pre–post design, the small convenience sample, experimental mortality, lack of use of inferential statistical procedures to determine chance occurrence of findings, and limited control over the experimental condition restrict the knowledge derived from this work.

Corrigan and Storzbach (1993) discuss several efforts to evaluate the outcome of cognitive rehabilitation with individuals with schizophrenia and identify both the strengths and the limitations of quasi-experimentation. One of the studies reviewed by these two authors evaluates the cognitive and social outcomes of an Integrated Psychological Therapy (IPT) program (Brenner, Roder, Corrigan, 1992). The program comprised five hierarchical steps: cognitive differentiation, social perception, verbal communication, social skills, and problem-solving skills. Although we classify the program as general stimulation, it also had a behavioral component to it and exemplifies an approach to cognitive rehabilitation in which a systematic behavioral intervention is specified and investigated along with the use of other techniques. To examine the efficacy of this program, three outcomes studies were conducted. The first was a repeated time series experiment in which participants in the program improved in attention tasks but not in more complex cognitive functions. In the second study, which was designed as a modified time series design over three weeks, concept formation improved but social and cognitive functions did not. As stated by Corrigan and Storzbach (1993), methodological limitations that characterize occupational therapy and other outcome research in cognitive rehabilitation were present in this research agenda as well, including small sample size and inadequate control. Yet, despite its limitations, the study by Brenner et al. (1992) is an excellent effort to specify and investigate how clients changed over time.

In efforts to mediate against the difficulties encountered by quasi-experimentation in drawing conclusions about the efficacy of general stimulation techniques, other researchers have selected varied designs to attempt to link outcome to intervention. For example, DePoy et al. (1990) used a multiple case study design, integrating qualitative and quantitative strategies to compare traditional and computerized general stimulation intervention, while also examining executive function and activity preference. The research was conducted in a clinical setting over a period of 3 weeks. The researchers found that while formal testing did not reveal changes, qualitative strategies allowed the investigators to view clinical phenomena from which to suggest principles for future testing and intervention. Unfortunately the actual outcome of either intervention was not ascertained. While such a study provides the foundation for future study, it was seriously limited by time constraints to yield support for intervention selection.

Using a broader approach than the conduct of a single study, Neistadt (1992) demonstrated the application of previous research to the development of a general stimulation technique. She examined the literature on constructional deficits, with particular emphasis on adult performance on block design tasks. Synthesizing research that indicated that the nature of the disability and the individual combined with the design complexity and presentation could influence performance, Neistadt developed a graded block treatment protocol. While Neistadt did not examine outcome and gave minimal attention to the generalizability of skills learned on this task to functional activity, her arti-

cle is an excellent example of how a broad body of research was applied to the development of a cognitive rehabilitation protocol.

As evidenced in the examples provided above, the quasi-experimental designs typically used to investigate the efficacy of general stimulation techniques are not capable of revealing direct cause and effect relationships between intervention and outcome. Case studies, while capable of investigating causal questions, frequently are constrained by limited time as a result of controlled length of stay for inpatients and other clinical realities. Many critics of these methodologies suggest that occupational therapy researchers should be implementing true-experimental designs. However, the increasing emphasis on short hospitalization and community-based intervention interferes with a researcher's ability to structure and conduct a controlled experiment. Why then, should occupational therapy researchers conduct and read research that cannot use true-experimental designs? Two principles give us the answer to this frequently asked question. The first principle relates to the use of literature to support intervention choice. As so skillfully illustrated by Neistadt (1994), literature can provide the theoretical and empirical rationale for intervention choice. Second, combined with a sound approach to intervention, quasi-experimental and case study designs provide the vehicles for systematic scrutiny of client progress.

Substitution Techniques

Investigating the efficacy of substitution techniques is a complex undertaking for several reasons. First, the use of substitution as a treatment modality can be based on a spectrum of views of cognition. On one extreme, scholars suggest that cognitive skill cannot change and thus an individual needs to adapt to his or her static deficits (Wechsler, 1981). Conversely, others assert the position that practice of substitution and cognitive remediation techniques are dynamic and have the capacity to change internal cognitive processes (Toglia; Hadas-Lidor & Katz, in this book). Moreover, Josman (in this book) and Toglia suggest that substitution techniques, in themselves, are useful, but only when used with other types of intervention approaches.

Their suggestions are based on research that high-lights the interactive nature of cognitive skills and the concomitant inability to identify, isolate, investigate, treat, and assess the cortical location and relocation of specific cognitive skills (Toglia, in this book).

Considering the two tenets advanced above, it is therefore not surprising that clinical research has not been successful in ascertaining the degree to which an intervention is responsible for a desired outcome. Not unexpectedly, investigation into the efficacy of substitution techniques is fraught with the same methodological difficulties addressed above. That is to say, nomothetic designs structured as true experiments are not feasible in the current health care systems, leaving researchers with limited options when attempting to link outcomes to interventions.

Thus, similar to the literature on general stimulation techniques, research investigating the efficacy of substitution techniques relies in large part on quasi-experimentation and case study designs. Yet, in this genre of intervention, case study is particularly valuable for examining substitution techniques, since substitution techniques are frequently developed to meet idiosyncratic individualized styles of clients.

The study by DePoy et al. (1990) is one example of the application of multiple case study design to the evaluation of substitution. In their study of executive function, the researchers found that compensatory strategies in the presence of an executive functional deficit may be insufficient to assist persons to improve daily function.

Substitution has been used widely for clients with static and progressive dementia. As high-lighted by Levy (1989, 1992, in this book), an adaptive approach is most useful in promoting optimum occupational function for elders with dementia.

In their chapter in this text, Hadas-Lidor and Katz have illustrated the value of case examination of cognitive modifiability. In each of the four cases they present, these authors specify assessment techniques, report assessment findings, follow individual cases through their instrumental enrichment treatment over a time, and then reassess each client. While no certain claims can be substantiated about the causal link between the intervention and the outcome, the systematic and rigorous illustration of each case provides evidence to suggest that the intervention, at least in part, produced the observed outcome.

Unfortunately, however, even in clinical comparisons such as the study by Hadas-Lidor cited in Hadas-Lidor and Katz's chapter in this text, while researchers may come to know which intervention was followed by the most desired outcome, the inability to provide control limits our ability to infer causal relationships between treatment and outcome. As suggested by Hadas-Lidor and Katz, Abreu, Toglia (all in this book), and DePoy et al. (1990), integrating qualitative inquiry strategies with quantitative measures of outcome would yield valuable insight and evidence about the use of substitution techniques. Qualitative inquiry is particularly valuable in this domain of inquiry, in that its epistemological foundation supports complexity rather than reductionism.

Systemic Intervention

Systemic interventions target the social and living environments of clients rather than focusing intervention on remediating a cognitive deficit. These strategies traditionally have been underpinned by the principle that adapting the environment to meet the needs of clients with cognitive challenges is essential to improve overall function. This area of intervention emerged formally in psychiatric occupational therapy when the deinstitutionalization movement began in the 1960s and 1970s. In the treatment of cognitive deficits, while occupational therapists have practiced systemic intervention informally, few scholarly works have been found that formally identify systemic intervention for persons with cognitive challenges. Levy (1992) addressed the need for systemic support given by family members of individuals with dementia, but did not empirically test systemic interventions to ascertain changes in function following their implementation.

Not unexpectedly, because of the complex and holistic nature of systemic intervention, the limited research in this area of cognitive rehabilitation has relied on naturalistic study. The studies conducted by Schwartzberg (1994) and Schulz (1994) are two prime examples. Both researchers conducted what they called ethnographic inquiry to ascertain the helping factors that occurred in peer support groups with persons with TBI. The studies relied on observation of group process. Each was able to reveal the processes and changes that occurred within the groups. While some critics may be concerned with the inability to generalize the findings, the work done by these two researchers illustrates the strength of naturalistic research in revealing the complexity of a process.

The area of systemic intervention is ripe for occupational therapy research. Considering the shift from institutional to community living even for individuals with the most severe cognitive challenges, occupational therapists must be in the forefront of empirically documenting systemic approaches to intervention that have previously not been implied, tacit, and nonsystematically developed, assessed, or applied in intervention. At this early point in the development of such a research agenda, naturalistic methods and case study designs may be the most valuable approaches for this effort and for the generation of theoretical knowledge to be quantitatively tested in future inquiry.

Strengths and Limitations of the Research Literature on Cognitive Rehabilitation

As we have indicated throughout our discussion, there are many approaches to conducting research in cognitive rehabilitation. Each has its strengths and limitations.

The research on assessment of cognition and functional correlates thereof is growing and developing. Much of the inquiry in assessment is devoted to the validation of existing and new assessment techniques. This research is conducted easily within clinical and field settings since its mechanical requirements are consistent with the process of clinical assessment and intervention. Intervention research, however, is more complex and riddled with ethical and mechanical concerns and limitations.

First, let us begin with an analysis of quantitative intervention research. As depicted in most methodological texts, true-experimental design or mechanical or statistical variations thereof are the only methods that can investigate causal relationships. When we want to know about the extent to which our intervention has caused an outcome, true-experimental designs usually come to mind. However, in most if not all cases, implementation of the experimental conditions of control, manipulation, and random assignment (DePoy & Gitlin, 1994) cannot be achieved easily in the field or clinical setting. As discussed above, ethical and field constraints are the most frequent deterrents to implementing true-experimentation. Thus, researchers must rely on quasi-, pre-, and nonexperimental designs to conduct their research. While these designs engender much debate regarding their utility for supporting the efficacy of interventions, we believe that they are extremely valuable contributions to occupational therapy knowledge, provided that the investigators limit their claims to those that can be supported by the design and the findings. Systematic inquiry and a sound theoretical base for interventions render this type of research extremely useful in guiding clinicians in their choices of interventions. Moreover, while the designs may not be able to say definitively that an intervention was responsible for an outcome, quasi-experimental, pre-experimental, and nonexperimental inquiry can determine what does not occur as a result of intervention. What happens after intervention can certainly be ascertained by these designs. In the pursuit and development of knowledge, the quantitative research to date has provided a foundation upon which further research can be grounded.

The increasing acceptance of naturalistic inquiry, particularly in occupational therapy research, is an empirical blessing. Such research, while limited by its context-bound nature, can generalize to theory and provide the opportunity to ascertain a comprehensive picture of intervention, including the capacity to determine the outcome of interventions for those observed. Case study methodology is similar in its strengths to naturalistic design, in that it can yield causal findings (Radomski, 1994). Critics of case study and naturalistic research underscore the inability of both genres to address the important clinical concern of external validity. How is a clinician to know if the findings of single cases or phenomena in unique contexts can inform his or her intervention choices? The answer to this question is twofold. First, while both naturalistic design and case study research cannot be generalized to populations, both types of inquiry can generalize to theory for future testing. Second, the assessment of applicability of findings to one's clinical needs is essential. That is to say, while claims regarding external validity are not relevant to these designs, research that is limited by its context can inform clinicians who are facing similar challenges in similar contexts.

In addition to the methodological issues raised above, additional criticism of existing research provides more detailed guidance for future research. First, the acknowledgment of interaction among the diversity of individual conditions, intervention choice, and outcome has raised important considerations for occupational therapy research in cognitive rehabilitation. The severity and nature of the injury must be considered in any study. As Pepin et al. (1995) suggest, nomothetic designs cannot account for the interaction of individual attributes with treatment. They remind us that cognitive rehabilitation is not done with a homogeneous population. Thus, techniques that yield specific outcomes for some do not for others.

Moreover, as revealed in the research literature (DePoy et al., 1990; Katz & Hartman-Maeir, in this book), the separation of metacognition from other cognitive skills is difficult at best. For example, if attention and memory are the skill targets, it may not be possible to implement a program without cueing the patient to initiate the task (Pepin et al., 1995). How to reduce cognition to its components is a research agenda to consider when working on performance skills.

Generalization of gains made in the clinic to environments in which clients function is critical to study and has not always been addressed in occupational therapy research in the field of cognitive rehabilitation. As we asserted in our introduction, generalization of cognitive skill improvements must be linked to functional outcomes, since occupational function is the domain of occupational therapy practice. Research designs capable of examining the link between clinical improvement and occupational function are therefore essential

to include in the epistemological foundation of occupational therapy (see Table 12-1).

Principles Guiding Research on Cognitive Rehabilitation in Occupational Therapy

We now turn our attention to future research. Critical analysis of current knowledge and its generation provides excellent guidance for future inquiry. Considering the strengths and limitations of existing studies, we suggest the following principles as guidelines for occupational therapy research in cognitive rehabilitation:

1. Language should be uniform, with the use of the term occupation to describe and examine what humans do in the domains of work, play, or daily living (Kielhofner, 1995), and with cognitive performance components being carefully identified and named when possible.
2. Quantitative assessment should rely on standardized instrumentation when possible. When not possible, efforts to investigate the properties of instrumentation should be undertaken to ensure methodological rigor.
3. Claims and conclusions about findings should be limited to the capacity of the design.
4. The nature of the research question and purpose should guide design selection. Nomothetic designs can be used to reveal norms and group outcomes, while idiopathic designs can be used to examine individual phenomena.
5. Researchers should keep in mind that there are practical and ethical constraints in occupational therapy research.
6. Use of integrated designs should be considered to examine the process and outcomes of cognitive rehabilitation intervention.
7. The link between cognitive intervention, context, and occupational function should be an essential area for occupational therapy research in the field of cognitive rehabilitation.

More specifically, as intervention moves into community settings within managed care, occupational therapy research in cognitive rehabilitation should be developed to examine community-based inter-

Table 12-1

Research Designs, Properties, and Suggested Applications

Methods	Strengths	Limitations	Suggested Applications
True-experimental design	has capacity to support cause and effect can isolate and examine interventions can be structured to be externally valid can quantify outcomes can test theory can isolate interactive and main effects of treatment on outcome	has limited feasibility in clinical settings and ethical considerations cannot examine complexity	carefully controlled examinations of the effect of behavioral interventions on behavioral outcomes carefully controlled testing of effect of general stimulation techniques on defined outcomes identification of interactive effects of treatment and other tested variables on outcomes
Quasi-, pre-, and nonexperimental designs	are feasible in clinical settings can quantify outcomes are capable of showing change following interventions are capable of comparing changes following more than one intervention can be structured to be externally valid can investigate and describe interactive relationships among treatment and other variables	cannot support cause and effect relationships cannot examine complexity	all clinical interventions in which standardized assessment is used description of change following general stimulation techniques and behavioral interventions description of interactive relationships among treatment, identified variables, and expected outcomes
Naturalistic designs	can describe complexity may support cause and effect relationships can identify unexpected influences on outcomes can examine uniqueness can examine multiple influences on occupational function generalize to theory	cannot be applied beyond the natural boundary of the inquiry does not rely on standard measures of outcome cannot compare individuals against normative data	useful for describing the process and outcomes of systemic intervention useful for revealing unexpected influences on occupational function

continued

Methods	Strengths	Limitations	Suggested Applications
integrated designs	can capture the strengths of qualitative and quantitative designs triangulation	can suffer from the weaknesses of qualitative and quantitative designs may be criticized for philosophical contradictions work and time intensive	useful in all areas of research on cognitive rehabilitation process and outcome
case study	can investigate single subjects longitudinal use of multiple measures and data collection strategies can capture complexity can use integrated methods can be generalized to theory	no external validity time intensive may be limited to insufficient length of time	can be useful in investigating the process and outcome of single systems and/ or subjects

Table 12-1—*Continued.*

Research Designs, Properties, and Suggested Applications

vention strategies and techniques to ensure generalization of functional gains to an individual's occupational function in his or her living environments and to define the unique contribution of occupational therapy to the health care team and to the system of managed care.

A Proposed Ideal for Occupational Therapy Research in Cognitive Rehabilitation

By now, it may be apparent that we have approached occupational therapy research from a flexible and purposive perspective. The availability and increasing acceptance of multiple approaches to research provide excellent opportunities for occupational therapy researchers to implement studies that contribute to our knowledge base on many different levels. We therefore propose an ideal research agenda for occupational therapists in the field of cognitive rehabilitation that includes the following purposes:

1. Descriptive investigation of phenomena
2. Theory generation
3. Advancement of theory-based cognitive interventions
4. Testing the efficacy of theory-based cognitive interventions in improving occupational function.

Accomplishment of these research purposes requires the skillful planning and use of diverse methodologies. Let us look at an example.

Consider the scenario of the development of a new community-based program to address the maintenance and improvement of occupational function for individuals with closed head injuries in their home communities. A first step would involve a full review of the literature. However, as revealed in this chapter, evaluation research has yielded equivocal findings about which strategies are most productive in promoting occupational function. The first task of the researcher might be to examine "what is." This examination would involve assessment of the unique and common elements of occupational function in the client group, assessment of the needs and resources offered in the community, and consideration of the other providers on the rehabilitation team. Integrated designs relying on standardized assessment of client occupational function (e.g., Allen's battery, LOTCA, AMPS), coupled with qualitative inquiry, would be extremely valuable in providing a full picture of the occupational function of the client group within the community context. Qualitative inquiry might include interview and observation of the unique resources to support individuals with closed head injury in their communities. The conduct of a focus group of significant others to ascertain what social and family supports are available for individuals with closed head injury would provide the therapist with necessary information about the client's social environment. Theoretical support and guidance would be sought from similar conditions explicated in the literature. Such depth and breath of information is critical for comprehensive, holistic intervention to promote occupational function in community-based settings. Use of standardized assessment data synthesized with empirical knowledge of community and social resources provides a solid foundation for program development and the specification of outcome goals and objectives. Integrated designs relying on quasi-experimental approaches and qualitative observation of clients as they participate in intervention would be the next essential component of a research agenda. This step would begin the process of describing change and assessing client outcome regarding cognitive and occupational performance. Cognitive gains and concomitant function in occupation could be ascertained by the use of standardized measures of cognition and functional skill acquisition in the context of formal intervention. Expanding the inquiry to client occupational function in varied contexts could be accomplished through naturalistic observation of clients in their work, play and self-care environments, by narrative strategies, and by interview with significant others who support and/or have contact with the client in the community.

Although context specific, the research described above could be generalized to theory. Theory-testing designs relying on measurement of expected outcomes would be implemented to test occupational performance outcomes in a broad cohort of clients with similar needs.

Summary and Conclusion

In this chapter, we have proposed a conceptual framework for occupational therapy research related to promoting occupational function through cognitive rehabilitation. We examined inquiry informing occupational therapy intervention in the areas of assessment, general stimulation techniques, behavioral intervention, substitution and transfer techniques, and systemic interventions. Critical analysis of existing research revealed that while limitations are imposed on occupational therapy research because of clinical and ethical constraints, the research that is available provides an empirical foundation not only for intervention choice but for future research design and substance. We have suggested principles to consider when embarking on research in cognitive rehabilitation and have illustrated an ideal research agenda in which occupational therapists would use multiple and diverse research approaches to answer questions about how to use cognitive rehabilitation techniques to promote occupational function in clients.

References

Allen, C. K. (1985). *Occupational therapy for psychiatric diseases: Measurement and management of cognitive disabilities.* Boston: Little, Brown.

Allen, C. K. (1992). Cognitive disabilities. In N. Katz (Ed.), *Cognitive rehabilitation: Models for intervention in occupational therapy.* Stoneham, MA: Butterworth-Heinamann.

Allen, C., Earhart, A., & Blue, T. (1992). *Occupational therapy treatment goals for the physically and cognitively disabled.* Bethesda, MD: American Occupational Therapy Association.

Arnadottir, G. (1990). *The brain and behavior: Assessing cortical dysfunction through activities of daily living (ADL).* Philadelphia: Mosby.

Averbuch, S., & Katz, N. (1991). Age level standards of the Lowenstein Occupational Therapy Cognitive Assessment (LOTCA). Israeli *Journal of Occupational Therapy, 1,* 1–15.

Brenner, H. D., Roder, V., & Corrigan, P. W. (1992). Treatment of cognitive dysfunction and behavioral deficits in schizophrenia: Integrated psychological therapy. *Schizophrenia Bulletin, 18,* 21–26.

Brown, C., Harwood, K., Hays, C., Heckman, J., & Short, J. (1993). Effectiveness of cognitive rehabilitation for improving attention in patients with schizophrenia. *Occupational Therapy Journal of Research, 13*, 71–86.

Burns, T., Mortimer, J., & Merchak, P. (1994). Cognitive performance test: A new approach to functional assessment in Alzheimer's disease. *Journal of Geriatric Psychiatry, 7*, 46–54.

Cermak, S. A., Katz, N., McGuire, E., Greenbaum, S., Peralta, C., Maser-Flanagan, V. (1995). Performance of Americans and Israelis with cerebrovascular accident on the Lowenstein Occupational Therapy Cognitive Assessment (LOTCA). *American Journal of Occupational Therapy, 48*, 500–505.

Corrigan, P., & Storzbach, D. (1993). The ecological validity of cognitive rehabilitation for schizophrenia. *Cognitive Rehabilitation, 11*, 14–21.

Cusick, A., & Harai, H. (1991). The Allen tests for cognitive disability: A cross cultural pilot study. *Occupational Therapy in Mental Health, 11*, 61, 75.

David, S. (1990). The relationship of the Allen Cognitive Level Test to cognitive ability. *American Journal of Occupational Therapy, 44*, 493–497.

DePoy, E., & Gitlin, L. (1994). *Introduction to research: Multiple strategies for health and human services.* St. Louis: Mosby.

DePoy, E., Maley, K., & Stanraugh, J. (1990). Executive function and cognitive remediation: A study of activity preference. *Occupational Therapy in Health Care, 7*, 101–115.

Fisher, A. G. (1993). The assessment of IADL motor skills: An application of many faceted Rasch analysis. *American Journal of Occupational Therapy, 47*, 319–329.

Giles, G. M. (1994). The status of brain injury rehabilitation. *American Journal of Occupational Therapy, 48*, 3, 199–205.

Green, M. F. (1993). Cognitive remediation in schizophrenia: Is it time yet? *American Journal of Psychiatry, 150*, 178–187.

Hartman-Maeir, A., & Katz, N. (1995). Validity of the Behavioral Inattention Test: Relationship with functional tasks. *American Journal of Occupational Therapy, 48*, 507–516.

Hopkins, R. W., Dixon-Medora, P., & Krefting, L. (1993). *Occupational Therapy Journal of Research, 13*, 241–252.

Katz, N. (1992). *Cognitive rehabilitation: Models for intervention in occupational therapy.* Stoneham, MA: Butterworth-Heinemann.

Katz, N., & Heimann, N. (1990). Review of research conducted in Israel on cognitive disability instrumentation. *Occupational Therapy in Mental Health, 10*, 1–15.

Katz, N., Itzkovich, M., Averbuch, S., & Elazar, B. (1989). Lowenstein Occupational Therapy Cognitive Assessment battery for brain injured patients: Reliability and validity. *American Journal of Occupational Therapy, 43*, 184–192.

Kielhofner, G. (1995). *A model of human occupation: Theory and application* (2nd ed.). Baltimore: Williams and Wilkins.

Levy, L.L. (1989). Activity adaptation in rehabilitation of the physically and cognitively disabled aged. *Topics in Geriatric Rehabilitation, 4*, 53–66.

Levy, L. L. (1992). The use of the cognitive disability frame of reference in rehabilitation of cognitively disabled older adults. In N. Katz (Ed.), *Cognitive rehabilitation: Models for intervention in occupational therapy.* Stoneham, MA: Butterworth-Heinemann.

Neistadt, M. E. (1992). The Rabideau Kitchen Evaluation-Revised: An assessment of meal preparation skill. *Occupational Therapy Journal of Research, 12*, 242–253.

Neistadt, M. E. (1993). The relationship between apraxia and meal preparation skills. *Archives of Physical Medicine, 74*, 144–148.

Neistadt, M. E. (1994). Using research literature to develop a perceptual retraining treatment protocol. *American Journal of Occupational Therapy, 48*, 62–72.

Nelson, D. L. (1988). Occupation: Form and performance. *American Journal of Occupational Therapy, 42*, 633–641.

Pepin, M., Loranger, M., & Benoit, G. (1995). Efficiency of cognitive training: Review and prospects. *Cognitive Rehabilitation, 14*, 8–14.

Prigatano, G. P. (1987). Recovery and cognitive retraining after craniocerebral trauma. *Journal of Learning Disabilities, 20*, 603–613.

Radomski, M. V. (1994). Cognitive rehabilitation: Advancing the stature of occupational therapy. *American Journal of Occupational Therapy, 48*, 271–273.

Ranchos Los Amigos Medical Center, Professional Staff Association (1986). *Rancho Los Amigos Cognitive Functioning Scale.* Adult Brain Injury Services of the Ranchos Los Amigos Medical Center. Downey, CA.

Royeen, C. (Ed.). (1993). *AOTA Self-Study series: Cognitive rehabilitation.* Bethesda, MD: American Occupational Therapy Association.

Schulz, C. H. (1994). Helping factors in a peer developed support group for persons with head injury. Part 2: Survivor interview perspective. *American Journal of Occupational Therapy, 48*, 305–309.

Schwartzberg, S. L. (1994). Helping factors in a peer developed support group for persons with head injury. Part 1: Participant observer perspective. *American Journal of Occupational Therapy, 48*, 296–304.

Shimelman, A., & Hinojosa, J. (1995). Gross motor activity and attention in three adults with brain injury. *American Journal Of Occupational Therapy, 49*, 973–978.

Spencer, J., Krefting, L., & Mattingly, C.(1993). Incorporation of ethnographic methods in occupational therapy assessment. *American Journal of Occupational Therapy, 47*, 303–309.

Thomas, K. S., Hicks, J. J. & Johnson, O. A. (1994). A pilot project for group cognitive retraining with elderly stroke patients. *Occupational Therapy in Geriatrics, 12*, 51–66.

Toglia, J. P. (1992). The dynamic interactional approach to cognitive rehabilitation. In N. Katz (Ed.), *Cognitive rehabili-*

tation: Models for intervention in occupational therapy. Stoneham, MA: Butterworth-Heinemann.

Toglia, J. P. (1993). Attention and memory. In C. Royeen, (Ed), *AOTA Self-Study Series: Cognitive rehabilitation.* Bethesda, MD: American Occupational Therapy Association.

Wechsler, D. (1981). *The measure of adult intelligence WAIS-R.* Baltimore: Williams and Wilkins.

Zemke, R. (1993). Task skills, problem solving and social interaction. In C. Royeen (Ed.). *AOTA Self-Study Series: Cognitive rehabilitation.* Bethesda, MD: American Occupational Therapy Association.

Index